PRIMARY CARE OF THE

Child with a Chronic Condition

PRIMARY CARE OF THE
Child with a Chronic Condition

Patricia Ludder Jackson, *RN, MS, PNP*
Associate Clinical Professor,
Pediatric Nurse Practitioner Program Coordinator,
Department of Family Health Care Nursing,
University of California, San Francisco,
San Francisco, California

Judith A. Vessey, *RN, PhD, DPNP*
Associate Professor,
College of Nursing,
University of Arkansas for Medical Sciences;
Research Facilitator,
Arkansas Children's Hospital,
Little Rock, Arkansas

With 62 illustrations

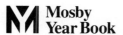 **Mosby Year Book**

St. Louis Baltimore Boston Chicago London Philadelphia Sydney Toronto

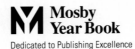
Mosby
Year Book
Dedicated to Publishing Excellence

Editor: Don Ladig
Developmental Editor: Winifred Sullivan
Project Supervisor: Barbara Merritt
Designer: Julie Taugner
Illustrator: Mark Swindle

Library of Congress Cataloging-in-Publication Data

Primary care of the child with a chronic condition / [edited by]
    Patricia Ludder Jackson, Judith A. Vessey.
        p.   cm.
    Includes bibliographical references and index.
    ISBN 0-8016-2396-0
    1. Chronic diseases in children—Treatment.   2. Chronic diseases
in children—Nursing.   I. Jackson, Patricia Ludder.   II. Vessey,
Judith A.
    [DNLM: 1. Chronic Disease—in infancy & childhood.   2. Primary
Health Care.   WS   200   P952]
    RJ380.P75   1992
    618.92—dc20
    DNLM/DLC
    for Library of Congress   91-28012
                                                                  CIP

92 93 94 95 96   GW/DC/DC 9 8 7 6 5 4 3 2 1

To the loving memory of my husband, Bruce;
To our children, Heather, Robert, and Scott,
  who taught me all I really know about parenting
  and the needs of all children;
To my father, for passing on his love of writing;
And to John, for his continued love and for being there
  when I needed him.

PLJ

To my parents, who encouraged me to reach for the stars;
And to Florence, who showed me the way.

JAV

Contributors

....

CATHERINE L. CASERZA, MS, RN
Graduate-Student,
University of California, Berkeley, School of Public
  Health;
Research Assistant,
Robert Wood Johnson Fellowship Program,
San Francisco, California

VIRGINIA H. CONTE, MSN, RN
Pulmonary Clinical Nurse Specialist,
Alfred I. duPont Institute,
Wilmington, Delaware

ELIZABETH H. COOK, MS, RNC, PNP
Pediatric Cardiovascular Clinical Nurse Specialist,
Children's Hospital Oakland,
Oakland, California

BEVERLY CORBO-RICHERT, MS, RN, CCRN
PhD Candidate,
Assistant Professor,
Parent-Child Nursing Graduate Program,
University of Pittsburgh School of Nursing,
Pittsburgh, Pennsylvania

ELIZABETH SHURTLEFF DAWES, MSN, RN,
  CPNP
Altos Pediatrics Associates,
Los Altos, California

MARY ALICE DRAGONE, MS, RNC, PNP
Hemophilia Nurse Coordinator,
Children's Hospital Oakland,
Oakland, California

MARY JO DUNLEAVY, BSN, RN
Level II Staff Nurse,
Nurse Coordinator Myelodysplasia Program,
The Children's Hospital,
Boston, Massachusetts

RITA FAHRNER, MS, RN, PNP
Clinical Nurse Specialist,
Occupational Infectious Disease Program,
HIV Prevention Service,
San Francisco General Hospital,
San Francisco, California

JUDITH A. FARLEY, MSN, RN, CNRN
Clinical Nurse Specialist,
Pediatric Neuroscience,
The Children's Hospital,
Boston, Massachusetts

DIANE J. GOLDMAN, MS, RN, PNP
Assistant Clinical Professor,
University of California, San Francisco, School of
  Nursing,
Department of Family Health Care Nursing,
San Francisco, California

STEVEN L. GOLDMAN, MD
Associate Clinical Professor of Pediatrics,
University of California, San Francisco;
Director, Neonatal-Perinatal Fellowship Program,
Children's Hospital of San Francisco,
San Francisco, California

MARGARET GREY, DrPH, FAAN, CPNP
Associate Professor of Nursing,
Program Director, Primary Care Program,
University of Pennsylvania School of Nursing,
Philadelphia, Pennsylvania

RANDI J. HAGERMAN, MD
Associate Professor of Pediatrics,
University of Colorado Health Services Center and
    Child Development Unit,
The Children's Hospital Denver,
Denver, Colorado

SARAH S. HIGGINS, PhD, RN
Pediatric Cardiovascular Clinical Nurse Specialist,
Children's Hospital Oakland,
Oakland, California

GAIL M. KIECKHEFER, PhD, RNC, PNP
Research Assistant Professor,
University of Washington,
Department of Parent and Child Nursing,
Seattle, Washington

ELIZABETH A. KUEHNE, MSN, CPNP
Director, Foster Care Health Services,
The Children's Aid Society,
New York, New York

NANCI L. LARTER, MSN, RN
Pediatric Pulmonary Clinical Nurse Specialist,
Pediatric Pulmonary Center at the University of Wash-
    ington and Children's Hospital and Medical Center,
Seattle, Washington

MARYANN E. LISAK, MSN, RN, PNP
Nurse Practitioner,
Sickle Cell and Thalassemia Program,
Children's Hospital of Los Angeles,
Los Angeles, California

MARGARET M. MAHON, MSN, RNC
Lecturer,
University of Pennsylvania School of Nursing,
Philadelphia, Pennsylvania

ANN HIX McMULLEN, MS, RN
Assistant Professor of Clinical Nursing,
University of Rochester School of Nursing,
Pediatric Pulmonary and Cystic Fibrosis Center,
University of Rochester Medical Center,
Rochester, New York

ROBERTA S. O'GRADY, DrPH, RN
Lecturer and Field Program Supervisor,
Program in Maternal and Child Health,
School of Public Health,
University of California, Berkeley,
Berkeley, California

VERONICA E. PERRONE, MSN, RN
Clinical Nurse Specialist, Pediatric Gastroenterology,
Yale New Haven Hospital;
Program Instructor, Yale University School of
    Nursing,
New Haven, Connecticut

PATRICIA M. REILLY, MSN, RN, PNP
Oregon Health Sciences University,
Pediatric Department Outpatient Clinic,
Portland, Oregon

JUDITH A. RUBLE, MS, RN, PNP
Endocrinology Clinical Nurse Specialist,
Children's Hospital, Oakland
Oakland, California

ELIZABETH SAN LUIS, MS, RN, PNP
Administrative Nurse II/PNP, Pediatric Primary Care,
University of California, San Francisco,
San Francisco, California

KATHLEEN ANN SCHMIDT, MS, RN
Coordinator of the Newborn Screening and Inborn Er-
    rors of Metabolism Programs,
Department of Pediatrics,
Division of Medical Genetics,
University of California, San Francisco,
San Francisco, California

JANICE SELEKMAN, DNSc, RN
Chair,
Department of Advanced Nursing Science,
College of Nursing,
University of Delaware,
Newark, Delaware

AMY CRONISTER SILVERMAN, MS
Genetic Counselor,
Sewall Child Development Center,
Denver, Colorado

SHIRLEY STEELE, PhD, RNC, PNP
Nursing Consultant,
United Cerebral Palsy of Greater Birmingham,
Birmingham, Alabama

MARIANNE WARGUSKA, MSN, CPNP
Director of Health Services,
The Children's Aid Society,
New York, New York

KAREN E. ZAMBERLAN, PhD, RN
Clinical Nurse Specialist, Transplant Surgery,
Children's Hospital of Pittsburgh;
Faculty, University of Pittsburgh School of Medicine
Pittsburgh, Pennsylvania

Reviewers

GAIL McILVAIN-SIMPSON, MSN, RN, C
Clinical Nurse Specialist,
Pediatric Rheumatology,
Alfred I. duPont Institute,
Wilmington, Delaware

CINDY A. NELSON, BSN, RN, MPH, CPNP
Pulmonary Nurse Specialist,
Children's Hospital Oakland,
Pulmonary Medicine Department,
Oakland, California

SUSAN N. PECK, MSN, RN, CPNP
Clinical Nurse Specialist,
Children's Hospital of Philadelphia,
Division of Gastroenterology and Nutrition,
Philadelphia, Pennsylvania

CATHY QUIDES, MSN, RN, C
Pediatric Nurse Practitioner,
Children's Hospital Medical Center,
Oakland, California

PATRICIA RIESER, BSN, FNP-C
Nurse Specialist,
Division of Pediatric Endocrinology,
University of North Carolina at Chapel Hill,
Chapel Hill, North Carolina

JUDITH A. RUBLE, MS, RN, PNP
Endocrinology Clinical Nurse Specialist,
Children's Hospital Oakland,
Oakland, California

MARY SMELLIE DECKER, MSN, RN
Clinical Nurse Specialist,
Neurosurgery,
Children's Hospital of Michigan,
Detroit, Michigan

DONNA STANLY-PAGE, MN, BSN, RN, PNP
Kaiser Permanente Medical Group,
Assistant Clinical Professor,
University of California, San Francisco,
San Francisco, California

MARJORIE E. STIRM, MS, RN, PNP, MPH
Clinical Nurse Specialist,
Department of Pediatrics/Rheumatology, Immunology,
University of California, San Francisco,
San Francisco, California

MARY W. TRUSKIER, MS, RN, PNP
Assistant Clinical Professor,
Department of Family Health Care Nursing,
School of Nursing,
University of California, San Francisco,
San Francisco, California

VICTORIA A. WEILL, MSN, RNC, CPNP
Pediatric Nurse Practitioner/Lecturer,
University of Pennsylvania, School of Nursing,
Philadelphia, Pennsylvania

LINDA M. WELLS, BA, RN, CNA
Head Nurse,
Children's Center for Cancer and Blood Disorders,
Children's Hospital at Richland Memorial,
Columbia, South Carolina

PHILIP R. ZIRING, MD
Chairman, Department of Pediatrics,
Pacific Presbyterian Medical Center,
San Francisco, California

Foreword

· ·

Historically and traditionally, nurse practitioners are well positioned to serve as both primary care providers and full partners on the primary care team delivering health services to chronically ill children and their families. Since nursing practice encompasses "life processes, well-being, and optimal function of human beings,"[1] experienced, as well as novice, nurse practitioners and nurses in schools and other areas of advanced practice will find this fully documented and nicely organized book a comprehensive and complete resource.

Part I defines issues in primary care and describes the impact of chronic illnesses on children and their families and on the nation's resources. Part II provides epidemiological and clinical information on specific chronic diseases, including contemporary problems such as Fragile X syndrome, prenatal drug exposure, and HIV infections.

Each chapter in Part II focuses on a specific chronic condition from the perspective of the child's physical, social, and psychological development; functional daily living; special family concerns; community resources, including support and voluntary health organizations; child care; and schooling. Additionally, charts, tables, and summaries set forth the unique primary care needs of the child with a specific chronic condition. Management options give the nurse practitioner a broad range of therapeutic and preventive choices. Scientific content and practical suggestions will help practitioners assist children and their families to understand, cope, and thrive under the complex stresses of normal growth and development and chronic conditions.

Primary, secondary, and tertiary prevention strategies are detailed for each condition. From these strategies nurse practitioners can formulate plans to empower families to maximize their child's development through nurturing, education, and the self-care process.

Nurse practitioners will find this work has many uses—for their own continuing education; as a quick reference; to summarize teaching points with parents, teachers, and others; for guidelines to record pertinent notes; and for understanding the complex issues in the delivery and financing of health care to children with chronic conditions and their families.

To carry on their tradition of primary care nursing, which began more than 25 years ago, nurse practitioners will value this major contribution to the literature. It improves access, fosters the provision of high quality care to chronically ill children and their families, and may encourage policy makers to initiate much-needed reforms in the delivery and financing of health care for this very special group in our society.

L.C. Ford, RN, EdD, FAAN
Professor and Dean Emeritus
School of Nursing
University of Rochester

Approximately 7.5 million children in the United States have chronic conditions. These children are becoming a more important part of pediatric practice and use a disproportionate amount of resources, including physicians' time. Also, the numbers of children surviving conditions such as HIV infection and low birth weight are expected to increase significantly.

The primary care of these children must integrate their fundamental biological and psychological needs with the specific needs related to their chronic conditions and must be provided in the context of their families and communities. Although a wealth of facts are available in medical journals and books to help the specialist deal with the biomedical aspects of specific illnesses, little coherent information is available to help the primary care provider care for these children. The information most helpful to the primary care practitioner is fragmented throughout the medical literature. Jackson and Vessey have taken those fragments and ordered them into a practical, comprehensive guide.

The introductory chapters of this book afford a clear understanding of the issues common to children and families with chronic conditions. The lucid, detailed, and practical guidelines in subsequent chapters serve as a reference that will greatly improve the daily care of children with chronic conditions. Each of these chapters discusses the medical management of the condition, its relation to fundamental traits of childhood such as growth and development, and the implication for primary care management, including screening and anticipatory guidance. This book should be used by all primary care physicians who care for children, including pediatricians, family specialists, general practitioners, and house officers working in pediatric clinics.

Gregory S. Liptak, MD, MPH
Associate Professor of Pediatrics
University of Rochester
Medical Center

Preface

GROWING UP

I've got shoes with grown up laces,
I've got knickers and a pair of braces,
I'm all ready to run some races.
 Who's coming out with me?

I've got a nice new pair of braces,
I've got shoes with new brown laces,
I know wonderful paddly places.
 Who's coming out with me?

Every morning my new grace is,
"Thank you, God, for my nice braces:
I can tie my new brown laces."
 Who's coming out with me?

 A.A. Milne

"Growing up" is not easy. Seemingly limitless potential is juxtaposed with devastating possibilities. Medical advances over the past 50 years have dramatically decreased the mortality and morbidity rates in children, especially from infectious diseases that in previous decades annually killed thousands. With many devastating illnesses controlled, pediatric health care providers shifted their focus of care from illness management to prevention with the goal of maximizing each child's potential through health promotion, disease and injury prevention, and growth and development counseling.

During this same period, however, a new childhood morbidity profile has emerged. Children with chronic conditions who decades ago would have died as a result of their condition are now surviving. Their medical care is often complex, frequently requiring multiple treatment modalities. In addition, treatments that were previously only provided in acute care hospitals by professionals are now being provided in the home by family members, shifting medical responsibilities from hospital professionals to community providers.

In an attempt to keep pace with the rapid developments in medical and surgical treatment for children with chronic conditions, care has often become specialized, focused on the disease process instead of holistic care for the child. In part, this has happened because primary care providers are hesitant to care for a child with a serious chronic condition for fear of not knowing how to manage the chronic condition well, and the specialist is reluctant to provide care above and beyond care needed for the chronic condition for fear of not knowing how to competently manage the child's primary health care needs. Consequently, children with chronic conditions often do not receive the primary health care provided their nonaffected peers.

"Growing up" with a chronic condition or disability is inherently more difficult; a child's growth and development may be compromised by the stress of the illness and treatments; a child's susceptibility to common childhood illnesses, behavioral dysfunctions, and injuries may be increased as a result of the chronic condition; and many children with chronic conditions also come from improvised families with little or no access to preventive health care, further increasing the potential morbidity from the chronic condition, as well as general health risks. The purpose of this book is to provide pediatric health care professionals with the knowledge necessary to provide comprehensive primary care to these children with special needs.

Part I addresses the major issues common to care of all children with chronic conditions: the role of the primary care provider, the impact of a chronic condition on the family and the child's development, and the financial resources, or lack thereof, available and needed to support the care of a child with a chronic condition. This knowledge is generic in that it is not condition specific but forms the framework for delivery of care to all children with chronic conditions.

Part II identifies 24 chronic conditions found in children that necessitate alterations in standard primary care practices as a result of the chronic condition. Each condition-specific chapter was written and reviewed by health care professionals with extensive experience in caring for the complex needs of children with the identified chronic condition. The information provided briefly covers etiology and clinical manifestations of the chronic condition but mainly focuses on how these affect the primary care needs of the child. The emphasis is on the need for and provision of primary care. Each chapter follows the same format for ease of reading, and the primary care needs are summarized at the end of each chapter for quick reference.

Decisions as to which chronic conditions were to be included in this text were based on two criteria. First, the prevalence of the condition needed to be at least 1 in 10,000 or would likely reach this

level if underreporting were not a problem. For conditions that are relatively new in children, such as organ transplantation or HIV infection, the decision to include them was based on how rapidly the incidence was increasing. The second criterion for inclusion was that the condition require significant adaptations in primary care.

Whenever possible, inclusive language regarding the health care provider has been used throughout the text. We have extended this terminology to include nurse practitioners, physicians, and other health care providers as individuals with a variety of professional preparations provide primary care to children with chronic conditions. The reader will also note that the terms, *patient* and *chronic illness*, are not used and whenever possible, the wording "the child with (condition name)" rather than the "(condition name) child" has been used. Although we recognize that this sometimes makes for awkward grammar, it reflects our philosophy that children be children first rather than be defined by their condition and that wellness and illness are relative.

It would be presumptuous to edit such a text without acknowledging its scope and limitations. First, it is assumed that the reader has a basic knowledge of growth and development and of common pediatric conditions and their management. Second, it is impossible to provide detailed information on treatment options for all secondary problems that may occur in conjunction with those highlighted. Wherever possible, the reader is referred to another chapter of this text. If this was not feasible, the reader should consult the general pediatric literature for management protocols. Third, a decision was also made to exclude pediatric mental health conditions despite the fact that over 40% of these are treated in the primary care arena. In part, this was due to the broad range of conditions and the disparity in treatment regimens currently used.

The preparation of this text has been a professionally challenging and personally rewarding endeavor for us. As with any text, its successful completion depended on the help of numerous others. We wish to extend our gratitude to the contributors and reviewers for their excellent careful and timely work. Our sincere thanks is also extended to our research assistants, Catherine Caserza and Katrina Liu, and our secretarial support staff, Marjorie Duncan, Maggie Pena, Nancy Stewart, and Rebecca Weber. The contributions of the University of California, San Francisco Departments of Family Health Care Nursing and Physiological Nursing, the University of Arkansas for Medical Sciences College of Nursing, the Arkansas Children's Hospital, and the Center for Ambulatory Research and Education are also recongnized. The assistance and support of the Mosby–Year Book staff—editors, Don Ladig and Winnie Sullivan and project supervisor, Barbara Merritt—are also gratefully acknowledged. We would also like to recognize the support for this project that has been provided through the Robert Wood Johnson Foundation's Clinical Nurse Scholars' Program and the Maternal Child Health Training grant #MCJ:000937-17-0.

In summary, we hope the information provided in this book will help children with chronic conditions to receive more holistic primary care that will promote their growth and development and maximize their potential in all areas. This can only be done if health care professionals are willing to say "I will come out with you" and to assume the challenge of assisting these children in "growing up."

Patricia Ludder Jackson
Judith A. Vessey

Contents

PART I
ISSUES IN PRIMARY PEDIATRIC CARE

1   **The Primary Care Provider and Children with Chronic Conditions**, 3

Patricia Ludder Jackson

2   **Chronic Conditions and the Family**, 12

Margaret M. Mahon

3   **Chronic Conditions and Child Development**, 26

Judith A. Vessey
Catherine L. Caserza

4   **Financing Health Care for Children with Chronic Conditions**, 45

Roberta S. O'Grady

PART II
CHRONIC CONDITIONS — Primary Care of the Child with . . .

5   **Asthma**, 63

Nanci L. Larter
Gail M. Kieckhefer

6   **Bleeding Disorders: Hemophilia and von Willebrand's Disease**, 81

Mary Alice Dragone

7   **Bronchopulmonary Dysplasia**, 101

Virginia H. Conte

8   **Cancer**, 117

Elizabeth Shurtleff Dawes

9   **Cerebral Palsy**, 148

Shirley Steele

10   **Congenital Adrenal Hyperplasia**, 169

Judith A. Ruble

11   **Congenital Heart Disease**, 187

Elizabeth H. Cook
Sarah S. Higgins

12   **Cystic Fibrosis**, 210

Ann Hix McMullen

13   **Diabetes Mellitus (Type I)**, 229

Margaret Grey

14   **Down Syndrome**, 245

Judith A. Vessey

15   **Epilepsy**, 268

Judith A. Farley

16   Fragile X Syndrome, 286

Amy Cronister Silverman
Randi J. Hagerman

17   Hydrocephalus, 303

Patricia Ludder Jackson

18   Inflammatory Bowel Disease, 318

Veronica E. Perrone

19   Juvenile Rheumatoid Arthritis, 336

Patricia M. Reilly

20   Learning Disabilities, 355

Janice Selekman

21   Myelodysplasia, 373

Judith A. Farley
Mary Jo Dunleavy

22   Organ Transplants, 389

Beverly Corbo-Richert
Karen E. Zamberlan

23   Pediatric HIV Infection and AIDS, 408

Rita Fahrner

24   Phenylketonuria, 426

Kathleen Ann Schmidt

25   Prematurity, 446

Diane J. Goldman
Steven L. Goldman

26   Prenatal Cocaine Exposure, 465

Elizabeth A. Kuehne
Marianne Warguska

27   Chronic Renal Failure, 480

Elizabeth San Luis

28   Sickle Cell Disease, 495

Maryann E. Lisak

Appendix — Additional Resources, 517

PART *I*

ISSUES IN PRIMARY PEDIATRIC CARE

....

The Primary Care Provider and Children with Chronic Conditions
Chronic Conditions and the Family
Chronic Conditions and Child Development
Financing Health Care for Children with Chronic Conditions

1

The Primary Care Provider and Children with Chronic Conditions

··

Patricia Ludder Jackson

A chronic health condition is defined as one that is long term and is either not curable or has residual features that result in limitations in daily living requiring special assistance or adaptation in function (Jessop and Stein, 1988). Jessop and Stein (1988) further define chronic conditions in children as lasting 3 months or more in 1 year or requiring at least 1 month of hospitalization. If this definition is used, an estimated 7.5 million children less than 18 years of age in the United States have chronic health conditions, with 10% to 15% of these conditions classified as severe (Hobbs, Perrin, and Ireys, 1985).

Estimates of the prevalence of chronic childhood conditions vary greatly but fall generally between 10% and 20% of the pediatric population (Butler, Rosenbaum, and Palfrey, 1987; Gortmaker and Sappenfield, 1984; U. S. Department of Health and Human Services, 1987). The percentage of the pediatric population with a chronic condition is increasing as the patterns of childhood morbidity and mortality have changed with advanced technology, improved treatment of previously fatal infectious diseases, and implementation of public and preventive health measures that have saved the lives of infants and children who previously would have died (Coupey and Cohen, 1984; Jessop and Stein, 1988).

Gortmaker and Sappenfield (1984) found the overall incidence of most childhood disorders had not changed significantly over the past 20 years. But in contrast to these relatively stable incidence rates, estimates of survival of children with a variety of chronic conditions have shown considerable change during the same time period. Dr. James Perrin (American Academy of Pediatrics Special Report, 1989) estimates that 20 years ago 80% of children with chronic illness died. Today most of these children survive, requiring continued, often complex, care. For example, children with cystic fibrosis now frequently survive into early adulthood (see Chapter 12). Improved surgical intervention and control of urinary tract infections have greatly prolonged the life expectancy of children with spina bifida (see Chapter 21). Newborn screening programs and early dietary intervention have dramatically improved the quality of life and reproductive capability of children with phenylketonuria (see Chapter 24).

New categories or groupings of childhood chronic conditions are also emerging. Infants surviving extreme prematurity or very low birth weight are posing new medical and management problems (see Chapter 25). A large population of infants and children with prenatal drug exposure present new challenges to the health care and educational systems (see Chapter 26). The number of children with acquired immune deficiency syndrome (AIDS) is projected to increase dramatically during the next 10 years (see Chapter 23). The health care system, with its advanced technology, has created a spectrum of children with chronic iatrogenic conditions, such as infants with bronchopulmonary dysplasia (see Chapter 7), children with immune suppression as a result of drug therapy following organ transplantation (see Chapter 22), and survivors of childhood leukemia who later suffer the residual effects of treatment (see Chapter 8). Decreased mortality rates, accompanied by an increased awareness of the functional limitations of children with chronic conditions, may be the reasons the National Health Interview Survey found a near-doubling of the reported number of children with limitations of activity due to chronic conditions between 1960 and 1980 (Newacheck, Budetti, and Halfon, 1986).

Many children with chronic conditions receive the majority of their medical care in specialty clinics that do not provide routine health care management (Palfrey, Levy, and Gilbert, 1980; Pless, Satterwhite, and Van Vechten, 1976; Stein, Jessop, and Riessman, 1983). Shuffled from specialist to specialist, the child often misses the screening, developmental assessment, anticipatory guidance, and even immunizations that healthy children of the same age receive (Palfrey, Levy, and Gilbert, 1980). This lack of routine health care appears to cross disease categories. Stein, Jessop, and Riessman (1983) interviewed mothers of children with a variety of chronic conditions and found that only 10% of the mothers had a health care professional to turn to when their child had minor illnesses, and only 20% said a professional was available to discuss normal growth and development, eating patterns, and so forth.

The development of medical specialization, which has improved the disease control and life expectancy of these children, has also resulted in fragmentation of health care delivery and increased medical costs (Liptak and Revell, 1989). The families of these children, far more than other families, have to interact with multiple institutions providing some aspect of care for their child, such as early intervention programs, equipment vendors, social services, special education programs, and federal, state, or private financial providers of care. In ad-

dition, there are often multiple medical subspecialists whose expectations may or may not be realistic for the family or child and whose demands are sometimes conflicting, uncoordinated, and incomprehensible to the family (Jessop and Stein, 1988).

BARRIERS TO OPTIMAL HEALTH CARE

Children with chronic conditions have unique health and social needs. Chronic illness in children is often not stable but subject to acute exacerbations and remissions that occur superimposed on the child's changing growth and development. If the impact of the chronic illness is to be minimized and the child allowed to develop to his or her maximum potential, comprehensive and coordinated care must be provided (Fox and Newacheck, 1990).

Many barriers have to be overcome to provide comprehensive quality health care to children with chronic conditions. The American Academy of Pediatrics (AAP Special Report, 1989) identified three categories of barriers for families: financial barriers, system barriers, and knowledge barriers. Liptak and Revell (1989) surveyed community physicians and found they identified similar barriers to providing complete care to children with chronic conditions. The barriers identified were lack of payments, lack of time, lack of knowledge regarding resources, and unfamiliarity with new techniques.

Financial barriers

The 1984 census indicated approximately 16 million children less than 21 years of age have no health insurance (AAP, 1989). Children with disabilities who are covered by health insurance are more likely to receive physician care than those children not covered by insurance (Butler et al., 1987). The U.S. Department of Health and Human Services (1984) estimates that approximately 40% of the nations disabled children are impoverished but not eligible for Medicaid, falling into the category of the uninsured poor. The National Association of Children's Hospitals and Related Institutions found uninsured children received 40% less health care than their insured peers (Sealing, 1989). In children with chronic conditions, this lack of regular care frequently results in aggravation of the chronic condition.

Although public programs such as Medicaid

and Supplemental Security Insurance have improved access to health care for many poor families during the past two decades, Medicaid eligibility regulations and benefits remain restrictive and vary significantly from state to state (Butler, Rosenbaum, and Palfrey, 1987). In 1986 Medicaid covered medical needs for only half of the children living below the poverty level, 400,000 fewer children than a decade ago, despite a one-third growth in child poverty during the same time period (Hughes and Johnson, 1988). In addition, families receiving Medicaid have limited access to providers, having to depend on publicly financed clinics where continuity of care is almost nonexistent. This lack of continuity frequently results in poor identification of disabilities and subsequent lack of appropriate referrals (Butler, Rosenbaum, and Palfrey, 1987).

If the child is covered by private insurance, access to care is usually improved, but out-of-pocket medical expenses may still have a significant impact on family finances. A recent national survey of group health insurance policies (Fox and Newacheck, 1990) found widespread coverage for inpatient hospital care, outpatient physician services, medical supplies, prescription medications, and laboratory services but less frequent coverage for services such as physical therapy, speech therapy, occupational therapy, and mental health services. More than two thirds of the insurance policies offered limited comprehensive home health services in lieu of more expensive inpatient care. Long-term skilled nursing care was covered by only one third of the insurance policies. In addition, the proportion of insurance policies requiring copayments by families for nonhospital expenses and substantial individual or family deductible payments has increased dramatically in the past 5 years, resulting in greater medical costs for families (Fox and Newacheck, 1990).

The cost of caring for a child with a chronic condition is not limited to medical expenses (Hobbs, Perrin, and Ireys, 1985). Additional expenses may include transportation costs, special diets, clothing, day care or respite care, dental and visual services, or home remodeling. Frequently the care required by the child necessitates that one parent be at home with the child, reducing time at work with subsequent loss of income and possibly insurance coverage. The cost to the family in terms of medical expenses, time, and psychosocial stress is just beginning to be identified (Bloom, Knorr, and Evans, 1985; Gale, 1989; Hobbs, Perrin, and Ireys, 1985).

Because of limitations of insurance coverage, the increased needs and complexities of health care for these children can also financially affect the primary care provider (Liptak and Revell, 1989; Shoemaker, 1989; Wissow et al., 1988). Adequate reimbursement schedules that compensate the primary care provider for additional training and for the time they must spend to provide health care maintenance to children with complex needs does not currently exist. It is more cost effective for the practitioner to see two or three well children with minor acute illnesses than it is to see one child with a chronic condition. Subspecialists receive reimbursement at a much higher rate than primary providers, and this may be one reason care is often shifted to the tertiary care centers.

System barriers

System barriers to optimal health care include the complex maze of federal, state, and private agencies designed to provide services, each with its own confusing bureaucracy and set of limitations and regulations (see Chapter 4) (Gale, 1989). Unfortunately, access to needed services is generally more dependent on geographic availability and the active involvement of medical personnel or disease-oriented voluntary organizations than it is on the needs of families (Hobbs, Perrin, and Ireys, 1985). Living in a rural or inner-city community where few appropriate services are available requires the family to travel great distances for care and may result in a major barrier to obtaining adequate health care. This lack of available appropriate health care has resulted in a population of medically homeless children who are at greater risk for poor health outcomes (Sealing, 1989).

Health care providers also find the maze of bureaucratic regulations overwhelming. When a child in their practice develops special needs, it may take an inordinate amount of time to identify and refer him or her to appropriate agencies in the community for needed services. Agencies and regulations keep changing, making it difficult to keep abreast of resources unless the provider has other clients with similar chronic conditions or access to a community social worker who can identify and make the appropriate referrals for the provider. In addition, many practices or health maintenance organizations routinely schedule brief visits with inadequate time for the provider to assess a child with complex needs. If the practitioner has little control over the practice schedule or support from the agency for this type of complex care, seeing children with chronic conditions may be very frustrating.

Knowledge barriers

Knowledge barriers to optimal health care can be present for both the family and the practitioner. Not knowing the need for or value of early intervention may delay initiation of care. Not knowing how to access services with proper referrals and eligibility identification may prevent the family from obtaining care they are entitled to receive. And not being sensitive to the families cultural heritage may inadvertently undermine the use of resources available to the family (Anderson and Fenichel, 1989).

Because of the explosive growth of medical knowledge and technology, it is difficult for practitioners to keep abreast of the current management techniques for children with chronic conditions. This recognition of knowledge limitations, possibly coupled with concern over potential legal consequences if subtle but important changes in a chronic condition are not recognized early, is frequently cited as the reason practitioners do not wish to assume medical or health care responsibilities for children with chronic conditions (Hobbs, Perrin, and Ireys, 1985; Liptak and Revell, 1989; Stein and Jessop, 1984).

ROLE OF THE PRIMARY CARE PROVIDER IN CARING FOR CHILDREN WITH CHRONIC CONDITIONS

Hobbs, Perrin, and Ireys (1985) discuss the issue of who should be responsible for health care of children with chronic conditions in light of the current disease-focused medical model that centers on specific conditions versus the general problems of management of childhood chronic conditions. Very few professionals would argue that the specialist, with advanced training and skills gained from caring for many children with similiar conditions, is

not the best professional to deal with the medical complexities of many chronic conditions. On the other hand, if the broader needs of the child and family are seen as the major focus of care—the common needs of education, support, advocacy, and health promotion, needs that families have regardless of the specific chronic condition—there is an obvious role for the primary care provider.

The primary care provider should be an integral part, if not the leading force, in the care of children with chronic conditions for multiple reasons. First, holistic health care of the child requires the child be viewed first, and primarily, as a child, with all the normal health care and developmental needs of any child. Second, the family must be seen as an integral part of the child's growth and development and recognized for its individual strengths and weaknesses (McDaniel, Campbell, and Seaburn, 1990). Third, health promotion, disease prevention, and anticipatory guidance have even greater significance when the child already has a condition that puts him or her at increased risk. Subspecialists are experts in their area of disease management but frequently have limited knowledge of normal growth and development and standard health care practices for health maintenance. Fourth, the primary provider most likely knows the family's community resources better than a subspecialist who may have a practice in a tertiary center many miles from the family's home (McInerny, 1984). This knowledge of community resources is extremely important in helping families receive optimal care and support for their child.

Caring for children with chronic conditions is a challenging, rewarding, and time-consuming proposition. It requires a commitment to service beyond that required for routine ambulatory pediatric care, increased knowledge about children with chronic conditions, and additional interpersonal communication and organizational skills necessary to provide optimal patient and family care.

Levels of intervention in the primary care of children and the knowledge base and skills needed by the primary care provider at each level of intervention are outlined in the box on pp 7-8. These levels of intervention are cumulative; that is, level 3 intervention cannot be attained until the knowledge base and skills of levels 1 and 2 are mastered. As the levels increase, so do the commitment of

HIERARCHICAL INTERVENTION FRAMEWORK FOR PRACTITIONERS CARING FOR CHILDREN WITH CHRONIC CONDITIONS

Level 1

Ongoing health care and illness management for children without chronic conditions

Knowledge base needed

- Routine health care maintenance and common illness management for children without chronic conditions and their families

Skills needed

1. The ability to collect subjective and objective data related to child health maintenance and common pediatric illnesses
2. The ability to elicit relevant family data related to family structure, medical history, and current health problems and concerns
3. The ability to listen effectively
4. The ability to assess the information obtained
5. The ability to identify a treatment plan for an individual nondisabled child and family
6. The ability to effectively communicate the treatment plan to the child and family
7. The ability to identify those children with more complex needs requiring additional services

Level 2

Task-oriented care for children with chronic conditions; primary care needs and specialty care needs managed by other professionals

Additional knowledge base needed

- Task-related knowledge

Additional skills needed

1. Performance of task in efficient correct manner

Level 3

Management of routine health care needs for children with chronic conditions; collaboration or referral for care related to the chronic condition

Additional knowledge base needed

- Basic pathophysiology of chronic conditions
- Child and family reactions to the stress of chronic conditions

- Collaborative role function
- Community agencies, tertiary care centers, and other professionals assuming responsibility for care of child's chronic condition

Additional skills needed

1. The ability to work with family members in their efforts to manage the child's normal growth and development
2. The ability to assess the child with a chronic condition identifying change requiring consultation or referral
3. The ability to identify family dysfunction requiring referral
4. The ability to communicate physical or psychosocial changes in the child or family to the appropriate professional

Level 4

Primary care of children with chronic conditions and their families

Additional knowledge base needed

- In-depth pathophysiology of chronic conditions
- Unique primary care needs of children with chronic conditions
- Common associated problems found in chronic conditions
- Differential diagnosis for common pediatric illnesses occurring in children with chronic conditions
- Community resources available to assist child and family
- Specific stressors for child and family of chronic condition

Additional skills needed

1. The ability to systematically assess the medical condition and health care needs of the child with a chronic condition
2. The ability to plan and implement primary health care, including common illness management, that is individualized for the child, the family, and the chronic condition
3. The ability to identify complications of the chronic condition requiring more complex care and make appropriate referrals

Continued.

HIERARCHICAL INTERVENTION FRAMEWORK FOR PRACTITIONERS CARING FOR CHILDREN WITH CHRONIC CONDITIONS — cont'd

4. The ability to educate the family on special complex needs of the child with a chronic condition
5. The ability to work with families to plan short- and long-term care consistent with medical needs and family function
6. The ability to assist parents and child in problem solving both medical and family concerns
7. The ability to help families recognize the needs of individual members and balance these needs during times of family stress and assist families in planning services and activities to reduce stress during these periods
8. The ability to make interdisciplinary referrals communicating child and family needs and expectations
9. The ability to provide consistent, available, long-term care

Level 5

Case management of families and children with chronic conditions

Additional knowledge base needed

- Service network available to child and family
- Cost-effective use of resources
- Service planning and systems coordination

- Eligibility requirements, referral process, and utilization measures for agencies or services that might benefit the family and child

Additional skills needed

1. The ability to develop an alliance with family and child to work together to provide optimum care
2. The ability to actively involve the family and child in the decision-making process for comprehensive care
3. The ability to make a comprehensive needs assessment for child and family
4. The ability to plan and initiate appropriate and successful referrals for services
5. The ability to coordinate services and personnel working with the family and child
6. The ability to monitor family and child progress
7. The ability to evaluate services used and make changes as necessary
8. The ability to communicate findings from multiple interdisciplinary sources to family, child, and other involved personnel or agencies
9. The willingness to function as child and family advocate

---

the provider and the completeness of care for the child and family. This model of care was inspired by work done in the area of family-centered care by Doherty and Baird (1987).

Level 1 care is defined as the provision of routine health care maintenance and common illness management to healthy children and their families. Some health care providers may elect not to care for children with chronic conditions because of practice restrictions, a knowledge base limited to the care of normal children, or the lack of skills necessary to adequately manage more complex medical and psychosocial problems. Optimal care can be provided at level 1, but only to children and families without complex health care needs.

Level 2 care is task-oriented care requiring minimal interaction with the child or family and no

commitment to continuity care. Level 2 care is not primary care but may be used to supplement primary care when a certain task needs to be accomplished. The knowledge base and skill level needed for this task-oriented care is limited to that which is necessary to complete the task efficiently, effectively, and safely. Examples of this level of care would include the primary care provider administering immunizations, ordering laboratory tests, or performing a prehospitalization physical examination, all at the request of the managing subspecialist.

Level 3 care is provided when the health care professional offers routine primary care to children with chronic conditions recognizing the unique health care needs of the child and family. The provider is able to assess the child's chronic condition but refers this care to other individuals or agencies. Because of the complexity of some conditions, personal interest or knowledge base of the provider, or practice restriction, the primary care provider may elect to manage some children with chronic conditions at this level while he or she manages children with other conditions at a higher level.

Level 4 care represents comprehensive primary health care incorporating the unique complexities of the chronic condition, the child, and the family. At this level the practitioner assumes the primary health care responsibilities of the child and family and uses consultation or referral for complex situations. He or she works collaboratively with the subspecialist to manage the chronic condition, common childhood illnesses, and routine health care maintenance. The practitioner does not abdicate care to the specialist but works with the specialist and the family to provide optimal care. As the health professional with the greatest knowledge of the family, the child, and the community, the primary care provider assumes a leadership role in providing comprehensive continuity care.

Level 5 care takes the role of the primary provider one step further, to that of case manager. A case manager is a person who assumes ongoing responsibility for service planning, assuring access to services, monitoring service delivery, advocating for child and family needs, and evaluating service outcomes, all while being concerned about cost effectiveness (Weil and Karls, 1985). It is the responsibility of the case manager to enhance the coordination, continuity, integration, and communication of services and to actively engage the family and child in this process (Harbin, 1989). The case manager must be able to perform a needs assessment of the child and family, plan and arrange for medical and nonmedical services, facilitate and coordinate services including the education and training of community providers, assume responsibility for follow-up to monitor services and client progress, and facilitate empowerment of children and their families through counseling, education, training, and advocacy (Liptak and Revell, 1989).

NEED FOR CASE MANAGEMENT

As the complexity of medical management increases with knowledge and technology and the health care financial system becomes overtaxed

with health care costs, service efficiency and cost effectiveness will be central concerns. In the past practitioners have been more likely to emphasize the quality of services and intensive care needs of clients, whereas administrators and funding sources often viewed service efficiency and cost effectiveness as more important (Weil and Karls, 1985). Primary care providers, functioning as case managers, must learn to assess and document the effectiveness of treatment programs used by their clients to support the continuation of these programs in this era of shrinking health care dollars and rising incidence of chronic conditions in children.

The case manager role has been incorporated into Public Law 99-457, the Early Intervention Program for Infants and Toddlers with Handicaps (Liaison Bulletin, 1986). Reimbursement for these services will be provided, but the extent of reimbursement and the funding service source will vary from state to state. This formal federal recognition of the benefits and necessity of case management for children with chronic conditions and the need for reimbursement for those services hopefully portends more movement in this direction.

SUMMARY

Primary care providers working with children with complex needs must identify their role and the roles of other health care professionals working with the child and family and communicate this role to all concerned, including the family. If they plan to intervene only at levels 1 to 3, the family must be informed of this decision and an appropriate professional identified to provide level 4 and 5 care.

If the chronic condition is medically complicated, uses complex technology, or requires prolonged use of resources housed in a tertiary care center, the primary specialist (often more than one specialist is working with a child) may be the appropriate professional to assume the leadership role in total health care management for the child. In this situation the specialist would be required to consult with or refer to a primary practitioner for normal health care maintenance appropriate for the child. Many specialty clinics are now using advanced nurse practitioners knowledgeable in both the specialty area and primary care to help facilitate communication and care between the specialty clinic, primary provider, and family (Frauman and Morton, 1988; Koop, 1985; Liptak and Revell, 1989; Wissow et al., 1988; Ziring et al., 1988).

But most chronic conditions of childhood are not so complex that the general practitioner, with additional knowledge about the chronic condition, its implications for primary care, and a commitment to effective communication, cannot assume a leadership role in health care management. Providers of pediatric health care have long embraced the philosophy that pediatric health care encompasses much more than disease management (AAP, 1988; American Nurses Association, 1983). Care rather than cure assumes greater meaning when one is working with children with chronic conditions, and there is much care to be provided that is common with the care needed by all children and their families.

The goal of health care maintenance for these children is to promote normal growth and development, to assist in maximizing the child's potential in all areas, to prevent or diminish the behavioral, social, and family dysfunctions frequently accompanying a chronic condition, and to confine or minimize the biologic disorder and its sequelae (Stein and Jessop, 1984). The primary care provider who knows the child and family well, knows the resources of the community, and is a specialist in health care maintenance is most often the appropriate health care professional to assume leadership in the often complex care and case management of these children.

REFERENCES

American Academy of Pediatrics: *Guidelines for health supervision*, Elk Grove, Ill, 1988, The American Academy of Pediatrics.

American Academy of Pediatrics Special Report: *Barriers to care: why millions of children live in the shadows, unable to receive appropriate health care*, Elk Grove, Ill, 1989, The American Academy of Pediatrics.

American Nurses Association: *Standards of maternal and child health nursing practice*, Kansas City, Mo, 1983, Division of Maternal and Child Health Nursing Practice.

Anderson PP and Fenichel ES: *Serving culturally diverse families of clinical infants and toddlers with disabilities*, Washington, DC, 1989, National Center for Infant Programs.

Bloom BS, Knorr RS, Evans AE: The epidemiology of disease expenses, *JAMA*, 253:2393-2397, 1985.

Butler JA, Rosenbaum S, Palfrey JS: Ensuring access to health care for children with disabilities, *N Eng J Med* 317:162-165, 1987.

Butler JA Singer JD, Palfrey JS, et al: Health insurance coverage and physician use among children with disabilities: findings from probability samples in fill metropolitan areas, *Pediatrics* 79:89-98, 1987.

Coupey SM and Cohen MI: Special considerations for the health care of adolescents with chronic illness, *Pediatr Clin North Am* 31:211-219, 1984.

Doherty W and Baird MA: *Family centered medical care: a clinical casework*, New York, 1987, Guilford Press.

Fox HB and Newacheck PW: Private health insurance of chronically ill children, *Pediatrics* 85:50-57, 1990.

Frauman AC and Morton JL: Well child care for the chronically ill child, *J Pediatr Health Care* 2:288-294, 1988.

Gale CA: Inadequacy of health care for the nation's chronically ill children, *J Pediatr Health Care* 3:20-27, 1989.

Gortmaker SL and Sappenfield W: Chronic childhood disorders: prevalence and impact, *Pediatr Clin North Am* 31:3-19, 1984.

Harbin G: Issues in case management: a national perspective, *Early Childhood Update* 5(2):6, 1989.

Hobbs N, Perrin JM, and Ireys HT: *Chronically ill children and their families*, San Francisco, 1985, Jossey-Bass.

Hughes D and Johnson K: *The health of America's children: maternal and child health data book*, Washington, DC, 1988, Children's Defense Fund.

Jessop DJ and Stein RK: Essential concepts in the care of children with chronic illness, *Pediatrician* 15:5-12, 1988.

Koop E: Our commitment to the disabled child, *Caring* 23-25, 1985.

National Association of State Directors of Special Education: EHA amendments of 1986 become law: establishes new partnership for early intervention programs, *Liaison Bull* 12(12): 1986.

Liptak GS and Revell GM: Community physician's role in case management of children with chronic illnesses, *Pediatrics* 84:465-471, 1989.

McCubbin MA: Family stress, resources, and family types: chronic illness in children, *Fam Relations* 37:203-210, 1988.

McDaniel SH, Campbell TL, and Seaburn DB: *Family-oriented primary care: a manual for medical providers*, New York, 1990, Springer-Verlag New York.

McInerny T: The role of the general pediatrician in coordinating the care of children with chronic illness, *Pediatr Clin North Am* 31:199-209, 1984.

Newacheck PW, Budetti PP, and Halfon N: Trends in activity-limiting chronic conditions among children, *Am J Public Health* 76:178-184, 1986.

Newacheck PW and McMarus MA: Financing health care for disabled children, *Pediatrics* 81:385-394, 1988.

Palfrey JS, Levy JC, and Gilbert KL: Use of primary care facilities by patients attending specialty clinics, *Pediatrics* 65:567-572, 1980.

Pless IB, Satterwhite B, and Van Vechten D: Chronic illness in childhood: a regional survey of care, *Pediatrics* 58:37-46, 1976.

Sealing PA: *Profile of child health in the United States*, Alexandria, Va, 1989, National Association of Children's Hospitals and Related Institutions.

Shoemaker FW: Are pediatricians intimidated by children with disabilities? *Calif Ped* 30:30 1989.

Stein RE and Jessop DJ: General issues in the care of children with chronic physical conditions, *Pediatr Clin North Am* 31:189-198, 1984.

Stein RE, Jessop DJ, Riessman CK: Health care services received by children with chronic illness, *Am J Dis Child* 137:225-230, 1983.

Surgeon General's Report: *Children with special health care needs*, Washington, DC, 1987, US Department of Health and Human Services.

US Department of Health and Human Services: *Report of the workshop on financing health care for handicapped children*, Washington, DC, 1987, USDHHS.

Weil M and Karls J: *Case management in human service practice*, San Francisco, 1985, Jossey-Bass.

Wissow LS, Warshow M, Box J, et al: Case management and quality assurance to improve care of inner-city children with asthma, *Am J Dis Child* 142:748-752, 1988.

Ziring PR, Kastner T, Friedman DL, et al: Provision of health care for persons with developmental disabilities living in the community: the Morristown model, *JAMA* 6:1439-1444, 1988.

2 Chronic Conditions and the Family

Margaret M. Mahon

THE FAMILY

Defining family is not as easy as it once was because there is no longer a majority that defines "traditional." Although certainly there are still nuclear families, a variety of family structures are now common, including single-parent families as a result of divorce, death, or because the parent never married, blended families, multigenerational families, children raised by gay or lesbian parents, children in foster or adoptive homes, and children living with grandparents, aunts or uncles, older siblings, or nonrelatives. In working with a child and family, one must ascertain who they define as their family and work within those parameters. One must also update this information over time, recognizing the high rate of flux within families today.

The definition of family and expectations of family members vary from culture to culture. Because the provider cares for families from varying ethnic and cultural groups, the role of each family member must be identified, as well as the family's perceived strengths and weaknesses.

The function of the family is nurturance. "The family generally creates an environment in which the basic needs necessary to sustain life and growth are met. When a family functions in a manner supportive of, or enabling the growth of its members, it is said to be functioning well" (Thomas, 1987, p. 30). Thomas describes five ways in which families differ from other societal groups: (1) their bonds are of affection, (2) they include a variety of ages and genders, (3) they are a group of virtual permanence, (4) there is a culture of previous and future generations, and (5) love and loyalty for family members will be stronger than extrafamilial bonds (Thomas, 1987).

These unique aspects of family might be considered ideal. They do not apply to some families, and not just those in which a child has a chronic condition. The bonds that tie can be those of obligation or ambivalence (Yost, Hochstadt, and Charles, 1988) rather than affection. For example, the ever-increasing numbers of infants abandoned in newborn nurseries by substance-abusing mothers represent parents who do not feel this bond or who are drawn more strongly by other forces.

Stability of family life is not ensured. Death, divorce, and separation of legally or nonlegally sanctioned relationships all lead to stress within family members (Johnson, 1986). Children may also experience instability if their parent or parents are substance abusers, are emotionally or physically abusive, or suffer from other chronic conditions (Blackford, 1988; Dura and Beck, 1988). Some children removed from their biologic families and adopted or placed in foster care experience a lack of cultural continuity associated with family life.

Changes in family structure do not necessarily mean weaker families, but these changes do require of the practitioner a greater awareness and sensitivity to differences within individual families and within society.

FAMILY CRISIS AND THE CHILD WITH A CHRONIC CONDITION

All families experience crises. Generally crises can be categorized into two types: developmental crises and situational crises. Developmental crises are experienced as an expected part of the developmental process of individuals and families, for example, marriage, the birth of a child, toilet training, starting school, or leaving home. Situational crises are not universal in that even though all families experience situational crises, they do not necessarily experience the same ones. Having a child with a chronic condition can be considered a situational crisis. With any crises, the equilibrium of the family is disrupted and usual problem-solving measures are inadequate to handle the situation (Aguilera and Messick, 1990). Any crisis, whether developmental or situational, changes the family. The attempt to regain equilibrium can leave the family stronger, weaker, or dissolved (Hymovich, 1981).

In assessing the impact of a chronic condition on a family, one must consider the situational crisis in the context of any concomitant or proximal developmental crisis. For example, the family whose newborn has a condition necessitating surgery or other treatment is dealing with the birth of a child and the child's chronic condition.

It is also essential that a practitioner not assume the family's functional level will be static; rather, it may fluctuate over time. Highs and lows relate presumably to those stresses that impinge on the system and to crisis resolution (Kazak, 1989). These stresses are not solely the result of a chronic condition. Families in which a child has a chronic condition are subject to the same stresses as other families. "The additions of other children to the family, divorces, deaths of grandparents, financial problems, relocation, and inclusion of nonblood kin in the family system are all 'normal' events families experience that will affect the way in which the child's illness is perceived and handled over time" (Kazak, 1989, p. 26).

Much of what is known about chronic conditions of childhood is from disease-specific studies (Feetham, 1984). This complicates the task of drawing broad conclusions about the effects of chronic childhood illness on family functioning. But some generalizations are possible, which, together with the disease-specific information, can help to explain the range of responses to chronic conditions.

A problem in any member of a family has an effect on all other members of the family system. A chronic condition in a child does not affect only the child but has ramifications for all members of the family system (Kazak, 1989). Having a child with a chronic condition is stressful (Hobbs, Perrin, and Ireys, 1985; Jessop, Reissman, and Stein, 1988; Kazak, 1989; Thomas, 1987). What has been relatively neglected in research until recently is the stress of a child with a chronic condition relative to other stresses. "Even a seemingly objective stressor like chronic illness in childhood cannot be fully understood apart from the larger context in which this event is embedded" (Jessop, Reissman, and Stein, 1988, p. 154). Other developmental and situational stressors are always happening not only to this child but to other members of the family system.

The term "chronic condition" is appropriate because it recognizes that children with a variety of deviations from the norm are not always "ill children." Families often define their children as "normal" even though to observers this is not the case (Anderson, 1981). Despite a history of morbidity, parents consider most of their children to be in good to excellent health (McCormick et al., 1988). Moreover, ratings by the health care provider of the burden of care of the child has no relationship to the psychologic status of the mother (Jessop, Reissman, and Stein, 1988). It is essential, then, as with the definition of family, to work within the framework given by the family.

The definition of chronic illness as developed by the 1949 National Commission on Chronic Illness (and as used in Chapter 1) reveals that a wide range of conditions qualify as chronic. The condition need not be permanent, serious, or obvious. On the other hand, some chronic conditions are nonreversible, are serious, and require comprehensive care.

The reality is that a child may be seriously impaired from birth, may have a transitory condition from which recovery is complete, or may have any degree of severity in between. Furthermore, a diagnosis is not always indicative of the severity of a child's condition. For example, asthma, the most common chronic condition of childhood, may severely affect a child's ability to function on a daily basis or may cause only occasional short-term disability.

FAMILY REACTION TO THE DIAGNOSIS OF A CHRONIC CONDITION

The diagnosis of a chronic condition is a time of extreme distress (Goldberg and Simmons, 1988) and disequilibrium (Thomas, 1987) for a family. Many factors affect a family's reactions. The identification of a diagnosis might cause a reaction not necessarily congruent with presenting symptoms, health of the child, or interventions required as a result of the diagnosis (Goldberg and Simmons, 1988). This suggests that family reaction, especially parental reaction, is based more on preconceived ideas about a chronic condition. A child previously thought of as healthy may now be thought of as ill.

Chronic conditions in newborns are either congenital (e.g., cleft lip or palate), genetic (e.g., trisomy 21), or a function of prematurity. In each of these situations, the parents are likely to grieve the healthy child they envisioned (Solnit and Stark, 1962). Initial reactions may include shock, disbelief, and denial (Holaday, 1984), which may translate to thoughts that the child is not their child but that there has been some kind of mix-up or mistake. If the condition is genetic, some parents will feel guilt that they caused this condition in their child (Goldberg and Simmons, 1988). For some parents, this grieving might mean that they are not immediately able to respond to the child who has been born or that their response is one of distancing themselves. This temporary distancing is not necessarily inappropriate and should not be treated as maladaptive.

As with newborns, the diagnosis of a chronic condition in a child usually results in disequilibrium (Thomas, 1987). The response may also include shock, disbelief, denial (Holaday, 1984), disgust, relief, guilt, despair, hate, rage, or confusion (Hobbs, Perrin, and Ireys, 1985). "Disruption of the family depends on the nature, severity, length, prognosis of illness and parental coping: support systems, fiscal resources, educational background,

previous experience with illness and a variety of individual definitions" (Andrews and Nielson, 1988, p. 112). One major difference that occasionally occurs with the diagnosis of a chronic condition in older children is a sense of relief at finally having a diagnosis. The suspicions of the parents are confirmed, the uncertainty is over, and interventions are begun. The child and family may also become eligible for a range of services for which they previously were not eligible (Goldberg and Simmons, 1988).

The diagnosis sets some parents on a search for causes of the condition, whether physiologic or environmental (Lipman, 1988). This quest for information is usually very appropriate. The parent or parents are obtaining knowledge about the condition, which is the first step in having some control over the situation (Hobbs, Perrin, and Ireys, 1985). In some parents, however, the search for information is a denial of the reality of their child's situation. For example, some parents will read medical books and talk with a variety of specialists and subspecialists. It can allow them to make informed choices or can be the beginning of a search exclusively for a cure, resulting in the child not receiving the immediate medical care needed.

Besides looking for facts about the condition, some parents search for religious or philosophic reasons for what has happened (Holaday, 1984). This sometimes takes the form of "why me" questions. Parents also worry about the health of their other children and begin to search for means of preventing the condition in them (Lipman, 1988).

The prognosis of the condition may affect the reaction of the parents, especially if the condition is potentially life threatening (Goldberg and Simmons, 1988). Other factors that affect the reaction of the parents and others are the visibility of the condition, the presence or absence of mental retardation, the expectation of pain for the child, the parents' experience with others who have chronic conditions, and preconceptions about the condition, whether correct or incorrect (Burr, 1985).

RESPONSES TO TREATMENT AND CHRONICITY
Role of the primary care provider

When a diagnosis of a chronic condition is made, the focus of the family often becomes narrow and very disease oriented. Whether caring for a newborn or an older child, the health care provider should consider several important guidelines. First, be concrete. Provide as much information as is immediately needed but not much more. Answer specific questions. If possible, provide information in writing or tape record discussions about the condition so the parents and child can hear the explanation repeated. Second, provide resources, such as the primary care provider, a subspecialist, a clinical nurse specialist, or a resource group. The family should be supplied information about "what comes next." Again, if possible, do this in writing. Third, help the family put the diagnosis in perspective. This is hard to do but can be very helpful for families. The first step is to ascertain what expectations the parent or parents already have. If there are misconceptions, they can be clarified. In addition, find something normal and positive about this child. For example, comment on the alertness of an infant born with myelomeningocele or the child's strong grasp. This is not an attempt to minimize the seriousness of the situation but to focus on the child as an individual with the same needs as other children.

There are no right or wrong reactions for family members at the time of diagnosis. The primary care provider should look for cues from the family concerning their readiness to learn, their difficulty accepting the diagnosis, or their unique fears or stressors and should respond to these cues in a supportive manner. Every interaction at this critical juncture should be ended with a statement concerning what to expect next and when the family will be seen again.

When the diagnosis of a chronic condition is made by someone other than the primary care provider, the family will often turn to the primary care provider for information, help, or advice. In some cases the practitioner is available but inaccurate (Hobbs, Perrin, and Ireys, 1985) concerning the details or treatment of the condition. It is important for the practitioner to consult with the specialist to facilitate the family's understanding of the diagnosis and treatment. The practitioner needs to help establish a team approach to care that includes the family because the ultimate responsibility for care of the child lies with the family (Horner, Rawlins, and Giles, 1987). This requires knowing and building on family strengths and considering potential stressors in planning for care. Most important, it means using the knowledge the family has acquired not only about the condition but also about the child and his or her individual responses.

Family roles and responsibilities

The management of a chronic condition rarely falls equally on familial care givers. The mother is usually identified as the one primarily responsible for the day-to-day care and management of the child (Howlin, 1988; Jessop, Reissman, and Stein, 1988; Kazak, 1989; Moyer, 1989). Some mothers give up their jobs to care for the child perhaps because of the demands of medical treatment (Stein et al., 1989). Because of limited day care for children with chronic conditions, some mothers who might otherwise be employed outside the home are forced to stay at home (Hobbs, Perrin, and Ireys, 1985; Stein et al., 1989). The chronic condition or resultant treatments may bring about behavioral changes that affect the parental relationship with the child. Such changes have been observed in response to the blood testing and insulin injections required for a child with diabetes (Goldberg and Simmons, 1988). While there can be many stressors, it is essential to note that many women evaluate this experience very positively.

Parents may also be negatively affected by these care demands. Some parents of children with chronic conditions are depressed and have decreased self-esteem, psychologic pain (Schlomann, 1988), and somatic conditions (Sabbeth and Leventhal, 1984). Some mothers experience depression, fatigue, headaches, insomnia, and loss of appetite, whereas fathers have experienced depression, fatigue, ulcers, headaches, and obesity (Hobbs, Perrin, and Ireys, 1985). Mothers may have more symptoms than fathers (Jessop, Reissman, and Stein, 1988), but this might be because mothers are more frequently the subject of research. Although it has been suggested that the functional status of the child is correlated with the mother's symptoms, maternal symptoms may be more related to stress than to the child's actual functional level (Jessop, Reissman, and Stein, 1988).

Many mothers report it very helpful to have someone with whom they can talk (Jessop, Reissman, and Stein, 1988). Because this person may not necessarily be a family member (Kazak, Reber, and Carter, 1988), support groups may be very helpful in meeting this need (Horner, Rawlins, and Giles, 1987). These groups are often most helpful to families near the time of diagnosis, probably because of the need for concrete information that is shared among the relatively small number of people who are in a similar situation. Mothers may perceive and use social supports differently from fathers (Kazak, Reber, and Carter, 1988). In one study, fathers and older parents were less likely to want to join support groups than mothers and younger parents (Winkel, 1988).

Normalization. Normalization is a management process employed by some families of children with a chronic condition. Normalization involves acknowledging the chronic condition, defining the life of the family as normal, defining the social effects of having a child with a chronic condition as minimal, and engaging in behaviors that demonstrate to others that this is a normal family (Knafl and Deatrick, 1986). Normalization is an ongoing process of actively accommodating the child's evolving physical, emotional, and social needs (Deatrick, Knafl, and Walsh, 1988). The child is integrated into the mainstream to the greatest extent possible (Holaday, 1984).

Acknowledging the condition is essential as the foundation of normalization. There is no denial involved, rather, the family is making a statement that "this child is a part of our family, and our family is just like every other family." The age of the child, as well as the severity of the condition, affects the ability of the family to use the process of normalization (Knafl and Deatrick, 1986).

Krulik (1980) described several antecedent principles necessary for the normalization process: (1) those involved in the care of the child, as well as the child, are prepared for the effects of the condition and treatment; (2) the child is involved in self-care and the decisions made about that care; (3) the child with a chronic condition is treated as a part of the family, not differently; (4) the child's condition is not treated as something to be kept secret, rather, information is shared; and (5) recognition of the parents' preexisting role in managing care decreases feelings of passivity and uncertainty.

Normalization is important because it focuses on the child, not the condition. Most parents who have used normalization techniques have discovered them on their own. The process, however, involves some concrete steps that can be taught. The health care provider can demonstrate some of these steps by recognizing the normalcy, the strengths, and the weaknesses of the family system, being open and supportive concerning the child's condition and treatment, and actively involving the family in all aspects of care. Reinforcing the family's successful use of these tactics can improve self-esteem and motivate further development.

Siblings. The impact of the chronic condition on siblings can be analyzed in much the same way as other childhood stressors. Having a sibling with a chronic condition may elicit feelings of isolation, rejection, anxiety, helplessness, resentment, guilt, or depression. These frequently stem from emotional realignment within the family, where there are periods of physical and emotional separation, a lack of information, and disrupted communication (Kramer, 1981; Krener and Adelman, 1988). A lack of balance between the needs of the affected child and of siblings is also disrupting (Krener and Adelman, 1988).

Parents may have difficulty accurately perceiving how their children are coping with the additional family stress. It is often very helpful for the primary care provider to ask how the sibling or siblings are doing and what they understand about recent changes in the family. Siblings may be uninformed about the nature of the condition for several weeks (Kramer, 1981). Parents may not have been able to take the time to explain the recent changes to the sibling.

Siblings are directly and immediately affected by the diagnosis of a chronic condition but are often without power to have any impact on the many and perhaps serious changes within the family. What makes this more difficult is that siblings often guess about the chronic condition and the resulting health status, in part because of the absence of the affected sibling or parents and the influx of visitors or increased number of telephone calls. What they overhear or piece together is often much worse than the reality. If the parents are unable to talk to the siblings, it is important to find someone else, such as the primary care provider, who can speak with the siblings in a developmentally appropriate way.

Worries or fears of the siblings can to a certain extent be predicted based on developmental level. Children in the preoperational stage of development are likely to have fears based on causality and contagion (Mahon, 1985). They must be told specifically that they were not responsible for the condition. Siblings whose conceptual ability is at the level of concrete operations are likely to be afraid of catching the condition. A sibling of a child who was being treated for cancer began to scrub the toilets in the house thoroughly. When asked about this by his mother, he explained that because the cancer cells were coming out in the urine, he did not want to catch it when he went to the bathroom. In this case, some very appropriate teaching had been done with this sibling, but he took the information and integrated his fears at his current level of understanding.

Siblings also often imagine gruesome things about the experiences associated with illness, hospitalization, and treatment. If possible, siblings should be allowed to see the hospital, treatment rooms, and perhaps treatments if it is acceptable to the affected sibling.

The effects of a condition or treatment, such as hair loss, flatulence, or copious secretions, may be embarrassing for siblings of school age and older. At the same time, children also want to protect the affected sibling from the derisive statements or stares of others (Trahd, 1986). These feelings of shame and embarrassment are usually not severe (Howlin, 1988).

Siblings often feel that the discipline for the affected child is not as strict as it is for them (Howlin, 1988), and, in fact, this is often the case. Some parents are not aware that they are treating their children with different standards. It is appropriate for the primary care provider to question families about methods and consistency of discipline.

Siblings are usually very aware of their negative feelings, which may include anger, feelings of being neglected, fears of causality, contagion, or responsibility, as well as other founded and unfounded feelings (Howlin, 1988; Kramer, 1981). As a result, they may experience guilt. Children need to be told that their emotions are acceptable,

but at the same time misconceptions need to be clarified. This may be a time-consuming process calling for self-realization, a difficult task for some families. For example, a sibling's perception that he or she has been receiving less attention can be confirmed. The child should also be told that it is okay to feel angry about it. This can be very difficult if sharing emotions such as anger is not usually done by a particular family.

The developmental level of siblings, both physical and psychosocial, must be considered in the plan for care of the affected child at home. If a child is to be cared for at home and needs the use of equipment and medications, recognizing and planning for sibling safety are required. Andrews and Nielson (1988) reported several cases of children injuring or potentially injuring themselves or siblings by changing intravenous flow rates or not understanding the danger of electrical equipment.

Siblings have also described many positive effects from having a sibling with a chronic condition, including being well adjusted, having a positive self-concept, being more mature, being more tolerant, and being capable of handling greater responsibility than their peers (Howlin, 1988; Kramer, 1981; Lynn, 1989). Siblings of children with a chronic condition have been reported to be cooperative and cognitively able to master situations earlier than their peers (Lynn, 1989).

Several factors predict adjustment. The most important factor is parental attitude about the child (Howlin, 1988). Siblings in a two-child family may be at greater risk because the bond with the affected child forms the sole sibling relationship (Trahd, 1986).

Relative birth order and gender are also significant. In one study among siblings younger than their affected brother or sister, boys were more impaired than girls, whereas among siblings older than their affected brother or sister, girls were psychologically more distressed (Breslau, Weitzman, and Messenger, 1981). These authors believed this was most likely to be the case if the condition were congenital. The possibility of more difficult adaptation by older sisters is congruent with the finding of Howlin (1988) because girls were more likely to have care-giving demands placed on them. Older sisters might be called on more often than younger sisters to perform these tasks.

There is some disagreement about the degree to which siblings should be involved in the care of a child with a chronic condition. One hallmark is to consider "what would be expected of siblings if a chronic condition were not involved." Two areas should be considered: the developmental abilities of the siblings and their desire to be involved. Gender-biased expectation of siblings does occur but should be avoided if possible. The most important consideration is consistency: are demands being made regardless of whether a chronic condition is present or absent in any particular child? For those siblings who want to be involved in the care of the child with the chronic condition, this altruism should not be discouraged (Howlin, 1988).

Throughout the course of the chronic condition, information for the siblings needs to be updated for two primary reasons. First, what is known about the condition changes, both as the affected child and parents learn more about the condition and because the manifestations of the condition in this particular child might change. Second, the developmental level of the siblings changes, thereby changing their ability to integrate information. Primary care providers are often in an ideal position to provide the impetus for further teaching, both as more is known about the condition and as the siblings progress developmentally.

Finances. Some chronic conditions place large financial demands on the family (Jacobs and McDermott, 1989), though costs vary a great deal depending on the condition and even among individuals with the same condition (Hobbs, Perrin, and Ireys, 1985). There are many additional expenses beyond those directly involved in the care of the chronic condition.

Additional costs for families include food required by special diet, transportation, baby-sitters for siblings while a child receives treatment or other care, time lost from work or school, cosmetics, wigs or clothing to hide the effects of the disease or treatment, and incidentals such as bandages, test kits, diapers, and bed pads, the cost of which adds up quickly (Hobbs, Perrin, and Ireys, 1985). Other financial requirements arise because of structural modifications to the home, counseling and mental health services, and respite homemaker services (Gale, 1989). Not all of these are covered by most third-party payers, and if they are, there is likely to be a limitation on the amount of reimbursement (see Chapter 4).

Two to five percent of children with chronic conditions are candidates for home health services, which might include monitoring equipment, phototherapy, oxygen and tracheostomy care, enteral and parenteral therapy, artificial ventilation, and dialysis (Andrews and Nielson, 1988). Primary care providers are likely to be caring for a child and family who are the recipients of such services. It is usually parents who deliver care at home (Edwardson, 1983). Home care teaching is usually done by nurses or a representative from a home care agency while a child is hospitalized. Many families have found that the teaching they received does not meet their needs once they are home. This may be a reflection not of inadequate teaching but of the lack of a frame of reference for the parent or parents who are learning the care. Also, the anxiety associated with providing care at home might interfere with parents' ability to learn. The first 2 weeks at home are the hardest (Andrews and Nielson, 1988).

Because of some families' inability to provide care, some children with chronic conditions are in need of medical foster care. The need for families capable of providing this service has dramatically increased in recent years. When foster care is not found, these children often become boarder infants in hospitals at great financial cost to the hospital and the public and at significant personal risk to the child. These children do not need the level of care a hospital provides; instead, they require a family environment for nurturance (Yost, Hochstadt, and Charles, 1988). Placing children in medical foster care results in a 40% to 98% savings in monetary terms and provides a home environment (Yost, Hochstadt, and Charles, 1988).

Social support

A primary need of most families is emotional support and practical help (Holaday, 1984). At the time of diagnosis there is often an influx of concerned people, possibly too many. The family may have difficulty using these resources. Types of support that families have found very helpful include transporting siblings or having them stay with friends during hospitalizations or necessary travel, providing meals, doing the laundry, running errands, or baby-sitting in the home so that the parents can have some time for themselves. This latter form of assistance may entail learning care such as cardiopulmonary resuscitation (CPR), use of monitors, or emergency care. It is extremely important that someone in addition to the mother be able and willing to do this. Improved social supports have benefits for the entire family (Wallander and Varni, 1989).

After the initial crisis period, many parents find that they are without support from friends and family, which can result in social isolation (Andrews and Nielson, 1988). In one study, 49% of respondents said that they needed help in finding community resources, and 34% asked for help in finding recreational activities for their children with chronic conditions (Horner, Rawlins, and Giles, 1987).

If the condition the child has is relatively common or is well understood, the child with the condition is less likely to face societal prejudice (Garrison and McQuiston, 1989). This issue of familiarity with the condition is one reason some parents turn to support groups; they do not have to explain and reexplain the condition, because the support group members experience similar situations.

School

The transition to school can be a difficult time for families. Although it is an indication that the child is "like other children" and well enough to attend school, many obstacles may need to be overcome in starting and maintaining school participation. Families often feel that teachers and others in the school system are not ready for the challenge of school attendance (Johnson, Lubker, and Fowler, 1988). Teachers support this, reporting that they feel inadequately prepared to care for children with chronic conditions.

The implications for teachers of having a child with a chronic condition in their class range from minimal to overwhelming. For example, the teacher of a child with diabetes should know what to give a child who is having a hypoglycemic reaction. The teacher of a child with heart disease should know CPR, the teacher of a child with epilepsy should know what to do if the child has a seizure. It is unrealistic to expect that care of children with chronic conditions can be handled by a school nurse; often a

school nurse divides time between several schools and would be unable to respond to an emergency without loss of precious time.

Families in which a child has a chronic condition are thus left in a very difficult position. Optimally their child should be in school, but often the school, and specifically the teacher, is inadequately prepared to care for the student. From the teacher's point of view, caring for the student would, at the least, take time away from other students and, at worst, could result in a dangerous situation for those students left unattended while the teacher is caring for the affected student. Because there is no ideal solution at this time, each situation should be planned for in advance, before the child begins in the classroom. This planning stage offers an ideal opportunity for the school nurse and primary care provider to cooperate with the family and teacher so that all concerned feel comfortable with the child being in the classroom.

LONG-TERM ADAPTATION

Initial responses of the family system to a chronic condition are often much like those of an acute illness. After living with the condition and learning its nuances and management, the family has a more thorough understanding of chronicity. The depth and breadth of understanding usually do not extend beyond the immediate family. For example, relatively simple things such as going out for a meal become difficult, require a great deal of planning, and may be time limited if a child cannot be away from suctioning and oxygen for an extended period.

The amount of time that has elapsed since diagnosis is directly related to the family's involvement in all aspects of care. The longer the child has had the condition, that is, the greater the duration of the chronicity, the more the family is involved in all aspects of the care. Over time family members gain greater understanding of the interplay of the condition with the individuality of the child. The expectations of the family become more realistic as experience with the condition is acquired (Goldberg and Simmons, 1988).

Selected aspects of some chronic conditions are frequently viewed by the parents as disruptive to their relationship with their child (Goldberg and Simmons, 1988). Examples include parents of children with cystic fibrosis (CF) who must perform postural drainage, the decreased physical contact that might be required as a result of osteogenesis imperfecta, or the blood testing and insulin injections required by children with diabetes too young for self-care. Parenting a child with a chronic condition "involve[s] qualitatively different work than parenting a child" without a chronic condition (Deatrick, Knafl, and Walsh, 1988, p. 21). There is often the assumption that "different" has negative connotations. It is essential to differentiate between assuming that having a child with a chronic condition is inherently negative and specifying what aspects of the situation are problematic (Knafl and Deatrick, 1987).

Parental concerns are often the same as those of families without a child who has a chronic condition. In a study of the concerns of parents of children with diabetes, the parents needed information about diet, the affected child marrying and having children, diabetes, care of minor illnesses, normal growth and development, and management of child behavior (Moyer, 1989), all concerns readily addressed by the primary care provider. All parents worry. The extent to which the parent of a child with a chronic condition worries cannot be predicted from the severity of symptoms (Stein et al., 1989).

Many parents are concerned not only about the effect of a chronic condition on the family as it exists at the time of diagnosis but also about the implications for future children. A major factor is whether or not the chronic condition has a genetic component. If, for example, a family has a child with Tay-Sachs disease, they might choose not to have more children or might choose to use prenatal screening to assess if the fetus is affected. If the condition is genetic but not a mendelian inheritance, such as trisomy 21 with a translocation defect that might have a 10% to 15% recurrence rate, the family might be more willing to risk having another child. In this case as well, the family can avail themselves of prenatal diagnosis. Parents who felt guilty about having a child with a genetically transmitted chronic condition will need to deal with this again if they consider having another child (Goldberg and Simmons, 1988) and later in life when their children have children.

Another common concern for parents is that of parental (usually maternal) workload: can they

physically and fiscally care for another child? Again, these concerns are often the same as those families in which there is no child with a chronic condition.

As the affected child gets older, the concerns about the ability to have children become his or her own. For example, with the increased survival time of people with CF, more women are surviving to childbearing age. Fertility for some of these women is unaffected by CF (MacMullen and Brucker, 1989), which has implications for these women but also for the family and primary care provider in regard to education and contraceptive counseling.

Marital relations

Some have assumed that because the presence of a chronic condition increases the stress in a family, the rate of family dissolution is greater. In fact, there is "no difference in divorce rates or marital adjustment with carefully controlled studies" (Kazak, 1989, p. 28). Although divorce is not more prevalent, tension and stress are more common than in families without a child who has a chronic condition (Hobbs, Perrin, and Ireys, 1985). All families have issues and stressors, and when families have a child with a chronic condition, it is easier to overemphasize the causal role of the child's condition in any problems that do exist (Howlin, 1988).

Chronic sorrow. Olshansky (1962) first described the phenomenon of chronic sorrow as an ongoing process differing from grief. Olshansky's description came as a result of working with children with mental retardation. Chronic sorrow refers to the recurrence of parental feelings engendered by the recognition that their child is "different." These feelings include sadness, anger, guilt, and failure. Chronic sorrow persists throughout the life of the child. This does not mean parents are always sad or that the family does not feel happiness or satisfaction and pride from the child with the chronic condition. Those positive feelings are present, sometimes with great intensity, just as they are for parents whose child does not have a chronic condition.

Parents are likely to experience the surges of emotion associated with chronic sorrow at times of expected developmental milestones such as walking or starting school, when younger siblings surpass the affected child, and when the child turns 21 years of age. Chronic sorrow also resurges at unpredictable times, which might be described as times the family would have shared had the child not had a chronic condition (Wikler, Wascow, and Hatfield, 1981).

Other researchers have generalized the use of the term "chronic sorrow" to apply to children with chronic physical alterations (Jackson, 1985; Lawson, 1977; Neill, 1979; Tenbrinck and Brewer, 1976; Young, 1977). Much of the work that has been done is not founded in research but has been adopted because clinicians sense an intuitive fit with the responses of families who have a child with a chronic condition.

Chronic sorrow does not necessarily occur uniformly within families. Damrosch and Perry (1989) found "clearcut differences in maternal and paternal patterns of overall adjustment. While 83% of the fathers depicted their adjustment as steady, gradual, and timebound, 68% of the mothers perceived their own adjustment as chronic, periodic crises" (p. 28). The authors stress the need to assess family functioning and adaptation not just as a unit but to recognize the responses of individuals within that unit as well.

THE DYING CHILD AND FAMILY

Most pediatric primary care providers do not frequently deal with the death of a child. Because trauma is the leading cause of death in children, pediatric primary care providers are likely to have more experience with survivors (parents and siblings) than with a terminally ill child. Primary care providers might be called on to provide care for a child with a terminal condition who has been treated at a tertiary care facility but is returning home to die. For the health care provider the death of a child can be a painful and awkward situation.

Parents often turn to the practitioner for advice on communicating with the ill child or the siblings concerning death. A good guideline to use in working with families is to answer the question the child asks, though it also is important to understand why the child is asking. Often the subtext is "who will take care of me?" or "does it hurt to die?" The inclination of parents and primary care providers may be to inundate children with information. If one is open to questions, that is, takes the time to

listen and is clearly willing to respond, the child will most often ask what he or she is ready to hear.

One exception is in the area of blame. Children of all ages often inappropriately assume some responsibility for the death or feel guilty about their responses to the death. If this is the case, the child should be told that he or she had no responsibility for the death. As is true with all crucial issues of development, the information will probably have to be repeated several times.

Parents

Once a child's condition has reached the terminal phase, the focus of care should switch from cure to amelioration of symptoms and provision of comfort (Edwardson, 1983). Often by this time in the condition the parents have become expert in providing complete care for their child. With time the focus switches from cure to facilitating a good death. The actual care that is given is likely to be based on several areas of input, including objective information, the wishes of the child, options the parents are given about the child's death, and personal and professional support they receive (Edwardson, 1983). When the decision as to whether the child should die at home or in the hospital is being made, it is essential to get the input of the child who is dying (Martinson, 1983).

Children who have been sick for a long time often have an understanding of sickness and death well beyond their chronologic age. These children are also well able to judge who is comfortable dealing with their impending death and who is not. Dying children may use the way care givers have handled other deaths as a test. For example, if a child and family are seen regularly in a clinic, they get to know other children and families. This bond is increased if simultaneous hospitalizations occur. If a friend dies, the child is likely to use the response of staff and other families as a gauge for how his or her own death will be handled and to measure how helpful others are likely to be in the process of preparing for death. The dying child, then, individualizes interactions based on an assessment of those with whom he or she is interacting. Children "maintain an open awareness with those who can handle it, and at the same time maintain mutual pretense with those who want to practice it" (Bluebond-Langner, 1978, p. 235).

To be honest with the child and family does not mean to take away hope; it should be interwoven throughout the course of the illness. The focus of hope, however, changes in the same way that increased knowledge and varying patient responses result in modification of plans of care (Gyulay, 1989). As the inevitability of death becomes clearer, the focus of the hope changes, perhaps from cure to minimal pain and control in the process of dying.

Pain control is an extremely important issue as a child is dying. Pain control in children is not as well understood as in adults largely because of underestimation of and misconceptions about the child's ability to feel pain. The guideline should be to treat the symptoms (Meehan, 1989). It is important to realize that symptoms and coping are likely to be different in children than in adults. Assessment of pain must also be different from techniques used with adults. Because a child is able to play with a video game for 30 minutes without complaining does not mean the child is not in pain. It is more likely that the child has excellent self-distraction abilities.

It is important to maintain the usual activities of childhood, such as playing and reading. Play is important because it enhances the child's feelings of control (Gray, 1989; Vessey and Mahon, 1990). Though the dying child may be less able to participate in familiar and favorite activities, usually modifications can be made if this is something the child really wants to do. For example, someone else can roll die and move a game piece. If the child is no longer able to read his or her own books, many children love to have books read to them. These are both ideal ways to involve siblings. Music is also a favorite distraction for children. Even very young children of 1 or 2 years have favorite tapes.

Older children may want to be involved in planning their own funeral. This is often very difficult for the family, but it is the last act of control for some children. Children have chosen particular readings or music for their funerals. One child asked that balloons be released in the church "to go up in the same way his spirit would go."

Dying children often seem ambivalent about the role of those around them. They may be adamant about not being left alone, but they are also likely to be selective about who they want to be with them. It may seem that their world is becoming progressively smaller. The child is likely to become less verbal because of decreased energy and perhaps because of a physical inability to talk. The child might also be in a coma, depending on the condition. If the latter is the case, parents can be encouraged to continue physical and verbal contact with the child. The presence of a few people and physical contact when possible are very important to the child.

The death of a child is the most painful loss one can experience. It is likely to take 3 years before parents regain the energy level they had before the child's death (Arnold and Gemma, 1983). Parents are likely to be preoccupied. There is not one specific right thing to say to support parents, but there are wrong responses. Parents should never be told "at least you have other children"; "at least he was young enough so you didn't have time to know him well"; "You're young. You can have more children"; or worst, "I know how you feel." Even those who have experienced the death of a child will not experience the same responses.

Within families there will also be variation in response to the death of a child. Mothers are more likely to receive social support and recognition of the depth of their loss. Fathers are expected to support the mother. This may help to explain why fathers do not heal with the passage of time as mothers do (Hogan, 1988).

Many families have found it helpful to have contact with the care provider about 1 month or more after the death. By this time, friends and relatives may be expecting the family members to better manage their grief, but their pain is still fresh. Not uncommonly, many parents want to learn more about their child's death. The primary care provider might be the person best able to answer any questions the parents have about the death, especially any last words, or whether or not the child was in pain, particularly if it was a sudden death or the parents were not present at the time of death.

Meeting with parents serves another purpose. It shows the family that someone does remember how recent the death was and how acute the pain is. Even with the death of a newborn, it is increasingly common for a parent to have found a pediatric care provider before their child's birth. With the death of an infant, the mother is likely to feel guilt or even rejection (Novak, 1988). These feelings must be acknowledged and realistic explanations given for the death. They might not immediately ameliorate negative feelings the mother has, but the information can serve as an accurate standard against which incorrect or irrational beliefs can be checked and can ultimately facilitate the grieving process.

Siblings

Siblings are likely to feel extremely isolated while the child is dying, especially if that child is hospitalized. If the child is hospitalized, it is very important that the sibling be kept apprised of the child's condition. Again, hospital visits are ideal but should not be forced.

If the child is dying at home, it is possible for the siblings to have a more active role in the dying process. This does not necessarily mean a task orientation, though helping out is likely to make siblings feel less isolated. Siblings should be prepared for what is likely to happen at the time of death. Home hospices or visiting nurse agencies can be very helpful in this concrete preparation.

After the child dies, the siblings' reactions are not based just on their own feelings but also on the grief reactions of their parents. Children are used to depending on their parents, and to see them in such pain exposes a vulnerability not previously evident. This is in turn painful for the child and can even evoke fear. As a result, siblings might act cheerful in an effort to spare the parents pain. Parents may misinterpret this response and feel the sibling is not grieving, which can increase tension at an already difficult time (Hogan, 1988).

The primary care provider may be very helpful during this time of crisis. Parents are often so overwhelmed with grief it is difficult for them to support and understand the grief work of their surviving children. Children are often reluctant to talk to their parents about their deceased sibling or matters related to the death for fear of causing them more pain. The practitioner can offer support and guidance for parents and concrete information and reassurance for the surviving children. Counseling services should be offered to all family members and are often available through the local hospice agency.

SUMMARY

The family unit, varied in structure and composition, is the primary unit of care and support for the child. A chronic medical condition in a child alters the roles and expectations of all family members by creating a situational crisis. The primary care provider can be instrumental in assisting the child and family to cope with a chronic condition by supporting individual coping strategies, providing accurate, understandable information on the condition and all aspects of the child's care, implementing preventive health measures to minimize complications of the condition and promote optimal well-being, accessing needed services for the family, and offering support for the long term emotional needs of each family member.

REFERENCES

Aguilera DC and Messick JM: *Crisis intervention. Theory and methodology,* ed 6, St Louis, 1990, Mosby–Year Book.

Anderson JM: The social construction of illness experiences: families with a chronically ill child, *J Adv Nurs* 6:427-434, 1981.

Andrews MM and Nielson DW: Technology dependent children in the home, *Pediatr Nurs* 14:111-114, 151, 1988.

Arnold JH and Gemma PB, eds: *A child dies: a portrait of family grief,* Rockville, Md, 1983, Aspen.

Blackford KA: The children of chronically ill parents, *J Psychosoc Nurs Ment Health Serv* 26:33-36, 1988.

Bluebond-Langner M: *The private worlds of dying children,* Princeton, NJ, 1978, Princeton University Press.

Breslau N, Weitzman M, and Messenger K: Psychologic functioning of siblings of disabled children, *Pediatrics* 67:344-353, 1981.

Burr CK: Impact on the family of a chronically ill child. In Hobbs N and Perrin JM, eds: *Issues in the care of children with chronic illness,* San Francisco, 1985, Jossey-Bass, pp 24-40.

Damrosch SP and Perry LA: Self-reported adjustment, chronic sorrow, and coping of parents of children with Down syndrome, *Nurs Res* 38:25-30, 1989.

Deatrick JA and Knafl KA: Management behaviors: day-to-day adjustments to childhood chronic conditions, *J Pediatr Nurs* 5:15-22, 1990.

Deatrick JA, Knafl KA, and Walsh M: The process of parenting a child with a disability: normalization through accommodations, *J Adv Nurs* 13:15-21, 1988.

Dura JR and Beck SJ: A comparison of family function when mothers have chronic pain, *Pain* 35:79-89, 1988.

Edwardson SR: The choice between hospital and home care for terminally ill children, *Nurs Res* 32:29-34, 1983.

Feetham SL: Family research: issues and directions for nursing, *Annu Rev Nurs Res* 2:3-25, 1984.

Gale CA: Inadequacy of health care for the nation's chronically ill children, *J Pediatr Health Care* 3:20-27, 1989.

Garrison WT and McQuiston S: *Chronic illness during childhood and adolescence*, Newbury Park, Calif, 1989, Sage Publications.

Goldberg S and Simmons RJ: Chronic illness and early development, *Pediatrician* 15:13-20, 1988.

Gray E: Emotional and play needs of the dying child, *Issues Compr Pediatr Nurs* 12:207-224, 1989.

Gyulay J: Home care for the dying child, *Issues Compr Pediatr Nurs* 12:33-69, 1989.

Hobbs N, Perrin JM, and Ireys HT: *Chronically ill children and their families*, San Francisco, 1985, Jossey-Bass.

Hogan NS: The effects of time on the adolescent sibling bereavement process, *Pediatr Nurs* 14:333-335, 1988.

Holaday B: Challenges of rearing a chronically ill child, *Nurs Clin North Am* 19:361-368, 1984.

Horner MM, Rawlins P, and Giles K: How parents of children with chronic conditions perceive their own needs, *MCN* 12:40-43, 1987.

Howlin P: Living with impairment: the effects on children of having an autistic sibling, *Child Care Health Dev* 14:395-408, 1988.

Hymovich DP: Assessing the impact of chronic childhood illness on the family and parent coping, *Image* 13:71-74, 1981.

Jackson PL: When the baby isn't perfect, *Am J Nurs* 85:396-399, 1985.

Jacobs P and McDermott S: Family caregiver costs of chronically ill and handicapped children: method and literature review, *Public Health Rep* 104:158-163, 1989.

Jessop DJ, Riessman CK, and Stein REK: Chronic childhood illness and maternal mental health, *J Dev Behav Pediatr* 9:147-156, 1988.

Johnson JH: *Life events as stressors in childhood and adolescence*, Newbury Park, Calif, 1986, Sage Publications.

Johnson MP, Lubker BB, and Fowler MG: Teacher needs assessment for the educational management of children with chronic illnesses, *J Sch Health* 58:232-235, 1988.

Kazak AE: Families of chronically ill children: a systems and social-ecological model of adaptation and challenge, *J Consult Clin Psychol* 57:25-30, 1989.

Kazak AE, Reber M, and Carter A: Structural and qualitative aspects of social networks in families with young chronically ill children, *J Pediatr Psychol* 13:171-182, 1988.

Knafl KA and Deatrick JA: How families manage chronic conditions: an analysis of the concept of normalization, *Res Nurs Health* 9:215-222, 1986.

Knafl KA and Deatrick JA: Conceptualizing family response to a child's chronic illness or disability, *Fam Relat* 36:300-304, 1987.

Kramer RF: Living with childhood cancer: healthy siblings' perspective, *Issues Compr Pediatr Nurs* 5:155-165, 1981.

Krener P and Adelman R: Parent salvage and parent sabotage in the care of chronically ill children, *Am J Dis Child* 142:945-951, 1988.

Krulik T: Successful "normalization" tactics of parents of chronically ill children, *J Adv Nurs* 5:573-578, 1980.

Lawson BA: Chronic illness in the school-aged child, *MCN* 2:49-55, 1977.

Lipman TH: What causes diabetes? *MCN* 13:40-43, 1988.

Lynn MR: Siblings' responses in illness situations, *J Pediatr Nurs* 4:127-129, 1989.

MacMullen NJ and Brucker MC: Pregnancy made possible for women with cystic fibrosis, *MCN* 14:196-198, 1989.

Mahon M: The chronically ill child and family. In Hayman L and Sporing E, eds: *The nursing of children clinical handbook*, Bethany, Conn, 1985, Fleschner Publishing.

Martinson I: Home care for the child with cancer. In Schoewalter JE, Patterson PR, Tallmer M, et al, eds: *The child and death*, New York, 1983, Columbus University Press.

McCormick MC, Athreya BH, Bernbaum JC et al: Preliminary observations on maternal rating of health of children: data from three subspecialty clinics, *J Clin Epidemiol* 41:323-329, 1988.

Meehan J: Pain control in the terminally ill child at home, *Issues Compr Pediatr Nurs* 12:187-197, 1989.

Moyer A: Caring for a child with diabetes: the effect of specialist nurse care on parents' needs and concerns, *J Adv Nurs* 14:536-545, 1989.

Neill K: Behavioral aspects of chronic physical disease, *Nurs Clin North Am* 14:443-456, 1979.

Novak S: In moments of crisis, *MCN* 13:349-351, 1988.

Olshansky S: Chronic sorrow: a response to having a mentally defective child, *Soc Casework* 43:190-193, 1962.

Sabbeth BF and Leventhal JM: Marital adjustment to chronic childhood illness: a critique of the literature, *Pediatrics* 73:762-768, 1984.

Schlomann P: Developmental gaps of children with a chronic condition and their impact on the family, *J Pediatr Nurs* 3:180-187, 1988.

Solnit A and Stark M: Mourning the birth of a defective child, *Psychoanal Study Child* 16:523-536, 1962.

Stein A, Forrest GC, Woolley H, et al: Life threatening illness and hospice care, *Arch Dis Child* 64:697-702, 1989.

Tenbrinck M and Brewer P: The stages of grief experienced by parents of handicapped children, *Ariz Med* 33:712-714, 1976.

Thomas RB: Family adaptation to a child with a chronic condition. In Rose MH and Thomas RB, eds: *Children with chronic conditions: nursing in a family and community context*, Orlando, Fla, 1987, Grune & Stratton, pp 29-54.

Trahd GE: Siblings of chronically ill children: helping them cope, *Pediatr Nurs* 12:191-193, 244, 1986.

Vessey JA and Mahon MM: Therapeutic play and the hospitalized child, *J Pediatr Nurs* 5:328-333, 1990.

Wallander JA and Varni JW: Social support and adjustment in

chronically ill and handicapped children, *Am J Community Psychol* 17:185-201, 1989.

Wikler L, Wascow M, and Hatfield E: Chronic sorrow revisited: parent vs. professional depiction of the adjustment of parents of mentally retarded children, *Am J Orthopsychiatry* 51:63-67, 1981.

Winkel MF: Juvenile rheumatoid arthritis—parent support groups: do parents perceive a need? *Pediatr Nurs* 14:131-132, 1988.

Yost DM, Hochstadt NJ, and Charles P: Medical foster care: achieving permanency for seriously ill children, *Child Today* 17(5):22-26, 1988.

Young RK: Chronic sorrow: parents' response to the birth of a child with a defect, *MCN* 2:38-42, 1977.

3 Chronic Conditions and Child Development

Judith A. Vessey and *Catherine L. Caserza*

DEVELOPMENT does not exist in a vacuum; children's developmental domains are often significantly influenced by their physiologic states. Children with chronic conditions may experience developmental lags in acquiring cognitive, communicative, motoric, adaptive, and social skills compared with their unaffected peers. These maturational alterations may range from minor to all encompassing, transient to permanent. The presence of a chronic condition does not necessarily connote the presence of developmental disturbances, however. The development of many children with chronic conditions progresses without interruption.

The maturational alterations that accompany chronic conditions may be characterized in several ways (Finn, 1982). Some alterations are manifested within a single area of development, such as motoric difficulty seen in a child with mild cerebral palsy. Other developmental alterations, such as those seen in a child with Down syndrome, are more global in nature. Alterations may also be classified as delayed or deviant. Children with delayed development will advance through the normal sequence of milestones but at a rate slower than that of their peers of the same chronologic age. Such is the case of a child with an uncorrected congenital heart defect. Deviant development, occurring from unevenly developed or damaged neurologic processes, involves a disruption in the normal developmental sequences (Cohen and Vessey, 1985).

The child with poorly managed phenylketonuria is one such example. The risks of children experiencing significant negative developmental sequelae increase exponentially for those with conditions of greater severity or multisystem involvement. Variables that contribute to the occurrence and severity of maturational alterations associated with chronic conditions include the natural history of the condition, personal characteristics of the child, and the larger social support networks.

CONDITION'S NATURAL HISTORY

The severity, pathophysiology, and prognosis of the condition, as well as any iatrogenic insults that may have occurred, all influence a child's developmental outcome.

Severity and pathophysiology

Numerous specific pathophysiologic mechanisms, including chronic hypoxemia, swings in serum glucose levels, and malabsorption, are known to alter development, although the correlation between disease severity and developmental consequences is not very robust. Many pathophysiologic changes lack sufficient severity or are ameliorated by treatment so that the child readily adapts to them, and the potential for developmental insult is minimized. The existence of conditions marked only by occasional exacerbations or limited visibility or that appear to cause only marginal problems may be ignored or denied by children and their families.

This denial is often motivated by an effort to normalize the child's condition. Unfortunately, data suggest that these children may have poorer developmental outcomes if these behaviors interfere with symptom recognition or ongoing management regimens (Stein and Jessop, 1984).

Developmental sequelae secondary to prolonged disease states are also emerging. As research continues to advance health care technology, the mortality previously associated with many chronic conditions has been reduced. All too often, reductions in mortality initially result in escalating morbidity. For example, in the recent past many children with acquired immunodeficiency syndrome survived only for several months after diagnosis, dying before developmental lag could occur or was of significance. Today their life expectancy has doubled, and increasingly negative developmental sequelae are surfacing.

Other developmental limitations are secondarily imposed by the condition's pathophysiology and management. Tremendous exertion may be needed to cope with intensive treatment protocols or time-consuming activities of daily living. Children with cystic fibrosis, for example, may spend more than 3 hours each day receiving pulmonary care. Additional energy is also required in adjusting to new or exacerbated symptoms. Such expenditures of time and energy may limit children's opportunities to engage in recreational activities or predispose them to significant fatigue as participation requires too much effort (Mearig, 1985).

Prognosis

Maturational progression is superimposed on the natural course of the condition. In conditions associated with increasing symptoms leading to a poor prognosis, children may initially achieve milestones but lose them as the condition worsens. It is always noted when there is progressive degeneration of the neurologic system, as with Tay-Sachs disease, but it is also a problem with any seriously compromised physiologic state. Even in nonprogressive conditions, developmental lags often become noticeable as children mature and developmental expectations are higher. In part the ability to sustain development is dependent on managing the disease's symptoms effectively and promoting the child's functional status and psychosocial adjustment when deterioration cannot be curtailed.

Another area of concern is for children who have a limited or uncertain future or whose significant others (family, teachers, etc.) consider the child's prognosis for reaching adulthood poor. These children may be deprived of a past-present-future perspective of learning about one's cultural heritage or forming goals and personal aspirations. This longitudinal perspective plays an integral role in shaping cognitive processes (Mearig, 1985). If individuals are misguided into thinking that such information is not worth transmitting or would be unduly upsetting, especially for the child who recognizes his or her potentially diminished longevity, this lack of information limits the child's ability to learn. Predicting prognoses is a risky business in light of rapid advances in medical science; the life expectancies for children with cystic fibrosis, organ transplantation, cancer, and many other conditions continue to increase at dramatic rates. If a poor prognosis is communicated to the family in the absence of a broader perspective for the child's future, it may become a self-fulfilling prophecy.

Iatrogenic insults

Selected treatment protocols may cause temporary or permanent developmental changes. Developmental iatrogeny refers to those health care interventions that hinder children from progressing through their normal developmental milestones (Vessey, Farley, and Risom, in press). Therapeutic interventions commonly associated with developmental iatrogeny are the associations between aminoglycosides and hearing loss (McCracken, 1986), cancer therapy and late effects (Moore and Klopovich, 1989), and oxygen administration and retinopathy of prematurity (Groenendaal et al., 1989). Numerous other interventions, however, directly or indirectly influence development. Many classes of drugs, such as anticonvulsants and asthma preparations, have been shown to alter cognitive performance and behavior.

CHARACTERISTICS OF THE CHILD
Age

The limitations imposed by chronic conditions have definite implications for each age group (Perrin and Gerrity, 1984). The age of onset of a condition will affect progression from one stage of development to the next. Achieving a developmental task that has never been acquired is very different from regaining a skill previously mastered and now lost. Overall, children with congenital conditions have greater developmental plasticity; they adjust more readily to condition-imposed limitations as greater adaptive mechanisms come into play (Pless, 1984).

The major developmental tasks of infancy include establishing trust and learning about the environment through sensorimotor exploration. For infants with congenital chronic conditions, these tasks may be difficult to accomplish. These infants may be very wearisome to care for, and parents may find little gratification in trying to meet their basic needs despite their best efforts. A poor prognosis may also lead some parents to emotionally divorce themselves from their infants in an effort to insulate themselves from further emotional hurt. Infants subjected to prolonged or frequent hospitalizations may encounter repeated separations, the unpredictability associated with numerous care givers, potentially unreliable or inadequate care, and painful experiences. All of these factors can inhibit attachment and subsequent development of a trusting relationship. For infants whose condition is physically limiting, they are unable to explore and interact with their environment. This too can curtail development.

The major developmental tasks of toddlerhood include acquiring a sense of autonomy, developing self-control, and forming symbolic representation through the acquisition of language. If a child's chronic condition requires careful limit setting and control of activities of daily living, parents may not be able to encourage their children's independence in tasks such as toileting, feeding, or acquiring larger social networks. For example, toddlers who are immunosuppressed need to be restricted in their social contacts and play arenas. Mandatory prolonged dependency can create difficulty in separating and contribute to a tenuous self-image. Developmental tasks that have just been mastered are often easily lost in toddlers experiencing acute exacerbations of disease, with or without hospitalization. This behavioral regression is a means of social and emotional adaptation whereby children revert to earlier, previously abandoned stages when they do not have the necessary psychic energy to maintain functioning at already achieved

developmental levels (Freud, 1966, Oremland and Oremland, 1973). Although regression can happen at any point along the developmental continuum, it is most commonly noted in this age group.

Acquiring a sense of initiative to successfully meet the challenges of their ever-expanding worlds is the primary developmental task for preschoolers. Preschoolers with chronic conditions may not have the physical energy or resources to design and perform such activities; opportunities for cultivating self-confidence and a sense of purpose are diminished. Preschoolers are egocentric, engage in magical thinking, and use correlational rather than causal reasoning, all of which directly influence their interpretation of their condition. They are likely to think that some unrelated behavior that they engaged in has caused their condition and often tell elaborate stories to explain what has happened to them. If such misconceptions are not corrected and children are permitted to assume responsibility for their condition, their developing self-esteem and motivation to undertake new tasks may be compromised.

For school-aged children, increasing independence and mastery over their environment are important developmental landmarks. A lack of physical stamina may prevent children with chronic conditions from participating in school and extracurricular activities. Such activities are known to contribute to gaining social skills, developing a sense of accomplishment, learning to effectively cope with stress, and acquiring those skills that result in self-sufficiency (Weitzman, 1984). Children with a condition that is not highly visible may try to hide its existence when they recognize that it makes them different from their peers until forced by circumstances to admit otherwise. If not provided with the skills needed to communicate information about their conditions to peers, these children may withdraw and their self-concept diminish. Moreover, enforced dependency, whether required by the treatment regimen or instituted by overprotective parents, creates additional emotional barriers between children with chronic conditions and their nonaffected peers.

Adolescents, in the transitional period from childhood to adulthood, should be becoming increasingly independent of their parents and begin to make decisions about future career and personal goals. For an adolescent who requires complex care or who has a limited life expectancy, these developmental tasks may go unmet. Adolescents are prone to two dangers in planning for the future: (1) they may overemphasize the potential barriers that accompany their condition and succumb to a sense of futility or despair, or (2) they may deny realistic limitations and set themselves up for failure by holding forth unrealistic expectations (Perrin and Gerrity, 1984). Puberty, always a time of rapid change and uncertainty for adolescents, further confounds this complex period for teens with chronic conditions. Delayed puberty accompanies many conditions, emphasizing the differences between affected and nonaffected adolescents. Adolescence is a particularly difficult time to be viewed as different by one's peers, and some adolescents may withdraw from those social activities and relationships with the opposite sex that promote healthy psychosexual development.

Individualism

Despite great odds, many children have been bestowed with intrapsychic and interpersonal resources that allow them to conquer virtually any disability and excel in life. A child's individualism, or the rubric of those relatively stable emotional attributes that underlie a child's behavior — temperament, motivation, hardiness, attitudinal qualities, and interpersonal skills — influence developmental attainment.

Children with chronic conditions display the same scope of individual differences as children without chronic conditions. Some behavioral traits, such as temperament, are present at birth, whereas others, such as self-concept, develop over time. A child's individualism is influenced by environmental factors, although there is no direct correlation between familial attitudes and practices and the child's psychologic development. A strong self-concept, or a positive interpretation of one's own individualism, is developed through successfully mastering a variety of physical, intellectual, social, and emotional tasks. At a somewhat higher risk for developing a vulnerable personality secondary to a poor self-concept in the presence of a chronic condition, many children develop an appropriately positive self-concept and approach life's challenges with aplomb. They learn to rapidly identify threats to their integrity, respond with justifiable anger to those who are prejudiced against them, and reject biased individuals as inferior to themselves. Simultaneously, these children will often work to educate those around them, dispelling myths and inaccuracies that might interfere with their own developmental competence. Children with a poor self-concept will be overwhelmed by life's expectations. A vulnerable personality linked with critical developmental periods does not bode well for physical or socioemotional health.

The interrelationships of a child's positive self-esteem, perceived autonomy, easy temperament, internal locus of control, and an accurate cognitive appraisal of the condition in conjunction with environmental and family support all increase the child's therapeutic adherence (Pidgeon, 1989). For example, a child who has a low activity level, is given appropriate autonomy, and adapts easily to new situations is more likely to readily comply with a regimen of bedrest and nutritional restrictions than a very active child who has difficulty adapting to new situations.

ROLE OF FAMILY AND SOCIAL NETWORKS

Development depends on repeated and varied interactions between the growing child and the environment. Such reciprocity results in a spiral of mutually effective interactions. A child's parents are the most important influence on development during early childhood. Most parents are tremendously resilient despite the demands made by the child's condition and effectively assume their role in parenting the child and thus promoting his or her development. For a small minority of parents, the converse is also true. Parental guilt or despair or unfinished grief work over the loss of the fantasied child may negatively affect the child's development. Well-functioning families enhance their child's development, whereas those with discordant functioning curtail it (see Chapter 2).

Differing cultural orientations and social class also influence development in children with chronic conditions. As these orientations vary, so do the symbolic and semantic significance of the events, their perceived origins, and the potential consequences (Gaines, 1986). Although to date little research has been done in this area, practitioners working with children from varied circumstances need to recognize the variations in intrafamily communication patterns, temporal orientation, religiosity, and the value placed on childhood because these are known to influence children's development.

As children mature, there is a natural expansion of their environment and social network, and extended family members, teachers, friends, and acquaintances influence their developmental attainment. Individuals who offer practical tangible support, provide intellectual stimulation, plan activities that help the child excel, and take pride in the child's accomplishments truly serve as the child's advocates. Unfortunately, many individuals have had few experiences with children with special needs, and they may be overcompensating for or rejecting of the child's limitations. For children whose conditions are associated with disfigurement, their development may be unwittingly at risk because of the reactions of others. Many uninformed individuals automatically assume that physical handicap is associated with cognitive impairment. Children may be spoken about as if they were not present, or questions may be addressed to nearby family members or peers. The damage that can be done to a child's sense of self-worth is inestimable. The family can be helped to educate significant others about the child's strengths and limitations and offered suggestions about effective methods for working with insensitive individuals.

DEVELOPMENTAL PERSPECTIVES OF THE BODY, ILLNESS, MEDICAL PROCEDURES, AND DEATH

Children's perspectives about their bodies, illness, and death differ depending on their age. These perspectives need to be taken into account when children are taught about their condition and their help is enlisted in therapeutic adherence.

Understanding of the body

By the preschool period children have well-defined concepts of their external body and the relationships between its parts. Their understanding of the internal body's structure and function, however, remains primitive and is in keeping with cognitive and perceptual abilities. Early school-aged children can name three to six body parts, with the heart,

brain, bones, and blood the most common. Their descriptions of the parts and how they function tend to be global, undifferentiated, and laced with fantasy, although there is a great deal of variation among children about their specific ideas. Interrelationships among the parts and their functions are equally hazy. Physiologic processes are seen as a series of static states, with each organ having a singular, autonomous function. By middle to late school age, when children's causal reasoning and ability to differentiate matures, they begin to understand the complexities of anatomy and physiology. Levels of the body's organization are differentiated and hierarchically integrated with each other (Crider, 1981).

Children with chronic conditions hold a slightly different, though not more sophisticated, view of their internal bodies than that of their unaffected peers. They tend to focus on the affected part of the body but identify fewer other organ systems. Evidence also indicates that these children do not develop the increasing differentiation seen in children without chronic conditions but remain more fixated on their defective part (Offord and Aponte, 1967). Children's use of advanced terminology often confounds others into thinking that their comprehension far exceeds what normally would be expected. For example, one 4-year-old stated that he was receiving "methotrexate intravenously" yet thought his blood filled an empty body cavity, because blood vessels remained an unknown entity.

Understanding of illness

Children's self-concepts, interpersonal abilities, and therapeutic adherence to treatment regimens are related to the beliefs they hold about illness. For those who perceive their chronic condition as totally negative and restricting, functional status, school performance, and psychosocial competence are more likely to be compromised. If children are considered to be sick by their parents, their developing views and personalization of illness will significantly influence how they interpret their condition. As children mature and their view of illness evolves, the primary care practitioner along with significant others are in the position to assist the child in developing a positive image of his or her condition (Burbach and Peterson, 1986).

Infants are concerned about illness only as it

directly interferes with their comfort and attachment to their parents. By the toddler period, children begin to have an understanding of the concept of illness. For children with chronic conditions, this is usually interpreted by how the condition interferes with desired activities. Many condition-specific tasks such as injections of insulin or wearing a seizure helmet are particularly onerous for this population.

As children mature, they begin to form and articulate their feelings about illness. Preschoolers' cognitive processes remain dominated by prelogical thought, which is manifested in their views of illness. Phenomenism, the most simplistic form, occurs when illness is attributed to any external concrete phenomenon regardless of its relationship to illness. It is later replaced by contagion, or ascribing the causes of illness to other temporally occurring events (Bibace and Walsh, 1981). Recently diagnosed preschoolers, for example, will often view their condition as punishment for having misbehaved.

As children reach school age, their view of illness begins to reflect their evolving causal thought. Illness is initially perceived as occurring from contamination or physically coming in contact with the causal agent. Over time this view matures, and the cause of illness is believed to be external, such as germs that enter the body. With the development of formal operations in adolescents, illness causation is seen as a complex, multifaceted process. Physiologic explanations initially emerge as the basis for illness. These later evolve into psychophysiologic explanations, and the relationship of behavior and emotion to illness are acknowledged.

Understanding of medical procedures

Children's misconceptions of medical procedures closely parallel their thoughts about the body and illness. Initially infants and young children have no specific understanding of procedures; they are interpreted only in light of how they intrude on personal comfort. By preschool age, children's comprehension of medical procedures is marked by magical thinking, transductive reasoning, and overgeneralization. A procedure's purpose is independent of a child's health status, and no discrimination as to its diagnostic or therapeutic purpose is made. All procedures are designed to make you "better" or "sicker." Health care personnel are identified by their clothes, and curative powers are attributed to their actions (Steward and Steward, 1981).

As children mature, their view of medical procedures evolves from overgeneralization, through overdiscrimination, to correct identification of their functions. Multistep procedures and their purposes can be comprehended by school age; school-age children are able to classify and order variables. Information, however, is usually interpreted quite literally, and misunderstandings can occur if the content taught is not validated. Children of school age respect health care personnel and their hierarchical position, but expressions of affection are often ambivalent. School-aged children, often intrigued with understanding medical procedures, are usually pleased when asked to participate in their own care (Steward and Steward, 1981).

Adolescents are capable of understanding the efficacy of specific medical procedures and the relationships between procedures and their health status. Informed decisions about alternative treatments are possible. Adolescents view the health care provider's authority as extending only as far as their willingness to adhere to the therapeutic regimen. Although the need for therapeutic adherence is understood, treatments are not automatically affectively and behaviorally assimilated into an adolescent's daily activities (Steward and Steward, 1981).

Understanding of death

Death is the ultimate experience in separation and loss for children and their families. Children's understandings of death are formed along a developmental progression and reflect their cognitive maturation (Koocher, 1981). Infants do not comprehend death itself but react to those phenomena, such as pain and separation, that are associated with death. By late toddlerhood and preschool age, children may talk freely about death but may describe its occurrence and attributes with magical thinking and from an egocentric viewpoint. The permanence of death is not realized until the school-aged period, when the concepts of reversibility and irreversibility are learned. Children in this age group tend to personify death as the bogeyman or some kind of monster. Adolescents, with their new metacognitive abilities, conceptualize death as a process of the life cycle, readily comprehending the emotional, social, and financial implications of the loss that occurs from death for themselves and their families.

Children with chronic conditions are often subjected to numerous intrusive and painful experiences and may have experienced the death of friends in the hospital. These experiences often exacerbate their anxieties about death. Depending on individual experience, a child's understanding of death may not follow the projected trajectory. Although information as to how affected children's views of death differ from their nonaffected peers is limited, it appears that the fears associated with death are remarkably similar to the fears of hospitalization and intrusive procedures (Waechter et al., 1986). Even in preschool-aged children, fear of separating may be expressed despite the fact that death may not yet be conceptualized as irreversible.

For the dying child, how issues such as separation, mutilation, and loss of control are handled play an important role in their personal conceptualization of death. Care must be taken to help these children maintain their autonomy, sense of mastery, and other developmental skills whenever possible.

PRIMARY CARE PROVIDER'S ROLE IN PROMOTING DEVELOPMENT

Because cure is not possible for many chronic conditions, the practitioner must focus on care. The goal of care is to minimize the manifestations of the disease and maximize the child's physical, cognitive, and psychosocial potential. No tested management protocols are available for meeting this objective. The practitioner must draw on information from a variety of sources. Planning for care is augmented if a noncategorical approach is adopted. A noncategorical approach focuses on those commonalities that selected groups of children with chronic conditions share. This approach, incorporated with discrete dimensions of the disease, such as its onset, course, and manifestations, provide a nexus on which to develop a holistic management plan. A good maxim to follow is to generalize developmental information across diagnostic groups, then individualize it for each child and family (Stein and Jessop, 1984).

Assessment and management

Maturational alterations are rarely immutable and should not be thought of as such. Children with chronic conditions require comprehensive habilitation if they are to achieve their optimal level of functioning. This requires long-term management and repeated assessments by interdisciplinary groups of professionals. The composition of the group is dynamic and will vary depending on the child's age, disability, level of impairment, familial involvement, and environmental resources. Coordination is critical if omissions and duplications of services are to be prevented (Cohen and Vessey, 1985). Involvement of the primary care provider will help ensure consistency across the disciplines.

Ideally, children at risk for developmental lags should be identified as soon as possible and followed closely. The goal for the primary care provider is to anticipate and, whenever possible, vigorously intervene before significant aberrations occur. This is best accomplished by identifying and initiating treatment in the preclinical period, that time when slight indications of developmental impairment may be detected, but gross manifestations are not yet evident (Stangler, Huber, and Routh, 1980). A "wait and see" attitude is not warranted because these children are known to be at developmental risk. Early intervention may prevent or ameliorate many secondary problems or those that result from neglect or mistreatment of the original condition. Although a child may suffer hearing loss from aminoglycosides, for example, subsequent language and cognitive delays may be prevented with aggressive intervention. Because a chronic condition generally persists throughout a child's lifetime, ongoing periodic evaluations of physical development and psychosocial adjustment are helpful.

Assessment of the child's physical development normally consists of evaluating basic indicators of health including growth measures and vital signs, performing a comprehensive physical examination, and noting any changes in the status of the chronic condition. An additional dimension, rating the child's functional status, should also be an integral part of the assessment (Pless, 1984). Functional status evaluation provides information about the child's ability to engage in activities of daily living known to heavily influence developmental outcomes.

Although the tendency may be to focus attention on the child's physical status, assessment of the child's psychosocial adjustment is of critical importance. Not all of the psychosocial stresses experienced by children with chronic conditions are caused by their condition, nor do only affected children experience stress. This population, however, has a higher percentage of psychologic difficulties, much of which can be attributed to the child's condition (Pless, 1984). It is estimated that 1½ to 3 times as many children with chronic conditions have behavioral problems as their nonaffected peers. Moreover, 30% to 40% of these children also have school-related problems, only one half of which are directly related to their condition (Goldberg and Simmons, 1988).

Assessment has traditionally focused on identifying how the child with a chronic condition differs from nonaffected peers. This information is useful for developing explanatory theory about the effects of chronic conditions but does little to help the child. Evaluating whether the child is effectively coping with the condition and successfully adjusting to school, peer groups, and the like provides guidelines on which interventions can be based.

Standardized assessment instruments are useful necessary adjuncts to a complete history and physical examination for a comprehensive developmental evaluation. When used at regular intervals, they provide objective data so that small developmental changes can be detected. Considering the ever-growing number of children with special needs being cared for in the community, the primary care practitioner needs to have a compendium of readily administered standardized instruments from which to draw (Table 3-1) and not rely only on the Denver Developmental Screening Test (DDST). Although considered the gold standard for developmental assessment by many primary care providers, the DDST has a limited place in assessing high-risk children. It has excellent specificity with few over referrals, but the DDST's sensitivity or ability to correctly identify children with abnormal findings has been demonstrated to be poor (Meisels, 1989).

Care must be taken in choosing instruments and interpreting results because most of these did not include children with chronic conditions when the norms were determined. Others are invalid if they are measuring one developmental construct based on the performance in a different arena of development. For example, the cognitive development of a child with a tracheostomy should not be assessed by an instrument requiring verbal responses. Timed tests may also bias results, particularly if a child has a motor or learning deficit. If a child fatigues easily, it is best to perform developmental assessments in short intervals so as not to obscure the child's true capabilities.

In general children with chronic conditions who are at risk for developmental deviations but where no indications of developmental deviation are apparent should undergo periodic screening and monitoring at the same intervals as their nonaffected peers. For those who are evidencing warning signs of developmental problems, more frequent assessments are appropriate. Too frequent assessments of at-risk but nonsymptomatic children, however, may alter parents' perceptions so that they believe their child is unduly vulnerable, creating a self-fulfilling prophecy (Chamberlin, 1987). The practitioner needs to walk the fine line between errors of commission and omission on deciding the frequency and intensity of assessment. The best defense is to place efforts on prevention rather than detection.

When untoward developmental manifestations are detected, the primary care provider can either provide treatment or, more likely, refer the child to specialists with expertise in the area of concern. Ideally referrals would be made to such individuals who are a part of the specialty team or within the child's school setting. However, additional local referrals may be necessary if the specialty team is geographically distant or school services are inadequate. Adding another layer of care providers requires exquisite coordination of services if the child is to receive appropriate care free of overlaps or gaps and avoid becoming fatigued by too many demands.

Obtaining services often requires that the child's condition and associated problems be diagnostically labeled. Providing a label also helps validate the concerns of children and families and provides direction for future interventions and activities. However, it must be done judiciously. Labeling often sets the child apart from his or her peers and may result in different treatment by fam-

Text continued on p. 41.

Table 3-1. Developmental tools used to assess children with chronic conditions

Type of screening tools	Test/source	Age level	Method	Comments
General development (social, emotional, cognitive, and co-ordination)	AAMD Adaptive Behavior Scale (school edition) Authors: K Nihiro, R Foster, M Shellhaas, H Leiland, N Lambert, and M Windmiller Source: CTB/McGraw-Hill Book Co	3-16 yr	Observation	• Used as a screening tool and for instructional planning • Can be an indicator in assessing children whose adaptive behavior indicates possible mental retardation, learning handicaps, or emotional disturbances
	Bayley Infant Scales Author: N Bayley Source: The Psychological Corp Harcourt, Brace, Jovanovich, Inc	2-30 mo	Observation/demonstration	• Evaluates motor, mental, and behavior of the infant and toddler • Diagnoses normal vs retarded development • Requires a qualified practitioner to examine and evaluate the infant
	Bender Visual Motor Gestalt Test Author: L Bender Source: American Orthopsychiatric Association	≥ 3 yr	Demonstration	• Used as an evaluation tool for developmental problems in children, learning disabilities, retardation, psychosis, organic brain disorders
	Carey Infant Temperament Questionnaire Author: WB Carey Source: WB Carey, MD 319 West Front St Media, PA 19063	4-8 mo	Interview	• Provides an objective measure of the infant's temperament profile • Fosters more effective interactions between parent and infant
	Carey and McDevitt Revised Temperament Questionnaire (95 items, 6-pt frequency scale) 1. Toddler Temperament Scale Authors: W Fullard, SC McDevitt, and WB Carey Source: W Fullard, PhD Dept of Educational Psychology Temple University Philadelphia, PA 19122	1-3 yr	Interview	• Provides an objective measure of the child's temperament profile • Fosters more effective interactions between parent and child

	Age	Method	Comments
2. Behavior Style Questionnaire Authors: SC McDevitt and WB Carey Source: SC McDevitt, PhD Devereux Center 6436 E Sweetwater Scottsdale, AZ 85254	3-7 yr	Interview	• Provides an objective measure of the child's temperament profile • Fosters more effective interactions between parent and child
Child Behavior Checklist Author: TM Achenbach Source: Center for Children, Youth, and Families University of Vermont 1 S Prospect St Burlington, VT 05401	2-3 yr	Observation/interview	• Provides an overview of the child's behavior • Parent and teacher forms available
Children's Depression Inventory (CDI) Author: M Kovacs Source: *Acta Paedopsychiatr* 1981; 46:305-315 M Kovacs, PhD Assistant Professor of Psychiatry 3811 O'Hara St Pittsburgh, PA 15261	8-13 yr	Paper/pencil inventory	• Used for clinical research in childhood depression • Advisable for individual administration with the psychiatric population
Denver Developmental Screening Test Authors: *Manual/Workbook for Nursing and Paramedical Personnel* (1978 ed) WK Frankenberg, JB Dodds, and A Fandal Source: LADOCA Project and Publishing Foundation E 51st Ave and Lincoln St Denver, CO 80216	Birth-6 yr	Observation and parental reporting	• Screens for developmental deviations • Minimal training required • Available in Spanish
Developmental Profile II Authors: GD Alpern, TJ Boll, and MS Shearer Source: Western Psychological Services 12031 Wilshire Blvd Los Angeles, CA 90025	Birth-9½ yr	Interview	• Provides information on physical, self-help, social, academic, and communicative abilities • Requires a qualified practitioner skilled in interviewing
McCarthy Scales of Children's Abilities Source: The Psychological Corp 7500 Old Oak Blvd Cleveland, OH 44130	2½-8½ yr	Observation and demonstration by the child	• Measures 6 aspects of children's thinking, motor, and mental abilities • Requires qualified practitioner to administer and evaluate the child

Continued.

Table 3-1. Developmental tools used to assess children with chronic conditions—cont'd

Type of screening tools	Test/source	Age level	Method	Comments
General development—cont'd	Minnesota Infant Development Inventory Authors: H Ireton and E Thwing Source: Behavior Science Systems PO Box 1108 Minneapolis, MN 55458	Birth-15 mo	Observation/interview	• A developmental guide • Measures the infant's development areas: gross motor, fine motor, language, comprehension and personal-social • Can be done by parent
	Minnesota Child Development Inventory Authors: H Ireton and E Thwing Source: Behavior Science Systems PO Box 1108 Minneapolis, MN 55458	1-6 yr	Observation/interview	• Provides a profile of the child's strengths and weaknesses • Can be done by a parent, also available on audiocassette for parents who have difficulty reading
	Pediatric Examination of Educational Readiness at Middle Childhood Author: MD Levine Source: Educators Publishing 75 Moulton St Cambridge, MA 02138	5-10 yr	Observation/demonstration	• Can be done by parent • Measures school readiness and academic achievement • Allow 1 hr for testing time • Administered by a certified practitioner
	Rapid Developmental Screening Checklist Authors: Committee on Children With Handicaps, American Academy of Pediatrics Source: MJ Giannini, MD Director, Mental Retardation Institute New York Medical College Valhalla, NY 10595	1 mo-5 yr	Checklist	• Requires minimal time allotment • Administered by any adult capable to make required observation
	Riley Motor Problems Inventory (RMPI) Author: GD Riley Source: Western Psychological 12031 Wilshire Blvd. Los Angeles, CA 90025	≥ 4 yr	Performance tasks by the child	• Provides a quantified system for observation and measurement of neurologic signs that lead to problems in speech, language, learning, and behavior • Needs to be administered by a qualified clinician

	Age	Method	Features
Vineland Adaptive Behavior Scales Authors: SS Sparrow, DA Balla, and DV Cicchetti Source: American Guidance Service Inc. Circle Pines, MN 55014-1796	Birth–adult	Semistructured interview with parent or care giver	• Assesses adaptive behavior in four sectors: communication, daily living skills, socialization, and motor skills • Used with mentally retarded and handicapped individuals
Vineland Social Maturity Scale Author: EA Doll Source: American Guidance Service, Inc Circle Pines, MN 55014-1796	Birth–adult	Interview	• Used to measure normal development or individual difference that may be significant in children with mental deficiencies and emotional disturbances • Assists in planned therapy or specialized individual education
Wheel Guide to Normal Milestones of Development Author: U Hayes Source: *A Developmental Approach to Case Finding*, ed 2 US Dept of Health and Human Services Superintendent of Documents Washington, DC 20402	1–3 yr	Observation	• Assesses basic reflexes and developmental milestones • Reinforces the normal growth and development patterns of children
Vision — Allen Picture Card Test of Visual Acuity Source: LADOCA Project and Publishing Foundation E 51st Ave and Lincoln St Denver, CO 80216	3–6 yr	Observation	• Preschooler screening test for visual acuity • Trained volunteers/ screeners can conduct the testing
Denver Eye Screening Test (DEST) Source: LADOCA Project and Publishing Foundation E 51st Ave and Lincoln St Denver, CO 80216	3 yr	Observation	• Identifies children with acuity problems • Good for preschool-aged children unable to respond to the Snellen Illiterate E Test
Distance Visual Acuity Screening Test for Young Children Source: LB Holt, MD, FICS 195 Professional Bldg 2240 Cloverdale Ave Winston Salem, NC 27103	3–5 yr ≥ 6 yr	Interview/ observation	• Used in children to measure central visual acuity • Can be administered by any adult, professional, or nonprofessional capable of developing rapport with children

Continued.

Table 3-1. Developmental tools used to assess children with chronic conditions—cont'd

Type of screening tools	Test/source	Age level	Method	Comments
Vision—cont'd	Picture Card Test (Adaptation of the Pre-school Vision Test) Author: HF Allan Source: LADOCA Project and Publishing Foundation E 51st Ave and Lincoln St Denver, CO 80216	≥ 2½ yr	Interview/ "name the picture"	• Identifies children with acuity problems • Administered by a carefully taught adult who has an interest in working with children
	Snellen Illiterate E Test Author: H Snellen Sources: National Society for Blindness 79 Madison Ave New York, NY 10016 American Association of Ophthalmology 1100 17th St NW Washington, DC 20036	≥ 3 yr	Observation using 3 persons as a team in screening	• Intended as a screening measure for central acuity of preschool-aged children and of other children who have not learned to read • Administered by a carefully prepared adult
Speech and language	Bankson Language Screening Test (BLST) Author: NW Bankson Source: University Park Press Chamber of Commerce Bldg Baltimore, MD 21201	4-8 yr	Observation	• Identifies children in need of language assistance • Can be administered by a perceptive adult
	The Bzoch-League Receptive Expressive Emergent Language Scale (REEL) Authors: KR Bzoch and R League Source: University Park Press 360 N Charles St Baltimore, MD 21201	Birth-3 yr	Paper-pencil inventory	• Identifies children needing further follow-up in language
	Denver Articulation Screening Exam (DASE) Author: Reference manual (1971 ed) AF Drumwright Manual/workbook WK Frankenburg Source: LADOCA Project and Publishing Foundation Inc E 51st Ave and Lincoln St Denver, CO 80216	2½-6 yr	Observation	• Screening children who may be economically disadvantaged and have a potential with a speech problem (articulation)–pronunciation • Administered by a qualified professional; special training required for the nonprofessional
	Emergent Language Milestone Scale (ELM) (1984) Source: Education Corp PO Box 721 Tulsa, OK 74101	Birth-36 mo	Interview Observation	• Screening instrument for auditory expressive, auditory receptive, and visual components of language

	Instrument/Source	Age	Method	Comments
	Peabody Picture Vocabulary Test, Revised (PPVT-R) Authors: Lloyd M. Dunn Leota M. Dunn Source: American Guidance Service Publishers Bldg Circle Pines, MN 55014	≥ 2½ yr	"Point to" response test	• Measures hearing vocabulary for standard American English • Used with non-English-speaking students to screen for mental retardation or giftedness • Requires a qualified practitioner to administer
	Physician's Developmental Quick Screen for Speech Disorders (PDQ) Authors: SG Kulig and KA Baker	6 mo-6 yr	Interview/demonstration	• Designed to identify children in need of a diagnostic evaluation by a speech pathologist for disorders of language, voice, articulation, and rhythm with speech • Administered by any well-trained paraprofessional or health care professional
	Riley Motor Problems Inventory (RMPI) Author: GD Riley Source: Western Psychological 12031 Wilshire Blvd Los Angeles, CA 90025	≥ 4 yr	Performance tasks by the child	• Provides a quantified system for observation and measurement of neurologic signs that lead to problems in speech, language, learning, and behavior • Needs to be administered by a qualified clinician
School readiness and academic achievement	Child Behavior Checklist Author: TM Achenbach Source: Center for Children, Youth, and Families University of Vermont 1 S Prospect St Burlington, VT 05401	4-16 yr	Observation/interview	• Provides an overview of the child's behavior • Parent and teacher forms available
	Peabody Picture Vocabulary Test, Revised (PPVT-R) Authors: LM Dunn and LM Dunn Source: American Guidance Service Publishers Bldg Circle Pines, MN 55014	≥ 2½ yr	"Point to" response test	• Measures hearing vocabulary for standard American English • Used with non-English-speaking students to screen for mental retardation or giftedness • Requires a qualified practitioner to administer

Continued.

Table 3-1. Developmental tools used to assess children with chronic conditions—cont'd

Type of screening tools	Test/source	Age level	Method	Comments
	Peabody Individual Achievement Test (PIAT) Authors: LM Dunn and FC Markwardt, Jr Source: American Guidance Service Publishers Bldg Circle Pines, MN 55014 Authors: LM Dunn	≥ 5 yr	Interview	• Used to screen for areas of weakness requiring more detailed diagnostic testing in scholastic achievement
	Riley Preschool Developmental Inventory (RPDSI) Author: CMD Riley Source: Western Psychological 12031 Wilshire Blvd Los Angeles, CA 90025	3-5 yr	Observation	• For children who have the tendency for academic problems • Requires a qualified clinician to administer
	The Texas Pre-school Screening Inventory Authors: JS Haber and ML Noris	3-6 yr	Observation/demonstration	• Used as a screening tool to identify children with possible learning difficulties
	Wide Range Achievement Test (WRAT) Authors: JF Jastak and S Jastak Source: Jastak Assessment Systems Jastak Associates, Inc 1526 Gilpin Wilmington, DE 19806	≥ 5 yr	Observation; paper-pencil subtests	• Used for education placement, measurement of academic achievement, vocational assessment, and job placement training • Large print edition is available
Functional status	Health Interview Survey Source: National Center for Health Statistics B Bloom: *Current Estimates From the National Health Interview Survey United States, 1981* Vital and Health Statistics, Series 10–No 141 DHHS Pub No (PHS) 83-1569 Washington, DC Public Health Service US Government Printing Office October 1982	6-16 yr	Interview	• Assesses functional status

ily members, teachers, and significant others. Diagnostic labels assigned in childhood follow children into adulthood, possibly preventing them from pursuing selected careers, joining the military or being eligible for insurance. Although it is usually feasible to label specific disease entities, care should be taken in labeling associated developmental manifestations.

The ultimate long-term goal of care is for the child to reach and sustain optimal levels of functioning. Developing precise, measurable, short-term goals will help ensure that optimal functioning is obtained.

Education

Two objectives of primary care, in addition to providing health maintenance, are to help prepare children in self-care behaviors and develop self-advocacy skills for dealing with the health care community. This is particularly important for children with chronic conditions because they will likely engage the health care system frequently throughout their lives, and such education helps empower them to do so effectively.

For children to accomplish these objectives, they must initially have a basic understanding of the workings of their body, characteristics of their condition, and the intricacies of the health care system. Unfortunately, it is often assumed that children are well versed about these topics because they know the jargon, often appear quite comfortable with the health care environment, and have been diagnosed "for years." As mentioned earlier, however, on closer examination much of this apparent sophistication is superficial (Carraccio, McCormick, and Weller, 1987); children may merely be mimicking vocabulary they have heard repeatedly. Children may also misinterpret or forget information, or advanced material may not be presented as they mature.

Developmentally appropriate teaching guides need to be incorporated into the primary care of all children with chronic conditions because learning is more likely to occur in a nonthreatening environment when the child is in a comparatively good state of health than when sick and hospitalized. A comprehensive plan, to be managed by the primary care provider in conjunction with parents and specialty providers, will help ensure that this learning

occurs. Teaching methods need to be altered to fit the child's developmental age. Children will learn best when the material presented to them remains within one level above their current cognitive functioning (Perrin and Gerrity, 1981).

A multisensory approach, one that brings all of the child's senses to bear on the learning task at hand, is more likely to be effective with preschool and school-aged children than more traditional methods. For example, using anatomic rag dolls to explain anatomy and physiology (Vessey, 1988) or doll hospitals for explaining various procedures has been shown to be highly effective with this population. A variety of options, including books, discussion, and videos, are appropriate for use with older children who are free of cognitive deficits.

Many commercially available materials are excellent and useful adjuncts to the individualized teaching plan. The practitioner is cautioned to examine all materials in advance to ascertain whether the information presented will correspond to the child's own experiences. The language of all materials needs to be carefully evaluated for age appropriateness and content validity. There is little sense of providing cute, albeit inaccurate, information to a child, because these myths will only need to be dispelled as the child matures (Vessey, Braithwaite, and Wiedmann, 1990). For younger children who have not developed causal reasoning, who engage in fantasy, and who tend to interpret their environment from a singular perspective, this is of particular significance.

Advocacy

Numerous professions are called on to care for the complex needs of children with chronic conditions. Although all hold the same goal, to help the child reach maximum potential, conflicts may arise as to the best approach for realizing it. The primary care provider is in the unique position to advocate for the child, inform the child and family of available resources, and help coordinate these services.

Hospitalization. Hospitalizations are not uncommon with this population of children, and during this time care is usually transferred to the specialty team. The primary care provider can be instrumental in assisting in a smooth transition. In addition to communicating information about the child's physical condition, parents need to be encouraged to provide information to the specialty team about developmental stimulation programs or schooling that the child is receiving. If the hospitalization is planned, every effort should be made for hospital-based educators or tutors to confer with school officials before the child's admission so that schooling is not interrupted. Properly preparing the child and family, especially for new situations, also helps in adjusting to hospitalization. Preparation needs to include procedural information about situations they will encounter, definitions of medical jargon specific to their condition, and opportunities to process (either through play, role playing, or discussion) new situations they may experience. For families who are nonassertive or overly aggressive, the primary care provider can assist in appropriately empowering the child and family members for self-advocacy by working through these tasks.

Monitoring the child's adjustment to hospitalization and future effects it may have on the child's development is also an important component of advocacy. Children's individualism and the severity of their condition are known to affect their adaptation to hospitalization. For many children with chronic conditions, hospitalization is an unwelcome intrusion into their lives. Other children have positive memories of previous hospitalizations and may see the hospital as a safe environment. They may perceive the staff as friends and are frequently relieved to have a temporary respite from school stresses, harassment of other children, or the demands of daily activities. Although uncommon, the primary care provider needs to recognize children will occasionally try to become hospitalized to remove themselves from home or school situations that have become particularly onerous.

Schooling. The role of the educational arena should not be undervalued. Participating in school provides a measure of independence and opportunities for self-mastery and self-esteem building that are not readily achieved at home (Weitzman, 1984). The primary care provider can promote the benefits garnered from schooling in numerous ways. Suggestions for altering treatment protocols and medications that interfere with school activities may be offered. Attempts to schedule appointments around the school day should be made so unnec-

essary absenteeism does not occur. A careful history of absenteeism needs to be collected. If it seems excessive for the child's condition, an interdisciplinary conference should be called.

After hospitalization the primary care provider can facilitate the child's transition to school by providing information about the condition and its ramifications for school participation to school authorities. Suggesting methods for preparing classmates for the return of the child is equally important, especially for the child with noticeable physical changes. "Sanctioned staring," or encouraging classmates to preview the new appearance of the child without fear of recrimination or causing embarrassment, is conducive to a child's acceptance on returning to school. This can be facilitated by suggesting the child share hospital experiences with classmates by writing a letter and including his or her picture or making a videotape to send to school. Because many teachers have little knowledge of chronic conditions, offering the address and telephone number of specialty agencies such as the American Cancer Society initially provides an important source of useful information.

Counseling. Because children with chronic conditions have a higher percentage of psychosocial problems, careful attention must be paid to the child's emotional health. Growing up is hard to do, and the incidence of alcoholism, drug abuse, suicide, and other self-destructive behaviors among all children continues to climb. Some children with chronic conditions will likely engage in these behaviors and would benefit from counseling. Referral may also be appropriate in helping a child adapt to a new diagnosis or deteriorating prognosis to deal with school, family, and peer group issues or to clarify interpersonal and career goals. These are usually very private concerns for older children and adolescents. Seeking such help while maintaining their privacy may be difficult if their ability to move about the community is limited. The primary care provider can be instrumental in facilitating such help.

Dying. Some children will die despite everyone's best efforts. The primary care provider can be of great assistance in planning for and providing psychologic care during this difficult and poignant time. One of the key roles is to encourage and facilitate the family's ability to provide this care (Koocher and Berman, 1983). Children's emotional needs and fears need to be addressed from their perspective. The primary care provider can help family members with this by modeling ways to communicate these sensitive issues and offering insights as to how a child's developmental level affects their ability to conceptualize death. Many times children's questions are upsetting to parents, as when a 6-year-old requests detailed information about death rituals or a preschooler wants to know, "Who will read me stories after I die?" Helping family members and other significant individuals communicate effectively with the child and each other will make death easier to bear.

Many children want to die at home, where they are in familiar surroundings, separation is minimized, care is individualized, and they are able to remain in great control of their situations. Other children may feel insecure at home and prefer to be hospitalized, surrounded by professionals they trust. Home care and hospitalization both have advantages and disadvantages, and the decision of which to pursue needs to be made in concert with the child's wishes and the family's capabilities. The primary care provider can be instrumental in facilitating either of these options in conjunction with local hospice services.

SUMMARY

Children with chronic conditions are at a higher risk for negative developmental sequelae than their nonaffected peers. The severity of the condition, individualistic traits of the child, and the available network for social supports all influence the child's developmental outcomes. Comprehensive prospective care, however, can eliminate or significantly ameliorate negative outcomes. Careful assessment using a multidisciplinary approach will help identify potential or emerging problems associated with the child's disease progression, functional status, social interactions, or global development. Individualized intervention strategies including therapeutic management, education, counseling, and advocacy can then be designed and implemented to assist children with chronic conditions in reaching their developmental potential.

REFERENCES

Bibace R and Walsh ME: Children's conception of illness. In Bibace R and Walsh M, eds: *New directions for child development: children's conceptions of health, illness, and bodily functions,* San Francisco, 1981, Jossey-Bass, No 14, pp 31-47.

Burbach DJ and Peterson L: Children's concepts of physical illness: a review and critique of the cognitive developmental literature, *Health Psychol* 5:307-325, 1986.

Carraccio CL, McCormick MC, and Weller SC: Chronic disease: effect on health cognition and health locus of control, *J Pediatr* 110:982-987, 1987.

Chamberlin RW: Developmental assessment and early intervention programs for young children: lessons learned from longitudinal research, *Pediatr Rev* 8:237-247, 1987.

Cohen M and Vessey JA: Developmental disabilities. In Hayman LL and Sporing EM eds: *Handbook of pediatric nursing,* Bethany, Conn, 1985, Fleschner, pp 538-557.

Crider C: Children's conceptions of the body interior. In Bibace R and Walsh M eds: *New directions for child development: children's conceptions of health, illness, and bodily functions,* San Francisco, 1981, Jossey-Bass, No 14, pp 85-103.

Finn K: The hospitalization of children with developmental disorders, *Child Health Care* 10:131-134, 1982.

Freud A: *The ego mechanism of defense,* rev ed, New York, 1966, International Universities Press.

Gaines AD: Trauma: cross cultural issues, *Adv Psychosom Med* 16:1-16, 1986.

Goldberg S and Simmons RJ: Chronic illness and early development, *Pediatrician* 15:13-20, 1988.

Groenendaal F, van Hof-van-Duin J, Baerts W, et al: Effects of perinatal hypoxia on visual development during the first year of (corrected) age, *Early Hum Dev* 20:267-279, 1989.

Koocher GP: Children's conceptions of death. In Bibace R and Walsh M, eds: *New directions for child development: children's conceptions of health, illness, and bodily functions,* San Francisco, 1981, Jossey-Bass, No 14, pp 85-103.

Koocher GP and Berman SJ: Life threatening and terminal illness in childhood. In Levine MD, Carey WB, Crocker AC, et al, eds: *Developmental-behavioral pediatrics,* Philadelphia, 1983, Saunders, pp 488-502.

McCracken GH: Aminoglycoside toxicity in infants and children, *Am J Med* 80(suppl 6B):172-177, 1986.

Mearig JS: Cognitive development of chronically ill children. In Hobbs N and Perrin JM eds: *Issues in the care of children with chronic illness,* San Francisco, 1985 Jossey-Bass, pp 672-697.

Meisels SJ: Can developmental screening tests identify children who are developmentally at risk? *Pediatrics* 83:578-585, 1989.

Moore IM and Klopovich PM: Late effects of cancer treatment in children and adults, *Semin Oncol Nurs* 5:1-3, 1989.

Offord DR and Aponte JF: A comparison of drawings and sentence completion responses of congenital heart children with normal children, *J Project Techniques Personality Assess* 31:57-62, 1967.

Oremland EK and Oremland JD: *The effects of hospitalization on children: models for their care,* Springfield, Ill, 1973, Charles C Thomas, Publisher.

Perrin EC and Gerrity PS: There's a demon in your belly: children's understanding of illness, *Pediatrics* 67:841-849, 1981.

Perrin EC and Gerrity PS: Development of children with a chronic illness, *Pediatr Clin North Am* 31:19-31, 1984.

Pidgeon V: Compliance with chronic illness regimens: school-aged children and adolescents, *J Pediatr Nurs* 4:36-47, 1989.

Pless IB: Clinical assessment: physical and psychological functioning, *Pediatr Clin North Am* 31:33-46, 1984.

Stangler SR, Huber CJ, and Routh DK: *Screening growth and development of preschool children: a guide for test selection,* New York, McGraw-Hill, 1980.

Stein REK and Jessop DJ: General issues in the care of children with chronic physical conditions, *Pediatr Clin North Am* 31:189-209, 1984.

Steward MS and Steward DS: Children's conceptions of medical procedures. In Bibace R and Walsh M, eds: *New directions for child development: children's conceptions of health, illness, and bodily functions,* San Francisco, 1981, Jossey-Bass, No 14, pp 67-83.

Vessey JA: Comparison of two teaching methods on children's knowledge of their internal bodies, *Nurs Res* 37:262-267, 1988.

Vessey JA, Braithwaite KB, and Wiedmann M: Teaching children about their internal bodies, *Pediatr Nurs* 16:29-35, 1990.

Vessey JA, Farley JA, and Risom LP: Iatrogenic developmental effects and pediatric intensive care, *Pediatr Nurs* (in press).

Waechter E, Crittenden M, Mikkelsen C, et al: Concomitants of death imagery in stories told by chronically ill children undergoing intrusive procedures: a comparison of four diagnostic groups, *J Pediatr Nurs* 1:2-11, 1986.

Weitzman M: School and peer relations, *Pediatr Clin North Am* 31:59-70, 1984.

4 Financing Health Care for Children with Chronic Conditions

Roberta S. O'Grady

CARE for children with chronic conditions in the United States is financed by four different methods: (1) private health insurance, including prepayment arrangements; (2) public programs, such as Medicaid, Services for Children with Special Health Care Needs (formerly Crippled Children's Services), and other federal and state categorical programs; (3) private, philanthropic sources; and (4) the family's own funds (Hobbs, Perrin, and Ireys, 1985). A child may be supported by one or a combination of these methods, depending on the type of condition, family income, parent's employment, the state and county of residence, availability of a voluntary organization for the specific condition, and availability of persons in the health care system who have the knowledge to advocate for the child's rights to specific sources of financial assistance.

PRIVATE HEALTH INSURANCE

The role of private health insurance in paying the costs of care for children with chronic conditions is substantial but difficult to comprehend because of great variation in patterns of coverage and scope of benefits (Weeks, 1985). Private health insurance is generally categorized by the method of reimbursement. The fee-for-service plans are those that pay after the service is provided. Prepayment plans

offer services in exchange for regular fixed payments. Examples of fee-for-service plans are the nonprofit voluntary associations called Blue Cross and Blue Shield and commercial insurance. The prepaid health plans or health maintenance organizations (HMOs) include prepaid group practices and individual practice associations. The prepaid group practices provide hospital and physician services using salaried physicians, whereas individual practice associations contract with hospitals and physicians in private practice to deliver services to enrollees (Hobbs, Perrin, and Ireys, 1985).

Fee-for-service plans

Blue Cross–Blue Shield arose from nonprofit, voluntary prepayment programs to cover unexpected hospital expenses and physician fees for treatment of conditions in the office or hospital, laboratory tests, and other services. Commercial health insurance is provided by profit-making organizations that sell all types of insurance.

Benefits that are likely to be covered by Blue Cross–Blue Shield and commercial insurance are hospital room and board, miscellaneous hospital expenses, surgery, physician's nonsurgical services rendered in a hospital, and outpatient diagnostic x-ray and laboratory expenses. Room and board in an extended care facility may be included when it can be shown that continued medical care rather than custodial care is required (Health Insurance Association of America [HIAA], 1983).

The insured person generally may expect to pay a deductible fee before insurance benefits are realized and coinsurance of about 20% of physician, hospital, and other related fees. There may be a stop-loss provision, which is the amount that a family must pay out of pocket in a calendar year before the plan pays 100% of further covered charges. There may also be a maximum lifetime benefit. Two million dollars is a typical lifetime benefit for a commercial insurance company.

Major medical expense policies, separate from general health insurance policies, that cover a broad range of catastrophic medical expenses, are available. The cost of major medical insurance is controlled by a deductible fee ranging from $2000 to $15,000 or more and a coinsurance percentage of 20% of those medical expenses that exceed the deductible. Maximum benefits are usually limited to $250,000 per person within a benefit period of 1 to 3 years, but there may be no limit to coverage within the benefit period (HIAA, 1983). Major medical plans do not necessarily have advantages for children with chronic conditions. Their health care needs are likely to be long term and repetitive and not fit into a benefit structure of 1 to 3 years (Weeks, 1985).

The problems faced by families who depend on fee-for-service health insurance to finance care for a child with a chronic condition are evident by looking at the exclusions and limitations of these policies. The insurer usually does not pay for preexisting conditions. Thus if a family was not adequately covered before their child acquired the chronic condition, a fee-for-service plan often will not cover the medical expenses related to the chronic condition. Other common exclusions are payments for preventive health care (e.g., routine physical examinations), rehabilitation services, hearing aids, eye glasses, and expenses associated with the birth of an infant up to the first 30 days of life.

Health insurance was designed to cover medical expenses, consequently coverage for health needs defined as nonmedical, such as special education, mental health services, transportation to health care facilities, and home renovations to care for a child with a chronic condition is generally not included in Blue Cross–Blue Shield or commercial health insurance. A survey of 259 members of the American Spinal Injury Association demonstrated that requests for durable medical equipment deemed medically necessary for mobility and transfer, adaptations to bathrooms for toileting and bathing, functional equipment to enable persons to feed themselves or turn the pages of a book, and special seating for functional posture are routinely denied by most types of fee-for-service plans (Donovan, Carter, and Wilkerson, 1987).

Fox (1988) reviewed health insurance benefits for services of importance to children with special medical problems. These findings are based on a survey of 60 employers representing small, medium, and large firms. Of the 55 who provided health benefits, all covered basic hospital, surgical, inpatient and outpatient physician, x-ray, and laboratory services. Ninety-four percent covered medical equipment, and 91% covered prescription drugs. Benefits decreased to 87% to 81% for visiting nurse services, physical and speech therapy, and home health aid services. Comprehensive home care was offered by 64% of firms. Occupational therapy was covered by 60%, and skilled nursing home care was covered by 27%. Larger firms were more likely to offer a greater scope of benefits.

One way in which employers control their costs for health care coverage is to expand benefits for lower cost alternatives to hospitalization, such as the comprehensive home care benefit. This may include home-based services of social workers and physical, occupational, and other therapists in addition to nursing or home health aid care (Fox, 1988).

Other important cost-saving developments in the voluntary and commercial insurance field are the Preferred Provider Option, Confirming Second Surgical Opinion, and the Pre-Hospital Admission Review (Tibbitts and Manzano, 1984). Under the Preferred Provider Option, the family selects a provider recommended by the insurance company who agrees to provide care at a predetermined cost. In return for limiting provider selection, the insurance company agrees to reimburse 90% of covered charges rather than 80%. Families who use the Confirming Second Surgical Opinion and the Pre-Hospital Admission Review are also eligible to receive full benefits. These options may be satisfactory for a family with routine health care needs. However, a family with a child with a chronic condition may not be able to take advantage of these options because of the need for a specific physician, hospital, or team of health care providers with specialized knowledge and skill in the child's condition.

Prepaid health plans

In contrast with the fee-for-service plans, HMOs function as both insurer and provider of health care. One type of provider arrangement is the prepaid group practice in which hospital and physician services are provided by salaried staff members. Another type is the individual practice association that contracts for services with private providers in the community.

Families enroll in HMOs through an employee group if the employer offers it as a benefits option. Monthly premiums are generally paid for by the employer. Preexisting conditions are not excluded. There is no deductible or coinsurance provision. Services provided are similar to those offered in fee-for-service plans, including limited skilled nursing facility and home health service. In contrast to most private insurance, HMOs provide preventive health services as a covered benefit. They have a strong incentive to keep their enrollees healthy, because the agency is at financial risk if more costly health services are required (Weeks, 1985).

After joining an HMO, the family must select a primary care physician who authorizes care by any other physician or hospital within the plan. Prepayment plans discourage use of providers and services outside of the plan because the cost of these services is likely to be higher and unpredictable. If a child with a chronic condition requires a physician or health care team with special expertise who is not available in the HMO, this type of health coverage may not be adequate for the child. Other services that may not be covered by HMOs are long-term physical, occupational, speech, and rehabilitation therapies not expected to show benefit in less than 60 days, prosthetics, and rental or purchase of durable medical equipment (Weeks, 1985).

Advantages of the prepaid plan for the family are the coverage of primary care and access to a different mix of services that may include pediatric nurse practitioners and clinicians, nutrition, and social services with expertise in various problems of living with a chronic condition (Hobbs, Perrin, and Ireys, 1985).

Parents of children with chronic conditions must consider their options for health insurance coverage carefully to obtain the best coverage for their particular needs. A publication for parents that will help them understand these options is available through the Association for the Care of Children's Health (McManus, 1988). Once the policy is purchased or obtained through employment, careful attention must be given to accuracy in filling out claims and filing them promptly, working with the claims agent who understands the family's problems, and following up rejected claims with convincing evidence of the importance of the treatment or piece of equipment to the well-being of the child (Jones, 1985). The primary care provider can be of great help to the parents by supporting their legitimate insurance claims and completing insurance forms accurately and in a timely manner.

GOVERNMENT HEALTH CARE PROGRAMS

The federal government provides medical benefits directly to Native Americans and military personnel and federal civilian employees and their dependents. Other public health care financing programs are jointly administered by the federal government and the states and are mandated to provide health care for individuals and families who are not eligible for or cannot purchase private health insurance.

Persons without access to health insurance may be unemployed, employed in firms that do not offer health care benefits, or employed in positions that are ineligible for health care benefits (e.g., part-time positions). Undocumented residents who do not wish to be identified as working in the United States may accept positions without health insurance coverage or other work-related benefits. In 1987 the Employee Benefit Research Institute published characteristics of uninsured persons (HIAA, 1989). Nearly one half are workers, one third are children less than 17 years of age, and only 17% are nonworking adults. Thirty-nine percent of this group have incomes that are greater than twice the federal poverty level.* Oberg (1990) reports that 12.2 million children less than 18 years of age are uninsured and that another 7 million may be insured for only part of the year.

Civilian Health and Medical Program of the Uniformed Services

Medical treatment at any Department of Defense installation is available to all active military personnel and their dependents. The Civilian Health and Medical Program of the Uniformed Services (CHAMPUS) is a program of medical benefits provided by civilian health care professionals for military families who are unable to use government medical facilities because of distance, overcrowding, or unavailability of appropriate medical treatment (HIAA, 1989). CHAMPUS resembles a traditional health insurance plan in that beneficiaries must pay a deductible, may have out-of-pocket costs, and may also be limited to a preferred provider panel of physicians (Hosek et al., 1987). Military organizations provide families of children with chronic conditions with information, financial assistance, and health care within the military community or through local community, state, and federal agencies. Health benefits advisors located on military installations facilitate access to both military and public programs in coordination with the multidisciplinary medical and social service support from the Army's Exceptional Family Member Program, the Air Force's Children Have Potential Program, and the Navy's Family Support Program. Of importance to eligible families with children with chronic conditions are the extensive benefits for home care, including physician visits, skilled nursing care and visiting nurse services, and provision of durable medical equipment, drugs, supplies, and physical and occupational therapy (Helton, 1988).

Indian Health Service

The Indian Health Service is an organization within the U.S. Public Health Service. Its purpose is to ensure the availability of a comprehensive health care delivery system to Native Americans, including hospital and ambulatory medical care, preventive and rehabilitation services, and community and environmental health programs. The extent to which children with chronic conditions are well served in this system is dependent on the skill of the staff at the local Indian Health Service Unit in determining the family's eligibility for third-party payment for health services, in making appropriate referrals, and in providing culturally sensitive counseling and education. The Indian Health Service interacts with other federal and state agencies and public and private institutions in developing ways to deliver health services, stimulate consumer participation, and apply resources. These include Indian Health Service and tribally operated hospitals and health centers and rural and urban health programs that receive both state and federal funding and are subject to regulations of Medicaid and private health care insurance (U.S. Department of Health and Human Services [USDHHS], 1989). Information on eligibility, location, and range of health care programs at the local Indian Health Service Unit may be obtained from Indian Health Service Headquarters in Washington, D.C., Headquarters West in Albuquerque, New Mexico, or through 1 of 11 area offices. (See Resources for Indian Health Service Administrative Offices.)

Medicaid

Medicaid (Title XIX of the Social Security Act) is the largest public medical program in the United States. It is administered by the Health Care Financing Administration in the Department of Health and Human Services. Medicaid is a program of federal grants to states to pay for designated health services for eligible persons. Within this group are children with chronic conditions in eligible families. Medicaid was established in 1966 and soon surpassed any other public health care program serving children in federal expenditures, estimated in 1987 to be $5.5 billion, or 12.3% of total Medicaid expenditures (Oberg and Polich, 1988).

Eligibility and services received vary from state to state because states are free to add services and enhance eligibility over and above the requirements of the federal law. The primary criterion for eli-

---

*The poverty index is based on a determination by the U.S. Department of Agriculture that families spend approximately one third of their incomes on food. The poverty level is therefore set at 3 times the cost of the economy food plan, which includes specific amounts of meat, vegetables, and other commodities. As of March 1991, a family of four meets the federal poverty guideline (stated as 100% of poverty) if their income is $13,400.

gibility is being in a welfare category such as receiving Aid to Families with Dependent Children (AFDC) or Supplemental Security Income (SSI) for old age, blindness, or other disability. In 1988, income eligibility for AFDC expressed as a percent of the federal poverty level ranged from 14.6% (Alabama) to 85.8% (Utah), with a state average of 48.8%. That is, a family of three could earn up to $1416 per year in Alabama or $8316 in Utah, with a state average of $4738, to be eligible for AFDC and Medicaid (U.S. General Accounting Office, 1989). A state Medicaid program may also permit benefits to families with an incapacitated parent or two unemployed parents under a "medically needy" program (Hobbs, Perrin, and Ireys, 1985).

A full range of preventive and illness-related services are covered by Medicaid. These are inpatient hospital care, physician and other outpatient services, laboratory tests, and skilled nursing services. States may choose to cover the costs of dental care, eye glasses, drugs, inpatient psychiatric care, and home health. Of importance to children is the preventive health program added to Medicaid in 1972, the Early Periodic Screening Diagnosis and Treatment (EPSDT) Program. This brings Medicaid-eligible children into the program for health screening. If health problems are identified in an EPSDT screen, the law requires referral for diagnosis and treatment (Myers, 1986).

As the costs of Medicaid rise, states may adopt certain strategies to conserve funds (Hobbs, Perrin, and Ireys, 1985), including denying eligibility to the medically needy groups whose participation is not mandated by federal law and requiring eligible families to join prepaid medical plans or primary care case management systems. Joining a prepaid plan or case management system could be of benefit to children with chronic conditions in that a wider range of preventive health services and other therapies may be available and better coordinated than those under the traditional Medicaid fee-for-service plan.

Children who are dependent on ventilators, parenteral nutrition, or other technologies and cannot be discharged from the hospital without skilled nursing and other health services may be eligible for coverage of home care under the Medicaid model home- and community-based waiver, authorized in 1981 in the Omnibus Budget Reconciliation Act (OBRA), Section 2176 (Public Law 97-35).

The purpose of the program is to reduce the cost of care to Medicaid resulting from lengthy hospitalizations and to avoid unnecessary institutionalization of children. It includes case management, homemaker services, home modifications, and other therapies. Qualifying for coverage and services for home care varies among states. States may remove parental income and assets as an eligibility consideration or may raise the Medicaid income standard. Diseases designated eligible may differ, and some states require that the child be discharged from an institution immediately before application for the waiver (Leonard, Brust, and Choi, 1989). It is often difficult for potentially eligible families to find out about home- and community-based waivers authorized under Medicaid. States have failed to publicize the program or have delayed processing applications (USDHHS, 1987). Health care professionals wishing to determine if this program is appropriate for a Medicaid-eligible or medically needy client and available in their state should request information from the state agency responsible for implementation of the Medicaid program, usually the county Department of Social Services.

Children with chronic conditions who receive Medicaid benefits may be faced with limited access to hospitalization and a decrease in quality of care because of prospective hospital payment systems. The prospective system, called Diagnosis Related Groups (DRGs), was first introduced to control hospital costs for Medicare, a compulsory federal insurance program for persons more than 65 years of age. An average cost of care is determined (based on the patient's age and specific type of care received), and hospitals are reimbursed according to this cost. The present DRG definitions do not adequately classify the problems and costs of care of hospitalized children normally treated in specialized pediatric settings, and efforts are underway to develop pediatric modified DRGs to avoid a crisis in hospital reimbursement of seriously ill infants and children (Munoz et al., 1989; Lichtig et al., 1989).

The Medicaid law undergoes continual reform by Congress in the areas of eligibility, benefits, reimbursement, and administration. The OBRA of 1989 mandated the following changes that may make Medicaid more accessible to poor families with a child with a chronic condition (Children's Defense Fund, 1990).* Medicaid eligibility has been raised for pregnant women and infants and children less than age 6 years from approximately 75% of the federal proverty line to 133%. States must now include in their Medicaid benefit package all ambulatory health care services offered to Medicaid beneficiaries receiving care in community and migrant health centers funded by the federal Public Health Services Act. The new law also encourages the use of pediatric and family nurse practitioner services in rural health clinics by mandating states to cover their services as long as they are practicing within the scope of state law, regardless of whether they are under the supervision of or associated with a physician. Further changes in the law permit a raise in reimbursement to obstetricians and pediatricians to enlist enough providers to serve eligible families. Reimbursement for physician services has not been as high as that of private insurance for a given geographic area. This has forced some Medicaid-eligible children to be dependent on emergency rooms and hospital outpatient departments where families may not be able to establish a relationship with a single provider who understands their particular needs.

Administrative changes in 1989 include strengthening the referral of Medicaid-eligible mothers and infants at nutritional risk to the Special Supplemental Food Program for Women, Infants, and Children (WIC), funded by the U.S. Department of Agriculture (USDA). Some long-standing deficiencies in the EPSDT Program will also be corrected. Although many states have periodicity standards for all types of health screening, the law now requires that states establish these standards for medical, vision, hearing, and dental screening and further requires that services must be furnished at other than scheduled intervals when medically necessary to treat a suspected illness or condition. In addition, states must offer necessary health services to correct or ameliorate a condition found in

the EPSDT screen whether or not such services are covered by the state plan. With the changes in the EPSDT Program, formerly optional services such as durable medical equipment, physical and speech therapy, prosthetic devices, rehabilitation, and case management are made more accessible to Medicaid-eligible children with chronic conditions.

In most states eligibility for Medicaid for individuals and families is determined by the Department of Social Services in the counties. Social workers in hospitals, public health, child welfare, and other human services agencies can assist families with children with chronic conditions to determine if they are eligible for Medicaid coverage and can also help health care providers to be informed of health services that are covered by Medicaid. Receiving Medicaid coverage for health care does not preclude receiving assistance from other federal programs for services and equipment that are not covered by Medicaid.

Medicare's end-stage renal disease program

Medicare is authorized under Title XVIII of the Social Security Act. Children generally are not entitled to any health care benefits under Medicare because it provides health insurance protection for persons more than 65 years of age and persons less than age 65 years who are collecting Social Security or Railroad Retirement Benefits. However, children with end-stage renal disease may be eligible to receive health care benefits to cover costs of peritoneal or hemodialysis and related services in the hospital or home. This benefit does not extend to other organ transplants.

Maternal and Child Health Block Grant: Title V

The federal-state program for children with special health care needs was established by Title V of the Social Security Act of 1935. Title V provided three grants-in-aid programs to states: maternal and child health, children with special health care needs, and child welfare. The program for children with special health care needs was called Services for Crippled Children until approximately 1987.

Title V legislation grew out of increased recognition that the federal government should bear some responsibility for the well-being of mothers

---

*The OBRA of 1989 also contains significant reforms that affect women's access to prenatal care.

and children and that federal assistance to state health departments would enable the states to provide needed services on the local level. Data demonstrating poor maternal care, an infant mortality rate that exceeded other industrialized countries, and lack of access to health care for disabled children, particularly those in rural areas, gave further impetus to Congress to pass the act. These data were gathered by the U.S. Children's Bureau, established in 1912, and the Maternity and Infancy Act (Sheppard-Towner) of 1920-1929. Under the Sheppard-Towner Act, a precedent was set for federal assistance to states for services for pregnant women, infants, and crippled children. Although the Sheppard-Towner Act survived only 8 years, states had the opportunity to establish a public health unit for mothers and children, improve birth registration, and increase public health nursing services. These positive experiences with federal support of state public health programs helped to lessen resistance on the part of private practitioners of medicine to federal intervention in health care and enabled passage of Title V (Lesser, 1985).

In 1981, with passage of the OBRA (Public Law 97-35), Title V programs were continued in the Maternal and Child Health (MCH) Block Grant. The MCH Block Grant is administered by the Administration for Children and Families, DHHS. The MCH Block Grant as amended in 1989 (Public Law 101-239) continues the original purpose of the 1981 act but with provisions that strengthen linkages to health services offered through Medicaid and the EPSDT Program, immunization programs of the U.S. Public Health Service, Centers for Disease Control, and the WIC supplemental feeding program in the USDA (U.S. Code, 1989).

The purpose of the block grant is to improve the health of all mothers and children consistent with the applicable health status goals and national health objectives for the year 2000 (U.S. Department of Health and Human Services, 1990). For fiscal year 1990, $686 million was authorized to be appropriated to each state, based in part on the number of births in a state. A rural birth counts twice that of an urban birth, a concept going back to 1935 when rural children were more likely to be isolated from health services. Other determinants of a state's allocation are the amounts spent

on Title V and other maternal and child health programs prior to 1981. The goals of the program are as follows:

1. To assure mothers and children, in particular those with low income, access to quality maternal and child health services.
2. To reduce infant mortality, the incidence of preventable diseases and handicapping conditions among children, to increase the number of children immunized, and to increase the number of low-income children receiving health assessments and follow-up diagnostic and treatment services.
3. To provide rehabilitation services for blind and disabled individuals less than 16 years of age who are receiving benefits under Title XVI (SSI) and who are not eligible for Medicaid.
4. To provide and promote family-centered, community-based, coordinated care for children with special health care needs.
5. To support certain categoric or discretionary programs, referred to as Special Projects of Regional and National Significance (SPRANS) with 10% to 15% of MCH Block Grant appropriations, set aside at the federal level. These discretionary programs are (1) MCH research and training; (2) genetic disease testing, counseling, and information dissemination; (3) hemophilia diagnostic and treatment centers; and (4) other special projects.

Maternal and Child Health Block Grant: programs for children with special health care needs

The program for children with special health care needs mandated by the OBRA, Title V legislation, requires that federal funds in combination with state matching funds be used to provide services for locating these children and for providing medical, surgical, and other services, and facilities for diagnosis and treatment for chronic conditions or conditions that may become chronic. States have different service delivery systems funded by this program. They may provide services directly through program-funded clinics staffed by program providers or may be a source of reimbursement for services rendered in the private sector by medical specialists, selected by the state program as qualified to offer services on a fee-for-service basis. Many states have elements of both systems (Ireys and Eichler, 1989).

States are mandated to provide these services in cooperation with medical, nursing, vocational, and social welfare groups. Each state defines which children will be served (Wallace, 1988). These differences in definitions of conditions to be served persist because the wealthier states overmatch federal funds. For example, of the total budget in California for children with special health care needs, only about 10% comes from the federal government. In addition, the counties of California are required by state law to contribute to the care of children with special health care needs who live in their jurisdictions, and this amount is matched by the state in a ratio of $3 for every $1 of county funds (Policy Analysis for California Education, 1989). The larger counties administer their own programs, determining eligibility, providing case management, authorizing care, and processing claims. Thus, eligibility for this program varies not only by state but also may vary by county within a state.

In general children who are likely to be eligible for care under this program have chronic conditions that are able to be corrected, such as a broad range of orthopedic conditions, conditions requiring plastic or orthodontic reconstruction, eye and ear conditions, which if untreated would lead to loss of vision or deafness, and other congenital anomalies that can be corrected or ameliorated with medical and surgical intervention. In addition to the eligible condition, most states require that the family income not exceed a specified amount. This amount will vary according to family size and tends to be set at 100% to 200% of poverty. Another criterion for eligibility may be that the child's parents be legal residents of the county or state in which they apply for assistance. This makes some children of undocumented persons ineligible.

The covered benefits are diagnostic services; comprehensive treatment by the appropriate pediatric medical and surgical specialities, including nursing, social work, physical and other therapies; and case management to enable the child and family to benefit from the multidisciplinary services. Case management is the skilled services of a professional

who is able to evaluate the psychosocial needs of the family and approve authorized services and interpret these to the family. As states have received less money for this program, some case management has been taken over by persons trained on the job and supervised by the program administrator, nurse, or social work consultant. They are paid less than the health professionals and are able to approve authorized services and give advice on the location of such services. In general they do not provide other counseling.

Children with mental retardation or mental illness, those with illnesses for which there is little curative or corrective intervention available, and those with conditions that usually result in early death are generally not eligible for this program. In recent years, with the development of new therapies, some state programs have broadened the definition of a child with special health care needs to include those with neoplasms, conditions of the nervous system, and endocrine and metabolic disorders. Professionals must stay well informed about the types of conditions covered by the states in which they practice through consultation with the state office responsible for Title V programs. In most states, this office is located in the state health department. However, the agency may be found in a university medical center, the state welfare department, or the state education department.

A state or county can conserve funds in several ways. One method is to require that an eligible family repay part of the cost of treatment services. Another method is by billing Medicaid, if the child is eligible, or billing the family's private insurance policy for covered services. Medicaid and Title V agencies at the state level are required by regulation to develop interagency coordination agreements. An example of a benefit of these agreements is the provision of case management through the MCH Block Grant to a child with special health care needs who is also Medicaid eligible (Saunders, 1988).

The 1989 amendments to the MCH Services Block Grant have modified the states' programs of services to children with special health care needs. States are now required to use at least 30% of their MCH Block Grant allotment for services to these children. They are further required to provide rehabilitation services for blind and disabled children younger than age 16 years who receive benefits under Title XVI (SSI) and who cannot obtain medical assistance through Medicaid. A more significant change is the mandate to provide and promote family-centered, community-based, coordinated care for children with special health care needs and to facilitate the development of community-based systems of services for such children and their families (Children's Defense Fund, 1990). Families of children with chronic conditions are both providers and consumers of health care. Therefore programs will need to make a commitment to ensure that family members are partners on a health care team that includes all the providers of care. In addition, efforts will need to be made to create linkages between tertiary and community-based health services to avoid fragmentation of health care and unavailability and inaccessibility of health services (National Maternal and Child Health Resource Center, 1988).

It is evident that the MCH Block Grant funds allocated to states are small in relation to Medicaid funds. Relatively few children with chronic conditions are eligible, but federal regulations demand that the programs set high standards of care that may benefit many more children than those actually receiving financial coverage. The requirement for a team approach using nursing, social work, and various rehabilitative therapists is also a model for other programs serving children with disabilities. Families may get information on the Program for Children with Special Health Care Needs through a private provider of health care, a local health department, or the office of the state health department responsible for the federal MCH Block Grant program.

Maternal and Child Health Block Grant and other programs for children with chronic illness

Supplemental Security Income. The SSI Program, Title XVI of the Social Security Act, was established by Congress in 1972 for aged, blind, and disabled adults and in 1976 for children less than 16 years of age with disabilities. The children's program was incorporated into the MCH Block Grant in 1981. This is an income support program to help recipients become as self-sufficient as possible within the limits of their disability. It is not a program to pay directly for costs of health care of a child with a chronic condition. However, SSI recipients receive health care services through Medicaid, and this may relieve the family of seeking other sources of payment.

Eligible children are those with specific disabilities who live in very low-income households. The type of disability considered to meet SSI criteria has been contested in the courts, because it has been too restrictive in comparison with the criteria for defining disability in an adult (United Cerebral Palsy Association [UCPA], 1990a). Adults must show that they have an impairment that is on a federal list of impairments. If the adult's impairment does not meet or equal those on the list, an assessment may be made of the claimant's functional limitations. Children are less likely than adults who are disabled to be eligible for SSI because their impairments must meet or equal those on the list. No other assessment of residual functional capacity is made.

On February 20, 1990, the Supreme Court upheld a lower court ruling that the policy for determining eligibility for children was unfair and inconsistent with the statutory standards of comparable severity. At the present time, approximately 50,000 children with disabilities have been denied SSI. This ruling will enable lower courts to reopen cases where a child has been denied benefits.

The other criteria for eligibility is based on the individual's income. As of January 1, 1989, this must be less than $4416 per year. A house occupied by the recipient, an automobile used for essential transportation or modified for the handicapped driver, and personal household effects valued up to $2000 per year may be excluded from determining eligibility (U.S. Social Security Administration, 1989). However, the regulations must be studied carefully if one is to understand other factors affecting benefits. For example, the basic SSI payment is reduced by the amount of other income and support available to the recipient. Unearned income of more than $20 per month will reduce SSI payments dollar for dollar. However, work is encouraged by treating earned income differently; $65 of earned income in any month is excluded from countable income. Thereafter, SSI payments are reduced by $1 for every $2 earned. Income from some other sources, such as scholarships, some student employment, and impairment-related work expenses, is excluded when payment amounts are determined.

The amount of SSI paid to an individual and the administration of the program will vary by state, because states have the option of supplementing the payments. About one half of the states administer their own supplementary payments, and the recipients receive this payment separately from that of the federal program. The other states choose federal administration; the Social Security Administration issues the federal payment and state supplement in one check. Applications for SSI payments are made at district offices of the Social Security Administration where supporting documentation on age, income, and assets is examined (USSSA, 1989).

Genetic disease testing and counseling service. The MCH Block Grant incorporated the funding for screening, education, and counseling for persons at risk for or afflicted with sickle cell disease under Public Law 92-294, the National Sickle Cell Control Act of 1972, and education, counseling, and medical referral for all genetic disorders mandated by Public Law 95-626, Title XI of the Public Health Services Act, 1978. This program supports genetic service grants and sickle cell clinic grants in some but not all states. It supports a National Clearinghouse for Human Genetic Diseases for the collection and dissemination of informational materials; a laboratory support program in hematology, cytogenetics, and biochemistry to develop laboratory standards, provide training, and conduct proficiency testing; and a system to collect and analyze epidemiologic data on genetic disease. Regional genetic networks are also supported to promote coordination and communication among genetic service providers and to demonstrate ways to address emerging issues in genetic testing and service delivery.

There are no direct payments to families for genetic counseling, fetal diagnosis, and other services under this program. Clinics serving pregnant women and families of children with genetic diseases must seek third-party payment for their clients to be financially self-supporting (Bernhardt et al., 1987). States may support a genetic disease section in the state health department and be able to offer at no or low cost such services as α-fetoprotein (AFP) screening for neural tube defects, amniocentesis for follow-up of a positive AFP test result, and newborn screening for phenylketonuria, galactosemia, and congenital hypothyroidism. The staff of genetic clinics and centers, such as genetic counselors, nurses and social workers, and the genetic disease branch of the state health department can provide information to other health professionals and families on indications for genetic counseling, location of services, and private and public programs that help to pay costs of these services.

Hemophilia treatment centers. The purpose of this program is to establish comprehensive hemophilia diagnostic and treatment centers (see Chapter 6). Once the center is established, third-party payment for services to individuals must be sought to enable the center to be financially solvent. Some states also support counseling and treatment for hemophilia by paying for blood products and home care. Persons with hemophilia are also represented by the National Hemophilia Foundation, a nationally coordinated health agency with local chapters to promote education and to change the restrictive policies of third-party programs to better cover treatment (Hilgartner, Aledort, and Giardina, 1985).

Federal programs for mental retardation and developmental disabilities

Mental retardation is defined as significantly subaverage intellectual functioning with IQ at 70 or less existing concurrently with deficits in adaptive behavior and manifested during the developmental period from birth to 18 years (Cohen, 1987). The term "developmental disabilities" was introduced in the 1970s to enable children with cerebral palsy, epilepsy, autism, and learning disabilities to benefit from federal programs directed at children with mental retardation and other functional problems that inhibited entry into school, employment, and mobility in the community. By the 1980s the definition of developmental disabilities changed from these categories to a functional description. The new definition requires a limitation in at least three of seven areas of major life activity: self-care, receptive and expressive language, learning, mobility, self-direction, capacity for independent living, and economic self-sufficiency (Braddock, 1987).

Third-party payment for primary and illness care of children with mental retardation and developmental disabilities does not differ from that of other children with chronic conditions. Eligibility for private health insurance will depend on the parents' access to comprehensive health insurance through employment. Medicaid eligibility is determined on a state-by-state basis by household income in relation to the federal poverty guidelines and the Medicaid regulations. Eligibility for financial support of medical and surgical treatment through the MCH Block Grant, Title V, Program for Children with Special Health Care Needs, will depend on the state's definition of an eligible condition, family income, and access to other third-party payment of medical expenses.

The history of federal programs for the mentally retarded and developmentally disabled is reviewed by Braddock (1987). Care of children with these diagnoses was traditionally the responsibility of states and counties and voluntary associations. The programs for mothers and infants in Title V of the Social Security Act of 1935 contributed to the prevention of mental retardation. However, the care and rehabilitation of these children were considered to be beyond the scope of Title V. They have been excluded from these state programs to the present time unless they have an eligible condition in addition to mental retardation.

Funds for research in mental retardation and demonstration of services and personnel training was provided by several congressional bills throughout the 1950s. In the early 1960s President John F. Kennedy's panel on Mental Retardation contributed to the passage of Public Law 88-164, the Mental Retardation Facilities and Community Mental Health Centers Construction Act of 1963, beginning the modern era of the federal government's mental retardation and financial assistance programs. This law enabled the establishment of research centers, a mental retardation branch at the National Institute of Child Health and Human Development, and university-affiliated programs for the provision of clinical services and training of personnel in the care of children with mental retardation.

Public Law 91-517, the Developmental Disabilities Services and Facilities Construction Act of 1970, extended services to individuals with cerebral palsy and epilepsy in addition to those with mental retardation. To receive federal funds under this act, states were required to establish developmental disabilities councils to promote coordinated planning and service delivery. Other significant legislation during this decade included Public Law 92-603, the Social Security Amendments of 1972, which added Title XVI, Supplemental Security Income; Public Law 92-223, the Social Security Amendments of 1971, to permit reimbursement for active treatment of the developmentally disabled in intermediate care facilities (ICFs); Section 504 of the Rehabilitation Act of 1973, prohibiting discrimination against individuals with developmental disabilities in any activity or place of employment receiving federal assistance; Public Law 93-647, the Social Security Amendments of 1974, consolidating social services grants to states under a new Title XX of the Social Security Act to provide states with funds to develop alternatives to institutional care; and Public Law 94-142, Education for All Handicapped Children Act of 1975.

With passage of the OBRA of 1981, federal funding of all social programs was curtailed, and for several years there was no growth in developmental disabilities services. However, the Medicaid waivers program for home- and community-based care was included in the OBRA to discourage the use of the more expensive ICFs.

In the area of civil rights legislation for all persons with disabilities, including the mentally retarded, the Americans with Disabilities Act, passed in 1990, extends federal protection in the private and public sectors to include employment, transportation, public accommodations, and communication. This law requires changes in physical plants to accommodate employees with disabilities; accessible buses, trains and subway cars, hotels, retail stores, and restaurants; and telecommunications devices on ordinary telephones to enable hearing- and voice-impaired persons to place and receive calls (UCPA, 1990b).

Given the complexity of laws, both federal and state, governing the availabilitiy and accessibility of services for individuals with developmental disabilities, it is difficult for families to know their rights in regard to treatment, education, and employment of their child with developmental disabilities. Social workers in agencies serving the developmentally disabled, public health nurses in programs for children with special health care needs, teachers in special education programs in public schools, voluntary organizations for the mentally retarded and other diagnoses leading to developmental disabilities, and members of local developmental disabilities councils are all sources of information. Payment for services for an individual child will not necessarily come from any of the legislated programs. Their intent is to provide model services and training of staff.

Education of All Handicapped Children Act and amendments for handicapped infants and toddlers

Programs of interest to providers who care for children with chronic conditions that link health and educational benefits are Public Law 94-142, Education for All Handicapped Children Act of 1975, with provisions to encourage states to expand early intervention services for preschool-aged children 3 to 5 years old, and Public Law 99-457, the 1986 amendments to the law for handicapped infants and toddlers. The Education for All Handicapped Children Act resulted from legal decisions establishing that handicapped children have a constitutional right to a publicly funded education in the least restrictive environment. The act defines handicapped children as those who require special education and related services because they are learning disabled, mentally retarded, or emotionally disturbed or have specified physical handicaps. The handicap has to be serious enough to impede successful progress in a regular educational program (Walker and Jacobs, 1985; Gelman, 1989). Other services that must be provided if determined to be necessary to the educational program are transportation and developmental, corrective, or other support services required for the child to benefit from education. These services may include speech pathology and audiology, psychologic services, physical and occupational therapy, recreation, counseling, social work, and medical services. Parents have the right to participate in planning their child's educational program and the right to appeal a school system's decision about their child's education. State education agencies are responsible for implementing the law. By 1984, federal funds to support the program reached $1 billion, which is estimated to be 10% of per-pupil costs nationwide (Braddock, 1987).

Children served in this program must have an individual educational plan (IEP), which is re-viewed annually. The IEP includes a statement of the child's current educational performance, short-term objectives and long-term goals, and a description of services to be provided (Braddock, 1987). Health care providers are encouraged to participate in the development of the IEP, although the law does not specify the extent of health care providers' involvement (Walker and Jacobs, 1985).

The Education for the Handicapped Amendments of 1986, Public Law 99-457, offers states the opportunity to extend the benefits of Public Law 94-142 to children with handicapping conditions, birth through 2 years of age. This act designates funds for development of a statewide comprehensive, coordinated, multidisciplinary interagency system to provide early intervention services. Eligible infants are those who are identified as experiencing developmental delays in cognitive, physical, language and speech, psychosocial, and self-help skills development or who have a diagnosed physical or mental condition that has a high probability of resulting in developmental delay. States may also include in their definition children whom they determine to be at risk of developmental delay if early intervention services are not provided (National Association of State Directors of Special Education, 1987).

Services to eligible infants and toddlers must include family training, counseling and home visits; special instruction; speech pathology and audiology; occupational and physical therapy; psychosocial services; case management services; medical services, restricted to diagnosis or evaluation; early identification, screening and assessment; and health services necessary to enable the recipient to benefit from the other early intervention services. The services must be provided by qualified personnel in conformity with an individualized family service plan (Center for Policy Research, 1987).

During 1986 to 1988, $125 million was authorized for this program. States' allocations were based on the population of children birth through 2 years. The minimum state allocation was $244,375, and the maximum was $4.9 million, received by California. These funds may be used for the provision of direct services only if these services are not covered by other public or private sources. The main purpose of this program is not to fund direct services but to support interagency service coordination. States had to designate a lead agency to receive the funds and, in 4 years' time, were to have in place a policy to provide appropriate early intervention services to all handicapped infants and toddlers and those at risk for handicapping conditions in the state. Typical lead agencies are human services agencies, departments of education, or health departments.

The Education for the Handicapped Amendments of 1986 addresses the persistent and difficult problem of interagency service coordination for handicapped children and those at risk for handicapping conditions. One of the barriers to coordination is that payment of direct services, regardless of the extent to which they are coordinated and comprehensive, are generally under the control of public or private third-party payers. The method of payment for services ultimately determines what services are received. Bringing an interagency collaboration initiative to fruition under the present fragmented system of paying for health services entails a complex and labor intensive process. The benefits to be realized are not yet known (Center for Policy Research, 1987).

FUTURE NEEDS IN FINANCING HEALTH CARE FOR CHILDREN WITH CHRONIC CONDITIONS

Reviewing the benefits of private health insurance and public programs for children with chronic conditions reveals that there are gaps in funding for both specialty and primary care. Children with chronic conditions who are also medically uninsured have particular difficulty finding a regular provider for primary care. Oberg (1990) has examined the nature and extent of the problem of access to health care for uninsured children and recent public policy initiatives to address inadequate financial access. Recent Medicaid expansion has allowed states to separate eligibility for AFDC from Medicaid eligibility, enabling many uninsured women and children up to age 6 years, with incomes up to 133% of poverty to be eligible for Medicaid. Families who stop receiving AFDC benefits to begin employment may now continue to receive Medicaid benefits for an additional 6 months.

Alternatives are also being proposed in Congress to expand private sector alternatives for the employed uninsured (Oberg, 1990). The Basic Health Benefits for All Americans Act, introduced in 1987, is a proposal to require that employers, even in small businesses, offer a minimum level of benefits to their employees. This act, if passed, would extend benefits to 66% of the uninsured population. The Child Health Incentive Reform Plan, introduced in 1989, would require insurers who offer dependent coverage to include comprehensive well-child care at reasonable cost with appropriate cost-sharing requirements. This proposal has already been enacted by seven states.

The MCH Block Grant of 1989 is addressing the need to examine ways to insure children who are presently uninsurable. In Section 6508, $5 million is authorized to fund four demonstration projects to provide health insurance coverage through an eligible plan to medically uninsurable children. Eligible plans include those that are school based, operated by a not-for-profit entity such as Blue Cross, or offered by a nonprofit hospital. Federal funding of the projects will be set at 50% for the first year and will be reduced over the second and third year or subsequent years from 35% to 20%. The demonstration projects may not restrict insurance coverage on the basis of a child's medical condition or impose waiting periods or exclusions for preexisting conditions. The insurance premium imposed under the project shall be disclosed in advance and adjusted for family income. An evaluation of the project will also be required to determine whether health care coverage for previously uninsurable children has been improved (U.S. Code, 1989).

A Congressional Commission (the Pepper Commission) to investigate universal health care coverage through a job-based or public system has been established. This system would encourage small businesses to offer a minimum insurance package to all employees, require businesses with more than 100 employees to provide health insurance, and offer a public plan financed and administered by the federal government that would replace Medicaid. Services would be subject to cost sharing, with subsidies for low-income people and limits on out-of-pocket spending. System reforms would include measures to contain costs, assure quality, and initiate innovative delivery systems for the underserved. It is proposed that the plan be phased in, making coverage available for children first. At full implementation, all Americans would be required to have health insurance through their employer or through the public plan.

SUMMARY

Private and public programs for financing care for children with chronic conditions are complex and ever changing. They are marked by inadequacies and inequalities among counties within a state and among states. Federal programs are implemented by states that may choose to follow the law by providing just the required state match of federal funds or overmatch to enrich the program by adding services or broadening coverage to include more diagnoses. Access to private insurance favors those who are steadily employed in large businesses or who are members of strong labor unions that can negotiate comprehensive benefit packages.

Primary providers must be informed about how their young clients with chronic conditions are paying for care and informed about referral options for which the clients are eligible. Referral for help in purchasing appropriate insurance or in gaining access to a federal or state public benefit requires dedication and persistence on the part of the family and provider and is crucial to implementing the plan of care.

RESOURCES
Informational materials

National Center for Clinical Infant Programs (NCCIP): *Meeting the medical bill* [25-minute videotape], Washington DC 1988, NCCIP.

This videotape discusses Medicaid waivers that finance home care for children with special health needs, SSI and tells how parents can work with private insurance companies to obtain the best possible coverage for children. It is available from the National Information Center for Handicapped Children and Youth (NICHCY), PO Box 1492, Washington, DC 20013.

McManus MA: *Understanding your health insurance options: a guide for families who have children with special health care needs,* Washington DC, 1988, Bureau of Maternal and Child Health and Resources Development.

This guide is designed to help families who have children with special health care needs understand their health insurance options and select plans that are most suited to their needs. Also addressed are important concerns in private and public insurance plans. It is available from the Association for the Care of Children's Health, 3615 Wisconsin Ave, NW, Washington, DC 20016.

Gaylord CL and Leonard AM: Health care coverage for the child with a chronic illness or diability, Madison, WI, 1988, Center for Public Representation.

This book is for parents and others who are responsible for the health care of a child with a chronic illness or disability. Information is provided on private and public health care coverage to enable parents to make decisions on financing treatment and obtaining services. This guide is specific to health insurance and services in Wisconsin, but any interested reader would benefit from the discussion on legal rights, resolving disputes, accessing public programs and many other financial issues.

Russell LM: *Alternatives: a family guide to legal and financial planning for the disabled,*Evanston, Ill, 1983, First Publication.

This book is written for families of persons with mental and physical disabilities to help them understand financial planning for their child in regard to wills, guardianship, trusts, government benefits, taxes, and insurance. Of particular interest is the discussion of the way families may provide for their child or young adult with a disability without disqualifying them for government benefits.

Shelton TL, Jeppson ES, and Johnson BH: *Family-centered care for children with special health care needs,* Washington, DC, 1987, Association for the Care of Children's Health.

This book discusses the elements of family-centered care, reviews the research in this area, and provides checklists for implementing family-centered care. In addition, family-centered care technical assistance, programs, and audiovisual and written materials are listed. It is available from the National Maternal and Child Health Clearinghouse, 38th and R Sts, NW, Washington, DC 20057.

Organizations

Indian Health Service Administrative Offices
Headquarters:
    Indian Health Service
    Parklawn Building, Rm 6A-20
    5600 Fishers Ln
    Rockville, MD 20857
    (301) 443-4242

Headquarters West–Albuquerque
    Indian Health Service
    2401 12th St, NW, Rm 316
    Albuquerque, NM 87102
    (505) 766-5557

Areas:
    Aberdeen Area
    Indian Health Service
    115 4th Avenue, SE
    Aberdeen, SD 57401
    (605) 226-7521

Nashville Area
Indian Health Service
Oaks Tower Building, Suite 810
1101 Kermit Drive
Nashville, TN 37217
(615) 736-5104

Alaska Native Indian Health Service
P.O. Box 7-741
250 Gambell Street
Anchorage, AK 99510
(907) 267-1154

Albuquerque Area
Indian Health Service
505 Marquette Ave,
NW
Suite 1500
Albuquerque, NM
87102
(505) 766-2151

Oklahoma City Area
Indian Health Service
215 Dean A McGee St, NW
Oklahoma City, OK 73102
(405) 231-4796

Bemidji Area
Indian Health Service
PO Box 439
203 Federal Bldg
Bemidji, MN 56601
(218) 751-7701

Phoenix Area
Indian Health Service
3738 N 16th St, Suite A
Phoenix, AZ 85016
(602) 241-2052

Billings Area
Indian Health Service
PO Box 2143
711 Central Ave
Billings, MT 59103
(406) 657-6403

Portland Area
Indian Health Service
Federal Bldg, Room 476
1220 SW Third Ave
Portland, OR 97204
(503) 326-2020

California Area
Indian Health Service
2999 Fulton Ave
Sacramento, CA 95821
(916) 978-4202

Navajo Area
Indian Health Service
PO Box G
Window Rock, AZ 86515
(602) 871-4811

REFERENCES

Bernhardt BA, Weiner J, Foster EC, et al: The economics of clinical genetics services: a time analysis of a medical genetics clinic, *Am J Hum Genet* 41:559-565, 1987.

Braddock D: *Federal policy toward mental retardation and developmental disabilities,* Baltimore, Md, 1987, Paul H Brookes Publishing.

Center for Policy Research: Getting it together for handicapped and at-risk infants and toddlers. In *Capital Ideas* (HR 87.08), Washington, DC, 1987, National Governor's Association.

Children's Defense Fund: *Report on 1989 maternal and child health federal legislation,* Washington, DC, 1990, The Fund (unpublished).

Cohen HJ: Mental retardation. In Wallace HM, Biehl RF, and Oglesby AC, eds: *Handicapped children and youth: a comprehensive community and clinical approach,* New York, 1987, Human Sciences Press, pp 347-359.

Donovan WH, Carter RE, and Wilkerson MA: Profiles of denials of durable medical equipment for SCI patients by third party payers, *Am J Phys Med* 66:238-243, 1987.

Fox HB: Private health insurance coverage of chronically ill children. In *Fostering home and community-based care for technology-dependent children,* Report of the Task Force on Technology Dependent Children, 1988, vol 1, HCFA Pub No 88-02171, Washington, DC, US Department of Health and Human Services, US Government Printing Office, pp 116-156.

Gelman C: Suspensions and expulsions under the education for all handicapped children act, *Wash Univ J Urban Contemp Law* 36:137-165, 1989.

Health Insurance Association of America: *Individual health insurance,* Chicago, 1983, Health Insurance Association of America, Insurance Education Program, pp 47-69.

Health Insurance Association of America: *Source book of health insurance-data,* Washington, DC, 1989, Public Relations Division of the Health Insurance Association of America, pp 10-14, 30.

Helton JD: Comments before the task force of technology dependent-children. In *Fostering home and community-based care for technology-dependent children,* Report of the Task Force on Technology Dependent Children, 1988, vol 1, HCFA Pub No 88-02171. Washington, DC, 1988, Department of Health and Human Services, US Government Printing Office, pp 30-305.

Hilgartner MW, Aldedort L, and Giardina PJV: Thalassemia and hemophilia. In Hobbs N and Perrin JM, eds: *Issues in the care of children with chronic illness,* San Francisco, 1985, Jossey-Bass, pp 299-323.

Hobbs N, Perrin JM and Ireys HT: *Chronically ill children and their families,* San Francisco, 1985, Jossey-Bass, pp 189-230.

Hosek SD, Anderson M, Hartford A, et al: *Plan for the evaluation of the CHAMPUS Reform Initiative.* Santa Monica, Calif, 1987, Rand.

Ireys, HT and Eichler RJ: Program priorities of crippled children's agencies: a survey. *Public Health Rep* 103:77-83, 1989.

Jones ML: *Home care of the chronically ill or disabled child.* New York, 1985, Harper & Row Publishers.

Leonard BJ, Brust JD and Choi T: Providing access to home care for disabled children: Minnesota Medicaid model waiver program, *Public Health Rep* 104:465-472, 1989.

Lesser AJ: The origin and development of maternal and child health programs in the United States. *Am J Public Health* 75:590-598, 1985.

Lichtig DK, Knauf RA, Bartoletti A, et al: Revising diagnosis-related groups for neonates, *Pediatrics* 84:49-61, 1989.

McManus JA: *Understanding your health insurance options: a guide for families who have children with special health care needs,* Washington, DC, Bureau of Maternal and Child Health Resource Development. (Available from the Association for the Care of Children's Health, 3615 Wisconsin Ave, Washington, DC 20016.)

Munoz E, Chalfin D, Goldstein J, et al: Health care financing policy for hospitalized pediatric patients. *Am J Dis Child* 143:312-315, 1989.

Myers BA: Social policy and the organization of health care. In Last JM ed: *Maxcy-Rosenau public health and preventive medicine,* ed 12, Norwalk, Conn, 1986, Appleton-Century-Crofts, pp 1639-1667.

National Association of State Directors of Special Education: EHA amendments become law: establishes new partnerships for early intervention programs. *Liaison Bull* 12(12) 1987.

National Maternal and Child Health Resource Center: *Community based health services.* Paper presented at the US Surgeon General's Conference, Building community based service systems for children with special health care needs, University of Iowa, Sept 8, 1988. Iowa City, Ia.

Oberg CN: Medically uninsured children in the United States: a challenge to public policy. *Pediatrics* 85:824-833, 1990.

Oberg CN and Polich CT: Medicaid: entering the third decade. *Health Aff* 7:83-96, 1988.

Policy Analysis for California Education: *Conditions of children in California,* Berkeley, Calif, 1989, University of California Press, p 190.

Saunders S: Medicaid and maternal child health and programs for children with special health needs. In Wallace HM, Ryan G, and Oglesby AC, eds: *Maternal and child health practices,* ed 3, Oakland, Calif, 1988, Third Party Publishing, pp 123-134.

Tibbitts SJ and Manzano AJ: *PPO's: preferred provider organizations,* Chicago, 1984, Pluribus Press, pp 34-46.

United Cerebral Palsy Associations: *Word from Washington,* New York, February-March 1990a, The Associations, p 9.

United Cerebral Palsy Associations: *Word from Washington,* New York, April-May 1990b, The Associations, pp 3-5.

US Code: *Congressional and administrative news, 1st session public news,* St Paul, Minn, 1989, West Publishing.

US Department of Health and Human Services: *Fostering home and community-based care for technology-dependent children,* vol 2, Report to the Congress and the Secretary of the Task Force on Technology-Dependent Children, Washington, DC, 1987a, US Government Printing Office.

US Department of Health and Human Services: *Indian health service: a comprehensive health care program for American Indians and Alaskan natives,* Washington, DC, 1989, US Government Printing Office.

US Department of Health and Human Services, Public Health Services: Healthy people 2000, national health promotion and disease prevention objectives, Washington DC, 1990, Public Health Service, US Department of Health and Human Services.

US General Accounting Office: *Medicaid: states expand coverage for pregnant women, infants, and children,* GAO/HRD-89-90, Gaithersburg, Md, 1989, USGAO, pp 16-17.

US Social Security Administration: Social security programs in the United States. *Soc Secur Bull* 52:62-65, 1989.

Walker DK and Jacobs FH: Public school programs for chronically ill children. In Hobbs N and Perrin JM, eds: *Issues in the care of children with chronic illness,* San Francisco, 1985, Jossey-Bass, pp 615-655.

Wallace HM: Organization of services for handicapped children and youth. In Wallace HM, Ryan G, and Ogelsby AC, eds: *Maternal and child health practices,* ed 3, Oakland, Calif, 1988, Third Party Publishing, pp 103-122.

Weeks KH: Private health insurance and chronically ill children. In Hobbs N and Perrin JM, eds: *Issues in the care of children with chronic illness,* San Francisco, 1985, Jossey-Bass, pp 880-911.

PART II

CHRONIC CONDITIONS

Primary Care of the Child with . . .
  Asthma
  Bleeding Disorders: Hemophilia
    and von Willebrand's Disease
  Bronchopulmonary Dysplasia
  Cancer
  Cerebral Palsy
  Congenital Adrenal Hyperplasia
  Congenital Heart Disease
  Cystic Fibrosis
  Diabetes Mellitus (Type I)
  Down Syndrome
  Epilepsy
  Fragile X Syndrome
  Hydrocephalus
  Inflammatory Bowel Disease
  Juvenile Rheumatoid Arthritis
  Learning Disabilities
  Myelodysplasia
  Organ Transplants
  Pediatric HIV Infection and AIDS
  Phenylketonuria
  Prematurity
  Prenatal Cocaine Exposure
  Chronic Renal Failure
  Sickle Cell Disease

5 *Asthma*

Nanci L. Larter and Gail Kieckhefer

ETIOLOGY

The exact etiology of asthma remains equivocal. Although a familial tendency has long been recognized, environmental factors are now thought to contribute to the presence of clinically recognized asthma. It is well established that a relationship exists between viral infections and the induction of asthma. In studying healthy subjects with viral illness, Frick and Busse (1988) found that viral respiratory infections cause small airway obstruction and airway hyperreactivity. Children with viral bronchiolitis are reported to have additional wheezing episodes after the initial insult, although the number of episodes usually decreases over time. In those children with asthma, upper respiratory infections (URI) heighten bronchial hyperreactivity and increase air flow obstruction. In the past asthma has been characterized as obstructive airway disease caused primarily by bronchoconstriction (smooth muscle contraction); however, over the last decade the roles of inflammation and mucous secretion have become increasingly important (Ellis, 1988). The ability of viral illness to promote this inflammatory process has not been well established.

Asthma may have at least two response phases to stimuli that trigger an episode. Dolovich (1988) describes an early phase, or response, which begins immediately after exposure to a trigger. It is most likely an immunoglobulin E–triggered response to disassembled mast cells and the release of histamine and other substances that result in smooth muscle contraction and bronchospasm in the airway. The second phase is called a late phase response and occurs initially 2 to 4 hours after exposure to an irritant, peaks at 6 to 12 hours, and disappears 12 to 24 hours later. In the late phase there is an influx of inflammatory cells (e.g., eosinophils and neutrophils) resulting in inflammation with increased airway cell edema and mucous secretion. This inflammation can lead to hyperresponsiveness of the airways for days, weeks, or even months (Dolovich, 1988). Whether the child has an early, late, or dual (early and late) phase response will direct therapeutic modalities.

INCIDENCE

The Bureau of Maternal Child Health (1989) indicates that respiratory diseases were the major cause of hospitalization for children (ages 1 to 9 years) in 1987 and accounted for 35% of all hospital discharges. Although these statistics are not further differentiated into types of disease, asthma is represented within these numbers. Approximately 10% of all children in the United States have had signs and symptoms compatible with asthma (Goldenhersh and Rachelefsky, 1989a). Moreover, 80% of these children have signs and symptoms of the disease before 5 years of age (Blair, 1977).

Reports on the incidence of asthma indicate an increase in the diagnosis over the past decade, with an even greater increase in reported morbidity and mortality. Whether the increase in asthma is the result of a rise in the disease or improved diagnostic screening is unknown. Asthma is more common in boys than girls, with a ratio of 2:1.5 until puberty. The trend then reverses, and asthma becomes more common in women by middle age (Goldenhersh and Rachelefsky, 1989a).

CLINICAL MANIFESTATIONS AT TIME OF DIAGNOSIS

Many children with asthma initially have wheezing associated with or following a URI. Other manifestations that may lead to the diagnosis of asthma include recurrent pneumonia, sinusitis or otitis media, chronic cough in the absence of wheezing, and nocturnal cough or wheeze. In children and teenagers decreased ability to exercise with complaint of shortness of breath, chest pain or pressure, and a history of cough or wheeze after exercise are indicative of exercise-induced bronchospasm, or EIB (Anderson et al., 1975).

Because children have a variety of symptoms, other diseases must be ruled out. Children who have recurrent pneumonia or sinusitis even with no evidence of malabsorption should have a quantitative pilocarpine iontophoresis (sweat chloride test) for cystic fibrosis (see Chapter 12). In young children monophonic expiratory wheezing or expiratory stridor (sometimes difficult to distinguish from one another) may indicate tracheal compression, stenosis, or tracheomalacia. Referral to a pulmonologist or otolaryngologist for bronchoscopy may be necessary for diagnosis.

Usually the diagnosis of asthma is made when the child has been seen repeatedly for wheezing or coughing episodes, especially when there is a positive family history of asthma or the episodes are responsive to bronchodilator therapy. Many children seen during acute exacerbations of asthma have a history of URI. Symptoms typically include a 2- to 3-day history of rhinitis, watery eyes, and slight fever. As these symptoms persist, cough, wheeze, or both begin. Some children respond more quickly to asthma triggers, and thus exacerbations occur within a short period after exposure. These children may have tachypnea, increased use of accessory muscles (nasal flaring, retractions), and prolonged expiratory phase or wheeze (or both). Children with sternocleidomastoid contraction and supraclavicular indrawing most often have severe airway obstruction (Commey and Levison, 1976) and need rapid assessment of their cardiorespiratory status and interventions immediately initiated. Observations regarding degree of dyspnea, retractions, body position, use of abdominal muscles to push air out, and mental status should also be noted. Auscultation for adventitious sounds will elicit the following and represent increasing airway obstruction: prolongation of the expiratory phase, expiratory wheeze, inspiratory and expiratory wheeze, and finally absence or distancing of breath sounds, an ominous sign indicative of impending respiratory arrest.

TREATMENT

In the treatment of the child with asthma, the primary goal is to allow the child to live as normal a life as possible. The child should be able to participate in normal childhood activities, experience exercise tolerance similar to peers, and attend school to grow intellectually and develop socially. Treatments to obtain these goals should be blended into family schedules, and if possible, side effects should minimally interfere with achievement of goals.

Self-management education

Educating the family and maturing child to become effective partners in the day-to-day management of asthma is a primary treatment goal. Instruction in self-management is a complement to regular health care and requires age-appropriate sharing of responsibilities among family members and the health care professional. The purposes of self-management education are to help prevent episodes of asthma exacerbation, minimize the severity of episodes that cannot be prevented, enhance the family's ability to understand and implement treatment strategies, and respond to life changes that may be necessitated by asthma.

Family education in self-management should promote a sense of teamwork. The foundations for self-management should be laid early, with the health care provider drawing the family into treatment decisions as their basic knowledge increases.

Self-management programs are offered by individual providers or community organizations recruiting families from a variety of providers. Curricular guides for several self-management programs have been developed and extensively tested (Klingelhofer, 1987). Programs have been found useful, relatively inexpensive, and easy to implement (see Resources section, p. 79). Other approaches have successfully used computer games (Rubin et al., 1986) and camp experiences, most commonly coupled with one of the self-management programs listed at the end of this chapter (Frost, Kieckhefer, and Rubino, 1988).

Most self-management programs contain information on the basic physiology of asthma exacerbation and information on controlling triggers, knowing early warning signs that signal the onset of a problem, having a plan to manage an exacerbation (including when to contact the health care provider), and strategies for relaxation, controlled breathing, altering medications according to set guidelines, and problem solving. Programs have demonstrated effectiveness in reducing child and family anxiety, increasing asthma management behavior, improving school attendance, and reducing costly emergency room and hospital use. Before a program is implemented or a child is referred to a program, it is imperative that the provider review the program to ensure it is consistent with his or her treatment philosophy, know whether it is an individualized or group approach, and recognize the age, child, or type of family for whom the program has previously worked best. Published comparisons of the programs listed in the Resources section are available (Feldman, Clark, and Evans, 1987). When the provider is knowledgeable about the self-management program and can reinforce learning during routine health care visits with the family, a true child-parent-provider partnership is enhanced to ultimately improve the child's overall health status.

Specific treatment modalities will depend on the age of the child, severity of disease, medication tolerance, and ability of the child or family to implement the treatment regimen. When various medications and schedules are considered, a detailed history is necessary. The frequency and severity of the episodes will direct intermittent versus continuous treatment. Children who quickly develop severe airway obstruction when exposed to a trigger need a plan of treatment to initiate at once. Identification of triggers assists in development of a plan for avoidance, pretreatment with medications before exposure (e.g., exercise-induced asthma), or initiation of treatment with early symptomatology (e.g., begin bronchodilators with signs of respiratory tract infection). Clearly documenting presenting or persistent symptoms over time helps to identify specific components of asthma. Some children have primarily a bronchospastic component,

whereas others have more of an inflammatory response (similar to the early or late phase responses), and treatment modalities should be modified accordingly.

Medications

Basically three types of medications can be used in the treatment of asthma: (1) bronchodilators, which include methylxanthines (theophylline preparations) and β-adrenergic agents (β_2-preparation); (2) antiinflammatory agents such as cromolyn sodium or corticosteroids; and (3) anticholinergic agents such as ipratropium bromide or atropine. The box on p. 66 lists commonly used medications and their actions.

For most children the first medication chosen for treatment of cough or wheeze is a β-adrenergic agent such as albuterol, which inhibits the early phase asthmatic response. Oral syrups containing these agents may be helpful and easy to administer; but they cause hyperactivity in many children. Using an air compressor with an updraft nebulizer to deliver a β-adrenergic medication often decreases side effects. Children as young as 4 years may be able to use a metered dose inhaler (MDI, or puffer) if a spacer is used with the MDI. A spacer is a chamber that attaches to the MDI, allowing the medicine to be puffed into the chamber. The child can then inhale from the spacer to receive the medication, which avoids having to coordinate compressing the MDI while inhaling slowly. A new delivery device, the rotocap, is now being used for delivery of β-adrenergics. It involves inhaling a powdered form of the medication but does not require a coordinated effort like the MDI. All β-adrenergics can cause increased heart rate and may cause tremor of the fingers or hands. Hyperactivity, irritability, and sleeplessness are also noted by some parents of young children.

Nebulized treatments offer several advantages, including (1) direct deposition of aerosolized medication in the respiratory tract, (2) decreased side effects, (3) better delivery than MDI when the tidal volume is reduced during an acute episode, and (4) the ability to mix β-adrenergic medications with other medications such as cromolyn sodium or atropine.

Some older children prefer to take a pill rather than use an MDI for convenience, and compliance may be improved if adolescents are given a choice

---

ASTHMA MEDICATIONS

Bronchodilators
Methylxanthines

Quick release
  Theophylline (Elixophyllin, Theolair, Slo-
    Phyllin, and Quibron)
Sustained release
  Theophylline (Slo-Bid Gyrocaps, Slo-Phyllin
    Gyrocaps, Theo-Dur, Theo-Dur Sprinkles,
    and Theolair-SR)
Ultra-sustained release
  Theophylline (Uniphyl, Theo-24)

β-Adrenergic agents

Metaproterenol (Alupent and Metaprel)
Albuterol (Proventil and Ventolin)
Terbutaline (Brethaire, Bricanyl and Brethine)
Isoetharine (Bronkosol)

Antiinflammatory agents

Cromolyn sodium inhalation aerosol (Intal)

Corticosteroids

Prednisone
Prednisolone (Prelone and Pediapred)
Methylprednisolone
Triamcinolone acetonide (Azmacort)
Beclomethasone dipropionate (Vanceril)

Anticholinergics

Ipratropium bromide (Atrovent)
Atropine

μ/ml. For children in the ambulatory setting, a level of 15 μ/ml should be the upper limit because theophylline metabolism is affected by many factors and this level provides a safe buffer should the theophylline level rise. Some children have a therapeutic response with a level lower than 10 μ/ml and will not need an increase in their maintenance dose.

Theophylline levels should be obtained every 6 to 12 months (Redding et al., 1989) and each time the theophylline dose is significantly adjusted, when there are signs of toxicity, or when the child experiences persistent or recurring asthma episodes on maintenance medications. Side effects of theophylline include nausea, hyperactivity, and restlessness. Signs of toxicity that indicate an immediate need to determine the theophylline level include severe headache or abdominal pain, vomiting, or any combination of these. Seizures are a sign of severe toxicity and require immediate intervention and hospital admission.

Cromolyn sodium is an antiinflammatory agent that has few side effects and is increasingly being used as a first choice medication for asthma because it inhibits both the early and the late phase response (Goldenhersh and Rachelefsky, 1989b). It is best known as a mast cell stabilizer, but there may be other inhibitory effects on inflammatory cells (Murphy, 1988). Cromolyn delivered by nebulizer, spinhaler, or MDI is given 2 to 4 times per day. One treatment per day is not sufficient for maintenance therapy. Cromolyn is compatible for up to 60 minutes when mixed with β-adrenergics for delivery by a hand-held nebulizer.

Corticosteroids inhibit the late phase asthmatic response and are used to treat inflammation and edema associated with asthma. Approximately 10% to 15% of children with asthma will require long-term corticosteroid therapy. Children on maintenance asthma therapy of methylxanthines, β-adrenergics, and cromolyn will probably require corticosteroid treatment when asthma is exacerbated by exposure to triggers such as upper URI, irritants, or allergens (e.g., smoke, air pollution, pollen). Those who need corticosteroid therapy more than once every 6 weeks probably require a continuous, every other day treatment program with corticosteroids (Ellis, 1988). Reevaluation is needed every 3 to 4 months. Children by 4 to 6 years of age may be able to use aerosolized cor-

between a pill or an inhaled bronchodilater by either nebulizer or MDI. For those choosing oral therapy, β-adrenergic tablets can be prescribed.

Some children will require the addition of theophylline (see the box above) if asthma is not controlled by daily β-adrenergic treatments. Methylxanthines in combination with β-adrenergics work synergistically to produce bronchodilation and may improve control of asthma symptoms. Metabolism of theophylline varies greatly among individuals and age groups; therefore the dose must be individually adjusted by monitoring theophylline blood levels. Usual therapeutic levels are 10 to 20 ticosteroids via MDI with a spacer and reduce their need for systemic treatment. During exacerbations, however, oral corticosteroid therapy is often necessary.

When a child is receiving continuous corticosteroid therapy, complications may occur. These include the development of cushingoid appearance, growth suppression, eye abnormalities (e.g., glaucoma or cataracts), osteoporosis with development of pathologic vertebral fractures, hypertension, glycosuria, menstrual disturbances, and peptic ulceration (Ziment, 1986). A thorough history is necessary to determine any adverse effects from corticosteroid therapy. In addition, growth and blood pressure should be monitored at each well child visit. Other tests such as a urinalysis or ophthalmic examination are indicated when a child is on long-term corticosteroid therapy. Referral to the pulmonary/allergy specialist is warranted when adverse side effects of corticosteroid therapy are detected.

Anticholinergic agents such as ipratropium bromide and atropine block cholinergic reflex bronchoconstriction and may be most useful in children with bronchitic symptoms of increased mucous secretion. They are not particularly helpful against allergic challenges, do not block late phase response, and do not inhibit mediators from mast cells (Barnes, 1989). Ipratropium bromide is the only anticholinergic drug currently approved for treatment of airway disease. Delivery of ipratropium is by MDI, and side effects such as dry mouth and drying of airway secretions have not been cited as problems. Atropine sulfate is absorbed rapidly when given via aerosol and can be mixed with albuterol and cromolyn sodium for the convenience of providing three medications with one aerosol treatment. Symptoms of overdose include dry mucous membranes, dilated unresponsive pupils, cutaneous flush, and fever. Bizzare mental and neurologic symptoms occur with central nervous system toxicity (Gross et al., 1988).

PROGNOSIS

Many children have mild to moderate asthma that is well controlled. Some will have refractory asthma, which may be caused by poor implementation of the treatment plan, extremely severe asthma, or corticosteroid resistance. Psychosocial difficulties in families also can complicate asthma

and its management. Chronic uncontrolled asthma may lead to persistent airway inflammation and fibrosis. Although some children seemingly outgrow their asthma, many who experience a disappearance of symptoms during the teen years or early adulthood will have symptoms return and increase in severity with increasing age (Woolcock, 1988).

Mortality from asthma is increasing. Between 1979 and 1983 the asthma death rate in all age groups increased between 10% and 47%, with the highest mortality occurring in black males (Friday and Fireman, 1988). Many factors may contribute to the increased rate of reported mortality, including increased severity of the disease, drug therapy and its abuse, failure to recognize severity of asthma symptoms or delay in initiating treatment, and psychosocial factors.

ASSOCIATED PROBLEMS
Allergies

All children who have allergies do not have asthma, but approximately 50% to 75% of children with asthma have allergies (Smith, 1988). Allergic triggers may include foods, animal dander, pollens from trees, grasses, or weeds, or a variety of other substances (e.g., feathers, lamb's wool, and house dust mites). If there is a strong history of allergic reactions associated with respiratory symptoms, testing to determine specific problematic allergens may be beneficial. Avoidance techniques and allergy immunotherapy may then be helpful. Antihistamines for treatment of allergic rhinitis also may help relieve postnasal drip or sinusitis symptoms, which can trigger an asthma episode.

Medications

Aspirin and to a lesser extent acetaminophen may precipitate an asthma episode in some children. These substances should be avoided and parents taught about reading over-the-counter drug labels because aspirin or acetaminophen can be combined with other substances in certain drugs, particularly cold remedies.

Gastroesophageal reflux

Gastroesophageal reflux (GER) can be found in many children with chronic lung disease. Reflux of gastric secretions into the esophagus can initiate a vagal response with an increased production of airway secretions. Theophylline is known to increase gastric secretion and decrease esophageal pressure and thus may aggravate GER in some children (Johannesson et al., 1985). Management of GER includes upright positioning following feedings for infants and use of medications that reduce acidity or increase gastric motility.

PRIMARY CARE MANAGEMENT
Growth and development

There is evidence that asthma is not outgrown; persistent changes remain in the pulmonary tract of adults with asthma who have been free of symptoms for many years. Therefore asthma must be considered a chronic condition that may affect growth and development throughout the life span (Creer, Marion, and Harm, 1988). As always, it is essential that the practitioner consistently measure height and weight and record these measurements on the child's National Center for Health Statistics growth grid. Any major deviation from the population norms (less than the tenth percentile) or departure (two or more zones) from the child's individualized curve should be noted and assessed in further detail. Smaller alterations may need to be monitored. During a series of acute exacerbations of asthma, the practitioner may note a plateau or small drop in weight; however, with improvement in health status, catch-up growth should occur. If it does not occur, the cause of the weight loss should be further explored. Genetic, social, and nutritional factors potentially unassociated with asthma must be considered.

There is evidence that asthma affects height attained. The age of greatest incidence for reported short stature is during adolescence, and it is seen most clearly in those with severe asthma (Schwam, 1987; Solé, Castro, and Naspitz, 1989). Growth retardation is currently thought to be primarily a function of the illness with its associated hypoxemia, appetite suppression during exacerbations, and sleep disruption. However, medications used in the treatment of asthma may also diminish growth. Of asthma medications, corticosteroids are most frequently associated with delayed growth. The least impact is seen with inhaled corticosteroid therapy or oral early-morning alternate-day administration (Nassif et al., 1987). Further research is needed in this area, but multicenter studies have shown significant dose-related suppression of unstimulated diurnal glucocorticosteroids even with inhaled corticosteroids (Zora, 1989).

Although the adolescent growth spurt may be slightly delayed, maximal height attainment is thought to be possible in children with asthma, given optimal management of the disease. The better the control of daily management and acute exacerbations, the more likely full height will be obtained at the age-appropriate time.

Chest deformities, such as pectus carinatum, can result from poorly controlled asthma with repeated and severe exacerbations. Early treatment of exacerbations will avert the problem. Even when present, chest deformities rarely lead to additional problems (Creer, Marion, and Harm, 1988).

Standard infant, child, and adolescent assessment tools are appropriate for use in assessing development (see Chapter 3). Research has documented both normal and delayed development, with delayed development related not necessarily to the physiologic severity of the asthma but to the imposed limitations placed on the child's experiences (Bruhn, 1983; Ellis, 1983; Walsh, 1984). Limitations typically involve reductions in physical activity and social experiences, including day care and school attendance. Therefore, the practitioner should encourage normalization of experiences whenever possible to reduce the unnecessary negative impact on development.

If there are instances where normal experiences must be discouraged to avoid specific asthma triggers, the practitioner should assist the parent and child to identify alternative experiences that could provide developmental stimulation. For example, if the child cannot play competitive soccer because of grass allergy, the child and family should be assisted in identifying an alternative sport, such as basketball or swimming. Either allows the child to exercise and participate in a competitive team sport, and the opportunity to engage in an age-appropriate social and skill-building activity. Without normalized experiences the child's self-image, self-esteem, perception of bodily control, and overall level of health are likely to be reduced and anxiety, fear, and dependency behavior increased (Bruhn, 1983; Ellis, 1983, Khampalikit, 1983; Walsh, 1984).

Parents and children may limit strenuous activity because of repeated exacerbations or fear of exacerbations. If this is done frequently, the practitioner should assist the family in building an exercise habit into their daily routine. This will help avoid a sedentary life pattern, which may lower the child's sense of physical accomplishment and results in unwanted weight gain.

Unnecessary limitation of the child's activity may be particularly harmful because children connect activity and health (Kieckhefer, 1988) and may limit activity even further, possibly producing a downward spiral in self-perception. Integration of children into sports programs has been associated with positive clinical outcomes even up to 12 months following the program (Huang et al., 1989). Helping the child find an enjoyable sport should be a significant goal for the primary practitioner.

There are reports of impaired cognitive development in children with repeated brief school absences. Similar impairment has been linked to some medications used to manage asthma. However, the demonstrated negative effect of medications on cognitive capabilities is not universal and is still being investigated (Furukawa, et al., 1988; Rappaport et al., 1989; Suess et al., 1986). Clearly, prevention and swift, adequate management of exacerbations will reduce the number and length of school absences and thus limit what is thought to contribute most to the impairment of cognitive development.

Immunizations

Although it has been suggested by some that vaccination with live virus vaccines may lead to airway inflammation and therefore increased hyperresponsivity in the child with asthma (Vermere, Demedts, and Yernault, 1988), the standard schedule of immunizations is recommended. If the child has egg sensitivity, vaccines using alternative media must be considered, even though some vaccines grown in chick embryo have been found devoid of allergenic components. Skin testing may be warranted. Treatment equipment for anaphylactic reactions should be readily available in the office.

Although infants and children with asthma may have signs of respiratory infection more frequently, these signs should not alone, in the absence of fever, be the basis for deferring immunizations. Inadequate immunization with subsequent risk of

infection is of great concern. Individualized assessment of the child with respiratory symptoms, including the progression of signs of pulmonary dysfunction, should guide decisions regarding immunization. Delayed immunizations should be rescheduled as soon as possible. Special, brief appointments when the child is afebrile may be needed to ensure adequate immunization during early childhood.

Children with asthma may experience more complications with influenza, such as increased wheezing, fluctuating theophylline levels, bronchitis, pneumonia, increased school absences, and increased medical care visits, than children not having asthma. Therefore it is recommended that children with moderate to severe asthma annually receive an influenza vaccine after the age of 6 months (Committee on Infectious Diseases, 1991 [CID]). Multicenter trials and controlled studies have shown that those given killed influenza vaccine had no increase in bronchial responsivity, reduction in pulmonary function test results, or increase in leukocyte histamine release (CID, 1991). Typically the subviron (split) vaccine is given to children less than 13 years of age. Children without prior vaccination may require two doses to develop a satisfactory antibody response. If the child has had a related strain vaccine previously, one dose is thought adequate to confer protection.

For influenza vaccine grown in chicken egg media, skin testing of allergic children is indicated, with one study suggesting that an immediate-reacting IgE skin test using a dilution of influenza vaccine is a more reliable indicator of allergy than is history (CID, 1991). Before 6 months of age and in the presence of contraindications to influenza vaccination, alternative treatment methods should be considered. These include immunization of contacts or treatment of influenza with amantadine if the child is more than 1 year of age (CID, 1991).

Influenza vaccine may be given at the same time as measles-mumps-rubella (MMR) and oral polio vaccine. A different site and separate syringe are needed if two vaccines are given parenterally. Three days should elapse between the influenza vaccination and diphtheria-pertussis-tetanus (DPT) immunization.

There is no research on the efficacy of giving children with asthma pneumococcal vaccine, even though children with asthma may be more susceptible to complications that would follow a pneumococcal infection (CID, 1991). Thus pneumococcal immunization is not currently recommended. The practitioner will need to keep informed of new research in this area as it becomes available.

Screening

Vision. Routine screening is recommended unless the child is taking high-dose corticosteroids daily because these drugs are known to cause inflammatory changes, cataracts, and glaucoma. If abnormal findings are identified during an eye examination the child should be referred to an ophthalmologist.

Hearing. Routine screening is recommended.

Dental. Routine screening is recommended.

Blood pressure. Blood pressure should be evaluated at each visit because sympathetic stimulation secondary to medications may occur, especially with β-adrenergic agents.

Hematocrit. Routine screening is recommended.

Urinalysis. Routine screening is recommended unless the child is taking high-dose corticosteroids daily, which may cause glycosuria. If glycosuria is present the child should be referred to a pulmonary allergy specialist for evaluation.

Tuberculosis. Routine screening is recommended.

Condition-specific screening

Lung function. Monitoring lung function is essential to assess immediate function as well as to identify long-term trends. Pulmonary function testing should be done to establish lung function baseline levels when the child is well. Referral to a lung specialist for this additional information is especially warranted if the child has moderate to severe asthma. Spirometry for children with moderate or severe disease should be completed with each visit to objectively monitor lung function and thus direct appropriate treatment. Spirometry recording the forced vital capacity (FVC) and the forced expiratory flow in 1 second (FEV_1) assess severity of airway obstruction. (Table 5-1 lists pulmonary function norms.) When spirometry is unavailable, peak flow meters can be used to measure

Table 5-1. Pulmonary function norms

Height		FVC (L)			
cm	in	Boys	Girls	FEV$_1$ (L)	PEFR (L/mn)
100	39.4	1.00	1.00	70	100
102	40.2	1.03	1.00	75	110
104	40.9	1.08	1.07	82	120
106	41.7	1.14	1.10	89	130
108	42.5	1.19	1.19	97	140
110	43.3	1.27	1.24	1.01	150
112	44.1	1.32	1.30	1.10	160
114	44.9	1.40	1.36	1.17	174
116	45.7	1.47	1.41	1.23	185
118	46.5	1.52	1.49	1.30	195
120	47.2	1.60	1.55	1.39	204
122	48.0	1.69	1.62	1.45	215
124	48.8	1.75	1.70	1.53	226
126	49.6	1.82	1.77	1.59	236
128	50.4	1.90	1.84	1.67	247
130	51.2	1.99	1.90	1.72	256
132	52.0	2.07	2.00	1.80	267
134	52.8	2.15	2.06	1.89	278
136	53.5	2.24	2.15	1.98	289
138	54.3	2.35	2.24	2.06	299
140	55.1	2.40	2.32	2.11	310
142	55.9	2.50	2.40	2.20	320
144	56.7	2.60	2.50	2.30	330
146	57.5	2.70	2.59	2.39	340
148	58.3	2.79	2.68	2.48	351
150	59.1	2.88	2.78	2.57	362
152	59.8	2.97	2.88	2.66	373
154	60.6	3.09	2.98	2.75	384
156	61.4	3.20	3.09	2.88	394
158	62.2	3.30	3.18	2.98	404
160	63.0	3.40	3.27	3.06	415
162	63.8	3.52	3.40	3.18	425
164	64.6	3.64	3.50	3.29	436
166	65.4	3.78	3.60	3.40	446
168	66.1	3.90	3.72	3.50	457
170	66.9	4.00	3.83	3.65	467
172	67.7	4.20	3.83	3.80	477
174	68.5	4.20	3.83	3.80	488
176	69.3	4.20	3.83	3.80	498

Data from Polgar G, and Promadhat V: *Pulmonary Function Testing in Children: Techniques and Standards,* Philadelphia, 1971, WB Saunders.

Table 5-2. Factors affecting serum of theophylline levels

	Factors increasing serum levels due to decreased clearance	Factors decreasing serum levels due to increased clearance
Age	Infants	12 mo-12 yr
Medications	Erythromycin	Phenobarbital
	Cimetidine (Tagamet)	Phenytoin (Dilantin)
	Oral contraceptives	Rifampin (Rifadin)
	Propranolol (Inderal)	
	Carbamazepine (Tegretol)	
Illnesses	Liver or heart dysfunction	
	Acute viral illnesses	
	Fever for over 24 hrs	
Other	Obesity	Cigarette or marijuana smoking

the greatest rate of air flow during a forced exhalation. This peak expiratory flow rate (PEFR), however, is effort dependent. Thus, if the child is obviously in respiratory distress, a PEFR may not be obtainable. Measurements of PEFR over time will establish an individual's baseline for continuous assessment and may or may not reflect average PEFR values as listed in Table 5-1.

Children who cannot or will not recognize airway obstruction or those with very labile asthma can use a home peak flow meter to monitor their asthma. These meters are inexpensive, are fairly easy to use, and provide a detailed record of airway reactivity through the day and night. These objective data are used to individualize the child's treatment plan. In some treatment plans, individualized baseline levels are established at which the parent or child should start or increase medications or call their health care provider.

Theophylline levels. Since theophylline preparations come in quick-release (every 6 to 8 hours) sustained-release (every 8 to 12 hours) or ultra-sustained-release (every 24 hours) forms, monitoring theophylline levels will be determined by the preparation or reason for the level. In general it is best to follow the manufacturer's guidelines for measuring theophylline levels. The level should be drawn at the same time (e.g., always 4 hours after the dose of a sustained-release preparation) to assure continuity in level monitoring. In the case of suspected theophylline toxicity, levels should be ordered immediately.

Allergic history. A biannual review of possible allergens and irritants in the home is helpful. In addition to identification of asthma triggers, it provides a time to discuss other health issues such as smoking, avoidance of triggers, dust control, or the need for allergy skin testing. Asthma self-management education can also be provided at this time.

Drug interactions

Several factors cause theophylline levels to rise or fall and should be considered when the child's overall health care plan is assessed (Table 5-2). Medications that affect theophylline clearance should be avoided or the theophylline dose appropriately adjusted and levels monitored.

Cough suppressants should generally be avoided because they may mask asthma signs or symptoms and delay diagnosis and appropriate treatment. Occasionally cough suppressants are helpful to control nighttime or continuous postviral cough where coughing itself is a trigger for increased cough because of irritation of the trachea and bronchi. In these cases over-the-counter cough medicines will probably be inadequate for cough control.

Antihistamines are now available without medical prescription and may be helpful in relieving allergic rhinitis. Antihistamines are thought not to contribute to drying or inspissation of secretions in the well hydrated child. A history of use by the child is important in planning a treatment regimen.

DIFFERENTIAL DIAGNOSIS
Wheezing

It is well known that all wheezing is not asthma so when a child presents with recurrent or persistent cough or wheeze, other diagnoses should be considered. These include foreign body aspiration (particularly in the infant or toddler), infections such as bronchitis, bronchiolitis, or pneumonia, other underlying airway diseases such as cystic fibrosis or bronchiectasis, structural abnormalities such as a vascular ring, or aspiration due to a primary swallowing disorder or secondary to underlying neuromuscular disease.

Respiratory infections

Viral respiratory infections are the most common cause of asthma exacerbations in children. Treatment is usually supportive and parents will need to know to give antipyretics for fever, provide extra fluids, and that a change in asthma therapy medications may be necessary. For example, the child who only receives cromolyn sodium via nebulizer for asthma control may need albuterol added to the nebulized treatments for control of cough or wheeze during an exacerbation.

Vomiting and diarrhea

Children with asthma who present with vomiting should be evaluated for theophylline toxicity if they are on theophylline preparations especially if the vomiting is associated with headache or stomachache. When gastroenteritis occurs in the child with asthma, the usual supportive care is required. The child should remain on the usual asthma therapy but may have difficulty with oral medications because of vomiting and may be at increased risk for mucus plugging if dehydration occurs. Controlling symptoms with nebulized medications and providing extra fluids should be considered. Hospitalization may be necessary if the child's asthma worsens, medications cannot be tolerated orally or by nebulizer, or fluid intake is extremely reduced.

Headache

If the child with asthma (on a theophylline preparation) presents with complaint of headache, theophylline toxicity should be ruled out especially if gastrointestinal upset, stomachache and/or vomiting are also occurring.

Sinusitis can present as a headache especially if associated with complaints of purulent nasal drainage, fetid breath odor, or nighttime cough. Since sinusitis can trigger an asthma episode, there may also be increased wheezing.

Fever

Asthma exacerbations are not associated with fever unless there is an underlying infection such as sinusitis, pneumonia, or otitis media. The cause of the fever needs to be evaluated by the usual methods. Increased fluids should be given to keep the child well hydrated to avoid mucus plugging which can occur with asthma.

DEVELOPMENTAL ISSUES
Safety

All age-appropriate safety precautions must be similarly considered for the child with asthma. The primary practitioner furnishes anticipatory guidance in this area and should be familiar with age-typical risks. Equipment and medications that are used to prevent or treat asthma exacerbations in the home may present additional concerns for safety.

During acute episodes of asthma the family may be advised to provide additional humidity to air in the room where the child sleeps. Parents need to be warned about the hazard of burns from warm steamers. Burns may result from direct contact with the steam, pulling the heated water down on the body, or tampering with the electrical cord or socket. Some clinicians recommend only cold humidifiers because of the hazards, the fact that warm water increases the probability of bacterial growth in the equipment, and the fact that efficacy of warm moisture is lost by the time it reaches the child's airway.

Electrical burns are possible when equipment such as steamers or nebulizers are run in the child's presence. Infants and young children should never be left alone where they can reach the equipment, cord, or open socket. School-age children and adolescents should be properly instructed in the safe use of electrical equipment and should demonstrate their use of equipment to parents or provider before being encouraged to use it independently.

Medications kept in the home must be safely stored in their original containers, in a locked location, inaccessible to the infant and young child. Since the child will ultimately need to become responsible for self-medication, the family should be assisted in making an age-appropriate plan to help the child with the medication regimen.

Practitioners can help parents identify their child's developmental capabilities and limits for safely assisting in the medication regimen by providing age-normative suggestions. For example, when the child is an infant or toddler, the parents need to speak about the medications as such, not as candy. With maturation, the toddler can be taught how to help take medicine from a spoon or hold the nebulizer mask to assist in therapy. The preschool-age child typically has the manual dexterity to increasingly take part in the medical therapy by helping the parent pour the medication or, in the parent's presence, taking the capsule from the container. The young school-age child may be asked to get the medication and take it in the presence of the parent. When older school-age children can tell time, they can assume greater responsibility to prompt the parent when the medication is needed, get the medication, take the medication in the parent's presence, and return it to its proper storage place. The school-age child should also become increasingly responsible for taking needed medication while at school. Parents can monitor and encourage safe and knowledgeable use by discussing or having the child count and record on a calendar the number of times medication was taken as required. As the child grows to adolescence, more autonomy should be given for independently purchasing, taking, and replenishing both routine and prn medication. However, parents need to be reminded that one consistent finding in successful adolescent compliance with prescribed medicines is the continued support and age-appropriate assistance of their parents. This support is not shown by "doing for" or "nagging" the adolescent but by demonstrating faith in their capabilities and offering assistance with any problems that arise. Thus parents can maintain an interested, interdependent attitude to best assist the adolescent in growing self-management of asthma.

Over the past 10 years there has been concern about the safe use of MDIs by persons of all ages. This concern is greatest for children too young to fully appreciate temporal relationships. Although MDIs are considered safe and uniquely effective in delivering a therapeutic dose of medication directly to the target organ, their use by children must be monitored. The child's skill in using the inhaler should be observed at each visit with the practitioner. Even many adults have difficulty in this maneuver. Up to 50% of children who do not receive such monitoring and corrective prompting for proper technique do not use the inhaler effectively.

With age and increasing time spent away from parents, children need to independently recognize when their treatment is not as effective as expected and to seek the assistance of their parent or another adult. An episode that does not respond to treatment in the manner expected may herald a particularly severe exacerbation requiring medical assistance. Simple mnemonic devices have been found helpful in this regard. A rhyme of "twice is nice but three needs more than me" could be a mnemonic device used to teach a child that he or she can try the inhaler twice, but if symptoms persist and the child feels the need to use it a third time, he or she should discuss it with an adult.

Child care

Most families will find it necessary to use child care services on either a regular or sporadic basis. Having a child with asthma should not prohibit use of this service. With proper communication and explanation, child care can be safely used with a responsible, interested caretaker. Whether child care is at a center or is home based, provided by a relative, neighbor, or professional, information must be shared by the parent to ensure success.

Parents must be responsible for providing all relevant information to the caretaker: what triggers the child's asthma, early warning signs of an impending asthma episode, what the caretaker should do first and what should be done next if the last action is not effective, how the parent and other responsible party (including health care provider) can be reached, and what information must be passed on to emergency personnel should they need to be called. The best way to provide this information is in a written format. A laminated card with detailed instructions on one side and the primary care provider's name and telephone number on the reverse side has proved helpful for many families.

If the child care provider is to give any treatments, the parent must demonstrate the procedures and observe the provider's repeat performance. In addition, center-based programs may require written prescriptions from the health care practitioner and written permission of the parent for the child care provider to perform the treatment. Parents must maintain close contact with the child care provider to learn about changing triggers, medications, or early warning signs. Anyone in repeated contact with the child who observes responses to treatments should also relay that information to the parent. The information can then be integrated into the overall routine reevaluation of the treatment plan. Any treatment changes should be relayed immediately to the child care provider so that a consistent approach is provided to the child regardless of setting. Frequent and open communication is the key to successful child care arrangements.

Diet

Sulfites, used to enhance the appearance of many fresh foods, have been implicated in severe asthma exacerbations in some children and therefore should be avoided. There are no other special dietary requirements for the child with asthma unless the child has concurrent food allergies. When food allergies are present, the practitioner needs to be familiar with alternative sources of the nutrients in the eliminated foods. If local grocery stores do not carry the alternative food sources, health food stores, dairy councils, or American Lung Association affiliates may be of assistance in locating the necessary items. Alternatively, the primary health care provider may refer the family to a local nutritionist for consultation. When the child has multiple food allergies, this referral is critical.

Discipline

Parents frequently report they find it difficult to deal with discipline for fear of upsetting the child and initiating an asthma exacerbation. Given current estimates that up to 40% of the children with asthma will experience some degree of bronchospasm with intense crying (Schwam, 1987), parental concern is realistic and understandable. Crying probably cannot be entirely avoided, but the parent should be reassured that most discipline can be implemented by rewarding desirable behaviors if this is done routinely and begun early in the child's life. Inconsistent limit setting for undesirable behavior only confuses the child and makes it more difficult to learn and internalize the limits chosen by the parents.

Another parental concern is that the child's irritability, refusals, or acting-out behavior is caused by illness or medications. Medications and illness may influence the child's behavior, but consistency of expectations is of greater importance. Blaming the illness or medication does not remove the necessity to assist the child to develop behaviors desired by the family and social networks.

Ultimately the child will need to develop a strong sense of internal control to participate effectively in self-management. Early consistent positive expectations set by the parents will form the foundation for the child's later self-discipline and sense of mastery and control. Avoiding discipline early in the child's life will not make the ensuing years more pleasant for the parent or aid the child in learning socially expected behaviors. Thus practitioners should initiate discussion regarding positive discipline early during an infant's first year of life, assuring parents that with time this issue should become less burdensome as the child is able to verbally express emotion without excessive crying leading to bronchospasm.

Toileting

Toileting needs typically are not altered by the child's asthma. Bowel and bladder training is achieved at the expected ages. Clinicians have noted that a small proportion of children experience problems with enuresis when taking theophylline preparations, possibly because of its diuretic action. However, the exact incidence remains undocumented. If standard behavioral interventions are not effective in eliminating enuresis, most practitioners seek an alternative medication regimen to manage the asthma.

Sleep patterns

The sleep of young children is often disrupted during asthma exacerbations. Even when an exacerbation is not evident, the child may routinely awaken with wheezing and coughing during the night or early morning hours. This tendency for early morning problems probably represents the normal circadian rhythm in airway caliber and steroid production. Because the symptom pattern represents an exaggeration of existing bronchial hyperresponsivity, optimizing daytime control and reducing environmental irritants in the sleeping room minimizes the symptoms. Persistent difficulty may necessitate an evening dosage of a short-acting theophylline preparation (Canny and Levison, 1987) or use of a long-acting time-release preparation in school-age children or adolescents.

Parents have reported that some medications disrupt their children's sleep, but systematic documentation is scarce. Most providers attempt an alternative medication regimen if the sleep disturbance does not resolve within 1 or 2 weeks of beginning a medication. Young children find a nighttime ritual soothing. This is accentuated in the child with asthma. Thus the practitioner should help parents establish a bedtime ritual that is relaxing and can be easily implemented in their family. A consistent bedtime is also helpful because frequent deviation of more than 30 minutes may cause difficulty in both settling the child and bringing on sleep.

School issues

Surveys of children with asthma report an average of 18 days lost from a typical 180-day school year (Creer, Marion, and Harm, 1988). Often these days are scattered throughout the year. This pattern of frequent, brief absences appears more harmful to academic progress than infrequent long absences, and efforts should be made to avoid this tendency.

There is current interest in the possibility of learning difficulties caused by asthma medication, but there are few firm conclusions. Factors that have been associated with specific learning difficulties or lowered school performance include corticosteroid-inclusive regimens (Suess et al., 1986), corticosteroids taken orally every other day for more than 12 months; presence of emotional and behavioral problems (Gutstadt et al., 1989), and theophylline regimens (Furukawa et al., 1988). One contradictory report demonstrates improvement in memory while children were taking theophylline (Rappaport et al., 1989). Practitioners are advised to keep current with research in this area as patterns may begin to emerge in the near future that might influence treatment regimens. In

all cases, individualizing the regimen to the child's unique response is necessary.

Parents report that communicating with school personnel is essential but often difficult. Many fears and misconceptions regarding children with asthma still exist in the general public. Teachers and administrators may attempt to limit the child more than the parent or provider believes necessary. Scheduling an annual parent-teacher conference to discuss the child's current treatment regimen is essential. Teachers should have the same written information suggested for child care providers. In addition, the teacher should be informed of the skills the child has for self-management. The school nurse may provide support to the parent during annual conferences and should be informed of all emergency treatment requirements that might be needed. Provider-prescribed emergency medications that may be needed should be given to the nurse or designate. If the school personnel hesitate to assume this responsibility, the parents or provider should discuss with them their legal responsibility to allow all children access to medications they need to enable school attendance. Mutual problem solving is essential to finding a workable solution.

Fitting in with school peers and maintaining positive peer relationships are essential to the child's full development. The parent can actively arrange peer gatherings, encourage the child to join clubs or organizations, and allow the child age-appropriate independence in visiting friends to ensure social experiences. Friends may question why the child is taking medications or has special equipment in the home. Simple explanations about the child's asthma should be given with the assurance that asthma is not contagious. This might also be done in school as a class presentation with the teacher's assistance. Parents are encourged to discuss their child's asthma with parents of their child's peers so that all may have an honest understanding of the child's condition and abilities as well as any limitations.

Sexuality

Sexual development may be delayed if the asthma has not been adequately controlled to allow regular growth (Solé et al., 1989). Systemic corticosteroids historically have been associated with delay in sexual development because of their effect on the adrenal glands and corticosteroid production. Current treatment regimens that rely on inhaled corticosteroids or every other day, morning dosage schedules appear to have reduced the adverse impact on general and sexual growth patterns. These schedules show the least adrenal suppression (Canny and Levison, 1987). If the adolescent becomes sexually active and wishes to use contraceptives, drug interactions must be considered. It is known that oral contraceptives may interfere with the breakdown of theophylline, thus increasing the likelihood of toxicity. As new asthma management drugs continue to be developed, their impact on the efficacy of any pharmacologic means of birth control must be explored.

SPECIAL FAMILY CONCERNS

Because of the familial nature of asthma, some family members express guilt during the child's flare-ups. Parents should be reminded that there is nothing they could have done to prevent asthma and that in regard to acute exacerbations, hindsight is always better than foresight. It may be an ideal but impossible goal to eliminate all exacerbations. A more realistic goal is to limit the number and extent of flare-ups and to learn something about prevention or management from each episode.

If many family members have a history of asthma, the family may retain outdated beliefs and habits regarding the treatment of asthma. The practitioner needs to respect the family history but also stress new knowledge and discuss the development of new therapies. This should encourage the family to take advantage of current information.

Most parents express ambivalence regarding long-term medication regimens. Although most parents acknowledge the effectiveness of these regimens, the majority also hold the belief that long-term medication can be harmful to their child (Donnelly, Donnelly, and Thong, 1987). Acknowledging and discussing these common feelings while presenting the fact that the most detrimental effects of asthma seem to come from poor management are helpful approaches for supporting parents. It is also useful to reinforce that the program will continue to be tailored to their child trying to decrease medication to the minimum needed for control.

Asthma does cause disruption in the life of the child's primary caretaker, most often the mother. This disruption is most marked when the child is young but can be minimized by actively involving the other parent or another family member in concrete, daily management tasks (Wasilewski et al., 1988).

Smoking by a family member is associated with increased need for emergency room visits for asthma flare-ups (Evans et al., 1987), but changing smoking habits of family members is difficult. In one recent study, only 20% of parents believed they would stop smoking even if they could be shown it adversely affected their child's asthma (Donnelly, Donnelly, and Thong, 1987). This was in contrast to 85% who said they would get rid of a pet that adversely affected their child's asthma. When advising families to eliminate smoke from their child's environment, the practitioner should convey resources for smoking cessation.

SUMMARY OF PRIMARY CARE NEEDS FOR THE CHILD WITH ASTHMA

Growth and development

Small stature and delayed adolescent growth are associated with poor control with exacerbations or oral corticosteroids.

Delayed development is noted only when unnecessary limitations are imposed on child.

Impaired cognitive development is most clearly linked to repeated school absences. Effects of medications have also been implicated.

Immunizations

Routine immunizations are recommended.

If child has documented egg sensitivity, vaccines using other media must be considered.

Influenza vaccine is recommended for children with moderate to severe asthma who are more than 6 months of age.

Pneumococcal immunization is not currently recommended.

Screening
Vision

Routine screening is recommended.

Hearing

Routine screening is recommended.

Dental

Routine screening is recommended.

Blood pressure

Routine screening is recommended.

Hematocrit

Routine screening is recommended.

Urinalysis

Routine screening is recommended.

Tuberculosis

Routine screening is recommended.

Condition-specific screening

Corticosteroid Therapy: Additional assessments are necessary to monitor glycosuria, osteoporosis, cataracts, glaucoma, and growth delay.

Lung Function Tests: Testing should be done every 6 months on children more than 6 years of age with moderate to severe asthma.

Theophylline Levels: Should be monitored with change in therapy.

Allergy Testing: Skin testing may be indicated depending on history.

Drug interactions

Antihistamines are not contraindicated.

Medications such as erythromycin, cimetidine or oral contraceptives will raise theophylline levels.

Phenobarbital will decrease theophylline levels.

Cough suppressants may mask symptoms of asthma.

Differential diagnosis

Recurrent or persistent cough or wheeze: Rule out infection, aspiration, structural anomalies, and cystic fibrosis.

Viral respiratory infections: URI may require change in asthma therapy to prevent or modify exacerbation of asthma.

Gastrointestinal symptoms: Rule out theophylline toxicity.

Headache: Rule out theophylline toxicity and sinusitis.

Fever: Not associated with asthma alone. When fever present prevention of dehydration is important to prevent mucus plugs.

Developmental issues
Safety

Burns from hot water humidifiers are a hazard. Electrical burns are possible from nebulizers or steamers.

Medication safety varies with developmental age.

Caution is needed on repeated use of MDIs.

Child care

Child care workers need to be provided with information on asthma triggers, early warning signs of asthma, treatment, emergency contacts, and medications used in day care.

Diet

Children may have allergies to sulfites or foods.

Discipline

Concern over discipline initiating asthma attack.

Rewarding desirable behavior should be encouraged.

The influence of medication and illness on behavior is a concern.

Consistency of expectation is important.

Continued.

SUMMARY OF PRIMARY CARE NEEDS FOR THE CHILD WITH ASTHMA — cont'd

Toileting

Toileting is routine.
Few children experience enuresis while on theophylline.

Sleep patterns

Exacerbation may interfere with sleep.
It is important to reduce environmental allergens in sleep area.
If medications disturb sleep, an alternative regimen should be tried.

School issues

Repeated school absences may interfere with academic performance.
There is concern over medications causing learning problems.
School personnel must be educated to identify child's limitations and use of medications.
There is concern over peer acceptance of child with chronic condition.

Sexuality

Sexual development may be delayed in severe cases or with prolonged corticosteroid use.
Oral contraceptives may interfere with breakdown of theophylline.

Special family concerns

Familial nature of asthma may lead to outdated beliefs of treatment.
Parents may be ambivalent regarding long-term medication regimens.
Smoking in home detrimental to children with asthma. Parents who smoke need support and assistance in quitting.

RESOURCES

Practitioners should become familiar with the local offices of national organizations (see the list that follows) to identify community-based services in their client's local areas that can complement their health care services. Many of these community-based services have programs that are useful to children and parents in managing day-to-day effects of asthma. These programs typically offer education about asthma and training in self-management skills for the child and parents (Rubin, Bauman, and Lauby, 1989).

If the practitioner's practice is large enough, educational programs for age-similar children with asthma have been effectively implemented in private practices (Alexander et al., 1988). Having a well-stocked lending library of reading materials on asthma assists parents and children in learning how to manage asthma. It is imperative that the practitioner provide families with knowledge on how they may obtain these materials for their own use.

Information materials

Self-Management Curricular Guides
Available from National Heart, Blood, and Lung Institute:
AIR WISE, AIR POWER, Open Airways, and Living with Asthma.
Available from Asthma and Allergy Foundation of America: Asthma Care Training for Kids (ACT).
Available from the American Lung Association: Super Stuff.

Newsletters
Leonidas, L, ed: *Asthma today*, 412 State St, Bangor, ME 04401.
Sander, N, ed: *Mothers of Asthmatics Newsletter*, 5316 Summit Dr, Fairfax, VA 22030.

Books
Mendosa A: *Peak performance: a strategy for asthma self-assessment*, Hawthorne Community Medical Group, Los Angeles, 1987.

It is available from Hawthorne Community Medical Group, West Los Angeles Office, 2990 Supulveda Blvd, Los Angeles, CA 90064.

Mendosa G, Sander N, and Scherrer D: *A user's guide to peak-flow monitoring*, Mothers of Asthmatics, Fairfax, VA, 1988.

It is available from Mothers of Asthmatics, Inc, 5316 Summit Dr, Fairfax, VA 22030.

Plaut T: *Children with asthma: a manual for parents*, ed 2, Amherst, MA, 1988, Pedipress.

Sander N: *So you have asthma*, Glaxo, Fairfax, Va, 1988. Provided as a public service by Glaxo Inc.

It is available from Mothers of Asthmatics, Inc, 5316 Summit Dr, Fairfax, VA 22030.

Organizations

American Lung Association and local or state affiliates (Check your telephone book for the chapter nearest you.)

Asthma and Allergy Foundation of America
1717 Massachusetts Ave
Washington, DC 20036

National Heart, Blood, and Lung Institute
Bldg 31, Room 4A-21
Bethesda, MD 20205

National Jewish Center
1400 Jackson St
Denver, CO 80206

A variety of hospitals and clinics in your area may have ongoing support groups. Telephone their public relations department for information.

Telephone lines

Allergy Information Line 1-800-822-ASMA

National Jewish Center Lung Line 1-800-222-LUNG

REFERENCES

Alexander SJ, Younger RE, Cohen RM, et al: Effectiveness of a nurse-managed program for children with chronic asthma, *J Pediatr Nurs* 3:312-317, 1988.

Anderson SD, Silverman M, Konig P, et al: Exercise-induced asthma, *Br J Dis Chest* 1(69):1-38, 1975.

Barnes P: A new approach to the treatment of asthma, *Med Intell* 321:1517-1527, 1989.

Blair H: Natural history of childhood asthma: 20 year follow-up, *Arch Dis Child* 52:613-619, 1977.

Bruhn J: The application of theory in childhood asthma programs, *J Allergy Clin Immunol* 72:561-577, 1983.

Canny GJ and Levison H: The modern management of childhood asthma, *Pediatr Rev Commun* 1:123-162, 1987.

Commey JO and Levison H: Physical signs in childhood asthma, *Pediatrics* 58:537-541, 1976.

Committee on Infectious Diseases: Report of the committee on infectious diseases, ed. 22, Elk Grove Village, IL, 1991, American Academy of Pediatrics.

Creer TL, Marion RJ, and Harm DL: Childhood asthma. In Hassett V, Strain P, and Hersen M, eds: *Handbook of developmental and physical disabilities*, New York, 1988, Pergamon Press, pp 177-194.

Dolovich J: Early/late response model: implications for control of asthma and chronic cough in children, *Pediatr Clin North Am* 35:969-979, 1988.

Donnelly JE, Donnelly WJ, and Thong YH: Parental perceptions and attitudes toward asthma and its treatment: a controlled study, *Soc Sci Med* 24:431-437, 1987.

Ellis E: Asthma in childhood, *J Allergy Clin Immunol* 72:526-539, 1983.

Ellis E: Asthma: current therapeutic approach, *Pediatr Clin North Am* 35:1041-1052, 1988.

Evans D, Levison MJ, Feldman CH, et al: The impact of passive smoking on emergency room visits of urban children with asthma, *Am Rev Respir Dis* 135:567-572, 1987.

Feldman C, Clark N, and Evans D: The role of health education in medical management of asthma: some program applications, *Clin Rev Allergy* 5:195-205, 1987.

Frick W and Busse W: Respiratory infections: their role in airway responsiveness and pathogenesis of asthma, *Clin Chest Med* 9:539-549, 1988.

Friday G and Fireman P: Morbidity and mortality of asthma, *Pediatr Clin North Am* 35:1149-1162, 1988.

Frost L, Kieckhefer G, and Rubino C: Research utilization to plan, evaluate, and revise programs for families of children with asthma, *Pediatr Nurs* 14:197-200, 1988.

Furukawa C, Duhamel T, Weimer L, et al: Cognitive and behavioral findings in children taking theophylline, *J Allergy Clin Immunol* 81:83-88, 1988.

Goldenhersh M and Rachelefsky G: Childhood asthma: Overview, *Pediatr Rev* 10:227-233, 1989a.

Goldenhersh M and Rachelefsky G: Childhood asthma: Management, *Pediatr Rev* 10:259-267, 1989b.

Gross N, Boushey H, and Gold W: Anticholinergic drugs. In Middleton E, Jr, Reed CE, Ellis EF, et al: *Allergy: principles and practice*, ed 3, St Louis, 1988, CV Mosby.

Gutstadt LB, Gillette JW, Mrazek DA et al: Determinants of school performance in children with chronic asthma, *Am J Dis Child* 143:471-475, 1989.

Huang S, Veiga R, Sila U, et al: The effects of swimming in asthmatic children—participants in a swimming program in the City of Baltimore, *J Asthma* 26:117-121, 1989.

Johannesson N, Anderson K, Joelsson B, and Persson C: Relaxation of lower esophageal sphincter and stimulation of gastric secretion and diuresis by anti-asthmatic xanthines, *Am Rev Respir Dis* 131:26-31, 1985.

Khampalikit S: The inter-relationships between the asthmatic child's dependency behavior, his perception of his mother's perception of his illness, *Maternal Child Nurs J* 12:221-296, 1983.

Kieckhefer G: The meaning of health to children with asthma, *J Asthma* 25:325-333, 1988.

Klingelhofer E: Compliance with medical regimens, self-management programs and self-care in childhood asthma, *Clin Rev Allergy* 5:231-247, 1987.

Murphy S: Cromolyn sodium: basic mechanisms and clinical use, *Pediatr Asthma Allergy Immunol* 2(4):237-254, 1988.

Nassif E, Weinberger M, Sherman P, et al: Extrapulmonary effects of maintenance corticosteroid therapy with alternate-day prednisone and inhaled beclomethasone in children with chronic asthma, *J Allergy Clin Immunol* 80:518-529, 1987.

Rappaport L, Coffman H, Guare R, et al: Effects of theophylline on behavior and learning in children with asthma, *Am J Dis Child* 143:368-372, 1989.

Redding G, Larter N, Brown G: Guidelines for care of children with chronic lung disease, *Pediatr Pulmonol* 19(suppl 3):19, 1989.

Rubin D, Leventhal J, Sadock R, et al: Educational interpretation by computer in childhood asthma, *Pediatrics* 77:1-10, 1986.

Rubin DH, Bauman LJ, and Lauby JL: The relationship between knowledge and reported behavior in childhood asthma, *Dev Behav Pediatr* 10:307-312, 1989.

Schwam JS: Assisting the parent of a child with asthma, *J Asthma* 24:45-54, 1987.

Smith L: Etiology and pathogenic factors in allergic diseases. In *Allergic disease from infancy to adulthood*, ed 2, Philadelphia, 1988, Saunders.

Solé D, Castro A, and Naspitz C: Growth in allergic children, *J Asthma* 26:217-221, 1989.

Suess WM, Stump N, Chai H, et al: Mnemonic effects of asthma medication in children, *J Asthma* 23:291-296, 1986.

US Department of Health and Human Services, Bureau of Maternal Child Health: *Child Health, U.S.A., '87*, Washington, DC, 1989, US Government Printing Office.

Vermere P, Demedts M, and Yernault J, eds: *Progress in asthma and COPD*, New York, 1988, Elsevier North Holland.

Walsh M: The experience of asthma in children [doctoral dissertation, University of Illinois, Chicago], *Diss Abstr Int* 45:516B: 1984.

Wasilewski Y, Clark N, Evans D, et al: The effect of paternal social support on maternal disruption caused by childhood asthma, *J Community Health* 13:33-42, 1988.

Woolcock A, ed: Asthma — what are the important experiments? *Am Rev Respir Dis* 138:730-744, 1988.

Ziment I: Steroids, respiratory pharmacology, *Clin Chest Med* 7:341-354, 1986.

Zora J: The use of corticosteroids in childhood asthma, *J Asthma* 26:159-165, 1989.

6 *Bleeding Disorders: Hemophilia and von Willebrand's Disease*

Mary Alice Dragone

ETIOLOGY

Hemophilia and von Willebrand's disease are the most common inherited bleeding disorders resulting from deficiencies or abnormalities of specific coagulation proteins. The von Willebrand protein is a critical part of the primary or extrinsic hemostatic mechanism that is activated when tissues are damaged. It promotes formation of an initial platelet plug by enabling platelet adhesion. Multiple coagulation proteins, including those that are deficient in hemophilia, are critical components of the secondary or intrinsic hemostatic mechanism that is activated when blood comes in contact with a foreign surface. These proteins are required for the formation of the final fibrin clot (Corrigan, 1985).

Hemophilia

Hemophilia involves a defect in the intrinsic hemostatic mechanism (Fig. 6-1). Factor VIII deficiency (classic hemophilia, hemophilia A) accounts for approximately 80% of hemophilia cases, whereas factor IX deficiency (Christmas disease, hemophilia B) accounts for 20% (Kasper and Dietrich, 1985). Less common factor deficiencies exist, although they are not specifically discussed in this chapter. Severity of hemophilia is defined by the percent activity of the deficient coagulation protein as presented in Table 6-1.

Hemophilia is inherited in an X-linked pattern in which female carriers most frequently pass the disorder to their sons. The severity of hemophilia remains constant within families, although clinical symptoms may vary based on lifestyle and treatment regimens. As occurs in other X-linked disorders (Gitschier, 1988), up to one third of all cases of hemophilia are thought to be the result of spontaneous mutation and not directly inherited through a female carrier. A woman is considered to be an obligate carrier if hemophilia has been diagnosed in either her father, two of her sons, or in one son and one other relative. Elston and colleagues (Abildgaard, 1984) calculated that approximately 28% of hemophilia A carriers are estimated to have factor VIII levels lower than 40%, predisposing some to bleeding with trauma or surgery. This validates the need for laboratory testing even in obligate carriers.

von Willebrand's disease

Generally a mild bleeding disorder, von Willebrand's disease is closely related to hemophilia. The von Willebrand protein's primary action is to facilitate platelet adhesion in the extrinsic hemostatic mechanism (see Fig. 6-1). This protein also helps to stabilize factor VIII, and when it is deficient, the amount of circulating active factor VIII may also be reduced. Most affected children have prolonged bleeding times when they injure cutaneous tissue.

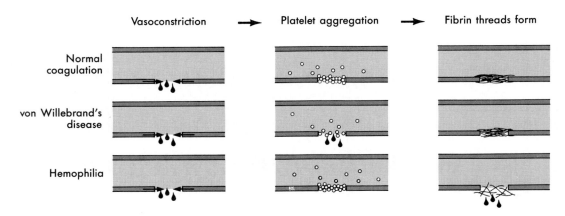

Fig. 6-1. Comparison of the defect in hemophilia and von Willebrand's disease with normal coagulation after a break occurs in a vessel wall.

Table 6-1. Severity of hemophilia

Severity	Factor VIII and IX coagulant activity (%)	Frequency and type of bleeding
Severe	<1	By school age, often several bleeding episodes occur each month that require treatment.
		Bleeding may be spontaneous or the result of injury.
Moderate	1-5	Frequency of bleeding is variable.
		Spontaneous bleeding is less common.
Mild	>5	Generally bleeding is excessive only as a result of trauma or surgery.

NOTE: Normal factor VIII and IX coagulant levels are generally >50% (>50 U/dl) but vary slightly between laboratories.

Three main variants of the disorder exist (Abildgaard, 1984; Corrigan, 1985). In the most common variant, type I, the total amount of the protein is decreased and both large and small forms (multimers) of the von Willebrand protein are present. Its inheritance is autosomal dominant. In type II the larger multimers are absent. Of note are the potential for thrombocytopenia with desmopressin use in type IIB (large multimers absent in the plasma) and the autosomal recessive inheritance of rarer type IIC (large multimers absent in plasma and platelets). Type III is a severe autosomal recessive form of the disorder marked by the absence of detectable von Willebrand protein.

INCIDENCE

Hemophilia occurs in all ethnic groups, with an incidence of 1 in 10,000 live male births for factor VIII hemophilia and 1 in 40,000 live male births for factor IX hemophilia (Miller and Lubs, 1986). In the past, reported incidence of von Willebrand's disease has been estimated at 3 to 7 in 100,000 live births (Coller, 1984). However, it is currently believed to be the most common inherited bleeding disorder, with an estimated prevalence as high as 1.6% in the general population (Miller, Lenzi, and Breen, 1989).

CLINICAL MANIFESTATIONS AT TIME OF DIAGNOSIS

By 18 months of age, approximately 70% of children with severe hemophilia are diagnosed because of positive family history or unusual bleeding (Baehner and Strauss, 1966). Often parents will have been questioned regarding child abuse as a result of excessive bruising. Diagnosis in infancy

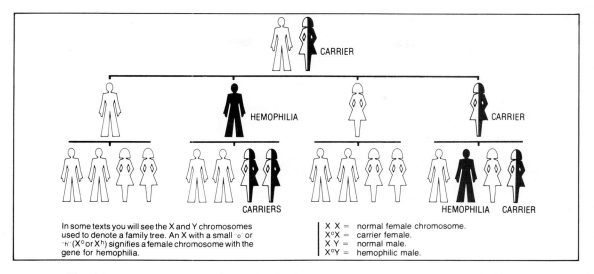

In some texts you will see the X and Y chromosomes used to denote a family tree. An X with a small "o" or "h" (X^o or X^h) signifies a female chromosome with the gene for hemophilia.

X X =	normal female chromosome.
X^oX =	carrier female.
X Y =	normal male.
X^oY =	hemophilic male.

Fig. 6-2. Inheritance pattern for hemophilia. From Eckert, EF: Your child and hemophilia, New York, 1990, © The National Hemophilia Foundation.

most commonly occurs because of a positive family history confirmed by cord blood coagulation assays, intracranial hemorrhage, excessive bruising with hematomas, cephalohematoma, bleeding following circumcision, or bleeding from the umbilical cord stump. Intracranial hemorrhage is life threatening and occurs in 1% to 4% of newborns with moderate to severe hemophilia (Kletzel et al., 1989; Olson et al., 1985). Olson and associates (1985) recommended that male newborns of known carriers be tested for hemophilia at birth by cord blood sampling. Those with factor VIII or IX levels less than 5% especially need careful observation for signs of intracranial hemorrhage during the first week of life. Some centers recommend screening on all such infants using computerized axial tomography (CAT) or ultrasound to diagnose early, small hemorrhages and provide factor replacement. Cesarean section is not routinely recommended in nontraumatic deliveries. Although factor VIII levels generally rise to greater than 50% during pregnancy, intrapartum and postpartum bleeding has been noted in some hemophilia carriers (Forbes, 1984).

Children who first show signs later in childhood or in adolescence more frequently have mild to moderate hemophilia. A frequent misconception is that children with hemophilia can "bleed to death" from a typical childhood cut or scratch. They may, however, demonstrate joint bleeding (hemarthrosis), muscle hematomas, excessive postoperative bleeding, or excessive or prolonged oral bleeding following frenulum tears, lost deciduous teeth, tooth eruption, and dental extractions.

von Willebrand's disease is commonly manifested by bleeding from the mucous membranes. Although epistaxis is most frequently noted, excessive oral, gastrointestinal (GI), and menstrual bleeding also occur. Additional findings may include excessive bruising with hematomas, oozing following circumcision, or excessive postoperative bleeding (Coller, 1984). Diagnostic testing is often requested in the presence of a positive family history of the disorder or when an increased partial thromboplastin time is obtained during routine preoperative screening. Because the level of the von Willebrand protein and factor VIII vary over time, coagulation testing may need to be repeated to establish a diagnosis (Abildgaard et al., 1980). Despite the relatively high incidence of this disorder, persons are frequently not diagnosed because the common symptoms of epistaxis and heavy menstrual bleeding are not brought to medical attention.

Table 6-2. Treatment products and general guidelines for use

Protein purification process and viral inactivation method	Manufacturer	Product
FACTOR VIII CONCENTRATES		
Recombinant DNA*	Cutter Biological/Miles	Kogenate
	Baxter Hyland	Recombinate
Monoclonal antibody		
Pasteurized	Armour	Monoclate P
Solvent-detergent	Baxter Hyland	Hemofil M
	American Red Cross	AHF-M
Solvent-detergent	Alpha	Profilate SD
	New York Blood Center	Factor VIII SD
Solvent-detergent and gel chromatography	Cutter Biological/Miles	Koate HP
Heated in aqueous solution	Armour	Humate P
	Cutter Biological/Miles	Koate HS

Dosage: To increase factor VIII activity by 2% (2 percentage points, or 2 U/dl) give 1 U/kg. Example: To treat an intracranial hemorrhage, 100% factor VIII activity is desired (dose 50 U/kg for a child with a baseline of <1% factor VIII).

FACTOR IX CONCENTRATES		
Solvent suspension	Alpha	Profilnine HT
Solvent suspension and affinity purified	Alpha	Alpha Nine
Dry heat	Cutter Biological/Miles	Konyne HT
	Baxter Hyland	Proplex T

Dosage: To increase factor IX activity by 1% (1 percentage point, or 1 U/dl) give 1 unit/kg. Example: To treat an intracranial hemorrhage, 100% factor IX activity is desired (dose 100 U/kg for a child with a baseline of <1% factor IX).

INHIBITOR TREATMENT PRODUCTS		
PCC†	Cutter Biological/Miles	Konyne HT
Activated PCC		
Vapor treated	Immuno	FEIBA
Dry heat	Baxter Hyland	Autoplex T
Porcine factor VIII	Portion	Hyate C
Factor VIII products	As listed above	

Dosage: Approximately 75-100 U/kg/dose is needed to override inhibitor.

Data compiled from Medical and Scientific Advisory Council of the National Hemophilia Foundation. *AIDS Update,* New York, December 1990, National Hemophilia Foundation and Hilgartner M and Montgomery R: *Understanding von Willebrand's Disease,* New York, 1985, National Hemophilia foundation.
*Product in clinical trials as of June 1990.
†PCC, prothrombin complex concentrate.

Table 6-2. Treatment products and general guidelines for use — cont'd

Protein purification process and viral inactivation method	Manufacturer	Product

DESMOPRESSIN ACETATE (DDAVP)

Dosage: 0.3 μg/kg IV in 30-50 ml of normal saline.

Administration: Give over 15-30 min. Take blood pressure and pulse every 10 min during infusion. Decreased response if given more frequently than every 48 hr.

Side effects:

Common: flushing, headache; enhancement of clot lysis (give with an antifibrinolytic agent when mouth or nose bleeding is being treated) (Bowie, 1986; Poole, 1987).

Less common: tachycardia, hypertension.

Uncommon: Hyponatremia and seizures (more common if <2 yr of age)(Smith et al., 1989).

ORAL ANTIFIBRINOLYTIC AGENTS

ε-Aminocaproic acid (Amicar)

Dosage: Approximately 50 mg/kg/dose by mouth every 6 hr until site of bleeding is healed (dose guidelines vary greatly; consult child's hematologist).

Supplied as 500-mg tablet and 250 mg/1 ml elixir.

Tranexamic acid (Cyklokapron)

Dosage: Approximately 25 mg/kg/dose by mouth every 6 hr as for Amicar.

Supplied as 500-mg tablet.

Interactions: Do not give in the presence of hematuria (enhances renal clot formation). Give at least 12 hr after or 6 hr before a factor IX or activated PCC dose (otherwise may induce hypercoagulation).

TREATMENT
Comprehensive care

The standard of care in hemophilia is a collaborative interdisciplinary approach facilitated by local hemophilia treatment centers (HTCs). These centers, funded in part by the federal government, provide comprehensive management of inherited coagulation disorders, namely hemophilia and von Willebrand's disease. The core team consists of a pediatric hematologist, nurse coordinator, and social worker. Other integral team members are the genetic counselor and physical therapist. Consultative services are provided by a pediatric dentist and orthopedic surgeon. With the advent of human immunodeficiency virus (HIV), HTCs have also been mandated by the government to either provide or procure comprehensive management for their clients exposed to HIV. Services of the HTC include interdisciplinary comprehensive evaluations, counseling and support services, carrier detection, access to new technology treatment products through clinical trials, and home infusion instruction for those with severe hemophilia.

All children and adolescents with hemophilia and von Willebrand's disease should receive regular comprehensive evaluations at the nearest HTC. The frequency of evaluations is every 1 to 1½ years, depending on the severity of the child's bleeding disorder. At these visits, children and their families are routinely seen by the members of the interdisciplinary team. Families and the primary care provider receive updated information on the status of the child's health and development, treatment options, and readiness for home therapy. The centers work closely with primary care providers to give care that is comprehensive, coordinated, and accessible and rely on them to provide day-to-day management of pediatric health care.

General guidelines

The goals of treatment are to rapidly initiate clotting when uncontrolled bleeding occurs and prevent bleeding during high-risk procedures.

The treatment product of choice should be decided in consultation with the child's hematologist (Table 6-2). This information should be updated yearly, incorporating rapid changes in available technology. Because of the limited availability of high-purity products in certain areas, many families keep a supply of the preferred concentrate in their home refrigerators to expedite treatment of their child in local emergency rooms. Factor concentrate need not be kept at school unless infusions are performed there.

Bleeding episodes frequently requiring hospital admission and hematologic consultation are significant head trauma or bleeding into the iliopsoas muscle (retroperitoneal), hip, GI tract, neck, or posterior pharynx. Consultation is also recommended for bleeding requiring more than two treatments and when there is any doubt as to the need to treat an injury or bleeding episode.

Providers are frequently asked by school personnel and families to recommend first-aid measures that can be instituted while the child is waiting for evaluation and possible infusion. For soft tissue, joint, and muscle bleeding, elevation of the affected area and the application of an elastic bandage and ice may help to reduce swelling. Crutches or a sling should be provided for lower and upper extremity bleeding, respectively. Firm pressure applied over a clean dressing is often sufficient to stop bleeding from surface lacerations in children with both hemophilia and von Willebrand's disease. Firm pressure applied to the nares is recommended for nosebleeding. Although ice may help to reduce the superficial swelling from a head hematoma, it should never replace a medical evaluation because intracranial bleeding is unaffected by its application.

Hemophilia

In the early 1970s clotting factor concentrates revolutionized the treatment of hemophilia because of their ease of administration, fewer allergic side effects, and ease of home storage compared with fresh frozen plasma and cryoprecipitate. Each vial of these same factor concentrates, however, contain the plasma of thousands of donors and at one time were produced by methods that did not fully inactivate HIV. Although there have been isolated cases of HIV seroconversion with the use of dry heat–treated products between 1985 and 1987 (Centers for Disease Control (CDC), 1988), there have been no seroconversions in viral safety studies of the newer factor concentrates (Brettler and Levine, 1989). Most products eradicated HIV and hepatitis B. Non-A, non-B hepatitis transmission, however, continues to be problematic for some solely dry heat–treated products (CDC, 1988).

Large amounts of extraneous proteins in earlier products first led to the development of higher purity products using monoclonal antibody techniques. The newest technologic advance in factor replacement is the use of recombinant DNA techniques to clone the human factor VIII gene (White et al., 1989); this synthetic factor VIII is theoretically free of all human viruses and is expected to be released from clinical trials by the early 1990s.

Advanced technologic products for factor IX generally become available a few years after introduction of similar factor VIII concentrates (see Table 6-1). The presence of larger amounts of extraneous proteins in factor IX concentrates and the resultant potential for uncontrolled clotting require providers to exercise caution when repeated doses are used (Abildgaard, 1984; Aledort, 1986). This is accomplished by monitoring the factor IX level and not allowing it to rise higher than necessary for hemostasis. Fibrinogen levels and prothrombin times should also be followed for evidence of hypercoagulability.

Desmopressin acetate (DDAVP) is also effective in raising the levels of factor VIII in many persons with mild to moderate factor VIII deficiency (De la Fuente et al., 1985; Mannucci, 1986; Warrier and Lusher, 1983). Its benefits include relatively few major side effects and the lack of viral contaminants, because it is not derived from human blood. It is discussed in greater detail in reference to von Willebrand treatment options.

Approximately 10% of persons with severe hemophilia develop antibodies to their deficient coagulation protein and are said to have inhibitors to factor VIII or factor IX (Kasper and Dietrich, 1985). Treatment options include the use of high doses of certain factor concentrates that can bypass part of the standard clotting cascade, porcine factor VIII, exchange plasmapheresis, immunosuppressive therapy, and γ-globulin given intravenously (Kasper, 1989).

Table 6-3. Assessment and treatment of common bleeding episodes*

Site of bleeding	Signs and symptoms	Treatment
Soft tissue	Mild: not interfering with ROM	Ice, Ace wrap
	Moderate: occurring in wrist, volar surface or forearm, plantar surface of foot; interferes with ROM	Ice, splint/Ace wrap FVIII 20-30 U/kg or desmopressin† FIX 30-40 U/kg
	Severe: pharyngeal; areas listed in "moderate" category accompanied by change in neurologic signs	Admit to hospital FVIII 50 U/kg FIX 80-100 U/kg
Joint	Early: tingling/odd sensation, warmth, stiffness	Rest FVIII 10-15 U/kg or desmopressin† FIX 20 U/kg
	Moderate: moderate swelling, mild-moderate pain, limited motion	Rest, splint/crutches FVIII 20-25 U/kg or desmopressin† FIX 30 U/kg
	Severe: tense swelling, moderate to severe pain, marked decrease in ROM; hip bleeding: limited abduction or adduction	Rest, splint/crutches PT plan May need repeat doses FVIII 30-40 U/kg FIX 40-50 U/kg Ultrasound follow-up for hip bleed
Muscle	Mild: swelling does not greatly affect ROM, mild discomfort	Rest, ±crutches, PT plan Ice, splint/Ace wrap FVIII 20-30 U/kg or desmopressin† FIX 20-40 U/kg
	Severe: swelling with neurologic changes	Rest, splint/Ace wrap PT plan FVIII 50 U/kg FIX 80-100 U/kg
	Iliopsoas (retroperitoneal): abdominal, inguinal, or hip area pain, limited hip extension, numbness from nerve compression	Strict bed rest/hospitalization May need repeat doses FVIII 50 U/kg FIX 80-100 U/kg
Nose	Mild: <10 min	Pressure to nares
	Severe: prolonged or recurrent	Collagen hemostat fibers and nasal pack vWd desmopressin, EACA/TXA FVIII 20 U/kg or desmopressin† FIX 20 U/kg

Continued.

Data compiled and modified from Warren M and McMillan C: Hemophilia. In Hockenberry M and Coody D, eds: *Pediatric Oncology and Hematology: Perspectives on care,* St. Louis, MO, 1986, Mosby–Year Book, pp. 252-272.

Note: Specific dosages may vary for individual patients, consult with child's hematologist.

*ROM, range of motion; FVIII, factor VIII hemophilia; FIX, factor IX hemophilia; U/kg, units of factor VIII or IX per kilogram (factor concentrate vials contain a given number of FVIII or FIX activity units); PT, physical therapy; vWd, von Willebrand's disease; EACA/TXA, antifibrinolytics: ∈-aminocaproic acid and tranexamic acid; cryo, cryoprecipitate.

†Desmopressin may be used if, after a test dose, the child with mild or moderate hemophilia has achieved a factor VIII coagulant level equal to the level that would be achieved after the recommended dose of factor VIII concentrate. Example: For a moderate soft tissue bleed in the calf, a dose of 20-30 U/kg should raise a child's factor VIII level to 40-60%. If after desmopressin the child reached a peak of only 25%, it is likely desmopressin would not be beneficial.

Table 6-3. Assessment and treatment of common bleeding episodes—cont'd

Site of bleeding	Signs and symptoms	Treatment
Oral areas	Dental extractions; regional blocks; frenulum, tongue, or lip bleeding	Topical hemostatic agents EACA/TXA (caution with FIX) vWd desmopressin FVIII 30 U/kg or desmopressin FIX 30 U/kg
Gastrointestinal system	Abdominal pain, hypotension, blood in emesis, tarry or red stools, weakness	Hospitalization likely vWd desmopressin/cryo/FVIII product with high level vWd FVIII 25-50 U/kg FIX 50-100 U/kg
Central nervous system	Head, neck, or spinal injury; presence of blurred vision, headaches, vomiting, unequal pupils, change in speech or behavior, drowsiness; if no symptoms yet significant injury, treat and observe	Hospitalization and/or rapid consult with hematologist depending on injury CT scan vWd desmopressin/cryo/FVIII product with high level vWd FVIII 50 U/kg FIX 80-100 U/kg
Urinary tract	Gross hematuria: bright red to brown; if clots present, more likely to infuse with factor concentrate	Push oral fluids, rest ± prednisone ± factor concentrate EACA/TXA *contraindicated*

FOLLOW-UP: By daily telephone contact or office visits through resolution of bleeding episode. If family is on home therapy, they should have telephone or office consultation if head, neck, or throat injury occurs, if >2 treatments are needed, or if bleeding occurs in hip, iliopsoas muscle, or urinary tract.

The unit of measurement for products that replace the deficient factor protein is calculated in international units of factor VIII or IX activity. Choice of a particular dose is based on the type of hemophilia, severity of the bleeding episode, the child's weight (Table 6-3), occurrence in a chronically affected joint, and the likelihood of follow-up by the child and family within 24 hours. Repeat doses may be given if significant improvement has not occurred.

Treatment is initiated as soon as a bleeding episode is identified. For joint bleeding, it may begin as early as a child who notices the onset of "tingling" in the joint. Many have come to know this as the first indicator of oozing blood in that area. For another child, loss of range of motion of a joint, mild swelling, or mild pain may be the first recognizable indicators. In still other children with high pain tolerances or little self-awareness of bodily changes, the bleeding episode may not be recognized until there is severe swelling, major limitation of joint motion, and severe pain. Treatment is usually given on demand as soon as bleeding is identified but may be given prophylactically to facilitate healing when bleeding is recurrent or severe or before high-risk procedures such as surgery, dental extractions, and physical therapy of a chronically affected joint.

Vials of factor concentrate come in various concentrations. The number of *whole* vials closest to the desired dose is always given because of the cost of wasted medication and the lack of adverse sequelae from a dose slightly higher than that originally prescribed. Most concentrates may be given by slow intravenous (IV) push over 5 to 10 minutes. Because these concentrates are blood products, those who reconstitute the lyophylized factor should always wear gloves and dispose of supplies contacting the factor in approved infectious waste containers.

High-purity products, such as the monoclonally separated factor VIII concentrates, cost 2 to 3 times as much as the lower-purity products (Pierce et al., 1989). For persons with severe hemophilia using at least 40,000 U/year, a 1-year supply of monoclonal product would cost more than $40,000.

von Willebrand's disease

The standard treatment for this disorder encompasses both synthetic and plasma-derived products. The provider is urged to consult with the child's hematologist and the National Hemophilia Foundation for the most current recommendations.

Desmopressin acetate, a synthetic analog of vasopressin, is the treatment of choice for most persons with von Willebrand's disease, excluding subtype IIB (De la Fuente et al., 1985). Although the mechanism of action is not completely understood, it is postulated that desmopressin releases stores of factor VIII and the von Willebrand protein from the endothelial lining of the blood vessels (Mannucci, 1986). Stores, however, may be depleted if treatment is repeated more frequently than every 48 hours (see Table 6-2).

Use of this medication for various bleeding episodes depends on the rise in coagulation protein activity or decrease in bleeding time after a test dose. Peak response is generally obtained 30 minutes after IV infusion is complete. Individuals tend to show consistency in the degree of response over time (Rodeghiero et al., 1989). Desmopressin has also been given subcutaneously with good results in some children (Köhler et al., 1989). A concentrated intranasal form is now being developed.

Cryoprecipitate, a traditional form of treatment for von Willebrand's disease, is obtained from the serum of single donors, screened for viruses, but not virally inactivated. Although not approved by the Food and Drug Administration for use in von Willebrand's disease, some virally inactivated factor VIII concentrates have been shown to contain significant amounts of the von Willebrand protein (Lawrie et al., 1989). Humate-P in particular has been clinically effective in controlling bleeding (Czapek et al., 1988). It is anticipated that purified, virally inactivated plasma products specific for von Willebrand's disease will be available in the near future.

Estrogens may be useful in the management of excessive menstrual and other types of bleeding because of their ability to increase levels of factor VIII and the von Willebrand protein (Bowie, 1984; Kasper and Dietrich, 1985).

Oral antifibrinolytic agents

Children with hemophilia and von Willebrand's disease often have oral bleeding requiring additional medication to keep the clot stable once it has formed. Because of the presence of digestive enzymes in the saliva that lyse fibrin clots, antifibrinolytic agents may be given orally every 6 hours for 7 to 10 days or until the site of oral bleeding has completely healed (Kasper and Dietrich, 1985). Two such medications are ε-aminocaproic acid (Amicar) and tranexamic acid (Cyklokapron) (see Table 6-2).

Topical hemostatic agents

Collagen hemostat (Avitene) fibers can be applied to nasal packing or at the site of frenulum tears or tooth extractions. When nasal packing is used, it is generally left in place for 24 to 36 hours to promote stable clot formation. Less conventional topical agents have been used successfully in the treatment of oral bleeding. Moistened tea bags that contain tannic acid provide local hemostasis, and commercially available superbonding glue has also been effective in sealing tongue lacerations without concurrent bonding between mucous membrane surfaces (Rothman, 1990).

Pain management

Uncontrolled bleeding into a joint or muscle can produce significant pain. Replacement of the deficient coagulation protein is the most effective way to prevent significant pain and to relieve current pain. Mild pain may be treated with acetaminophen, ice, and elevation of the affected extremity. If pain is moderate or severe, acetaminophen with codeine every 4 to 6 hours is recommended. Pain medication is generally not necessary after the first day of factor replacement. Continued pain may suggest ineffective control of bleeding because of inadequate dosing of the factor concentrate, development of an inhibitor, or synovitis. Pain caused by irritation of the synovial lining may be more effectively treated with a nonsteroidal antiinflammatory agent. These agents should be used with caution, however, because they can cause GI bleeding secondary to interference with platelet aggregation.

Physical therapy

Splinting and immobilization for 1 to 2 days after acute bleeding often aid resolution of the episode (Koch, 1985). A resting splint that maximally extends the extremity is recommended for night use for up to several days following a significant hemarthrosis to prevent further bleeding during sleep (Koch, 1985). Following severe bleeding or prolonged immobilization, a physical therapy program should be prescribed, enabling the child to achieve his or her baseline range of motion and to regain muscle mass.

Surgical intervention

Destruction of a joint from chronic bleeding can result in significantly decreased range of motion, making it impossible for the individual to have an acceptable quality of life. Theoretically, a synovectomy removes the source of bleeding. Removal of the synovium has been performed using an open surgical procedure, arthroscopy, and most recently injection of radioactive isotopes into a joint (Rivard, 1987).

PROGNOSIS

The major factors contributing to morbidity in hemophilia are neurologic sequelae of intracranial bleeding, disability from chronic joint disease (arthropathy), liver disease secondary to hepatitis, and HIV infection. Intracranial bleeding that occurs at or soon after birth may result in spastic quadriplegia and brain damage, whereas bleeding that occurs later in life may affect the achievement of developmental milestones. Because of the availability of clotting factor concentrates, disabling arthropathy in childhood is now much less common. However, those who are affected by it often have visible deformities, increased school absenteeism, and more difficulty finding suitable employment. Before the use of heat-treated concentrates, approximately 90% of those treated were exposed to hepatitis B, with 5% to 10% becoming chronic carriers (Brettler and Levine, 1989; Spero et al., 1979). It is also believed that 90% to 100% of those who received untreated products have been exposed to non-A, non-B hepatitis (Brettler and Levine, 1989). The incidence of liver disease should decrease with the use of more highly purified products. The rate of HIV infection among the 10,000 adolescents with hemophilia in the United States ranges between 22% and 75% depending on the type of clotting factor received and the treatment center surveyed (Brady and Humphries, 1990).

By the mid- to late 1970s, life expectancy of persons with hemophilia approached that of the general population (Hilgartner, Aledort, and Giardina, 1985). For those who are HIV antibody positive, life expectancy is already decreasing, although the final course cannot be accurately predicted. Johnson and colleagues (Pierce et al., 1989) have reported that acquired immunodeficiency syndrome (AIDS) has become the leading cause of death in persons with hemophilia. However, in those not affected with HIV, the leading cause of death remains bleeding, especially from intracranial hemorrhage.

Data regarding morbidity and mortality in von Willebrand's disease are not readily available; however, because of the generally mild nature of the disorder, life expectancy is postulated to be normal. The relatively small number who have been infected with HIV through infusions of cryoprecipitate have a decreased life expectancy.

ASSOCIATED PROBLEMS
Hematologic problems

Anemia is found in many persons with hemophilia in part because of sequestration of blood in joints and muscles during bleeding episodes. Significant anemia can also occur as a result of slow persistent oozing from oral bleeding or pooling of blood in muscle hemorrhages. In persons with von Willebrand's disease, excessive or prolonged menstrual bleeding or persistent or recurrent epistaxis can be problematic.

Neurologic problems

Intracranial hemorrhage is the most frequent cause of death related to bleeding in persons with hemophilia. If left untreated, it can result in spastic quadriplegia, developmental delay, or death. In as many as 50% of cases of intracranial bleeding, no known prior injury is identified (Eyster et al., 1978). For this reason, any injury or neurologically related symptom should be treated aggressively. There may be signficant intracranial bleeding without the presence of a "goose egg" because the most significant bleeding occurs from internal shearing of the brain and cranium. However, the presence of a hematoma indicates that the cranium may have met with significant force. Those with von Willebrand's disease also are at increased risk for this type of bleeding. Bleeding within or around the spinal column can also produce enough pressure to produce neurologic damage. Compartment syndrome resulting from nerve compression may occur following uncontrolled bleeding into the forearm or calf.

Respiratory problems

Posterior pharyngeal bleeding, increasing the potential for asphyxia, can result from a traumatic throat culture or from dental extractions or deep injection of anesthetic without pretreatment with factor concentrates or desmopressin.

Gastrointestinal problems

Exposure to non-A, non-B hepatitis (Pierce et al., 1989) through blood products is indicated by transaminases greater than 2 times normal and the absence of other positive serologic markers. Specific serologic testing for hepatitis C, thought to cause most cases of non-A, non-B hepatitis, has recently become available. Some persons exposed to hepatitis B may be chronic carriers of the disease. With the use of the hepatitis B vaccine series, the incidence of hepatitis B has been reduced.

Bleeding into the GI tract may occur in von Willebrand's disease as well as hemophilia. The fragile mucous membrane–lined digestive system is prone to bleeding that can result from ulcers, gastritis, hemorrhoids, rectal fissures, and endoscopic procedures (Mittal et al., 1985). This type of bleeding should be considered when there is either an unexplained drop in hemoglobin levels or abdominal pain.

Immunologic problems

Approximately 10% of persons with severe hemophilia can develop alloantibodies or inhibitors to factor VIII or IX. Inhibitors usually occur in early childhood but may occur at any age (White et al., 1982). Level of inhibitor severity is measured in Bethesda units. Bleeding episodes are much more difficult to control and treatment options more limited when alloantibody formation occurs. There appears to be a genetic predisposition to the development of inhibitors.

Although the incidence varies greatly from center to center, approximately 70% of those exposed to untreated factor concentrates between 1978 and 1985 have developed HIV infection (Brettler and Levine, 1989). Directed donor cryoprecipitate and female donor factor concentrate, used during the years before HIV was actually isolated, spared many children from exposure to the virus. The incidence of HIV infection in persons with von Willebrand's disease who were exposed to cryoprecipitate is much lower, however, because of the smaller size of the donor pool.

Musculoskeletal problems

The normally smooth synovial lining of a joint produces synovial fluid that with the cartilage serves as a shock absorber for the joint (Fig. 6-3). The synovium is also supplied with many blood vessels. When bleeding into a joint ceases with the administration of the deficient coagulation protein, enzymes clear away the blood from the synovial fluid. These enzymes, however, do not seem to focus their destruction solely on the unwanted blood cells; they begin to eat away at the smooth synovial lining, producing breaks in the surface that can make it easier for bleeding to recur in that joint. Eventually the cartilaginous surface of the bones may undergo destruction by these enzymes (Arnold and Hilgartner, 1977). The more blood that accumulates in the joint capsule, the more enzymes that are released. This destructive process can ultimately lead to fusion of the joint. A single hip hemarthrosis can produce aseptic necrosis of the femoral head if bleeding is not fully resolved. When bleeding recurs in a specific joint, it may be referred to as a "target joint." Thus a strong case is made for early detection and treatment of bleeding episodes.

The nonintact synovial lining can cause the synovium to produce abnormal amounts of fluid in an inflammatory response—synovitis. Even when actual bleeding into the joint does not occur, the joint may become swollen and stiff. Synovitis is differentiated from a hemarthrosis by its gradual onset, mild or absent pain, and fuller range of motion.

Genitourinary problems

If a boy has bleeding into the testicle that is not treated promptly, future fertility and maintenance of a patent urinary tract may be compromised. This type of bleeding can result from riding on an adult's

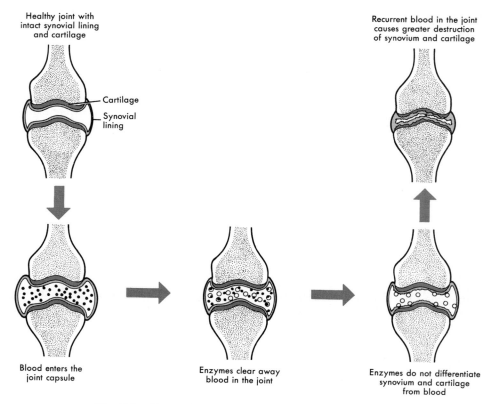

Fig. 6-3. Progression of joint destruction in hemophilia.

shoulders, bicycle stunts, or vigorous play on a rocking horse or playground toy.

Hematuria occurs most commonly in adolescents with hemophilia, is usually not a result of trauma, is of short duration, and often stops spontaneously (Forbes, 1984). Clots can sometimes cause renal or ureteral obstruction with temporary renal colic and, at times, hydronephrosis (Kasper and Dietrich, 1985).

PRIMARY CARE MANAGEMENT
Growth and development

Monitoring a child's weight is particularly important because obesity places added stress on joints and muscles. Limb length may be increased by bony overgrowth of the epiphysis from chronic arthropathy. Gait disturbances caused by scoliosis may predispose an individual with hemophilia to joint or muscle bleeding.

A thorough baseline and ongoing assessment of developmental parameters and neurologic status is useful in follow-up for head trauma and for screening of potentially undiagnosed or unreported intracranial bleeding. Normal development is anticipated unless there has been a history of intracranial bleeding.

Immunizations

All routine injectable vaccines should be given subcutaneously (Baehner and Strauss, 1966) with a 23-gauge needle because intramuscular injections may cause muscle bleeding. Applying firm pressure over the immunization site for 5 minutes can also decrease the incidence of hematoma development.

Before the oral polio vaccine is given, it is important to obtain a history of exposure to HIV and potential contact with others who are infected with HIV. Even if the child is not at risk for HIV infection, those with hemophilia are likely to have close family contacts who also have hemophilia and who may be infected with HIV. If a child or adolescent was exposed to blood products before 1985 and tests positive for the HIV antibody or has not yet been tested, he or she should receive the inactivated polio vaccine.

The recombinant hepatitis B vaccine series is recommended for all children likely to be exposed to blood products and may be given to newborns. The vaccine may be administered subcutaneously at birth and at 1 and 6 months of age. Hepatitis B surface antibody checked at 3 and 6 months after the final immunization should identify nonresponders who will need an additional vaccine. An accelerated series of injections at 0, 1, 2, and 12 months may be considered for those at high risk to receive blood products in the near future (Hollinger, 1989). There are currently no standard guidelines for booster innoculation for persons who respond to the initial series.

Screening

Vision. Following an eye injury, referral to an ophthalmologist is recommended, with follow-up until resolution is obtained. Otherwise, routine office screening and attention to the fundal examination are sufficient.

Hearing. Routine screening is recommended.

Dental. Invasive dental procedures can often be prevented through careful oral hygiene (including flossing under parental supervision) and regular dental evaluations. An initial dental evaluation is recommended by 1 year of age (Lancial, 1987), in part to impress upon parents the importance of preventive care. Pediatric dentists with expertise in the management of persons with bleeding disorders are often associated with the local hemophilia treatment center. If needed, local dentists can manage most procedures with consultation. Prophylactic treatment with desmopressin or factor concentrate is generally not necessary for routine dental cleaning or anesthetic infiltrates close to the gum line. For dental extractions and regional blocks, desmopressin, factor concentrate, an antifibrinolytic, or a combination of these is recommended (Poole, 1987).

Blood pressure. Routine screening is recommended.

Hematocrit. Annual screening for anemia is recommended. Nosebleeds, short in duration but occurring frequently, may not be regularly reported by families and may lead to significant anemia. If venipuncture is required, firm pressure should be applied for at least 5 minutes to prevent hematoma formation.

Urinalysis. An annual urinalysis is recommended to screen for microscopic hematuria.

Tuberculosis. Routine screening is recommended.

Condition-specific screening

Children who have received any blood products in the past year should have liver function studies performed. For those with hemophilia, a factor VIII or IX inhibitor screen should be administered as well, but these tests are usually performed during comprehensive evaluations at the hemophilia treatment center. HIV antibody testing with pre- and post-test counseling are recommended for children and adolescents exposed to blood products prior to 1986.

Drug interactions

All aspirin-containing products are contraindicated. Caution should also be exercised with prolonged use of other medications that can affect platelet aggregation, such as antihistamines, guaifenesin (cough medications), dextromethorphan (cough medications), and nonsteroidal antiinflammatory agents. Because of the proliferation of over-the-counter medications, a list of those that can affect bleeding may be obsolete soon after compilation. It is more helpful to educate parents about how to read medication labels (e.g., choosing those with acetaminophen rather than those with acetylsalicylic acid) and how to enlist the help of the pharmacist when they are in doubt as to the use of a particular product.

Oral antifibrinolytic agents (e.g., Amicar and Cyklokapron) and factor IX concentrates or prothrombin complex concentrates ideally should not be given within the same 24 hours because of an increased risk of hypercoagulation.

DIFFERENTIAL DIAGNOSIS AND MANAGEMENT OF COMMON PEDIATRIC CONDITIONS

Headaches and head injury. Intracranial bleeding must be ruled out whenever there is a history of injury within the past several days, focal headaches, or vomiting without GI distress. A computerized tomography (CT) scan is often helpful in ruling out intracranial bleeding. However, providers in consultation with the hemophilia team will often treat the child with factor concentrate or desmopressin prophylactically to achieve a factor VIII or IX level of 100% if there is either significant history or physical symptoms. This conservative approach is often adopted because of the serious implications of a delay in diagnosis. Therapy may cease after the resolution of symptoms if scans remain normal. If bleeding is documented, the child would need hospitalization and factor replacement regularly for several weeks.

Visual disturbance. In the presence of acute changes in visual acuity, it is necessary to rule out intraocular bleeding by performance of a thorough funduscopic examination. In the presence of documented bleeding, ocular injury, or persistent visual changes, referral to an ophthalmologist is warranted.

Sore throat. If a throat culture is indicated, extreme caution must be exercised because of the potential for posterior pharyngeal bleeding. A throat culture should not be attempted in an uncooperative child. If streptococcal pharyngitis is suspected, a course of penicillin should be initiated based on history and physical findings.

Mouth bleeding. Although oral bleeding may not appear profuse in these children, persistent slow oozing can cause a significant drop in hemoglobin levels. If bleeding is uncontrolled after the use of either topical measures or an antifibrinolytic agent, an infusion of factor concentrate or desmopressin is indicated.

Abdominal pain. In persons with hemophilia or von Willebrand's disease, the practitioner should have a high index of suspicion for GI bleeding in the presence of acute abdominal pain or significant drop in hemoglobin levels in the absence of other bleeding. Testing stool or emesis for blood can easily be done in the office as a screening tool. In hemophilia, iliopsoas bleeding (i.e., combination of the iliacus muscle [origin, iliac fossa; insertion, greater trochanter] and psoas muscle [origin, thoracic and lumbar vertebrae; insertion, lesser trochanter]) can cause abdominal or inguinal area pain. Hospital admission is often required for iliopsoas and GI bleeding.

Gait disturbance. Gait disturbance may be the result of scoliosis or bleeding in or around the ankle, knee, hip, or iliopsoas muscle. Inability to fully extend the hip and, later, leg paresthesias are characteristics of iliopsoas bleeding. Ultrasound is useful for confirmation. Bleeding into the hip socket is characterized by limitation of hip abduction and adduction. Hospital admission is often required for severe hip or iliopsoas bleeding.

Dysuria and hematuria. Pressure within the urinary tract can cause dysuria. It is necessary to rule out testicular bleeding. Frequently, bleeding into this area is quite pronounced, with obvious bruising and swelling. Hospitalization may be required for aggressive therapy and bed rest. Hematuria may be spontaneous and related directly to the bleeding disorder. However, whenever it occurs, the origin of bleeding within the urinary tract and potential infection should be considered. Increased fluid intake, bed rest, and avoidance of antifibrinolytic agents, as these may cause obstructive clots, are routinely recommended as part of a treatment plan. The benefits of treating with factor concentrate or corticosteroids, however, are debated among clinicians.

Numbness, tingling and pain. Compression of nerves caused by deep or superficial hematomas should be suspected in individuals with changes in sensation or focal pain. Bleeding in or near the calf, volar surface of the forearm, spine, buttock, and iliopsoas muscle can lead to neurologic changes.

DEVELOPMENTAL ISSUES

Safety. Protection against head injury is of primary importance. A protective helmet for children with hemophilia who are learning to walk may reduce the risk of head injury. Use should be discontinued when the child is walking well because it restricts peripheral vision and can also provide the child and parent with a false sense of security. In addition, knee pads may be used in the pants of toddlers prone to knee hematomas; high-top "leather" sneakers are suggested for children at risk for hemarthroses from the age of 2 or 3 years.

Contact sports such as football, soccer, hockey, wrestling, boxing, and vigorous competitive basketball are strongly discouraged because of the increased chance of head trauma. However, appropriate physical activity is encouraged to maintain strong muscles that promote joint stability and to promote normal social adjustment. Swimming is an ideal aerobic activity (Gilbert et al., 1985). Although recommended for all children, helmets are of particular importance for those with bleeding disorders when they are riding bikes or scooters or using rollerskates. Skateboarding is not recommended even with the use of a helmet.

Use of a medical identification emblem that includes diagnosis, treatment product, and blood type should be encouraged. Infants can have it pinned to their car seats or jackets when traveling. Older children who grow up wearing one become accustomed to it. A wallet identification card may be used if the child or adolescent refuses to wear the emblem. Medical information should be checked yearly and updated as necessary.

Families participating in a home infusion program should follow accepted guidelines for infection control, including use of gloves to mix and administer factor concentrates and disposal of infectious wastes in approved containers that are then disposed of at the hospital.

Child care. Contact with the proposed source of child care can clarify the caretaker's responsibilities with regard to prevention and management of bleeding episodes and trauma. Hemophilia treatment center personnel or the primary care practitioner may provide this service. For children with severe hemophilia it is helpful to emphasize that early recognition of bleeding (mild swelling or slight change in range of motion) and rapid access to medical evaluation and treatment are of primary importance. Spontaneous bleeding may occur, however, despite diligent safety efforts. Some facilities may be fearful of admitting children with bleeding disorders because of fear of liability or potential HIV infection. Disclosure of HIV status is at the parent's discretion.

Diet. Meeting the recommended requirements for protein and calcium intake is especially important because of their role in bone and muscle formation. A nonconstipating diet may prevent rectal bleeding that can occur when hard stools are passed. When a child has mouth bleeding, a soft diet and avoidance of foods of extreme temperatures, those with sharp edges (chips), and straws (sucking action can disturb the clot) are recommended.

Discipline. Some families tend to overprotect the child with the bleeding disorder and may be stricter with unaffected siblings. Age and developmentally appropriate, positive disciplinary techniques that do not include physical punishment should be recommended for all children. Pulling a child with a bleeding disorder by the arm is a specific action that may result in serious shoulder bleeding as well as radial head subluxation. The primary care provider should evaluate the disciplinary style of the parents and offer counseling on alternative discipline measures if potentially injurious methods are used.

Toileting. Standard developmental counseling is advised.

Sleep patterns. Standard developmental counseling is advised.

School issues. The teacher, school nurse, and athletic coaches should be informed of the child's bleeding disorder. Families and children may be reticent to disclose the diagnosis to others, fearing discrimination because of the connection between hemophilia and HIV. The most frequent concerns of school personnel are prevention of bleeding (which may not be possible), emergency management, and fear of HIV infection. Many HTCs offer school visits by the program's nurse coordinator and social worker. These educational visits are most helpful on entrance to a new school and should be done with the permission and, most ideally, the participation of the child and parent or parents. Children and adolescents with hemophilia may encounter peer disbelief that the disability created by an acute bleeding episode can resolve in 1 to 2 days and they are often thought of as "fakers".

Children with learning problems from intracranial bleeding must be fully evaluated and provided with appropriate support.

Sexuality. When a newborn has a family history of hemophilia or von Willebrand's disease and circumcision has been requested by the parents, the surgery should be delayed until screening of the infant is completed. This may be performed on cord blood. If a bleeding disorder is diagnosed, the options include canceling the planned circumcision, pretreating with factor concentrate before the procedure, or managing hemostasis using only local measures. The last option arises from the knowledge that not all boys with even severe hemophilia have bled excessively following circumcision.

Alterations in body image and self-esteem because of chronic joint arthropathy or limitations on physical activity may affect adolescent development. Safe-sex counseling, including decision-making skills, values clarification, instruction in the use of condoms to prevent transmission of HIV, hepatitis B, and other sexually transmitted diseases, should be offered to all adolescents. Some adolescents who test HIV antibody positive may avoid sexual relationships because of fear of rejection once their status is known to a potential partner.

The genetic counselor at the HTC interacts with children beginning with basic education regarding the inheritance of the bleeding disorder and eventually including a discussion of reproductive options. A single performance of carrier testing for hemophilia using the factor VIII coagulant/antigen ratio has an accuracy of 80% to 90%, which increases when the test is repeated (White and Shoemaker, 1989). The use of DNA testing to detect carriers has an estimated accuracy of 95% to 99%, depending on the number of probes used; however, it is expensive, is not available in many areas, and requires blood samples from multiple family members. Sophisticated carrier testing for factor IX hemophilia is less available than that for factor VIII hemophilia. Prenatal diagnosis may be performed by amniocentesis as early as 13 to 16 weeks' gestation, by chorionic villus sampling at 9 to 12 weeks' gestation, or by fetal blood sampling at 19 to 21 weeks' gestation (Pinheiro, 1990).

SPECIAL FAMILY CONCERNS

If the child with a bleeding disorder has excessive bruising before and after diagnosis, parents will frequently encounter questions regarding suspected child abuse from health care providers or accusatory stares from friends, relatives, teachers, and strangers. Compounding the distress of the parents may be guilt regarding the inheritance of the bleeding disorder.

It is difficult for parents to cope with their inability to prevent bleeding episodes despite diligent efforts to prevent injury. Fear of injury to the infant may even interfere with parent-infant bonding. When the child does require an infusion of blood products to stop bleeding, parents often continue to question the viral safety of the product despite current data on product safety. Although most children and adolescents exposed to HIV have been tested for the antibody, families may continue to fear future positive test results.

Reimbursement for factor replacement has reached crisis proportions as adults and in some cases children reach maximum lifetime amount of insurance reimbursement and medical providers debate the cost effectiveness of ultrapure products.

The scope of psychosocial needs related to HIV and the bleeding disorder can be overwhelming (see Chapter 23). Primary care providers are urged to use the resources of local HTCs.

SUMMARY OF PRIMARY CARE NEEDS FOR THE CHILD WITH BLEEDING DISORDERS: HEMOPHILIA AND VON WILLEBRAND'S DISEASE

If the child or adolescent with a bleeding disorder also has HIV infection, please see additional guidelines given in Chapter 23.

Growth and development

Obesity should be prevented to reduce stress on joints.

Developmental screening should be done as follow-up for head trauma or to screen for undiagnosed or unreported intracranial bleeding.

Immunizations

All injectable vaccines should be given subcutaneously with a 25-gauge needle.

Firm pressure should be applied over the immunization site for 5 minutes.

Because of potential contact with family members who may have hemophilia and HIV infection, Salk polio vaccine may be needed. Salk vaccine also is indicated when the child is untested for HIV yet has been exposed during at-risk years.

The hepatitis B vaccine (Recombinant) series is recommended for all likely to be exposed to blood products.

Screening
Vision

Examination by ophthalmologist for eye injury. Routine office screening with attention to funduscopic examination is recommended.

Hearing

Routine screening is recommended.

Dental

Initially teeth should be evaluated at 1 year of age, then routine regular examinations should be done. Hygiene should include flossing under supervision. Factor replacement or desmopressin is recommended for regional blocks; an antifibrinolytic should be added for dental extractions.

Blood pressure

Annual screening is recommended.

Hematocrit

Annual screening is recommended.

Urinalysis

Annual screening for microscopic hematuria is recommended.

Tuberculosis

Routine screening is recommended.

Condition-specific screening

If blood product has been received in the past year, a factor VIII or IX inhibitor screen (persons with hemophilia) and liver function studies are indicated. HIV antibody testing with pre- and post-counseling are recommended for those exposed to blood products prior to 1986.

Drug interactions

Aspirin-containing products are contraindicated.

Prolonged use of other substances that can affect platelet aggregation; such as antihistamines, guaifenesin, dextromethorphan, and nonsteroidal antiinflammatory agents, should be avoided.

Differential diagnosis
Headaches

Rule out intracranial bleeding, especially with concurrent vomiting and absence of GI symptoms.

Sore throat

Throat cultures present risk for posterior pharyngeal bleeding. Cultures should not be taken from an uncooperative child.

Gastrointestinal symptoms

Rule out GI bleeding. Rule out iliopsoas muscle bleeding with lower abdominal pain and decreased hip extension.

Mouth bleeding if uncontrolled by topical measures requires antifibrinolytic agents.

Gait disturbance

Rule out scoliosis and bleeding in and around the ankle, knee, hip, and iliopsoas muscle.

Continued.

SUMMARY OF PRIMARY CARE NEEDS FOR THE CHILD WITH BLEEDING DISORDERS: HEMOPHILIA AND VON WILLEBRAND'S DISEASE — cont'd

Dysuria and hematuria

Rule out testicular bleeding, renal or ureteral bleeding, and infection.

Numbness, tingling, and pain

Rule out nerve compression caused by bleeding.

Developmental issues
Safety

May recommend protective helmet for children who are learning to walk to reduce risk of head injury. Discontinue use when child is walking well because it restricts peripheral vision.

Knee pads in pants of toddlers may decrease knee hematomas.

Recommend high-top sneakers (not canvas type) for children at risk for hemarthroses from the age of 2 to 3 years.

Encourage participation in noncontact sports.

Recommend no bike riding without a helmet; skateboarding is not recommended even with a helmet.

Recommend wearing a medical identification emblem, including diagnosis, treatment product, and blood type. Update it yearly.

Discourage activities that increase the chance of testicular bleeding, particularly in boys with moderate or severe hemophilia.

Families participating in a home infusion program should follow accepted guidelines for disposal of infectious wastes.

Child care

Contact with the proposed source of care by provider or HTC staff is often useful to clarify responsibilities with regard to prevention and management of bleeding episodes and trauma.

Recognize that the provider may have fears regarding potential HIV infection.

Diet

Adequate protein and calcium intake is of particular importance because of their role in bone and muscle formation.

Avoid obesity because it places extra stress on joints.

Discipline

Recognize the potential for overprotection of the affected child and the use of deferential disciplinary methods when compared with unaffected siblings.

Discourage pulling the child by the arm because it may result in shoulder bleeding.

Toileting

Standard developmental counseling is advised.

Sleep patterns

Standard developmental counseling is advised.

School issues

School visits are most helpful on enrollment in a new school and ideally include the child and parent or parents as participants.

Because of the difficulty in understanding acute onset and resolution of bleeding episodes, peer acceptance is potentially poor.

Acknowledge potential fear of HIV infection among school personnel.

Sexuality

Delay circumcision until the child with a positive family history is screened for bleeding disorders.

Recognize potential alterations in body image and self-esteem because of chronic joint arthropathy or limitations on physical activity.

Safe sex counseling recommended to prevent sexually transmitted diseases.

Special family concerns

Child abuse may be suspected.

Parents may experience guilt regarding hereditary nature of bleeding disorder.

Fear of injury to infant may decrease parent/infant bonding.

Parents may fear the inability to prevent bleeding episodes despite attempts to prevent injury.

The potential for undiscovered HIV infection may be a concern.

The family may experience uncertainty regarding the viral safety of blood products.

Insurance crises may occur as children and adults reach lifetime maximum amounts of reimbursement.

RESOURCES
Organizations

The National Hemophilia Foundation* and its local chapters disseminate information regarding recent advances in therapy not only for hemophilia and von Willebrand's disease but also for HIV infection. Its active membership includes consumers, their families, and health care providers at hemophilia treatment centers (HTCs). The local chapters provide educational programs and support services to meet the members' needs.

HTCs also provide educational programs and support groups for children and adolescents with bleeding disorders and their families. A list of HTCs is available from the National Hemophilia Foundation.

REFERENCES

Abildgaard C: Progress and problems in hemophilia and von Willebrand's disease. In Barness L, ed: *Advances in pediatrics,* Chicago, 1984, Year Book Medical Publishers, pp 137-177.

Abildgaard C, Suzuki Z, Harrison J, et al: Serial studies in von Willebrand's disease: variability versus "variants," *Blood* 56:712-716, 1980.

Aledort L: *Current management in the treatment of hemophilia: a physician's manual,* New York, 1986, National Hemophilia Foundation.

Arnold W and Hilgartner M: Hemophilic arthropathy, *J Bone Joint Surg* 59A:287-305, 1977.

Baehner R and Strauss H: Hemophilia in the first year of life, *N Engl J Med* 275:524-528, 1966.

Bowie E: Von Willebrand's disease, *Clin Lab Med* 4:303-317, 1984.

Brady R and Humphries R: Pediatric HIV infection and AIDS: AIDS and adolescents, *Seminars Pediatric Infect Dis* 1:156-162, 1990.

Brettler D and Levine P: Factor concentrates for the treatment of hemophilia: which one to choose? *Blood* 73:2067-2073, 1989.

Centers for Disease Control: Safety of therapeutic products used for hemophilia patients, *MMWR* 37:441-450, 1988.

Coller B: Von Willebrand's disease. In Ratnoff E and Forbes C, eds: *Disorders of hemostasis,* Orlando, FL, 1984, Grune & Stratton, pp 241-269.

Corrigan J: *Hemorrhagic and thrombotic diseases in childhood and adolescence,* New York, 1985, Churchill Livingstone.

Czapek E, Gadarowski J, Ontiveros J, et al: Humate-P for treatment of von Willebrand disease, *Blood* 72:1100, 1988.

De la Fuente B, Kasper C, Rickles F, et al: Response of patients with mild and moderate hemophilia A and von Willebrand's disease to treatment with desmopressin, *Ann Intern Med* 103:6-14, 1985.

Eyster E, Gill F, Blatt P, et al: Central nervous system bleeding in hemophiliacs, *Blood* 51:1179-1188, 1978.

Forbes C: Clinical aspects of the hemophilias and their treatment. In Ratnoff E and Forbes C, eds: *Disorders of hemostasis,* Orlando, FL, 1984, Grune & Stratton, pp 177-239.

Gilbert M, Schorr J, Holbrook T, et al: *Hemophilia and sports,* New York, 1985, National Hemophilia Foundation.

Gitschier J: Maternal duplication associated with gene deletion in sporadic hemophilia, *Am J Hum Genet* 43:274-279, 1988.

Hilgartner M, Aledort L, and Giardina P: Thalassemia and hemophilia. In Hobbs N and Perrin JM, eds: *Issues in the care of children with chronic illness,* San Francisco, 1985, Jossey-Bass, pp 299-323.

Hilgartner M and Montgomery R: *Understanding von Willebrand's disease,* New York, 1985. National Hemophilia Foundation.

Hollinger F: Factors influencing the immune response to hepatitis B vaccine, booster dose guidelines, and vaccine protocol recommendations, *Am J Med* 87(suppl 3A):36S-40S, 1989.

Kasper C: Treatment of factor VIII inhibitors. In Coller B, ed: *Progress in hemostasis and thrombosis,* vol 9, Philadelphia, 1989, WB Saunders, pp 57-86.

Kasper C and Dietrich S: Comprehensive management of haemophilia, *Clin Haematol* 14:489-512, 1985.

Kletzel M, Miller C, Becton D, et al: Postdelivery head bleeding in hemophilic neonates, *Am J Dis Child* 143:1107-1110, 1989.

Koch B: Rehabilitation of the child with joint disease. In Molnar G, ed: *Pediatric rehabilitation,* Baltimore, 1985, Williams & Wilkins, pp 263-271.

Köhler M, Hellstern P, Tarrach H, et al: Subcutaneous injection of desmopressin (DDAVP): evaluation of a new, more concentrated preparation, *Haemostasis* 1:38-44, 1989.

Lancial L: Early dental intervention for the child with hemophilia. In Ridley K and Bergero L, eds: *Dental care of the hemophilia patient,* Ann Arbor, 1987, Hemophilia Foundation of Michigan, pp 45-52.

Lawrie A, Harrison P, Armstrong A, et al: Comparison of the in vitro characteristics of von Willebrand factor in British and commercial factor VIII concentrates, *Br J Haematol* 73:100-104, 1989.

Mannucci P: Desmopressin (DDAVP) for treatment of disorders of hemostasis. In Coller B, ed: *Progress in hemostasis and thrombosis,* vol 8, Orlando, FL, 1986, Grune & Stratton, pp 19-45.

Medical and Scientific Advisory Committee of the National Hemophilia Foundation: *AIDS Update* (December 1990), New York, National Hemophilia Foundation.

Miller C, Lenzi R, and Breen C: *Gene frequency in von Willebrand disease.* Abstract presented at the meeting of the American Society of Human Genetics, Baltimore, MD, November 1989.

*National Hemophilia Foundation, Soho Bldg, 110 Greene St, Suite 406, New York, NY, 10012 (212) 219-8180.

Miller C and Lubs M: *The Inheritance of Hemophilia,* New York, 1986, National Hemophilia Foundation.

Mittal R, Spero J, Lewis J, et al: Patterns of gastrointestinal hemorrhage in hemophilia, *Gastroenterology* 88:515-522, 1985.

Olson T, Alving B, Cheshier J, et al: Intracerebral and subdural hemorrhage in a neonate with hemophilia A, *Am J Pediatr Hematol Oncol* 7:384-387, 1985.

Pierce G, Lusher J, Brownstein A, et al: The use of purified clotting factor concentrates in hemophilia, *JAMA* 261:3434-3438, 1989.

Pinheiro S: Personal communication, April 10, 1990.

Poole A: DDAVP (desmopressin) in the dental management of patients with mild or moderate hemophilia and von Willebrand's disease. In Ridley K and Bergero L, eds: *Dental care of the hemophilia patient,* Ann Arbor, MI, 1987, Hemophilia Foundation of Michigan, pp 136-149.

Rivard G: Syniorthesis with radioactive colloids in hemophiliacs. In *Rehabilitation in hemophilia: proceedings of a conference,* New York, 1987, National Hemophilia Foundation, pp 29-37.

Rodeghiero F, Castaman G, DiBona E, et al: Consistency of responses to repeated DDAVP infusions in patient with von Willebrand's disease and hemophilia A, *Blood* 74:1997-2000, 1989.

Rothman D: Personal communication, April 23, 1990.

Smith T, Gill J, Ambruso D, et al: Hyponatremia and seizures in young children given DDAVP, *Am J Hematol* 31:199-202, 1989.

Spero J, Lewis J, Fisher S, et al: The high risk of chronic liver disease in multitransfused juvenile hemophiliac patients, *J Pediatr* 94:875-878, 1979.

Warren M and McMillan C: Hemophilia. In Hockenberry M and Coody D, eds: *Pediatric oncology and hematology: Perspectives on care,* St. Louis, MO, 1986, Mosby-Year Book, pp. 252-272.

Warrier A and Lusher J: DDAVP: a useful alternative to blood components in moderate hemophilia A and von Willebrand's disease, *J Pediatr* 102:228-233, 1983.

White G, McMillan C, Blatt P, et al: Factor VIII inhibitors: a clinical overview, *Am J Hematol* 13:335-342, 1982.

White G, McMillan C, Kingdon H, et al: Use of recombinant antihemophilic factor in the treatment of two patients with classic hemophilia, *N Engl J Med* 320:166-170, 1989.

White G and Shoemaker C: Factor VIII gene and hemophilia A, *Blood* 73:1-12, 1989.

7 *Bronchopulmonary Dysplasia*

··

Virginia H. Conte

ETIOLOGY

Bronchopulmonary dysplasia (BPD) was first described by Northway, Rosan, and Porter (1967) in a review of chest radiographs of premature infants who were treated with positive pressure ventilation and oxygen for respiratory distress syndrome (RDS). When they first described the disease, they used a four-stage classification. Stage 1 described the first 2 to 3 days, with a radiograph similar to that showing RDS. Stage 2 evolved over the next 4 to 10 days, with a chest radiograph revealing complete opacification of lung fields. Stage 3, from 10 to 20 days, was marked by small round cystic lesions on x-ray film. Stage 4, the final and most severe stage, showed small bubbles of radiolucency on x-ray film, enlarging to form a hyperaerated cyst. Infants in this group had mechanical ventilatory support for greater than 1 month.

Philip (1975) broadened the definition to include nonradiographic findings and management. They included (1) institution of positive pressure ventilation within the first week of life for a minimum of 3 days; (2) clinical findings of tachypnea, rales and retractions persisting beyond 28 days of life; (3) an oxygen requirement to maintain arterial oxygen pressure (PaO_2) greater than 55 mm Hg for more than 28 days; (4) and chest radiographs showing persistent strands of densities with areas of normal and hyperlucency in bilateral lung fields.

As advances in the study, diagnosis, and treatment of BPD have progressed, these early classification systems have become less frequently used. Today BPD is often classified as mild, moderate, or severe.

Conditions causing or contributing to the development of BPD include hyaline membrane disease (HMD), meconium aspiration, congenital heart disease (CHD), patent ductus arteriosus, and fluid overload in the newborn period (Bancalari and Gerhardt, 1986; Bancalari and Sosenko, 1990; Goldson, 1984).

Infants born with HMD that progresses to RDS are likely candidates for BPD because they generally require mechanical ventilatory support with oxygen because of respiratory distress and acute respiratory failure at birth (Bancalari and Gerhardt, 1986; Bancalari and Sosenko, 1990; Merritt, Northway, and Boynton, 1988). Infants born before 28 to 32 weeks' gestation have an insufficient amount of pulmonary surfactant. Surfactant is a lipoprotein that lowers the surface tension of the air-alveolar surface and allows lung expansion, thus maintaining the patency of alveoli and preventing atelectasis.

As the birth weight of the infant decreases, the risk for developing BPD increases because of the need for ventilatory support with oxygen. Initial lung injury from barotrauma combined with the surfactant deficiency causes a release of toxic oxidants and proteolytic enzymes (Bancalari and Gerhardt, 1986). Bancalari simplifies the development of BDP by the following equation: immaturity + oxygen + pressure + time = BPD (Merritt, Northway, and Boynton, 1988). Lung healing is abnormal and the course complicated with continued and recurrent episodes of hypoxia and inadequate nutrition (Merritt, Northway, and Boynton, 1988).

At a cellular level stretching and shearing from pressures of mechanical ventilatory support tear bronchial epithelium, exposing subepithelial connective tissue (Logvinoff et al., 1985; Merritt, Northway, and Boynton, 1988). Macrophages and polymorphonuclear cells invade the airways, causing airway edema. In addition, there are losses of cilia and denudation of airway lining, resulting in the loss of the normal cleansing abilities of the lung. The continued use of oxygen affects the growth and development of lung structures. The number of developing alveoli is reduced by one third to one half of the number within a normal lung.

Nutritional status has significant implications in the etiology and severity of this disease. Premature infants have little caloric reserve. If they are born before the third trimester, these infants are deficient

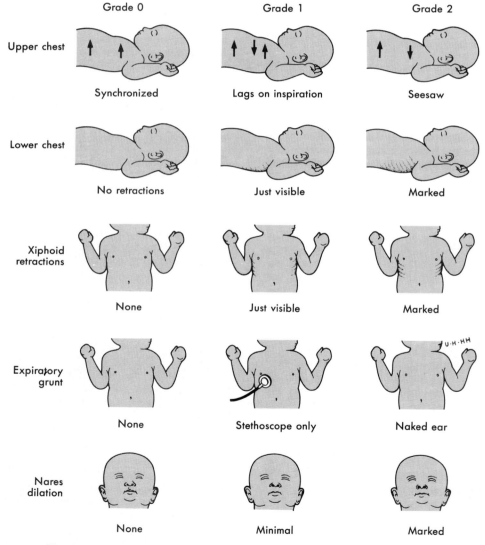

Fig. 7-1. Manifestations of respiratory distress in bronchopulmonary dysplasia.

in iron, zinc, and selenium (Bancalari and Gerhardt, 1986). These minerals help break down oxygen and facilitate lung repair. Adequate nutrition is difficult to achieve because of a combination of factors: the need to restrict fluids as a result of pulmonary and cardiac instability, the increased caloric needs required to promote lung healing and development, and the immaturity of the premature digestive system.

INCIDENCE

The reported incidence of BPD varies because of the lack of consistent definition of the disease. Goldson (1984) estimates that 2.4% to 68% of infants requiring mechanical ventilation develop BPD, whereas McElheney (1989) estimates that 20% to 25% of infants requiring mechanical ventilation develop BPD.

The population at greatest risk are low birth weight infants (Merritt, Northway, and Boynton, 1988). The incidence is 14% for infants weighing 501 to 1000 g, 6% for infants weighing 1001 to 1500 g, 4% for infants weighing 1501 to 2000 g, and 2% for infants weighing more than 2000 g at birth. If the need for mechanical ventilation is factored in, the incidence is 72% for infants weighing less than 1000 g and 22% for those weighing 1250 to 1500 g (Markestad and Fitzhardinge, 1981; Meisels et al., 1986; Meisels et al., 1987; Merritt, Northway, and Boynton, 1988).

CLINICAL MANIFESTATIONS AT TIME OF DIAGNOSIS

Clinical manifestation of BPD varies depending on the age at onset and disease severity. It can range from a child with some pulmonary symptoms requiring bronchodilator treatment and diuretics to a child requiring a tracheostomy and mechanical ventilatory support for prolonged periods in the hospital and at home.

An abnormal respiratory examination is the key finding in this diagnosis (Fig. 7-1). On visual examination, the respiratory rate may be elevated greater than baseline for age by as much as 20 to 30 breaths/min. A prolonged exhalation with increased use of abdominal and accessory muscles is seen with respiratory distress. Cyanosis and activity intolerance (feeding and handling) are common findings (Hagedorn and Gardner, 1989). A child

with mild BPD may be free of wheezes and rales. If fluid retention, increased airway reactivity, or infection occurs, wheezing, inspiratory rales, or exhalatory rales may be present. These adventitious sounds may be more easily identified after clearing of upper airway sounds by suctioning or by having the child cough because this facilitates the auscultation of breath sounds and eliminates the presence of referred upper airway noise. In a stable child secretions are clear to white, sparse, and thin. A change to yellow or green indicates the presence of infection.

Chest x-ray findings in children with BPD display a hyperinflated chest with flattened diaphragms and increased interstitial markings. These markings may persist up to age 9 years (Merritt, Northway, and Boynton, 1988). Pulmonary function tests demonstrate decreased compliance, abnormal airway reactivity, increased airway resistance, and increased dead space (Goldson, 1984; Koops, Abman, and Accurso, 1984; Logvinoff et al., 1985; Merritt, Northway, and Boynton, 1988).

TREATMENT

Infants with BPD are usually not discharged home until they have reached at least 40 weeks' gestational age, are able to feed adequately to support growth and lung tissue healing, need medications only 3 to 4 times per day, and can maintain a transcutaneous oxygen concentration of 55 mm Hg during routine activities such as feeding, bathing, crying, and sleeping.

The need for supplemental oxygen varies with the severity of lung dysfunction. Infants who require oxygen after hospital discharge rarely require more than 1 to 2 L/min delivered by nasal cannula. These children must be followed at frequent intervals to assess for hypoxia by physical examination and by oxygen and carbon dioxide readings. Ideally, these readings can be obtained via pulse oximeter or transcutaneous oxygen monitoring instead of arterial blood samples. Oxygen and carbon dioxide measurements must be done during periods of rest and activity to accurately determine the child's continuing supplemental oxygen needs (Bernbaum and D'Agostino, 1986). When the child appears clinically stable, is gaining weight, and is not anemic, gradual weaning from oxygen is initiated by the neonatal pulmonary team. A typical weaning schedule is presented in Table 7-1.

Table 7-1. Weaning a patient from supplemental oxygen: sample schedule

Time	Amount of oxygen (per min)
At hospital discharge	0.5 L at all times
1 mo after discharge*	0.5 L during feedings and sleep; 0.25 L when awake
2 mo*	0.25 L at all times
3 mo*	0.25 L during feedings and sleep; room air when awake
4 mo*	Room air at all times

From Bernbaum JE, Friedman S, Hoffman-Williamson M, et al: Preterm infant care after hospital discharge, *Pediatr Rev* 10:195-208, 1989.
*Assumes clinical stability, adequate weight gain, and proof of adequate oxygen saturation (intervals may vary).

Infants with the need for prolonged ventilatory support, tracheal malacia, or subglottic stenosis will require a tracheostomy. It is becoming quite common for these children to be cared for at home. The most frequent complications are infection of the tracheostomy, obstruction by secretions, or accidental decannulation (Bernbaum et al., 1989).

Nutritional support is vital for healing of damaged lung tissue and optimal growth and development of the infant. These infants are often poor feeders because of prematurity, hypoxia, oral defensiveness as a result of endotracheal tubes and suctioning, and deprivation of oral feeding experiences. Total parenteral nutrition early in treatment is often necessary, followed by supplementation of breast or bottle feedings with gavage feedings. In infants with severe BPD and feeding problems, a gastrostomy tube may be necessary. Caloric requirements are high, up to 150 to 200 kcal/kg per day, with most infants requiring formula with a caloric concentration of 24 kcal/30 ml (fl oz) or greater to achieve optimal catch-up growth (Hagedorn and Gardner, 1989). Formula may be fortified with vegetable oil, triglycerides, or glucose polymers to increase the calories per ounce (Bernbaum et al., 1989). The breast milk of mothers of premature infants has been found to be well suited for the nutritional needs of the premature infants (American Academy of Pediatrics, 1985).

Nutritional requirements must be balanced with

Table 7-2. Diuretics commonly used to treat bronchopulmonary dysplasia

Drug	Dosage (mg/kg/day)	No. of divided doses
Furosemide (Lasix)*	1-2	2
Chlorothiazide (Diuril)*	20-40	2
Spironolactone (Aldactone)	1.5-3	1-2

From Bernbaum JE, Friedman S, Hoffman-Williamson M, et al: Preterm infant care after hospital discharge, *Pediatr Rev* 10:95-208, 1989.
*Supplement with potassium chloride.

fluid restrictions so as not to overload the already stressed cardiopulmonary system. Diuretics are often necessary to decrease the amount of excess lung and total body water (Table 7-2). Because of the potential electrolyte imbalance associated with diuretic therapy, these children must have serum electrolyte values monitored frequently and are given potassium chloride supplements (Bernbaum et al, 1989).

PROGNOSIS

Survival rates and outcomes are steadily improving for children with BPD. Expert care is now available for these infants through easier access to tertiary care centers staffed with specially trained critical care personnel. Improvements in prenatal care and technologic advances in diagnostic and treatment techniques have greatly improved the outcome for these infants.

Even with these new advances, mortality ranges from 10% to 25% for infants with BPD. The latter figure is associated with the rising number of low and very low birth weight infants who survive the first few weeks, only to die of BPD (Koops, Abman, and Accurso, 1984). Morbidity figures vary depending on prematurity and severity of BPD. Mental retardation, development delays, learning disabilities, and cerebral palsy all have been reported. Sauve and Singhal (1985) reported that infants with BPD had a much higher incidence of upper and lower respiratory tract infection, rehospitalizations, and abnormal physical findings on examination than did infants of comparable maturity and birth weight without BPD. Most adolescents and young adults who had BPD as infants have been found to have some degree of pulmonary dysfunction, consisting of airway obstruction, airway hyperactivity, and hyperinflation (Northway et al, 1990).

ASSOCIATED PROBLEMS
Pulmonary problems

Structural damage to the infant's premature respiratory tree frequently occurs when the infant requires intubation and ventilation early in life. Subglottic stenosis, vocal cord damage or paralysis, and tracheobronchial malacia have been reported as a result of long-term use of artificial airways (Merritt, Northway, and Boynton, 1988). Insertion of the suction catheter beyond the end of the artificial airway can cause bronchial main stem stenosis and promote formation of granulation tissue. Denudation of cilia from suctioning further compromises the respiratory status by impeding the body's ability to effectively move mucus through the tracheobronchial tree.

It can be anticipated that almost half of the infants discharged home with BPD will require rehospitalization for respiratory problems in the first year of life (Koops, Abman, and Accurso, 1984). They are more susceptible to bacterial and viral illnesses, especially if there is an artificial airway in place.

Infants and children with BPD have an increased incidence of reactive airway disease when exposed to airway irritants or viral infections (Davis, Sinkin, and Aranda, 1990; Koops, Abman, and Accurso, 1984; Logvinoff et al, 1985; Nickerson and Taussig, 1980). Bronchospasms are controlled with bronchodilator therapy to lessen the wheezing, coughing, and increased use of abdominal muscles seen in this condition. Bronchodilators are administered either orally (e.g., theophylline, albuterol, or metaproterenol) or via an aerosolized route (e.g., albuterol, cromolyn sodium, or metaproterenol) (Table 7-3) (Davis, Sinkin, and Aranda, 1990; Koops, Abman, and Accurso, 1984; Logvinoff et al., 1985; Meritt, Northway, and Boynton, 1988).

During a viral or bacterial respiratory illness, airway function is further compromised by increased airway sensitivity, increased mucous production, and airway swelling. Methylprednisone (predisone), 2 mg/kg per day in two divided doses over 4 days, helps to decrease airway swelling, ease coughing and wheezing, and facilitate oxygenation and ventilation (Davis, Sinkin, and Aranda, 1990; Koops, Abman, and Accurso, 1984; Merritt, Northway, and Boynton, 1988).

Daily chest physiotherapy (CPT) and postural drainage facilitate the mobilization of secretions to allow for removal from the airway by coughing or suctioning if an artificial airway is present. During a viral or bacterial illness, secretion production increases and more frequent chest physiotherapy and drainage will probably be necessary.

Otorhinolaryngology problems

Often the same bacteria that colonize the lower airways also colonize the upper airways and precipitate upper respiratory infections. Recurrent otitis media is frequently seen in this population, resulting in the need for antibiotic prophylaxis, placement of bilateral myringotomy tubes, or both. Hearing loss can occur as a result of chronic infection and chronic intravenous use of furosemide and aminoglycosides.

Sinusitis is prevalent in children with chronic lung disease and children who have required or continue to require nasogastric tube feedings. There is a persistent unilateral or bilateral off-colored drainage from the nares. Postnasal drainage results in coughing and throat clearing, especially after waking from sleep. Severe sinusitus causes cough-

Table 7-3. Medications used to treat bronchopulmonary dysplasia

Drug	Dosage	Frequency of doses
Theophylline	4-6 mg/kg/dose	Every 6-8 hr
Metaproterenol (Alupent)	2 mg/kg/day	3-4 divided doses
Cromolyn disodium	20 mg	3 times/day

From Bernbaum JE, Friedman S, Hoffman-Williamson M, et al: Preterm infant care after hospital discharge, *Pediatr Rev* 10:195-208, 1989.

ing throughout the day and is unrelieved by bronchodilator therapy or frequent suctioning of an artificial airway. Radiographs of the sinuses confirm the presence of infection and degree of involvement. Antibiotics taken orally for a minimum of 3 weeks clear most infections, but prolonged therapy may be needed to treat severe cases.

Seizures

Hypoxic insults and intraventricular hemorrhages occurring in the newborn period predispose the infant to seizures. Even with anticonvulsant therapy the onset of new seizures can be triggered at any time by an infection with a high fever or a hypoxic insult. Children with BPD who have been free of seizures for a minimum of 1 year with electroencephalograms free of epileptiform activity can be considered for weaning of anticonvulsants (see Chapter 15).

Cardiac conditions

Chronic cardiac changes persist in children with BPD who have suffered numerous hypoxic insults or who have been maintained at a low PaO_2. Left and right ventricular hypertrophy and cor pulmonale can occur as the result of poor lung compliance. Systemic hypertension is seen in 50% of the children with BPD. If the systolic pressure reaches 150 to 200 mm Hg, the child should undergo further work-up for renal, pulmonary, and cardiac problems (Goldson, 1984; Koops, Abman, and Accurso, 1984; Merritt, Northway, and Boynton, 1988; Morray et al., 1981). Congenital heart disease complicates the course of BPD. Early diagnosis and treatment of CHD help improve lung function and decrease ventilatory support (Merritt, Northway, and Boynton, 1988).

Orthopedic anomalies

Infants with BPD often develop rickets secondary to prolonged parenteral nutrition and difficulty absorbing calcium and phosphorus. The population most at risk are those infants with a birth weight less than 1000 g. Long-term furosemide administration can also contribute to a negative calcium balance, inhibiting normal bone formation. This condition is reversible with dietary management and use of alternate diuretics such as spironolactone and hydrochlorothiazide (Merritt, Northway, and Boynton, 1988).

Renal conditions

Chronic furosemide treatment may cause hypercalcinuria, urolithiasis, and nephrolithiasis. Other medications contributing to these conditions are sodium bicarbonate and calcium gluconate. The incidence of renal stones is quite high in younger children with BPD (Merritt, Northway, and Boynton, 1988). Renal stones may be noted first radiographically but should be confirmed with a renal ultrasound. Treatment consists of decreased vitamin D intake in the diet. Calcilo-XD, a low calcium vitamin D free formula by Ross Laboratories is available for treating this population. It meets infants' and young children's nutritional needs yet has minimal calcium and vitamin D.

Cholelithiasis

Gallstones occur, but the cause is unknown. One theory is related to the use of total parenteral nutrition. These solutions contain a protein hydrolysate that promotes bile stasis and fat emulsions, resulting in bile crystalization. Stones are seen on chest x-ray film in the right upper quadrant of the abdominal area. Children may be diagnosed with gallstones from 11 days to 7 months of age, with an average age of 3 months. Diagnosis is confirmed with renal ultrasound. Spontaneous resolution usually occurs by 2 years of age. Long-term prognosis is unknown (Merritt, Northway, and Boynton, 1988).

Ophthalmologic problems

The incidence of retinopathy of prematurity (ROP) has decreased as the toxic effects of oxygen have become known. Central blindness can occur with repeated incidence of severe hypoxia and severe intraventricular hemorrhage. Strabismus is also a common finding and should be followed for consideration of surgical repair (Koops, Abman, and Accurso, 1984; Merritt, Northway, and Boynton, 1988).

Stoma problems

Children with tracheostomy tubes are at risk for irritation around the tracheostomy stoma. Secretions that ooze from tracheostomy stomas may irritate the skin. Meticulous regular care to the tracheostomy stoma will generally maintain skin integrity.

Skin lacerations on the neck can be caused by

fastening tracheostomy ties too tightly. A small premeasured protective patch of Stomahesive may be placed over the laceration to allow it to heal without continued direct contact with tracheostomy ties or the flange of the tracheostomy tube.

Some children may develop areas of granulation tissue on and around the tracheostomy stoma. If left unattended, it will continue to grow and can impede or block insertion of the tracheostomy tube into the stoma. Occasionally the tissue forms a tight band around the tracheostomy stoma. Application of silver nitrate to the site will promote shrinkage and eliminate tissue. In extreme cases the child will need to be referred to an otorhinolaryngologist for possible surgical excision under anesthesia.

Similar difficulties with granulation tissue occur with gastrostomy stomas and the same treatment applies. Leakage of feeding around the gastrostomy tube causes irritation of the skin on the abdomen. Usually the cause is mechanical. Some families are instructed to change gastrostomy tubes on a regular basis because over time the stomach acid alters the integrity of the tube within the stomach.

The primary care provider should examine the tube to determine its type and how it is inserted. Foley catheters, Malecot tubes, and gastrostomy button devices may be used as gastrostomy tubes. Some tubes may be placed securely with a fluid-inflated balloon. The amount of fluid in the balloon should be documented in the discharge plan. If the amount contained within the balloon is less than the prescribed amount, it can contribute to leakage. It is important to ensure that the internal balloon is pulled up close to the internal abdominal wall to prevent leakage.

When leakage is persistent, some practitioners insert a larger tube into the stoma. This technique is controversial because over time the stoma will only expand and the problem will recur. The less the tube is manipulated, the longer the stoma will remain intact. Secure fastening procedures can help minimize movement of the gastrostomy tube.

Gastroesophageal reflux

Gastroesophageal reflux (GER) is a common gastrointestinal dysfunction seen in children with BPD. Frequent emesis occurs during and after meals. Poor growth patterns despite adequate caloric intake, frequent episodes of aspiration pneumonitis, and multiple setbacks in pulmonary status are typical of GER. Moderate to severe GER causes irritation of the esophagus. Theophylline aggravates GER by decreasing the pressure of the lower esophageal sphincter. Ranitidine (Zantac) or an over-the-counter antacid helps buffer the acidity of the stomach after meals and decreases the episodes of bronchospasm caused by gastric content irritation. If these medicines are not effective in controlling symptoms, metoclopramide (Reglan) is considered. Metaclopramide promotes gastric emptying and eliminates residuals from refluxing. The last option considered if symptoms and the clinical picture do not demonstrate any improvement is Nissan fundal plication surgery (Merritt, Northway, and Boynton, 1988).

Delayed growth and development

Delayed initiation of oral feedings, prolonged oral intubation, recurrent emesis, fatigue, and aversion to food contribute to poor feeding abilities. Children with BPD demonstrate strong aversions to new tastes and textures as a result of prolonged parenteral hyperalimentation and enteral feedings. Nutritional needs are difficult to meet because of poor GI tolerance, restricted fluid intake, and increased caloric needs related to the increased work of breathing (Pridham et al., 1989; Schlomann, 1988).

Overall, growth patterns depend on the severity of the lung disease and nutritional status. Sixty-seven percent of the children are below the tenth percentile for weight and 53% are below the tenth percentile for height at 2 years of age (Meisels et al., 1986; Merritt, Northway, and Boynton, 1988). These children appear small with decreased amounts of subcutaneous tissue. The head appears long and boxy and falls at about the 50th percentile for head circumference (Merritt, Northway, and Boynton, 1987).

Figures as high as 34% (Vohr, Bell, and Oh, 1982) are quoted for the incidence of moderate to severe developmental delay in this population. Studies by Meisels and associates (1986) found boys to be more vulnerable than girls. Using the Bayley Scales of Infant Development, they found that 35% tested with delays greater than 1 standard deviation on the Mental Development Index and 47% on the Psychomotor Developmental Index.

Markestad and Fitzhardinge (1981) found poor growth patterns to be more severe with the infants small for gestational age. These children showed decelerated growth rates in the first 6 to 12 months of life because of persistent respiratory distress and environmental deprivation. In 6% to 19% of cases, late acceleration of skill development was seen as the child's health improved and the need for hospitalization lessened (Markestad and Fitzhardinge, 1981). Vohr, Bell, and Oh (1982) found spastic diplegia to be the most common neurologic diagnosis. Later assessments of these children often reveal attention deficit disorders, perceptual-motor integration problems, and language delays despite normal intelligence as measured by IQ tests (Bernbaum et al., 1989).

PRIMARY CARE MANAGEMENT
Growth and development

Height and weight measurements, corrected for gestational age, should be obtained and plotted monthly while hospitalized and with each subsequent ambulatory care visit. Growth measurements taken before discharge from the hospital will help establish growth trends in the newly discharged infant. Even minor illness in these children may result in a loss of weight because of their high caloric needs. The head shape of the premature infant often appears boxy, and the head circumference must be measured and recorded carefully on standardized growth curves for premature infants or corrected for gestational age and plotted on National Center for Health Statistics graphs. The corrected age should be used for 2½ years, or until the sutures are normally fused. Both macrocephaly and microcephaly have been reported in infants with BPD (Sauve and Singhal, 1985). A head circumference percentile that is significantly higher than weight or height percentiles suggests the possibility of intraventricular hemorrhage or poor nutritional status with head sparing (Bernbaum and D'Agostino, 1986). Careful physical examination and documentation of caloric intake should indicate if a cranial ultrasound is needed.

It is difficult to determine the relative importance of BPD versus prematurity when developmental outcome is projected. It is well accepted that the more premature the infant, the greater the chance of developmental abnormalities. A recent study comparing premature infants with and without respiratory distress found no significant differ-

ence in their cognitive ability at 12, 36, and 48 months of age (Ludman et al, 1987), but other studies indicate infants with BPD are at higher risk for developmental problems than their matched controls (Meisels et al, 1987). Prolonged ventilatory support related to moderate or severe BPD is believed to be associated with significantly poorer developmental outcomes (Bernbaum et al., 1989).

Developmental screening by the primary provider can be accomplished using the child's corrected age and standard screening tools. Even with correction for prematurity, these infants often exhibit developmental lag during the first year of life. Most infants with transient developmental delays will test normal after their first year. If developmental delays are significant or persist after the first year of life, referral for further assessment and therapeutic intervention is recommended. Early intervention for these high-risk children and control of secondary pulmonary problems offer the best prospect for optimal long-term prognosis.

Immunizations

Infants with BPD should receive all standard immunizations at the normal chronologic age. Because of prolonged hospitalizations and recurrent illnesses however, they are often delayed in their immunization schedule. Before immunizations are initiated in the primary care office, hospital records should be reviewed to determine if any immunizations were administered during hospitalization. If inactivated polio vaccine was given in the hospital, the practitioner may continue with this series or switch to trivalent oral polio vaccine. If the infant has a history of uncontrolled seizures, pertussis may be withheld until the seizures are controlled or diphtheria and tetanus vaccines may be given without pertussis (see Chapter 15). Infants and children with chronic BPD are at highest risk for serious morbidity with pertussis infection, so pertussis vaccination should not be withheld without cause.

The administration of subvirion influenza vaccine during the fall or early winter months is recommended for children more than 6 months of age with BPD and their caretakers (Committee on Infectious Diseases [CID], 1991). Pneumococcal vaccine trials have not been conducted on children with BPD so no formal recommendation to give pneumococcal vaccine has been made.

Screening

Vision. Evaluations for ROP should be done every 2 or 3 months by a pediatric ophthalmologist during the first year of life. If there is a question of blindness, a visual evoked response test can be requested. Routine eye examinations with Hirschberg, cover test, tracking, and fundoscopic examinations should be done at each primary care visit to follow the common problems of myopia and strabismus (Koops, Abman, and Accurso, 1984). Surgical correction for strabismus is often required.

Hearing. Infants with BPD are at risk for hearing loss as a result of prematurity and the IV administration of furosemide, corticosteroids, and aminoglycosides. A basal auditory evoked response (BAER) test should be completed before discharge from the hospital, and routine hearing screening should be conducted with each primary care visit (Koops, Abman, and Accurso, 1984). If recurrent otitis media is a problem, regular audiometry examinations should be conducted to identify hearing impairment and speech delays. Speech delays can be anticipated in children with long-term tracheostomies.

Dental. Routine dental care is recommended. Hypoplastic and discolored maxillary central and lateral incisors were found in more than 25% of infants with BPD in one study (Sauve and Singhal, 1985). Orally ingested ferrous sulfate may cause tooth staining, which can be remedied with good dental hygiene. Daily tooth brushing may be a challenge for parents because of the child's oral defensiveness. Primary care providers can recommend using toothettes or foam-tipped brushes, which are softer, and baking soda instead of toothpaste because of its milder taste.

Blood pressure. Measurements should be taken with every visit and routinely followed to detect early signs of progressive cardiac disease, pulmonary hypertension, or renal dysfunction.

Hematocrit. Premature infants are more susceptible to iron deficiency anemia than full-term infants and must be followed closely during the first year of life. Hematocrit values should be checked monthly for the first 6 months of life and bimonthly for the following 6 months (see Chapter 25). Anemia of prematurity may be further aggravated by erosive GER and frequent blood tests.

Children with chronic hypoxia may have an elevated hemoglobin and hematocrit values.

Urinalysis. Routine screening is recommended.

Tuberculosis. Routine screening is recommended.

Condition-specific screening

CHEST X-RAY FILMS. Chest x-ray studies should be ordered every 4 to 6 months while the child is symptomatic (Koops, Abman, and Accurso, 1984) to identify changes in the lung structure. If the child has remained free of infection, every 6 months is sufficient.

PULMONARY FUNCTION TESTS. Pulmonary function tests should be done every 6 months by a pulmonologist to document changes in the child's respiratory function. The results are available for the primary care provider.

Drug interactions

Cough suppressants are not recommended for the child with BPD; the cause of the cough should be evaluated and treated. Likewise, antihistamines are not recommended for the child with an artificial airway. The drying effect can cause thickening of airway secretions, presenting the potential for plugging of the smaller peripheral airways and the tracheostomy tube.

Theophylline is a commonly used bronchodilator. If doses are missed, the blood level and resulting effectiveness of the medication may be significantly altered. Theophylline may cause a number of adverse GI side effects, including gastric irritability, nausea, and vomiting. These can be prevented by administering certain preparations with food. If the child is already difficult to feed, this adds an additional challenge. Theophylline levels are altered by some commonly used medications (see Table 5-2), and serum levels must be checked often when these medications are prescribed.

DIFFERENTIAL DIAGNOSIS AND MANAGEMENT OF COMMON PEDIATRIC CONDITIONS
Respiratory tract infections

Respiratory tract infections, either bacterial or viral, are the most common illnesses that children with BPD will contract. Some will be associated with otitis media, sinusitus, or pneumonia. The physical examination focuses initially on the respiratory system. The child should be assessed for an elevated respiratory rate, increased work of breathing with substernal and intercostal retractions, nasal flaring, and a change in baseline breath sounds. Activity level and appetite may decrease. The child should also be assessed for other sources of infection, such as a viral illness. Children dependent on respiratory support, either oxygen, aerosolized bronchodilators, or mechanical ventilation, may require an increased level of support to reverse hypoxia and hypercarbia during this period of respiratory workload.

If a temperature greater than 101° F persists for more than 24 hours despite antipyretic administration, the primary care giver should consider further work-up with a complete blood cell count, secretion culture, and possibly a chest x-ray film. The outcome of the culture and sensitivity test will determine the antibiotic of choice and the route of administration, either enteral or intravenous. A chest x-ray film will determine if the child has atelectasis, an infectious pulmonary process such as pneumonia, or increased pulmonary fluid.

During the months of November to March, respiratory syncytial virus (RSV) should be considered as a possible cause for infection (Hall, 1986; Nederhand et al., 1989). Diagnosis is made via a nasopharyngeal wash done for viral isolation. Treatment involves supportive care. High-risk children with compromised pulmonary status and congenital heart disease may receive ribaviron (Virazole) pharmacologic therapy. Symptoms of RSV infection often persist even with respiratory support and antiviral treatment.

Gastrointestinal disturbances

Disturbances such as diarrhea, nausea, emesis, and feeding intolerances are common in this population. Gastrointestinal disturbances may be associated with a respiratory infection, antibiotic therapy, theophylline toxicity, feeding intolerance to formulas, or a change in osmotic load as a result of changes in caloric density of the formula. If the previous reasons have been reviewed and diarrhea persists, a stool specimen should be obtained to rule out bacterial or viral etiology. Hydration status must be monitored to avoid dehydration. The child may need to be hospitalized for fluid management.

Candida infections

Fungal infections are often contracted after a course of antibiotic treatment. Most sensitive are the warm, moist surfaces of the body, including diaper areas and tracheostomy and gastrostomy stomas. Practicing good skin hygiene and keeping the skin dry prevent the spread of the rash. Topical treatment with antifungal creams such as Nystatin is also indicated.

DEVELOPMENTAL ISSUES
Safety

Children with BPD who are tethered by oxygen or ventilator tubing require close supervision. Respiratory equipment should have alarm systems because free-spirited toddlers will wander beyond the length of the tubing. Restricted and supervised areas of play need to be set up so that there is a safe area for recreation. Children should be supervised at all times to prevent them from manipulating dials on their support equipment. Some devices have safety Plexiglas that covers control dials.

Children with tracheostomy tubes need virtually continuous observation. If they are not directly attended by care givers, a noninvasive monitoring system with an oxygen saturation or apnea monitor should be in place. An accidental decannulation can cause death or serious physical and developmental sequelae. Security of the tracheostomy tube ties should be assessed every 4 to 8 hours and readjusted if greater than one finger-breadth insertion is found between the tracheostomy ties and the child's neck.

Families with toddlers must be warned against the insertion of small toys into ventilator tubing and artificial airways. Playful siblings can contribute to accidental airway decannulations and equipment disconnections when they are insufficiently supervised or educated. Older school-aged and adolescent children can be instructed to observe and intervene with specified responsibilities in emergency or routine situations.

Oxygen is a highly flammable gas and must be used with caution in the home. Parents and caretakers must be taught the necessary safety precautions, and the implementation of these safety measures should be evaluated whenever a home visit is made (Table 7-4).

Table 7-4. Safe use of oxygen at home

Safety guidelines	Rationale
Secure oxygen tank in upright position.	
Keep oxygen tanks at least 5 ft from heat source and electrical devices (e.g., space heaters, heating vents, fireplaces, radios, vaporizers, and humidifiers).	Oxygen tanks are highly explosive; if a horizontally positioned tank explodes, the rapid release of oxygen can catapult it through animate (human bodies) and inanimate objects (walls).
Ensure that no one smokes in the room or in the area of the oxygen tank.	Smoking increases the risk of fire, which could cause the tank to explode; escaped oxygen would feed the fire.
Use lemon-glycerin swabs to relieve dryness around the child's mouth; avoid oil or alcohol-based substances (e.g., petroleum jelly, vitamin A and D ointment, baby oil).	Both alcohol and oil are flammable and increase the risk of fire.
Have the child wear cotton garments.	Silk, wool, and synthetics can generate static electricity and cause fire.
Keep a fire extinguisher readily available.	It is necessary to put out fire immediately.
Turn off both volume regulator and flow regulator whenever oxygen is not in use.	If the volume regulator is on when oxygen is turned on, the child might receive a rapid, forceful flow of oxygen in the face that could be frightening and uncomfortable. Oxygen leakage, which might not be detected because oxygen is odorless, can cause fire.

From Hagedorn MI and Gardner SL: Physiologic sequelae of prematurity: the nurse practitioner's role. part 1. Respiratory issues, *J Pediatr Health Care* 3:288-297, 1989.

The primary care provider should review use of aerosol cans and open flames in the home with the family. Fumes and smoke cause increased irritation to already sensitive airways and a fire hazard is present if oxygen is in use. Care givers and visitors should be warned against smoking in the home and around the child.

Consideration for safety with the use of electrical equipment should be part of the discharge preparation from the hospital. Reinforcement from the primary care provider will help ensure safety. All medical equipment should be electrically grounded. Extension cords should not be used unless approved by the home care equipment vendor.

Before discharge, contact with emergency services is established. These include fire, ambulance, police, electrical, and telephone services. A review of this with families helps reinforce required actions. Inadvertent omission of an essential contact may be identified, thus avoiding needless anxiety or lack of attention in a true emergency (Schreiner, Donar, and Kettrick, 1982; Steele and Morgan, 1989).

Child care

Children requiring mechanical ventilation often have the support of nursing care during the day that is reimbursed by third-party payers. Children who have an artificial airway may or may not have this coverage; this will depend on third-party payer guidelines.

Children who do not require technologic support may not qualify for supportive care through insurance. This can present a problem for families who have limited budgets and cannot afford private in-home baby-sitters. Regular day care services are not recommended because of the incidence of exposure to infections. The primary care provider can assist families in exploring child care options. Hospital discharge programs will often incorporate additional family members or neighbors into the teaching plans if requested.

The primary care provider should review the family support systems to determine if they are satisfactory to the well-being of the child and the family. Nursing care should be used to provide support for families during activity-intensive periods of the day (Donar, 1988). Time without nursing support can be scheduled to incorporate activities and responsibilities within the context of the family structure and routine (Hazlett, 1989).

Increasingly there is an awareness of the need for medical day care facilities that provide services for children requiring supportive treatments. Funding may be supported by insurance. The number of operating facilities is small, but the availability should increase as the need intensifies.

Diet

The high caloric requirements caused by prematurity and the increased work of breathing with BPD require creative ways of providing adequate nutrition in an appealing, tasteful manner that does not require high expenditure of energy to consume or create fluid overload in the compromised infant. It is important for the primary care provider to assess weight gain on a regular basis and evaluate nutritional needs. It is beneficial to maintain contact with the nutritionist from the discharging hospital for assistance in maintaining adequate caloric intake. As mentioned before, children with severe BPD or feeding problems may require supplemental feedings via gavage or gastrostomy tube.

The introduction of solid foods is generally initiated between 4 and 6 months of corrected age or when the infant weighs 6 to 7 kg (Bernbaum et al., 1989). Oral tactile hypersensitivity as a result of oral trauma from passage of nasogastric or orogastric tubes, endotracheal tubes, or repeated suctioning may make it difficult for the child to feed adequately. Early recognition of the problem and intervention by trained health care providers such as nurses, the speech pathologist, or occupational therapist can facilitate feeding and decrease parental frustration and feelings of failure.

Discipline

Children with technologic support learn quickly that the sounding of alarms and monitors immediately summons a care giver. Purposeful disconnections can easily become an attention maneuver. The child and family should be educated with regard to potential risks.

Parents need support and guidance from the primary care provider in recognizing that these children need reasonable consistent discipline. The primary care provider can assist the family in developing consistent responses and discipline approaches that can be used by numerous care givers, including parents, siblings, therapists, and nurses. Approaches should be based on the child's cognitive and developmental age, not chronologic age.

Toileting

Delayed bowel and bladder training may occur as a result of prolonged hospitalization, prematurity, or neurodevelopmental delay. The use of diuretics or theophylline may make bladder training more difficult because of increased frequency of urination. Parents must be assisted in identifying cues indicating the child's neurologic readiness for toilet training.

Sleep patterns

Most hospitals preparing to discharge children with BPD attempt to arrange the child's care to provide for several hours of undisturbed sleep at night. The primary care provider should determine if there has been any change in the child's status as a result of the schedule adjustment. For example, bronchodilator treatments and CPT may be extended from 6 to 8 hours to promote the child's and parents' sleep. If schedules for home life have not been restructured, this is an appropriate time to discuss the schedule with the family and gradually implement changes (Andrews and Nielson, 1988).

The infant's and parents' sleep patterns may be altered because of the monitors placed in the home for children who require mechanical ventilation, receive oxygen therapy, or have a history of apnea. The primary care provider should inquire about the frequency of alarms and determine what type of alarm is appropriate for the child's condition. Readjustment of alarm limits may be warranted if there is a frequent number of false alarms; the limits are set within the physiologic range of the child's heart and respiratory rate. With increasing frequency, the pulse oximeter is the preferred monitor because of the simplicity of use and accuracy of measurement.

It is important to determine how audible the monitor alarm is to the family. If the alarm is so loud that it is very disturbing, the monitor can be placed on a cloth to absorb sound. If the sound is not sufficiently audible, the primary care provider can recommend a commercially available intercom system.

School issues

All children with BPD should have had a thorough developmental evaluation while hospitalized. Plans should be established for outpatient follow-up either at a community-based education center or within the home (Koops, Abman, and Accurso, 1984; Markestad and Fitzhardinge, 1981; Raulin and Shannon, 1986). This is a provision of Public Law 99-457.

The potential for developmental delay, especially in language, in children with BPD is very high (Vohr, Bell, and Oh, 1982). Parents will require ongoing support as the child grows and develops. The primary care giver can assist the family with planning special education needs.

Sexuality

There are no specific problems related to BPD. The children with physical and developmental delays and handicaps will need referrals and follow-up appropriate to their needs. The earliest survivors are now entering their third decade, and to date there has not been any information documenting any difficulties in the area of sexuality.

SPECIAL FAMILY CONCERNS
Financial responsibilities

Most third-party payers fund the cost of equipment and rehabilitative and nursing needs. There are variations from state to state for children supported by Medicaid (see Chapter 4). Financial strains created by numerous visits from medical and rehabilitative care (Donar, 1988; Hazlett, 1989; Scheiner, Donar, and Kettrick, 1982) can stress family budgets. Equipment such as mechanical ventilators, compressors, and monitors increase the use of electricity. Calls to physicians, therapists, vendors, and nursing services increase telephone bills. Some utility companies have programs for families with special needs.

Privacy

The increased numbers of people within the home environment, including nurses, vendors, respiratory therapists, and rehabilitative therapists, can seriously limit family privacy. When the family appears capable of assuming care safely and voices concerns about the lack of privacy and the needs of the child are stabilized, the primary care provider in conjunction with the pediatric respiratory team can suggest decreasing some of this support (Andrews and Nielson, 1988; Donar, 1988; Schreiner, Donar, and Kettrick, 1982).

Once a child has been discharged from the hospital, the reality of the developmental delay may become apparent. Families will need ongoing emotional support to face and adjust to this. The primary care giver can assist with investigation of appropriate educational and rehabilitative programs (Schreiner, Donar, and Kettrick, 1982).

◆ ▬▬▬▬▬▬▬ ◆

SUMMARY OF PRIMARY CARE NEEDS FOR THE CHILD WITH BRONCHOPULMONARY DYSPLASIA

Growth and development

Height and weight are less than average in the majority of children even at 2 years of age.

Plot head circumference, height, and length corrected for gestation age with each visit.

Review caloric intake for adequacy.

Developmental delay is often seen during the first year of life. Continued delay may be seen in children of very low birth weight or with a history of severe BPD. Learning disabilities are often evident during school years.

Immunization

Many children are delayed in receiving immunization because of prolonged hospitalization.

Children should be immunized according to routine schedule based on the chronologic age, not gestational age.

Hospital records must be reviewed.

Pertussis vaccine should be withheld only with just cause because of the high risk of significant morbidity with active disease in this population.

Inactivated polio vaccine may be administered in the hospital before discharge.

Influenza vaccine is recommended yearly for children with chronic lung disease.

Pneumococcal vaccine trials have not been done with this population.

Screening
Vision

Evaluation by a pediatric ophthalmologist should be done every 2 to 3 months during the first year to rule out ROP. Cover test and tracking ability should be screened at each visit.

Myopia and strabismus are common and must be followed in the office and by a pediatric ophthalmologist.

Hearing

A BAER test should be done before discharge from the hospital.

There is a risk of hearing loss because of prematurity and medications.

Routine office screening should be done at each office visit.

Audiometry screening should be done with recurrent serous otitis media.

Speech delays are anticipated in children with tracheostomies.

Dental

Routine screening is recommended.

Hypoplastic and discolored teeth are common.

Oral defensiveness may make dental hygiene difficult.

Blood pressure

Blood pressure should be taken at each visit. Children with abnormal BP findings should be referred to pulmonologist.

Hematocrit

Because of prematurity, iron deficiency anemia is common.

Hematocrit screening must be done frequently during the first year of life.

Chronic hypoxia may cause elevated hemoglobin levels.

Urinalysis

Routine screening is recommended.

Tuberculosis

Routine screening is recommended.

Condition-specific screening
Chest X-ray studies

Radiographic examinations of the lung should be done every 4 to 6 months to document change in the lung structure.

Pulmonary function tests

Pulmonary function tests should be done every 6 months to document changes in the child's respiratory function.

Drug interactions

Theophylline interacts with other medications (see Table 5-2).

SUMMARY OF PRIMARY CARE NEEDS FOR THE CHILD WITH BRONCHOPULMONARY DYSPLASIA — cont'd

---

Cough suppressants may mask an underlying condition. They are not recommended.

Do not use antihistamines with children with tracheostomy tubes because of the thickening of airway secretions.

Differential diagnosis
Respiratory problems

Rule out bacterial or viral infection, atelectasis, pneumonia, and sinusitis. During November to March, consider RSV infections.

Fever

Rule out respiratory tract infection, otitis media, and viral infection.

Gastrointestinal disturbances

Consider feeding intolerances, bacterial and viral infections, GER, or theophylline toxicity.

Skin

For skin problems around tracheostomy and gastrostomy stomas, diaper areas, consider candida infection and cellulitis.

Developmental issues
Safety

Beware of accidental disconnections from respiratory support and accidental decannulations.

Use caution with oxygen use in home.

Electrical safety requires grounded equipment.

Establish emergency service contact before the child is discharged home.

Child care

Recommend that children not supported by oxygen and mechanical ventilation attend home or small day care centers to reduce exposure to infection.

Children with mechanical support may be eligible for nursing support from third-party payers.

Diet

Adequate caloric intake is important for optimal lung repair and growth and development.

Difficulties can be encountered with oral motor function. Oral feedings may need to be supplemented with enteral feedings.

Referral to a pediatric nutritionist early can prevent long-term problems.

Discipline

Children should receive discipline appropriate to their developmental level of understanding.

A consistent plan should be followed.

Toileting

Delayed bowel and bladder training may occur as a result of prolonged hospitalization and the use of diuretics and theophylline.

Sleep pattern

Attempt to evaluate the child's schedule of care to decrease disturbances and provide for the whole family.

Evaluate functioning of monitors.

School issues

Associated problems are covered by Public Law 94-142.

Assist family with developmental evaluations and planning early intervention programs.

Assist families with adjustment to developmental delays.

Sexuality

Care is routine unless associated problems warrant additional care.

Special family concerns

Financial responsibilities are great even with insurance coverage.

There may be a lack of privacy in the home because of the need for medical care givers.

Developmental outcome is uncertain. The potential for developmental delay and persistent medical problems result in great emotional strain on parents.

REFERENCES

American Academy of Pediatrics: Nutritional needs of low-birth weight infants, *Pediatrics* 75:976-986, 1985.

Andrews MM and Nielson DW: Technology dependent children in home, *Pediatr Nurs* 2:111-114, 151, 1988.

Bancalari E and Gerhardt T: Bronchopulmonary dysplasia, *Pediatr Clin North Am* 33:1-23, 1986.

Bancalari E and Sosenko I: Pathogenesis and prevention of neonatal chronic lung disease: recent developments, *Pediatr Pulmonol* 8:109-116, 1990.

Bernbaum J and D'Agostino J: The NICU graduate: managing the major complications, *Contemp Pediatr*, 3: pp 69-82, August 1986.

Bernbaum JE, Friedman S, Hoffman-Williamson M, et al: Preterm infant care after hospital discharge, *Pediatr Rev* 10:195-208, 1989.

Committee on Infectious Diseases: Report of the Committee on infectious disease, ed. 22, Elk Grove Village, IL, 1991, American Academy of Pediatrics.

Davis JM, Sinkin RA, and Aranda J: Drug therapy for bronchopulmonary dysplasia, *Pediatr Pulmonol* 8:117-125, 1990.

Donar ME: Community care: pediatric home mechanical ventilators, *Holistic Nurs Pract* 2:68-80, 1988.

Goldson E: Severe bronchopulmonary dysphagia in the very low birth weight infant: its relationship to developmental outcomes. *J Dev Behav Pediatr* 5:165-168, 1984.

Hagedorn MI and Gardner SL: Physiologic sequelae of prematurity: the nurse practitioner's role, part I, Respiratory issues, *J Pediatr Health Care* 3:288-297, 1989.

Hall CB: Get set for the yearly visitation of RSV, *Contemp Pediatr* 1:22-31, 1986.

Hazlett DE: A study of pediatric home ventilator management: medical, psychosocial, and financial aspects, *J Pediatr Nurs* 4:284-294, 1989.

Koops BL, Abman SH, and Accurso FJ: Outpatient management and follow-up of bronchopulmonary dysplasia, *Clin Perinatol* 2:101-118, 1984.

Logvinoff MM, Lemen RJ, Taussig LM, et al: Bronchodilators and diuretics in children with bronchopulmonary dysplasia, *Pediatr Pulmonol* 1:198-203, 1985.

Ludman WL, Halperin JM, Driscoll JM, et al: Birthweight, respiratory distress syndrome, and cognitive development: a four year follow-up of premature infants, *Am J Dis Child* 141:79-83, 1987.

Markestad T and Fitzhardinge PM: Growth and development in children recovering from bronchopulmonary dysplasia, *J Pediatr* 4:597-602, 1981.

McElheney JE: Parental adaptation to a child with bronchopulmonary dysplasia, *J Pediatr Nurs* 4:346-352, 1989.

Meisels SJ, Plunkett JW, Pasick PL, et al: Growth and development of preterm infants with respiratory distress syndrome and bronchopulmonary dysplasia, *Pediatrics* 3:345-352, 1986.

Meisels SJ, Plunkett JW, Pasick PL, et al: Effects of severity and chronicity of respiratory illness on cognitive development of preterm infants, *J Pediatr Psychol* 1:117-132, 1987.

Merritt T, Northway W, and Boynton B: *Bronchopulmonary dysplasia,* St. Louis, 1988, CV Mosby.

Morray JP, Fox WM, Kettrick RG, et al: Clinical correlates of successful weaning from mechanical ventilation in severe bronchopulmonary dysplasia, *Crit Care Med* 9:815-818, 1981.

Nederhand K, Solon J, Sweet J, et al: Respiratory synctial virus: a nursing perspective, *Pediatr Nurs* 4:342-345, 1989.

Nickerson BG and Taussig LM: Family history of asthma in infants with bronchopulmonary dysplasia, *Pediatrics* 69:1140-1144, 1980.

Northway, WH et al: Late pulmonary sequelae of bronchopulmonary dysplasia, *N Eng J Med*, 323: 1793-1799, 1990.

Philip AG: Oxygen plus pressure plus time: the etiology of bronchopulmonary dysplasia, *Pediatrics* 55:44-50, 1975.

Pridham KF, Martin R, Sondel S, et al: Parental issues in feeding young children with bronchopulmonary dysplasia, *J Pediatr Nurs* 4:177-185, 1989.

Raulin AM and Shannon KA: PNP's: case managers for technology dependent children, *Pediatr Nurs* 12:338-340, 1986.

Sauve RS and Singhal N: Long-term morbidity of infants with bronchopulmonary dysplasia, *Pediatrics* 76:725-733, 1985.

Schlomann P: Developmental gaps of children with chronic conditions and impact on their family, *J Pediatr Nurs* 3:180-187, 1988.

Schreiner MS, Donar ME, and Kettrick RG: Pediatric home mechanical ventilation. In Orlowski J, ed: *Pediatric clinics of North America,* Philadelphia, 1982, WB Saunders, pp 47-60.

Steele NF and Morgan J: Emergency planning for technology-assisted children, *J Pediatr Nurs* 4:81-87, 1989.

Vohr BR, Bell EF, and Oh WM: Infants with bronchopulmonary dysplasia, *Pediatrics* 5:443-447, 1982.

8 *Cancer*

••

Elizabeth Shurtleff Dawes

ETIOLOGY

An estimated 7600 children are diagnosed with cancer annually in the United States (American Cancer Society, 1990). Cancer results when there is a failure of the body to regulate cell production. A proliferation and spread of abnormal cells then occurs, which, if left unchecked, may lead to death of the host (Sutow, Fernbach, and Vietti, 1984). Common sites of malignancy in children include the blood and bone marrow, bone, lymph nodes, brain, central nervous system (CNS), kidneys, and soft tissues (Table 8-1).

Because of the relative rarity of childhood malignancies and the inconsistency in classification, the causes of childhood cancers are poorly identified. It is frequently hypothesized that genetic and environmental influences play a role in the expression of malignancies.

INCIDENCE

The overall incidence of malignancy in children less than 15 years of age is approximately 14:100,000 per year (Bleyer, 1990). The incidence of malignancy among children worldwide varies widely with the exception of Wilms' tumor, which is remarkably uniform. A comparison of the incidence rates of the various childhood malignancies in the United States (see Table 8-1) illustrates a wide variation depending on site.

CLINICAL MANIFESTATIONS AT TIME OF DIAGNOSIS

The signs and symptoms of a malignant disease will depend on the interval between time of origin and diagnosis, as well as the type and location of the tumor. In general, cancer may manifest in one of three ways: (1) as a mass lesion, (2) with symptoms directly related to the tumor, or (3) with nonspecific symptoms (Altman and Schwartz, 1983). The presence of a mass lesion should alert the health care practitioner to the possibility of a malignancy. The few mass lesions considered to be benign on the basis of location or physical appearance alone would include an inflamed lymph node, hemangiomas, thyroglossal duct cyst, fat necrosis, dermoid cysts of the eyebrow, prepubertal breast hyperplasia, lymphangiomas, and torticollis tumors (Altman and Schwartz, 1983). A biopsy of other lesions should be taken in a timely manner to rule out malignancy. Symptoms related directly to the tumor may include bony pain, unexplained bleeding, bruising or petechiae, neurologic signs resulting from brain or spinal cord lesions, hematuria, airway or urinary tract obstruction, or endocrinologic symptoms from hormone production by the tumor. Nonspecific symptoms would include weight loss, diarrhea, low-grade fevers, malaise, or failure to thrive.

Prompt referral to a pediatric cancer treatment

Text continued on p. 122.

Table 8-1. Common pediatric cancers

Type	Site	Incidence (<15 yr)	Etiology	Signs/symptoms	Treatment
LEUKEMIA					
	Bone marrow	40 per 1 million white children per year 24.1 per 1 million black children per year	Genetic factors Constitutional chromosomal abnormalities Familial predisposition (ALL)	Pallor Fatigue, headache Fever, infection Purpura, bruising Organomegaly Bone pain	Combination chemotherapy CNS prophylaxis Radiation therapy and intrathecal chemotherapy Combined intrathecal chemotherapy
Acute lymphoblastic leukemia (ALL)		29.4 per 1 million white children per year 13.7 per 1 million black children per year	Environmental factors Ionizing radiation Chronic chemical exposure Use of alkylating agents for treatment of malignant disease (ANLL) Possible viral infection		
Acute nonlymphoblastic leukemia (ANLL)		4.8 per 1 million white children per year 4.6 per 1 million black children per year			Combination chemotherapy CNS prophylaxis Single-agent intrathecal chemotherapy Bone marrow transplant in first remission
CENTRAL NERVOUS SYSTEM					
Brainstem/cerebellar Medulloblastoma	Brain/brainstem Midline cerebellar	24.3 per 1 million white children per year 21.3 per 1 million black children per year	Genetic factors Heritable disease Familial Environmental factors Chronic chemical exposure Ionizing radiation Other primary malignancies Exogenous immunosuppression	Early Decreased academic performance Fatigue Personality changes Intermittent headache Late Morning headache Vomiting and nausea Diplopia/visual changes Brainstem/cerebellar Deficits of balance/positioning	Anticonvulsants, if symptom present Treatment of hydrocephalus Corticosteroids Shunting Surgical resection (if operable) Radiation therapy
Ependymoma	Ependymal lining of ventricular system or central cord of spinal cord				

	Location	Etiology/Incidence	Signs and Symptoms	Treatment
Supratentorial			**Supratentorial**	
Astrocytomas	Ventricles, midline diencephalous, cerebrum		Nonspecific headache	
Craniopharyngioma	Sella turcica		Seizures	
Gliomas	Visual pathway		Hemiparesis	
Primitive neuroectodermal tumor or germ cell	Pineal region			
NON-HODGKIN'S LYMPHOMA		Multifactorial	Generally rapid progression	Treatment of emergent symptoms
	Usually generalized	Immunodeficiency	Lymphoblastic lymphoma	Multiagent chemotherapy
		Exogenous immunosuppression	Dysphagia	CNS prophylaxis
		9.1 per 1 million white children per year	Swelling of neck, face, upper extremities	
		4.6 per 1 million black children per year	Supradiaphragmatic lymphadenopathy	
Lymphoblastic lymphoma	Anterior mediastinum		Respiratory distress	
	Lymph nodes		Small noncleaved lymphoma	Multiagent chemotherapy
	Bone marrow		Abdominal pain or swelling	CNS prophylaxis
	Abdomen		Change in bowel habits	
Small noncleaved lymphoma Burkitt's lymphoma Non-Burkitt's lymphoma	Upper respiratory tract		Nausea/vomiting	
	Bone marrow (infrequent)		GI* bleeding	
	Mediastinium (rare)		Rarely, intestinal perforation	
Large cell lymphoma	Lymph ndoes		Inguinal/iliac/adenopathy	
	Cutaneous lesions		Intussception	
	Mediastinum			
	Abdomen			
	Head, neck			

Continued.

Data from Young JL, Reis LG, Silverberg E, et al: *Cancer* 58:598-602, 1986.
*GI, gastrointestinal.

Table 8-1. Common pediatric cancers—cont'd

Type	Site	Incidence (<15 yr)	Etiology	Signs/symptoms	Treatment
NON-HODGKIN'S LYMPHOMA—cont'd				Large cell lymphoma As cited earlier, depending on site	Multiagent chemotherapy
HODGKIN'S LYMPHOMA	Single lymph node or lymphatic chains Mediastinal mass Spleen	7.3 per 1 million white children per year 5.2 per 1 million black children per year	Genetic factors Familial predisposition Environmental influence Iatrogenic or acquired immunodeficiency Infectious etiology	Lymphadenopathy Organomegaly Fatigue Anorexia/weight loss/fever	Splenectomy, if surgical staging Multiagent chemotherapy Radiation therapy
NEUROBLASTOMA	Anywhere along the sympathetic nervous system chain Most commonly Abdomen Adrenal gland Paraspinal ganglion Other sites, including paraspinal area of thorax, neck, pelvis	8.7 per 1 million white children per year 7.4 per 1 million black children per year	Possible genetic factors Familial predisposition Associated with neurofibromatosis, Beckwith-Wiedemann syndrome, nisidiroblastosis, fetal alcohol syndrome Associated with fetal hydantoin syndrome	Dependent on primary site, site of metastases Presence of a mass (abdomen, thoracic, cervical, pelvic, liver) Symptoms from compression of mass (Horner's syndrome, edema of lower extremities secondary to vascular compression, hypertension caused by compression of renal vasculature, cord compression symptoms [paresis, paralysis, bowel/bladder dysfunction]) Skin or subcutaneous nodules (infants only) Nonspecific symptoms (fever, weight loss, failure to thrive, generalized pain) Rarely syndrome of opsoclonus-myoclonus	Treatment of emergent symptoms Surgery (staging excision of tumor, evaluation of treatment) Radiation therapy Combination chemotherapy

	Location	Incidence	Etiology	Signs/Symptoms	Treatment
SOFT TISSUE SARCOMAS					
Rhabdomyosarcoma / Undifferentiated sarcoma	Anywhere in body	8.0 per 1 million white children per year / 7.7 per 1 million black children per year	Environmental factors / Ionizing radiation / Possible viral etiology	Dependent on location and size of tumor	Surgical removal (if feasible) / Radiation therapy for residual tumor / Multiagent systemic chemotherapy
KIDNEY					
Wilms' tumor (nephroblastoma, renal embryoma)	Unilateral, bilateral	7.7 per 1 million white children per year / 10.0 per 1 million black children per year	Genetic factors / Association with specific chromosomal abnormalities / Familial predisposition / Environmental factors / Chronic chemical exposure (hydrocarbons/lead)	Asymptomatic mass / Malaise, pain / Microscopic or gross hematuria / Hypertension	Complete surgical excision (if bilateral, nephrectomy of more involved site, excisional biopsy/partial nephrectomy of smaller lesion in remaining kidney) / Multiagent chemotherapy / Radiation therapy
BONE TUMORS					
Osteosarcoma	Long bones of extremities	6.5 per 1 million white children per year / 4.8 per 1 million black children per year	Genetic factors / Familial predisposition (hereditary retinoblastoma)	Pain over involved area with or without swelling (often 3–6 mo or longer)	Multiagent chemotherapy / Surgical excision of tumor preserving as much function of primary site as possible
Ewing's sarcoma	Bones of pelvis, humerus, femur, generally axial skeleton	2.9 per 1 million white children per year / 4.0 per 1 million black children per year	Association with skeletal and genitourinary abnormalities / Genetic factors / Association with hereditary retinoblastoma	In presence of metastatic disease nonspecific symptoms (fatigue, anorexia, weight loss, intermittent fever, malaise)	Amputation may be necessary, if extent of disease or location does not allow complete excision / Localized radiation therapy (Ewing's sarcoma)

Continued.

Table 8-1. Common pediatric cancers—cont'd

Type	Site	Incidence (<15 yr)	Etiology	Signs/symptoms	Treatment
RETINOBLASTOMA	Eye	3.3 per 1 million white children per year 4.3 per 1 million black children per year	Genetic factors Familial predisposition Gene mutation (nonhereditary)	Leukokoria (cat's eye reflex) Squint Strabismus Orbital inflammation	Surgery (resection, enucleation with extensive disease; salvage of one eye attempted in bilateral disease) Radiation therapy Chemotherapy (usually palliative)

center ensures specimens for staging are properly obtained and the child is enrolled in multiinstitutional treatment studies. The initial work-up is crucial to the accurate and timely establishment of a diagnosis. It should include a thorough history and physical examination, laboratory tests, specific nuclear and radiologic examinations, ultrasonography, surgery, and frequently a bone marrow aspirate, bone marrow biopsy, lumbar puncture, or a combination of the three, depending on the type of tumor suspected.

TREATMENT

Cancer treatment involves the concurrent or sequential use of surgery, chemotherapy, radiation therapy, immunotherapy, and less frequently, bone marrow transplantation. Bone marrow transplantation is used both as an initial therapy of choice and as a salvage therapy when other therapies have failed.

A child's treatment protocol, determined by the type of cancer and the extent of disease, consists of a schedule and combination of therapies shown to be effective in treating the condition. A particular disease may have several treatment protocols ("arms") which are based on an accepted standard treatment. Because no protocol is known to be more effective than another, ongoing research investigates various therapies that maximize treatment efficacy while minimizing toxicity. Before a child is assigned to a particular protocol, informed consent is obtained from the parents and, if appropriate, the child. If a child is on an experimental therapy protocol, the family may elect to withdraw the child from the study at any time and have the child treated according to standard therapy (Fochtman et al., 1982).

Surgical intervention is used to (1) obtain a biopsy specimen, (2) determine the extent of disease, (3) remove primary or metastatic lesions, (4) evaluate previously unresectable tumors, and (5) relieve symptoms. Surgical procedures are also used in placing indwelling venous access devices and for displacing organs outside of the radiation field (e.g., ovaries during pelvic irradiation).

The goal of chemotherapy is to interrupt the cell cycle of proliferating malignant cells while minimizing the damage to normal cells. In combination chemotherapy, different drugs are used to

Text continued on p. 128.

Table 8-2. Summary of chemotherapeutic agents used in the treatment of childhood cancers*

Agent/administration	Side effects and toxicity	Comments and specific nursing considerations
ALKYLATING AGENTS		
Mechlorethamine (nitrogen mustard, Mustargen) IV, IT‡	N/V§ (½-8 hrs later) (severe) BMD‖ (2-3 wks later) Alopecia Local phlebitis	Vesicant†
Cyclophosphamide (Cytoxan, CTX,¶ Endoxan) PO, IV, IM‡	N/V (3-4 hrs later) (severe at high doses) BMD (10-14 days later) Alopecia Hemorrhagic cystitis Severe immunosuppression Stomatitis (rare) Hyperpigmentation Transverse ridging of nails Infertility	BMD has platelet-sparing effect Give dose early in day to allow adequate fluids afterward Force fluids before administering drug and for 2 days after to prevent chemical cystitis; encourage frequent voiding even during night Warn parents to report signs of burning on urination or hematuria to practitioner
Chlorambucil (Leukeran) PO	N/V (mild) BMD (7-14 days later) Diarrhea Dermatitis Less commonly may be hepatotoxicity	Usually slow onset of side effects; side effects related to high doses
ANTIMETABOLITES		
Cytosine arabinoside (Ara-C, Cytosar, Cytarabine, arabinosyl cytosine) IV, IM, SC,‡ IT	N/V (mild) BMD (7-14 days later) Mucosal ulceration Immunosuppression Hepatitis (usually subclinical)	Crosses blood-brain barrier Use with caution in patients with hepatic dysfunction
5-Azacytidine (5-AzaC) IV	N/V (moderate) BMD (7-14 days later) Diarrhea	Infuse slowly via IV drip to decrease severity of N/V
Mercaptopurine (6-MP, Purinethol) PO	N/V (mild) Diarrhea Anorexia Stomatitis BMD (4-6 wks later) Immunosuppression Dermatitis Less commonly may be hepatic dysfunction	6-MP is an analog of xanthine; therefore allopurinol (Zyloprim) delays its metabolism and increases its potency, necessitating a lower dose (⅓ to ¼) of 6-MP

Continued.

*Table includes principal drugs used in the treatment of childhood cancers. Several other conventional and investigational chemotherapeutic agents may be employed in the treatment regimen.

†Vesicants (sclerosing agents) can cause severe cellular damage if even minute amounts of the drug infiltrate surrounding tissue. Only nurses experienced with chemotherapeutic agents should administer vesicants. These drugs must be given through a free-flowing intravenous line. The infusion is stopped *immediately* if any sign of infiltration (pain, stinging, swelling, or redness at needle site) occurs. Interventions for extravasation vary, but each nurse should be aware of the institution's policies and implement them at once.

‡IV, intravenous; IT, intrathecal; PO, by mouth; IM, intramuscular; SC, subcutaneous.

§N/V, nausea and vomiting. Mild = <20% incidence; moderate = 20% to 70% incidence; severe = >75% incidence.

‖BMD, bone marrow depression.

¶Abbreviations stand for chemical compound.

Table 8-2. Summary of chemotherapeutic agents used in the treatment of childhood cancers — cont'd

Agent/administration	Side effects and toxicity	Comments and specific nursing considerations

Methotrexate (MTX, Amethopterin) PO, IV, IM, IT
May be given in conventional doses (mg/m^2) or high doses (g/m^2)
	N/V (severe at high doses)
	Diarrhea
	Mucosal ulceration (2-5 days later)
	BMD (10 days later)
	Immunosuppression
	Dermatitis
	Photosensitivity
	Alopecia (uncommon)
	Toxic effects include
	  Hepatitis (fibrosis)
	  Osteoporosis
	  Nephropathy
	  Pneumonitis (fibrosis)
	Neurologic toxicity with IT use — pain at injection site, meningismus (signs of meningitis without actual inflammation), especially fever and headache; potential sequelae — transient or permanent hemiparesis, convulsions, dementia, and death
		Side effects and toxicity are dose related
		Potency and toxicity increased by reduced renal function, salicylates, sulfonamides, and aminobenzoic acid; avoid use of these substances, such as aspirin
		High dose therapy:
		  Citrovorum factor (folinic acid or leucovorin) decreases cytotoxic action of MTX; used as an antidote for overdose and to enhance normal cell recovery following high-dose therapy; avoid use of vitamins containing folic acid during MTX therapy unless prescribed by physician
		IT therapy:
		  Drug *must* be mixed with preservative-free diluent
		  Report signs of neurotoxicity immediately

6-Thioguanine (6-TG, Thioguan) PO	N/V (mild)
	BMD (7-14 days later)
	Stomatitis
	Rarely
	  Dermatitis
	  Photosensitivity
	  Liver dysfunction
		Side effects are unusual

PLANT ALKALOIDS Vincristine (Oncovin) IV	Neurotoxicity — paresthesia (numbness), ataxis, weakness, foot drop, hyporeflexia, constipation (adynamic ileus), hoarseness (vocal cord paralysis), abdominal, chest, and jaw pain, mental depression Fever N/V (mild) BMD (minimal; 7-14 days later) Alopecia	Vesicant Report signs of neurotoxicity because may necessitate cessation of drug Individuals with underlying neurologic problems may be more prone to neurotoxicity Monitor stool patterns closely; administer stool softener Excreted primarily by liver into biliary system; administer cautiously to anyone with biliary disease
Vinblastine (Velban) IV	Neurotoxicity (same as for vincristine but less severe) N/V (mild) BMD (especially neutropenia; 7-14 days later) Alopecia	Same as for vincristine

Table 8-2. Summary of chemotherapeutic agents used in the treatment of childhood cancers—cont'd

Agent/administration	Side effects and toxicity	Comments and specific nursing considerations
VP-16-213 (Etoposide, Ve-Pesid)	N/V (mild to moderate) BMD (7-14 days later) Alopecia Hypotension with rapid infusion Bradycardia Diarrhea (infrequent) Stomatitis (rare) May reactivate erythema of irradiated skin (rare) Allergic reaction with anaphylaxis possible	Give slowly via IV drip with child recumbent Have emergency drugs available at bedside*
ANTIBIOTICS		
Actinomycin-D (Dactinomycin, Cosmegen, ACT-D) IV	N/V (2-5 hrs later) (moderate) BMD (especially platelets; 7-14 days later) Immunosuppression Mucosal ulceration Abdominal cramps Diarrhea Anorexia (may last few weeks) Alopecia Acne Erythema or hyperpigmentation of previously irradiated skin Fever Malaise	Vesicant Enhances cytotoxic effects of radiation therapy but increases toxic effects May cause serious desquamation of irradiated tissue

Doxorubicin (Adriamycin, Doxyrubicin) IV	N/V (moderate)
	Stomatitis
	BMD (7-14 days later)
	Fever, chills
	Local phlebitis
	Alopecia
	Cumulative-dose toxicity includes
	  Cardiac abnormalities
	  ECG changes
	  Heart failure
		Vesicant (extravasation may *not* cause pain)
		Use only sterile distilled water as a diluent
		Observe for any changes in heart rate or rhythm and signs of failure
		Cumulative dose must not exceed 550 mg/m²
		Warn parents that drug causes urine to turn red (for up to 12 days after administration); this is normal, not hematuria

Daunorubicin (Daunomycin, Rubidomycin) IV	Similar to doxorubicin	Similar to doxorubicin
Bleomycin (Blenoxane) IV, IM, SC	Allergic reaction—fever, chills, hypotension, anaphylaxis Fever (nonallergic) N/V (mild) Stomatitis Cumulative dose effects include Skin—rash, hyperpigmentation,	Should give test dose (SC) before therapeutic dose administered Have emergency drugs* at bedside Hypersensitivity occurs with first one to two doses May give acetaminophen before drug to reduce likelihood of fever

Continued.

Table 8-2. Summary of chemotherapeutic agents used in the treatment of childhood cancers—cont'd

Agent/administration	Side effects and toxicity	Comments and specific nursing considerations
	thickening, ulceration, peeling, nail changes, alopecia Lungs—pneumonitis with infiltrate that can progress to fatal fibrosis	Concentration of drug in skin and lungs accounts for toxic effects
HORMONES		
Corticosteroids (prednisone most frequently used; many proprietary names such as Meticorten, Deltasone, Paracort) PO; also IM or IV but rarely used	For short-term use, no acute toxicity Usual side effects are mild: moon face, fluid retention, weight gain, mood changes, increased appetite, gastric irritation, insomnia, susceptibility to infection	Explain expected effects, especially in terms of body image, increased appetite, and personality changes Monitor weight gain Recommend moderate salt restriction Administer with antacid and early in morning (sometimes given every other day to minimize side effects) May need to disguise bitter taste (crush tablet and mix with syrup, jam, ice cream or other highly-flavored substance; use ice to numb tongue before administration; place tablet in gelatin capsule if child can swallow it) Observe for potential infection sites; usual inflammatory response and fever are absent
	Long-term effects of chronic steroid administration are mood changes, hirsutism, trunk obesity (buffalo hump), thin extremities, muscle wasting and weakness, osteoporosis, poor wound healing, bruising, potassium loss, gastric bleeding, hypertension, diabetes mellitus, growth retardation	All of above; in addition, encourage foods high in potassium (bananas, raisins, prunes, coffee, chocolate) Test stools for occult blood Monitor blood pressure Test blood for sugar and urine for acetone Observe for signs of abrupt steroid withdrawal: flulike symptoms, hypotension, hypoglycemia, shock
ENZYMES		
L-asparaginase (Elspar) IV, IM	Allergic reactions (including anaphylactic shock) Fever N/V (mild) Anorexia Weight loss Arthralgia Toxicity: Liver dysfunction Hyperglycemia Renal failure Pancreatitis	Have emergency drugs at bedside* Record signs of allergic reaction, such as urticaria, facial edema, hypotension, or abdominal cramps Check weight daily Normally, BUN and ammonia levels rise as a result of drug—not evidence of liver damage Check urine for sugar and blood amylase

*Emergency drugs include oxygen and parenteral preparations of epinephrine 1:1000, diphenhydramine or similar antihistamine, aminophylline, corticosteriods, and vasopressors.

Table 8-2. Summary of chemotherapeutic agents used in the treatment of childhood cancers—cont'd

Agent/administration	Side effects and toxicity	Comments and specific nursing considerations
NITROSOUREAS		
Carmustine (BCNU) IV Lomustine (CCNU) PO	N/V (2-6 hours later) (severe) BMD (3-4 weeks later) Burning pain along IV infusion (usually due to alcohol diluent) BCNU—flushing and facial burning on infusion	Prevent extravasation; contact with skin causes brown spots Oral form—give 4 hours after meals when stomach is empty Reduce IV burning by diluting drug and infusing slowly via IV drip Crosses blood-brain barrier
OTHER AGENTS		
Hydroxyurea (Hydrea) PO	N/V (mild) Anorexia Less commonly Diarrhea BMD Mucosal ulceration Alopecia Dermatitis	Must be given cautiously in children with renal dysfunction
Procarbazine (Matulane) PO	N/V (moderate) BMD (3-4 wks later) Lethargy Dermatitis Myalgia Arthralgia Less commonly Stomatitis Neuropathy Alopecia Diarrhea	Central nervous system depressants (phenothiazines, barbiturates) enhance central nervous system symptoms Monoamine oxidase (MAO) inhibition sometimes occurs; therefore all other drugs are avoided unless medically approved; red wine, fava beans, and broad bean pods are avoided
Dacarbazine (DTIC-Dome) IV	N/V (especially after first dose) (severe) BMD (7-14 days later) Alopecia Flulike syndrome Burning sensation in vein during infusion (not extravasation)	Vesicant (less sclerosive) Must be given cautiously in patients with renal dysfunction Decrease IV rate or use warm moist towels on IV site to decrease burning
Cisplatin (Platinol) IV	Renal toxicity (severe) N/V (1-4 hrs later) (severe) BMD (mild, 2-3 wks later) Ototoxicity Neurotoxicity (similar to that for vincristine) Electrolyte disturbances, especially hypomagnesium, hypocalcemia, hypokalemia, and hypophosphatemia	Renal function (creatinine clearance) must be assessed before giving drug Must maintain hydration before and during therapy (specific gravity of urine is used to assess hydration) Mannitol may be given IV to promote osmotic diuresis and drug clearance Monitor intake and output Monitor for signs of ototoxicity (e.g., ringing in ears) and neurotoxicity; re-

Continued.

Table 8-2. Summary of chemotherapeutic agents used in the treatment of childhood cancers—cont'd

Agent/administration	Side effects and toxicity	Comments and specific nursing considerations
	Anaphylactic reactions may occur	port signs immediately; ensure that routine audiogram is done before treatment for baseline and routinely during treatment
		Do not use aluminum needle; reaction with aluminum decreases potency of drug
		Monitor for signs of electrolyte loss; i.e. hypomagnesium—tremors, spasm, muscle weakness, lower extremity cramps, irregular heartbeat, convulsions, delirium
		Have emergency drugs at bedside*

*Emergency drugs include oxygen and parenteral preparations of epinephrine 1:1000, diphenhydramine or similar antihistamine, aminophylline, corticosteroids, and vasopressors.

disrupt the cell cycle at different phases. This increases the exposure of the malignant cells to cytotoxic agents.

Chemotherapeutic agents may be either cell-cycle phase specific or nonspecific. Cell-cycle phase–specific drugs kill cells only in a certain stage of the cell's development and are most effective on rapidly growing cells. Along with malignant cells, the cells of the bone marrow, hair follicles, and intestinal epithelium are susceptible to damage from these drugs. Cell-cycle phase–nonspecific drugs kill cells regardless of their stage of development. They are most effective on slowly growing cells and have been effective in cells in the resting phase. Chemotherapeutic agents are further classified by their mechanism of action (Evans et al., 1989). The major classifications include alkylating agents, antimetabolites, vinca alkaloids, antibiotics, and corticosteroids. Side effects and toxicities vary depending on the specific agent (Table 8-2).

Radiation therapy often is used in conjunction with surgery, chemotherapy, or both. The goal of radiation therapy is to destroy the cancer cells while minimizing the high incidence of complications and long-term sequelae. The role of radiation therapy may be definitive, adjunctive, or palliative (Altman and Schwartz, 1983). Definitive treatment is given

with curative intent to a tumor on which a biopsy has been performed or that has been partially resected. In adjunctive radiotherapy, a primary tumor, although totally resected, is at risk for a local recurrence. This area is then treated with a lower dose of radiation than what would be given to control the tumor without surgery. Palliative radiotherapy is used to relieve symptoms of incurable disease after more conservative methods have proved ineffective.

The tumor's response to radiation is dependent on the type of tumor, type and dose of radiation delivered, and size of the area irradiated. These factors also influence the type and severity of side effects and long-term sequelae. Many side effects are similar to those of chemotherapy. However, rather than a systemic response, the side effects are generally related to the irradiated area. They include nausea and vomiting, diarrhea, mucositis, cataracts, and skin changes.

The goal of immunotherapy is to stimulate the body's natural immune system to selectively target and destroy malignant cells. The premise of immunotherapy is that cells undergoing neoplastic changes acquire new antigens. The normal immune system of the host recognizes these new antigens as a foreign body and mounts an immune response, resulting in the destruction of the tumor. Interferon and the use of monoclonal antibodies are examples of immunotherapeutic agents.

Bone marrow transplantation is used in treating relapsed acute lymphoblastic leukemia (ALL), acute nonlymphocytic leukemia (ANLL) (Wiley and House, 1988), non-Hodgkin's lymphomas, Ewing's sarcoma (Cogliano-Shutta, Broda, and Gress, 1985), Hodgkin's disease, and neuroblastoma. In some institutions, bone marrow transplantation is the initial therapy of choice for children with high-risk (having clinical and laboratory features at diagnosis that are known to have a poor prognosis) ALL and acute myelogenous leukemia (AML). Bone marrow transplantation allows for potentially lethal doses of chemotherapy and radiation to be given to rid the body of all malignant cells. The donor marrow replaces the child's destroyed marrow and after engraftment should produce the donor's nonmalignant functioning cells.

Four forms of bone marrow transplantation are syngeneic, allogenic, autologus and tissue-identical unrelated. Syngeneic transplantation uses genetically identical bone marrow from a twin. Allogenic transplantation uses marrow from a tissue-identical donor who is preferably related to the recipient. An autologus transplant is one in which the marrow is collected from the affected child. An autologus transplant may be used when the tumor is not in the marrow or the marrow can be purged (e.g., in AML) of all tumor cells. Tissue-identical unrelated transplantation uses a donor from outside the immediate family who meets very specific tissue typing criteria.

Bone marrow transplantation is a promising treatment modality for certain malignancies in children. However, it must be realistically viewed in terms of the potentially fatal toxicities, developmental sequelae, and psychosocial and financial impact on the child and family (Wiley and House, 1988). A second concern for the family is using an otherwise healthy sibling as the marrow donor. Although the marrow harvest itself entails little risk (Bortin and Buckner, 1983), the use of anesthesia has a small but increasing risk with decreasing age (Wiley and House, 1988).

PROGNOSIS

The prognosis of a malignancy is dependent on the age of the child, primary site, extent of the disease,

and cell type. Over the past 20 years dramatic advances have been made in the treatment and potential cure of children with cancer (Table 8-3). The current figures on ALL estimate a durable (defined as 5 years or greater) event-free survival to be 50% to 70%, with a slightly higher outcome for individuals treated on multiinstitutional studies (Chauvenet and Wofford, 1990). The outcomes for ANLL are estimated to be 35% to 40%. The prognosis for brain tumors is also steadily improving, with the 5-year survival rate approximating 59%. This is attributed to the combined therapy of surgical resection, radiation therapy, and multiagent chemotherapy (Sutow, Fernbach, and Vietti, 1984).

Non-Hodgkin's lymphoma constitutes a wide variation in tumors. The estimated overall survival rate for this group is approximately 68%. Hodgkin's disease boasts approximately an 85% to 90% cure rate, but there is controversy over what constitutes the optimal therapy. The issues center around striking a balance between aggressive treatment with lower relapse rates, higher potential for second malignancies, and long-term sequelae as opposed to less aggressive therapy, with potentially higher relapse rates but fewer late effects.

An overall survival rate for those who have neuroblastoma is approximately 56%. When the survival rates are viewed by age group, there is a significantly higher survival rate for children less than 1 year of age. For children more than 1 year of age with widely metastatic disease (constituting 40% of the total neuroblastoma population), there is less than 10% chance of survival (Chauvenet and Wofford, 1990). Those with Wilms' tumor have an estimated survival rate of 83%; the majority of these children have less advanced forms of the disease with a favorable histology. Likewise with rhabdomyosarcoma, childrens' overall survival rate is 65%, with 80% survival for children with less advanced disease compared with 25% for those with distant metastatic disease.

Those with bone cancers, including osteogenic sarcoma and Ewing's sarcoma, have an approximately 60% to 80% survival for the former and a markedly improved 74% for the latter. The improved prognosis for Ewing's sarcoma is attributed to the introduction of adjuvant chemotherapy. Long-term disease-free survival is a reality for the majority of children with a malignant disease, but

Table 8-3. Trends in survival of children with malignant disease

Site	Relative 5-yr survival rates (%)				
			Yr of diagnosis		
	1960-1963*	1970-1973*	1974-1976†	1977-1980†	1981-1986†
All sites	28	45	55.1	61.6	66.8‡
Acute lymphocytic leukemia	4	34	53.4	67.9	72.8‡
Acute myeloid leukemia	3	5	16.1	25.4§	24.3§
Wilms' tumor	33	70	74.1	79.6	83.3
Brain and nervous system	35	45	54.5	55.9	59.0
Neuroblastoma	25	40	48.6	52.3	56.4
Bone	20	30	51.9§	47.1	53.8§
Hodgkin's disease	52	90	80.4	87.5	85.0
Non-Hodgkin's lymphomas	18	26	42.3	50.1	68.3‡

From American Cancer Society: Cancer statistics. *CA*, Statistics Branch, National Cancer Institute.
*Rates are based on End Results Group data from a series of hospital registries and one population-based registry.
†Rates are from the SEER program. They are based on data from population-based registries in Connecticut, New Mexico, Utah, Iowa, Hawaii, Atlanta, Detroit, Seattle, Puget Sound, and San Francisco-Oakland. Rates are based on follow-up of patients through 1986.
‡The difference in rates between 1974-1976 and 1980-1986 is statistically significant ($p < 0.05$).
§The standard error of the survival rate is between 5 and 10 percentage points.

research needs to continue to focus on therapy for those with more advanced disease.

ASSOCIATED PROBLEMS
Vascular access

Children receiving prolonged, intensive treatment are required to endure frequent venipunctures for laboratory tests, chemotherapy, administration of blood products, antibiotic therapy, and nutritional support (Cameron, 1987). These children are often aided by the placement of a long-term indwelling venous access device, which helps minimize the trauma of frequent needle sticks and vein irritation from the chemotherapy. Access devices include right atrial catheters (Broviac, Hickman, Corcath) and a subcutaneous (SC) port or reservoir (Port-a-cath, Infus-A-Port, MediPort) (Marcoux, Fisher, and Wong, 1990).

The right atrial catheters are single or double lumen silicone catheters with a Dacron felt cuff that anchors the catheter under the skin and provides a barrier to infection (Hartman and Shochat, 1987). The right atrial catheter has an internal and external portion, whereas the SC port or reservoir is totally implanted below the skin. The catheter tip lies at the junction of the superior vena cava and the right atrium. The catheter is tunneled under the skin and attached to a port that lies in an SC pocket on the chest (Marcoux, Fisher, and Wong, 1990). Venous access is achieved by puncturing the skin above the reservoir and passing a specially designed needle through the silicone membrane into the port receptacle.

The patency of all long-term venous access devices is maintained through periodic flushing with heparinized saline. Care of these lines is taught to the child (when appropriate) and parents. Complications of the indwelling venous access devices include infection, occlusion of the catheter because of thrombus and fibrin formation, damage to the external portion of the catheter, and rarely, cardiac tamponade (Marcoux, Fisher, and Wong, 1990).

Because the child with cancer is at risk for profound neutropenia due to therapy, prompt and aggressive treatment of infection at the catheter site is necessary. Most external infections can be cleared with oral antibiotics; however, tunnel infections and septicemia require IV antibiotics and possible catheter removal.

Therapy-related complications

Nausea and vomiting. Nausea and vomiting are common side effects of chemotherapy and radiation. Nausea and vomiting can have a profound physiologic and psychologic impact on the child receiving therapy (Frick et al., 1988). Problems including dehydration, chemical and electrolyte imbalances, and decreased nutritional intake can lead to decreased compliance or termination of treatment.

The mechanisms involved in nausea and vomiting are complex, and no single drug will consistently control these side effects. The situation is further complicated by the wide variation in response by the individual child to both the chemotherapeutic agent and the antiemetic. The antiemetic should be given before nausea and vomiting occur and should be continued until the symptoms have resolved. Generally nausea and vomiting related to the chemotherapy will not last longer than 48 hours after chemotherapy administration (Noyes, 1986).

Anorexia and weight loss. During therapy, anorexia and weight loss are common and can be attributed to both the disease and its treatment. The psychologic impact of cancer and the tumor's metabolic influence can contribute to weight loss. Treatment-induced nausea and vomiting and changes in taste acuity may lead to food aversion. Therefore, it is imperative to closely monitor weight throughout treatment. Oral supplements and, in some cases, nasogastric feedings or hyperalimentation may be necessary.

Bone marrow suppression. Bone marrow suppression is another side effect of chemotherapy and radiation. With chemotherapy, leukopenia, thrombocytopenia, and anemia begin within 7 to 10 days after drug administration, and the nadir (the point at which the blood cell counts are the lowest) occurs at approximately 14 days. The marrow then recovers by 21 to 28 days. The exact time of the nadir will vary depending on the specific chemotherapeutic agent. Close monitoring is necessary to determine the extent of marrow suppression.

CALCULATION OF ABSOLUTE NEUTROPHIL COUNT (ANC)

White blood count (WBC) = 7400 (also expressed as 7.4 k/UL; $7.4 \times 10^3/mm^3$)
Neutrophils (poly. segs) = 40%
Nonsegmented neutrophils (bands) = 12%
Step 1: Determine total percent neutrophils (poly. segs + bands)
$$40\% + 12\% = 52\% \ (0.52)$$
Step 2: Multiply WBC by % neutrophils
$$ANC = 7400 \times 0.52$$
$$ANC = 3848 \ (normal)$$
WBC = 900 (0.9 k/UL; $0.9 \times 10^3/mm^3$
Neutrophils (poly. segs) = 7%
Nonsegmented neutrophils (bands) = 7%
Step 1: 7% + 7% = 14% (0.14)
Step 2: $ANC = 900 \times 0.14$
$$ANC = 126 \ (severely \ neutropenic)$$

Leukopenia refers to the presence of a low number of all white blood cells (WBCs), whereas neutropenia refers specifically to a low neutrophil cell count. Neutrophils are the body's main defense against bacterial infection. It is necessary to determine the absolute neutrophil count (ANC) (see the box above) because the incidence and severity of infection are inversely related to the ANC (Barson and Brady, 1987).

Infections represent the major cause of death in children with cancer (Albano and Pizzo, 1988). The use of good handwashing techniques by the child, the parents, and the care givers is paramount to reducing the spread of pathogens. Good personal hygiene by the child, including thorough dental care, is also important. The child with neutropenia should avoid individuals who are ill, crowded situations, and anyone with a communicable disease, especially chickenpox. Rectal temperatures and suppositories should also be avoided because abrading the rectal mucosa increases the risk of introducing bacteria into the bloodstream.

The child who is thrombocytopenic may require transfusions of platelets because of the risk of serious hemorrhage (Happ, 1987). If the platelet count is less than 20,000 or in the presence of

132

bleeding, cytomegalovirus (CMV)–negative, irradiated platelets should be administered.

A child whose hemoglobin level is less than 8g or who is symptomatic (i.e., shortness of breath, headache, or dizziness) may require a transfusion of CMV-negative, irradiated packed red blood cells (RBCs). Any child who is a potential bone marrow transplant candidate must receive CMV-negative products because they will be at greater risk of complications from CMV infection if they are CMV positive at the time of transplant.

Hair loss. A distinguishing therapy-related complication that is bothersome to children is alopecia. A temporary condition, it results from damage of the hair follicles by chemotherapy and radiation. The child can be reassured that the hair will grow back after therapy; however, initially the texture and color may be slightly different.

Late effects

As the survival rates continually improve, the long-term effects of therapy are becoming evident. The goal of current therapy is not merely improving survival but reducing physiologic and developmental morbidity as well. A growing body of knowledge indicates that both chemotherapy and radiation have adverse effects on normal tissues that may not be manifested for months or years after therapy. The development of second malignancies (Altman and Schwartz, 1983), impaired growth, diminished cognitive functioning, and organ damage are the areas of greatest concern (McCalla, 1985). Factors that appear to influence the development of late effects include the child's age and stage of development at the time of diagnosis, the primary tumor and extent of involvement, and the therapy used.

Evidence shows a second malignancy is more likely to develop if treatment consisted of both chemotherapy and radiation rather than either therapy alone. This is illustrated by the incidence of AML in children previously treated for Hodgkin's disease or in the increased incidence of osteosarcoma following treatment for retinoblastoma. Although it is possible the second malignancy is the result of a genetic predisposition, it is not clear to what extent the treatment of the first malignancy contributes to the development of the second neoplasm.

Growth is influenced by chemotherapeutic agents that affect the proliferation of all cells, and the radiation has a direct-kill effect on cells in the radiated areas. Radiation to bones or glands responsible for growth-related hormones can produce permanent damage (Waskerwitz and Fergusson, 1986).

Children receiving treatment directly to the CNS are at risk for negative neurologic and intellectual sequelae (McCalla, 1985; Moore, Glasser, and Albin, 1988). Neurotoxicity is related to the number and sequence of treatment modalities used. The use of radiation and intrathecal chemotherapy for CNS prophylaxis in the child with ALL has greatly increased survival. However, neurotoxicity and learning disabilities have been reported (Ochs and Mulhern, 1988; Waskerwitz and Fergusson, 1986). The impact of late effects on the various organ systems are described in Table 8-4.

Relapse

Despite the advances in treatment of childhood cancer, some children will experience a relapse of their disease. Relapse, like diagnosis, is a crisis period for the family. It poses a challenge for the oncology team because the best methods of treatment were used at diagnosis. Relapse often requires more experimental modes of treatment. The primary care provider in cooperation with the oncology team can support the family and especially the child through this difficult time.

Death

There may come a time when all possible viable treatment options have been exhausted. The care of the child moves from focusing on a cure to providing comfort and providing as much quality time as possible. The collaboration between the primary care provider and the oncology team can be invaluable during this time. Families frequently seek guidance and support in making decisions that they can live with long after the child's death. Knowledge of the community- and hospital-based hospice programs in their area can be beneficial in meeting many of the home care needs. All families need reassurance that they will not be abandoned at this time and that multidisciplinary resources will be made available to them as required.

Text continued on p. 137.

Table 8-4. Adverse effects of antineoplastic therapy upon body system

Body system	Adverse effects	Causative agent	Time interval	Signs and symptoms	Predisposing factors	Preventive therapeutic measures
Cardiovascular system	Cardiomyopathy	Anthracycline chemotherapy	Weeks to months	Abrupt onset of congestive heart failure; tachycardia; tachypnea; edema; hepatomegaly; cardiomegaly; gallop rhythms; pleural effusions	Anthracycline therapy, especially lifetime cumulative dose of 550 mg/m² Age <15 yr or >70 yr Radiation to heart	Careful patient monitoring with Chest x-ray film ECG Observation for shortness of breath, weight gain, edema
	Chronic constrictive pericarditis	Radiation to mediastinum	Few months to years	Chest pain; dyspnea; fever; paradoxic pulse; venous distention; friction rub; Kussmaul's sign	Most common with doses of 4000-6000 rad	Partial shielding of mediastinum Treatment with antiinflammatory agents Pericardiectomy
Pulmonary system	Pneumonitis	Pulmonary radiation; some chemotherapeutic agents	2-6 mo following radiation therapy	Dyspnea; nonproductive cough; fever	Increased risk with Large lung volume in radiation field Therapy during period of pulmonary infection Concomitant mediastinal radiation Chemotherapeutic agents that act as radiation sensitizers Doses >4000 rad	Careful monitoring of patient status with physical examination and chest x-ray film Most cases resolve spontaneously High-dose corticosteroids for severe cases
	Pulmonary fibrosis	Pulmonary radiation; some chemotherapeutic agents	9-12 mo following radiation	Increased dyspnea; decreased exercise tolerance; pulmonary insufficiency	Pneumonitis occurs first	Careful monitoring of patient status with chest x-ray film and pulmonary function tests Encourage frequent rest periods

Continued.

From McCalla JL: *Nurs Clin North Am* 20:117-130, 1985.
*CAT, computerized axial tomography.

Table 8-4. Adverse effects of antineoplastic therapy upon body system — cont'd

Body system	Adverse effects	Causative agent	Time interval	Signs and symptoms	Predisposing factors	Preventive therapeutic measures
Hematopoietic system	Long-term suppression of bone marrow function	Extensive radiotherapy to marrow-containing bones	Months to years following therapy	Fall in WBC and platelet counts; hypoplastic/aplastic bone marrow aspirates; diminished uptake of radioisotopes	Radiation doses: 3000-5000 rad Older patients Concomitant use of chemotherapy	Limitation of areas of marrow irradiated Monitoring of patient status with periodic bone marrow aspirates and peripheral blood cell counts
Hematopoietic system	Alterations in immune system	Radiotherapy to marrow-containing bones Chemotherapy	Months to years following therapy	Fall in WBC and platelet counts; hypoplastic/aplastic bone; marrow aspirates; diminished intake of radioisotopes; predisposition to infection	Radiation doses: 3000-5000 rad Chemotherapy: high dose/extended periods	Limitation of areas of marrow irradiated Monitoring of patient status with periodic bone marrow aspirates, peripheral blood counts, and tests of immune response
Gastrointestinal system	Hepatic fibrosis-cirrhosis	Chemotherapy	Months to years following therapy	Persistent elevation of liver function tests after cessation of therapy; hepatomegaly once cirrhosis is present	Daily low doses of methotrexate by mouth for long periods Long-term use of 6-mercaptopurine	Monitor patient status with liver function tests Perform liver biopsy if liver function test results remain persistently abnormal
	Chronic enteritis	Radiation therapy	Months to years following therapy	Pain, difficulty swallowing; recurrent vomiting; obstipation/constipation; bloody or mucus-containing diarrhea; malabsorption syndrome	Radiation doses >5000 rad Patients with previous abdominal surgery Chemotherapy with radiation sensitizers	Avoid concomitant use of radiation sensitizers Careful monitoring of patient's status Supportive therapy when symptoms develop, including low residue, low-fat, gluten and milk-free diet
Kidney and urinary tract	Radiation nephritis Acute and chronic	Radiation to renal structures	Acute: 6-12 mo following therapy Chronic: months to years following therapy	May appear as benign or malignant hypertension. Acute: rapid decrease in renal function with BUN, proteinuria, anemia, hypertension, signs of congestive heart failure	Renal radiation of 2000-3000 rad Combined use of radiation and chemotherapy	Periodically monitor patient's renal status during and after therapy, with blood pressure readings, urinalysis, and blood work Radiation-induced hypertension spontaneously resolves when damage is unilateral

			Once progressive renal failure develops, treatment is supportive	above or insidious development of anemia, proteinuria, azotemia, hypertension; may lead to chronic renal failure or cardiovascular damage	
Chronic hemorrhagic cystitis	Chemotherapy Pelvic radiation therapy	Months to years	Sterile, painful hematuria; urinary frequency	Pelvic radiation >4000 rad Inadequate hydration of chemotherapy patients	Sound radiotherapy techniques to reduce bladder exposure to radiation Adequate hydration before, during, and after chemotherapy Concomitant use of investigational drug with chemotherapy Treatment of bladder hemorrhage with formalin instillation and/or fulgration of bleeding sites
Skeletal system	Radiation to skeletal structures Chemotherapy	Months to years following treatment	Growth retardation; reduction in sitting height; scoliosis; altered growth of facial skeleton	Effect of spinal irradiation to vertebral bodies in doses 1000-2000 rad dependent on age of child; known damage >2000 rad Unilateral radiation results in asymmetric deformities Symmetric growth delay during periods of chemotherapy	Careful monitoring of patient status with growth charts and x-ray studies Dose radiation reduction during periods of rapid growth
Impaired skeletal growth					
Endocrine system	Radiotherapy to thyroid gland	Months to years	Hypothyroidism; may be asymptomatic and have abnormal thyroid function; nodular abnormalities	Reported with varying radiation doses: 2500-7000 rad	Monitor thyroid function with blood tests Hormonal replacement therapy for all patients with abnormal thyroid tests
Thyroid gland dysfunction					

Continued.

Table 8-4. Adverse effects of antineoplastic therapy upon body system—cont'd

Body system	Adverse effects	Causative agent	Time interval	Signs and symptoms	Predisposing factors	Preventive therapeutic measures
Endocrine system—cont'd	Injuries to gonads	Radiation field, including gonads Chemotherapy	Months to years	Infertility; sterility; hormonal dysfunction, azoospermia; teratogenic during first trimester of pregnancy	Testicular radiation; ovarian radiation Chemotherapy damage dependent on drug used, dose, duration of therapy, patient sex, and age	Protection of testes/ovaries from radiation field Gonadal dysfunction from chemotherapy may be reversible
Nervous system Peripheral and central	Peripheral Sensory or motor neuropathies	Radiotherapy to peripheral nerves; chemotherapy	Months to years	Deficit in function Pain Decreased tendon reflexes	Radiation doses: 5500-12,000 rad Chemotherapy with vinca-alkaloids	Careful monitoring of patient status during and after therapy Vinca-alkaloid damage may be diminished or reversed by reducing or withholding therapy
	Central Neuroendocrine dysfunction of hypothalamic-pituitary axis	Cranial radiation; chemotherapy	Months to years	Growth hormone deficiency Panhypopituitarism with short stature; hypothyroidism; Addison's disease	Dependent on dose of radiation, age of child, and concomitant use of chemotherapy Younger children who receive >2400 rad at greatest risk	Careful monitoring of patient status with growth charts and head CAT* scan Laboratory tests necessary for patients with questionable growth curves or CAT scan results Treatment with replacement of deficient hormones
	Encephalopathy	Cranial radiation; chemotherapy	Months to years	May be asymptomatic but demonstrate abnormalities on head CAT scans May have overt symptoms ranging from lethargy, somnolence, dementia, seizures, paralysis, and coma	Cranial radiation alone or with concomitant chemotherapy Frequency increased with chemotherapy Less damage with cranial radiation <1800 rad	Monitor patient status with careful physical examination, head CAT scans, psychometric testing Reduce chemotherapy dose when preclinical x-ray findings appear

Intelligence deficits and/or neuropsychologic dysfunctions	Radiation; chemotherapy	Months to years	Abnormal psychologic tests with deficits in perceptual behavior, language development, and learning abilities Personality changes	Younger children more vulnerable More common in younger patients, those who received cranial irradiation >1800 rad and concomitant chemotherapy Damage may occur in all patients who receive CNS prophylactic or therapeutic cranial radiation and/or chemotherapy	Careful monitoring with periodic head CAT scans and psychometric evaluations Early intervention with multidisciplinary approach and specialized education programs

PRIMARY CARE MANAGEMENT
Growth and development

Growth retardation secondary to chemotherapy appears to be temporary (Waskerwitz and Fergusson, 1986). The effect of radiation, however, can be permanent. The child's growth should be followed on a standardized growth curve, with growth patterns examined over time rather than as isolated measurements. Preferably both sitting and standing heights should be obtained (Blatt and Bleyer, 1989). Growth should be followed every 1 to 3 months during therapy and for the first year after therapy. Then measurements should be taken every 6 months until linear growth is completed. Because of the risk of significant weight loss, weight should also be monitored at each visit.

The primary care provider can play an invaluable role in providing anticipatory guidance for parents regarding the developmental changes the child with cancer will experience. Children with cancer are often limited in their opportunities for developing independence and autonomy. The limitations come from restrictions placed by treatment regimens, therapy-related complications, and protective parents.

Ongoing developmental assessment should be performed during and after therapy. Early identification and intervention is important in assisting the child in maintaining age-appropriate development. Neuropsychologic testing is recommended within the first 2 years after completion of therapy for children receiving cranial radiation or who were younger than 8 years at the time of diagnosis. Age-standardized tests should be used to measure intellectual ability, visual perception, visual-motor and motor skills, language, memory and learning, academic achievement, and behavior and social functioning (Blatt and Bleyer, 1989) (see Chapter 3). Neuropsychologic testing should be repeated every 2 to 3 years until young adulthood.

Immunizations

Because of the immunosuppressive nature of treatment, the child's immune system may not be able to mount a response to vaccinations. Normal immunologic response usually returns between 3 months and 1 year after discontinuing immunosuppressive therapy (Committee on Infectious Diseases, 1991). There is great variation in immunization recommendations; therefore, it is best to consult with the child's oncology team for specific recommendations. The child recovering from a bone marrow transplant presents a special situation. Immunizations should be given according to the schedules and protocols established by the transplant center.

Diphtheria, tetanus, and pertussis. The schedule for diphtheria, tetanus, and pertussis vaccines should be resumed after treatment at the discretion of the child's pediatric oncology team.

Poliovirus. Children should not receive the Sabin (live) oral polio vaccine once therapy has been initiated, but the Salk (inactivated) polio vaccine may be given at the discretion of the pediatric oncology team. Siblings of the child should receive the Salk polio vaccine because the polioviruses are transmissible to the immunocompromised child (Committee on Infectious Disease, 1991).

Measles, mumps, and rubella. The child's protection against these diseases must rely on herd immunity until after treatment when the measles, mumps, and rubella (MMR) vaccine may be given. If the child has a direct exposure to someone with a documented case of measles and the child is seronegative for the rubeola antibody, the child should receive prophylactic γ-globulin at a dose of 0.5 ml/kg, with a maximum dose of 15 ml (Committee on Infectious Disease, 1991). Siblings may receive the MMR vaccine without any special precautions.

Haemophilus influenzae type b. The *Haemophilus influenzae* type b vaccine may be given after therapy at the discretion of the child's pediatric oncology team. Children diagnosed with Hodgkin's disease who are 24 months or older should be immunized 2 weeks before starting chemotherapy or undergoing a splenectomy (American Academy of Pediatrics, 1990; Committee on Infectious Disease, 1988).

Varicella prophylaxis. If a child who is seronegative to the varicella virus has a direct exposure to someone who has active chickenpox or to someone who breaks out with lesions within 48 hours of the contact, the child must receive varicella-zoster immune globulin (VZIG). It is available with a physician's order through the regional distribution centers of the American Red Cross Blood Services. It should be administered within 72 to 96 hours of exposure (Feldman and Lott, 1987). The dose of VZIG is 125 units/10 kg, with a maximum dose of 625 units. Once a child is exposed to chickenpox, the child must be isolated from the 10th to the 28th day from other immunocompromised children. Immunization with the experimental live attenuated chickenpox vaccine in children with ALL on therapy has proved to be highly effective with a minimum of side effects (Arbeter et al., 1990; Lawrence et al., 1988).

Other immunizations. Children with Hodgkin's disease should routinely receive the pneumococcal vaccine before a splenectomy is performed. They should also be maintained on daily oral penicillin therapy (250 mg orally twice daily) because of the increased risk of postsplenectomy pneumococcal septicemia.

At this time there is limited research to validate the efficacy of giving routine influenza vaccines to either the child with a malignant disease or to the siblings of this population.

Screening

Vision. Routine vision screening is advised. A recurring brain tumor may manifest as impaired visual acuity caused by ocular nerve compression or increased intracranial pressure or as blurred vision caused by papilledema. There may be ptosis, visual disturbances, and sixth cranial nerve dysfunction with recurrent orbital rhabdomyosarcoma. Two classic signs of recurrent retinoblastoma are the white eye reflex in place of the normal red reflex and strabismus. Cataracts are also a late effect of radiation therapy.

Hearing. Routine hearing screening is advised. Unilateral hearing loss may be indicative of the presence of a mass. Children receiving radiation, cisplatin (Platinol), or both are at increased risk for hearing loss; evaluation by an audiologist every 6 months is recommended.

Dental. Routine dental care is advised during treatment and after therapy. Both radiation therapy and chemotherapy place a child at risk for stomatitis, dental caries, and periodontal disease. Dental work requiring manipulation of the oral tissues should be avoided if the ANC is less than 1000 or the platelet count is less than 50,000. Daily brushing with a soft-bristled brush and flossing are recommended when counts are not compromised and stomatitis is not present (Neihaus et al., 1987).

Daily fluoride rinses may be indicated in children with a high potential for caries. Good oral hygiene is important in preventing stomatitis and infection. In the presence of low blood cell counts or stomatitis, cleansing with a mild mouthwash (salt and bicarbonate of soda, half-strength hydrogen peroxide) and a gauze pad or sponge is recommended.

Blood pressure. Blood pressure should be measured every visit because of possible hypertension from corticosteroids and the potential renal toxicity of many chemotherapeutic agents.

Hematocrit. Because of frequent hematologic analyses, routine screening is not necessary while a child is on therapy. After therapy, routine screening is recommended.

Urinalysis. Routine screening is advised. Urinalysis may reveal RBCs in children with bladder or kidney tumors. Late effects of radiation therapy may include proteinuria. Children receiving cyclophosphamide (Cytoxan) may experience a mild transient hemorrhagic cystitis, although symptoms may occur months to years after the drug has been discontinued (Armstrong, Resnick, and Richards, 1979).

Tuberculosis. Routine screening of children off therapy is advised. Children receiving therapy may be anergic to skin testing. The placement of controls (e.g., *Candida* and diphtheria/tetanus [dT]) will help assess the individual's responsiveness. A chest x-ray film may be necessary if skin testing is unsuccessful.

Children receiving immunosuppressive therapy are at risk for tuberculosis. Children with documented tuberculosis should receive 9 to 12 months of therapy with at least two effective antituberculous agents (e.g., isoniazid [INH, Isoniazid] and rifampin [Rifadin]) (Hathorn and Pizzo, 1989).

Condition specific screening. The primary care provider must keep in mind the possibility of abnormalities because of disease recurrence or the long-term effects of treatment (see Table 8-4). Screening for these complications should be done in consultation with the pediatric oncology team or other subspecialty.

Drug interactions

Children receiving therapy need to avoid aspirin-containing products because of its impairment of platelet function. Acetaminophen is generally rec-

ommended; however, its use during periods of neutropenia is discouraged because it may mask a fever. Multivitamins high in folic acid should be avoided because of the interference of folate with methotrexate. Low folic acid–containing vitamins (e.g., Centrum Jr.) are acceptable. Because of the number of drugs a child may be taking for therapy and the possibility of interaction, it is advisable that the primary care provider contact the pediatric oncology team before prescribing additional medications.

DIFFERENTIAL DIAGNOSIS AND MANAGEMENT OF COMMON PEDIATRIC CONDITIONS
Fever

Children receiving therapy will experience the same illnesses as their peers. The presence of an infection, however, adds a critical dimension in the face of neutropenia. If adequate therapy is not initiated immediately, septic shock may occur and quickly progress to death (Mason, 1987). The first step in evaluating a fever is obtaining a complete blood cell count (CBC) with differential to determine if the child is neutropenic.

The evaluation of the febrile, nonneutropenic child involves a thorough history and physical examination. Blood and urine cultures, as well as a diagnostic work-up for any localized symptoms, should be obtained. Antibiotic treatment is not recommended unless there is an identified source of infection. However, close monitoring of the child is warranted. If the fever persists, a CBC should be repeated every other day because a decreased WBC count often occurs with a viral illness.

The febrile child with an indwelling venous access device should have aerobic and anaerobic blood cultures obtained peripherally and from each lumen of the catheter or port. A broad-spectrum oral antibiotic should be started and continued until the culture results are final. If after 48 to 72 hours the cultures are negative, the antibiotics may be stopped. If the cultures are positive, a full 10- to 14-day course should be administered.

If the ANC is less than 500 and a temperature is greater or equal to 38.5° C, the child must be admitted to the hospital. After cultures of the blood, urine, throat, sputum (with cough, tachypnea, or dyspnea), stool (in the presence of diarrhea), and any skin lesion and chest x-ray film are obtained, an IV form of broad-spectrum antibiotics should be started immediately (Mason, 1987). Two or three drug regimens commonly used include a semi-synthetic penicillin (e.g., carbenicillin [Geopen], ticarcillin [Ticar]), a cephalosporin (e.g., cefazolin [Kefzol, Ancef]), cefamandole [Mandol], cephalothin [Keflin], cefuroxime [Kefurox, Zinacef]), or both and an aminoglycoside (e.g., gentamicin [Garamycin], tobramycin [Nebcin], amikacin [Amikin]) (Albano and Pizzo, 1988).

Herpes viral infections

The human herpesviruses affecting the child with a malignant disease are herpes simplex virus (HSV), varicella-zoster virus (VZV), and CMV. Treatment of HSV infections in children with cancer is dependent on the site and severity of the infection. Mild lesions on the mucosal surface may resolve without intervention. Acyclovir (Zovirax) may be applied topically to speed the healing process of mild to moderate skin lesions (Committee on Infectious Disease, 1991).

In the event that the child contracts an active case of chickenpox, acyclovir (500 mg/m^2 every 8 hours) should be administered intravenously immediately and continued for 7 days (Grouse and Giller, 1988). The child is closely monitored for evidence of systemic involvement. A chest x-ray film is obtained to rule out pulmonary involvement. Aspartate aminotransferase (AST [SGOT]), alanine aminotransferase (ALT [SGPT]) and total bilirubin levels should be monitored for signs of liver involvement. Some institutions are studying the viability of using the oral form of acyclovir in mild cases of chickenpox or in those children off therapy less than 1 year; further research is needed in this area.

Cytomegalovirus infection is common at all ages, but antibody presence is significantly greater in children with cancer (Barson and Brady, 1987). Seroconversion following transfusions of non-treated blood may be responsible for this increased prevalence. Signs and symptoms of an acute CMV infection include fever, hepatosplenomegaly, retinitis, pneumonia, colitis, CNS manifestations, and a rash (Barson and Brady, 1987). Antiviral therapy for CMV infections has been more difficult than other herpesviruses. Vidarabine (Vira-A) and acyclovir have been shown to be less effective. Gancyclovir shows promise in treating CMV-associated pneumonitis, retinitis and GI infections (Barson and Brady, 1987), although it has significant toxicities.

Other infections

Candidiasis and aspergillosis are the two most common fungal infections in the child with a malignant disease. Candidiasis is more common and can involve the oral mucosa, GI tract, urinary tract, bone, lungs, and, less frequently, the blood. Aspergillosis is seen most frequently in the respiratory tract, GI tract, and brain. Amphotericin B (Fungizone) is the most effective drug for systemic fungal infection; however, it has potent side effects.

The immunocompromised child, at risk for *Pneumocystis carinii*, may take trimethoprim-sulfamethoxazole (Septra, Bactrim) prophylactically. The usual dose is 150 mg/m^2 divided and given twice daily for 2 or 3 consecutive days. The prophylaxis is continued for approximately 6 months after the completion of therapy. Parenteral or aerosolized Pentamidine given on a monthly or biweekly basis has been shown to be effective prophylaxis for the child with human immunodeficiency virus (HIV). Research is being conducted to evaluate its use in the child with cancer. Pneumonitis is the most clinical manifestation of *Pneumocystis carinii*. Symptoms include a dry cough, fever, tachypnea, cyanosis, and respiratory distress. Onset may be acute (few days) or insidious (months). All significant infections in immunocompromised children should be managed in consultation with the oncologist.

Gastrointestinal symptoms

Nausea, vomiting, and diarrhea, common side effects of cancer treatment, may be difficult to distinguish from viral or bacterial illness. The health care provider must establish the relationship of the symptoms to the administration of chemotherapy, radiation, or intrathecal medications during the history. During these periods, it is important to monitor fluid intake and avoid dehydration, especially in those children currently receiving chemotherapy. In some cases IV fluid replacement and antiemetics may be necessary. Blood chemistry values, especially BUN, creatinine, AST, and ALT, must be monitored closely to avoid damaging vital organs from concentrated levels of the chemotherapeutics from delayed excretion as a result of dehydration. Chemotherapy may be temporarily delayed or withheld because of GI illness.

Headaches

Headache pain, usually benign late in childhood and adolescence, is indicative of serious underlying difficulties in the young child. Morning headaches associated with vomiting and minimal nausea should always arouse suspicion of a brain tumor or CNS involvement. Headaches following a lumbar puncture, which resolve with lying down, may be caused by a slow cerebrospinal fluid leak. This type of headache is best treated by bed rest. While taking a thorough history, one should note onset, any precipitating factors or symptoms, location, severity, and what, if any, medication gives relief. A thorough neurologic examination is imperative. Many headaches may be treated at home with acetaminophen and rest. However, if the headache symptoms are unrelieved by medication, or there is any change in vision or neurologic function, immediate evaluation is necessary.

Pain

Pain in children is often difficult to assess and requires understanding of normal child development and age-appropriate verbal and behavioral cues. It is important to keep in mind that children rarely fabricate the presence of pain (Miser and Miser, 1989). The child with cancer poses additional challenges because of the multiple etiologies of pain. Pain may result from the malignancy, treatments, procedures (e.g., bone marrow and spinal tap), or incidental pain (e.g., trauma) (Miser and Miser, 1989).

Tumor-related pain occurs with direct tumor invasion of the bone, with impingement of the tumor on nervous tissue, or by metastatic lesions. Compression of the spinal cord by a tumor may result in back pain and is accentuated by maneuvers such as coughing, sneezing, and flexion of the spine (Pack and Maria, 1987). Immediate evaluation is imperative, because an untreated cord compression can rapidly progress to irreversible neurologic damage. Treatment-related pain can occur from mucositis, infection, radiation-induced dermatitis, abdominal pain, or phantom limb pain following the amputation of a limb.

DEVELOPMENTAL ISSUES
Safety

Safety issues for the child with a malignant disease involves balancing normal participation in daily activities with taking appropriate precautions imposed by the treatment of a malignant disease. For the safety of all children, chemotherapeutic agents must be stored securely out of reach. Thorough hand washing should follow the handling of any chemotherapeutic agent. Pregnant women should avoid contact with the chemotherapeutic agents. If circumstances make this impossible, gloves should be worn to avoid direct contact with the medication. Unused portions of chemotherapeutic drugs should be returned to the dispensing pharmacy for disposal with other potent chemicals.

Right atrial catheters must have a clean dressing applied to the exit site and the line secured to the chest to minimize any excessive tension of the catheter. Needles, syringes, and other supplies used in the maintenance of the line should be stored properly out of reach of children. Needles should be disposed of carefully, without recapping, in a "sharps" container.

If the child should have a fall or head injury, blood cell counts should be checked to determine the platelet count. Platelets should be given prophylactically if the level is less than 50,000. The child should be instructed not to roughhouse or play contact sports if the platelet count is less than 100,000.

Many of the chemotherapeutic agents will alter the skin's tolerance for sun exposure. It is important that children on chemotherapy take extra caution in using a *p*-aminobenzoic acid–free sun block whenever prolonged sun exposure is anticipated. It is best to avoid sun exposure during the time of day when the child's shadow is shorter than the child's height. If the child has alopecia, a hat and sun block should be worn to protect the scalp.

The primary care provider can play a key role in helping the child and family set realistic expectations and limitations on activities. Limitations are influenced by immunosuppression, hematologic compromise, or extremity dysfunction because of peripheral neuropathy induced by chemotherapy or as a result of amputation or limb salvage procedures.

Child care

The intensity of the initial phases of therapy may make day care impractical. However, when a child has begun less intensive therapy, a home or small group situation is recommended because it minimizes exposure to the various common pediatric illnesses. The caretaker must be educated about (1) the child's disease and instructed to notify the family immediately of any fever, signs and symptoms of infection, or increased bruising or bleeding; (2) reporting any communicable illness in the other children, especially chickenpox; and (3) any medication or oral chemotherapeutic agent that must be administered during child care hours.

Diet

Maintaining adequate nutrition while a child is receiving treatment is challenging because of the child's anorexia. Well-balanced, nutritious meals should be offered. Often small, frequent meals may be more appealing than the standard three meals each day. High-calorie, high-protein snacks may also be helpful.

Children receiving corticosteroids will often experience an increased appetite and weight gain, but because corticosteroids usually are administered for limited amounts of time, such symptoms generally are of short duration. Nutritious foods low in sodium should be encouraged.

Constipation and diarrhea are frequent side effects of chemotherapy. Constipation may be relieved by increasing the child's fluid intake and encouraging high-fiber foods and fruits. A stool softener or laxative may be necessary. Enemas should be avoided, especially if the child is neutropenic. Diarrhea should be monitored closely and the child evaluated for signs and symptoms of dehydration.

Often parents will inquire about the use of herbs, special diets, or other dietary interventions to speed the recovery of the blood cell counts or to combat the tumor. It is important to examine with the parents the intervention they desire to use. Herbs and vitamins must be viewed in terms of their potential for interacting with chemotherapeutic agents. The primary care provider can acknowledge and support the parents desire to help their child while also acting in the best interest of the child.

Discipline

Discipline for the child with a cancer should be managed as for all children. A consistent approach in establishing expectations and setting limits is important to the child's security. The parents should be supported in maintaining normal patterns of discipline, although they may initially be ambivalent about this. Consistency in discipline among siblings is also important.

Toileting

No special toileting measures need to be taken. Toilet training may be delayed or regression may occur if diagnosis occurs during the toddler or preschool period.

Sleep patterns

Disturbances in sleep patterns are common. The extent to which the child is affected will depend on the age at diagnosis, the frequency of hospitalizations, and the general coping patterns of the individual. Maintaining a consistent bedtime ritual whenever possible provides security during a time when many things are disrupted. Parents should also be encouraged to accept transitional objects, because these may help the child with sleep during periods of hospitalization.

School issues

With the advances in the treatment of children with cancer, more children are surviving into adulthood. The child who is too ill to participate in the regular classroom should be enrolled in a home study program. The role of health care providers, parents, and educators is to work as a team to assist the child in returning to school as soon after diagnosis as is medically possible. The return to school provides a sense of normalcy and contributes to the child's sense of hopefulness (Stevens et al., 1988).

The child's reentry must be carefully planned. Establishing an individualized educational plan (IEP) can help define and anticipate the special needs of the child (Deasy-Spinetta and Tarr, 1985). The teachers and the school staff must be informed of the child's illness and implications that will influence attendance, social interaction, educational capacity, and the restrictions or special needs dictated by medical care (Riley-Lawless, 1988). Early recognition of learning disabilities will enhance prompt assessment and intervention.

It is recommended that with the family's and child's permission the child's classmates be taught about the child's illness at an appropriate developmental level. The child will also need to be prepared to answer classmates' questions. The primary care provider can provide the family with support and resources to help ease the transition into school.

Sexuality

The child with cancer often struggles with an alteration in body image because of hair loss, weight loss or gain, or disfiguring surgery. A major task of these children is learning to deal with this change, be it temporary or permanent. This is especially true in the adolescent who, in addition to his or her treatment, may or may not be experiencing the normal pubertal changes. Ongoing monitoring of the child's development through the use of Tanner staging is important. Failure to progress through the stages warrants referral to a pediatric endocrinologist.

A young woman on chemotherapy may experience delayed development of secondary sexual characteristics and amenorrhea. Often after the cessation of therapy, development will occur and the menses begin. Fertility status of children surviving childhood malignancies is variable depending on the type and extent of treatment. Ongoing long-term follow-up is required.

Sperm banking should be offered to pubescent males before therapy because sterility and mutagenicity can occur from cancer treatment. Ongoing assessment of appropriate sexual development and functioning (e.g., libido, impotence) is important. Peer support groups are often helpful in assisting the adolescent to deal with issues of sexuality and body image.

SPECIAL FAMILY CONCERNS

The advances in medicine that have led to improved survival rates of children with cancer have also brought problems of chronic uncertainty. Chronic uncertainty "is experienced as an exquisitely heightened sense of vulnerability, accompanied by a compelling need to know the unknowable future." (Cohen and Martinson, 1988). The uncertainty faced by families centers around the basic issue of the child's survival. Family concerns will often reflect the phase of treatment they are experiencing. In the beginning, uncertainty is focused on whether or not remission will be obtained. If remission is achieved, will it be long term or will relapse occur? If relapse occurs, will the child enter remission again or will he or she die?

The goal of members of the health care team must be to help the families cope with uncertainty, not to focus on the unlikely goal of removing that uncertainty (Cohen and Martinson, 1988). Learning to cope with uncertainty is important to the health and well-being of all family members. Support for the child and family must be ongoing, not only at diagnosis but long after completion of therapy or death of the child.

The financial burden of a catastrophic illness is of monumental concern to the family. It not only affects the current financial status of the family but also has far-reaching implications for the child's future insurability. Insurance companies and health maintenance organizations vary in their reimbursement of medications and procedures they deem to be experimental. These factors all add up to a tremendous amount of stress on an already taxed family unit.

SUMMARY OF PRIMARY CARE NEEDS FOR THE CHILD WITH CANCER

Growth and development

Slowing of growth because of chemotherapy and radiation.

Closely monitored weight; child is at risk for significant weight loss because of disease and treatment.

Periodic developmental screening to assess for age-appropriate behaviors.

Neuropsychologic testing for children who received cranial radiation or who were less than 8 years old at the time of diagnosis.

Immunizations

No immunizations are recommended while child is receiving therapy.

Siblings and household contacts should not receive live polio vaccine because of transmissibility to immunocompromised individual. Siblings and household contacts may receive MMR vaccine.

Use of the varicella vaccine is under investigation; for the first year after therapy, however, recommendation will vary depending on the cancer treatment center.

Children recovering from bone marrow transplantation require special consideration in determining immunization schedule and protocol.

Children with Hodgkin's disease and non-Hodgkin's lymphoma should be vaccinated with the pneumococcal vaccine before splenectomy is performed. Children with Hodgkin's disease who are 24 months or older and immunized should receive *H. influenzae* type b conjugate vaccine.

Screening
Vision

Visual screening is routine. Thorough assessment is warranted if visual abnormalities are detected.

Hearing

Hearing testing is routine. Children receiving ototoxic drugs should have periodic evaluation by an audiologist.

Dental

Dental screening is routine. A CBC should be done before an appointment to verify adequate ANC, platelet count. Meticulous oral hygiene is necessary to prevent infections.

Hematocrit

Hematocrit testing is routine and is done off therapy. It is done as needed while the child is on therapy. Critical levels are ANC less than 500, platelets less than 20,000, and hemoglobin less than 8%.

Urinalysis

Urinalysis is routine. Protein may be observed after radiation therapy, or hematuria may be seen after cyclophosphamide therapy.

Tuberculosis

Tuberculosis screening is routine and is done off therapy. Most probably the results are inaccurate while the patient is on therapy.

Condition-specific screening

Close assessment is required for signs and symptoms of late effects of therapy or recurrence of malignancy (see Table 8-4).

Drug interaction

No aspirin-containing products should be given. Acetaminophen is recommended except in times of neutropenia to avoid masking a fever.

Low folic acid multivitamins should be taken. Consult with the oncology team before prescribing additional medication because of the risk of drug interactions.

Differential diagnosis
Fever

Rule out neutropenia; rule out infection. Do septic work-up as warranted. Prompt intervention is required with neutropenia.

SUMMARY OF PRIMARY CARE NEEDS FOR THE CHILD
WITH CANCER — cont'd

Herpesvirus

Treat mucosal lesions topically. Children without prior immunity should avoid exposure to chickenpox. Acyclovir is given intravenously for chickenpox in the immunosuppressed individual. Rule out dissemination of disease. Give *Pneumocystis* prophylaxis.

Gastrointestinal symptoms

For nausea and vomiting, determine the relationship to chemotherapy and intrathecal medications; rule out viral and bacterial infection.

Headache

Give a thorough neurologic examination. Consider the possibility of a brain tumor, CNS involvement, sinusitis, and spinal lumbar puncture.

Pain

Determine the source of pain; rule out cord compression.

Developmental issues
Safety

Assure proper handling of chemotherapeutic agents at home and proper maintenance and protection of indwelling venous access devices. Use platelet prophylaxis for head injury or fall if counts are low. Minimize roughhousing and contact sports if the platelet count is less than 100,000. Because of photosensitivity, protect the child from sun. Establish realistic expectations and limitations of activities because of disease or treatment.

Child care

Generally a small group setting is better than a large group to minimize exposure. The caretaker should know the signs and symptoms that pose a concern.

Diet

Maintain an adequate diet. Offer small frequent meals if the child is experiencing anorexia. Low-sodium foods should be given to children on corticosteroid therapy. Increase fluid intake and high-fiber foods for constipation. Monitor diarrhea closely. Offer support and education for alternative diets or therapy.

Discipline

Use normal patterns of discipline; it is important to maintain consistency for all family members.

Toileting

Standard developmental counseling is advised. Regression may occur.

Sleep pattern

Disturbances are common. Maintain consistent bedtime schedule and routine whenever possible. A transitional object may increase security during hospitalization.

School

The child should return to school as soon as possible. Ongoing communication between health care providers and teachers is necessary. Education of school staff and classmates is crucial. Assist the family in the development of an IEP. Periodically assess for school problems and learning disabilities. If the child is unable to participate in a regular school program, arrange for home tutoring.

Sexuality

Give support for altered body image. Assess for appropriate Tanner staging. Sperm banking is an option before the adolescent male begins chemotherapy or radiation.

Special family concerns

Dealing with chronic uncertainty.
Insurance and catastrophic financial impact.

RESOURCES

Numerous local, regional, and national organizations provide information and educational resources about childhood malignant diseases. Local hospitals and cancer centers will often provide support groups for family members. Informal parent-to-parent interactions based on the sense of having a common understanding of parenting a child with cancer can be a powerful source of support (Lynam, 1987). Identifying local resources will provide a much-welcomed service to these families.

Organizations

American Cancer Society
90 Park Ave
New York, NY 10016

> *This is a volunteer organization offering educational programs, patient services, rehabilitation support and referral to local and regional resources.*

Cancer Information Service
NCI, Bldg 31
National Institute of Health
Bethesda, MD 20892

> *This is a network of regional information centers that provides personalized answers to cancer-related questions from patients, families, the general public, and health care professionals. This organization also provides referral to local and regional resources.*

Candlelighters Childhood Cancer Foundation, Inc.
2025 I St, NW, Suite 1011
Washington, DC 20006

> *This is an international organization of parents whose children have had cancer. This organization provides guidance and emotional support through local chapters, information, and referral to local and regional resources.*

Leukemia Society of America
800 Second Ave
New York, NY 10017

> *This is a volunteer organization offering educational programs, information, financial assistance, and referral to local and regional resources.*

REFERENCES

Albano EA and Pizzo PA: The evolving population of immunocompromised children, *Pediatr Infec Dis J* 7(suppl):79-86, 1988.

Altman AJ and Schwartz AD: *Malignant diseases of infancy, childhood and adolescence,* Philadelphia, 1983, WB Saunders Co.

American Academy of Pediatrics: Policy statement: *Haemophilus influenzae* type b conjugated vaccines: Immunization of children at 15 months of age, *AAP News,* July 1990, p 10.

American Cancer Society: *Cancer facts and figures-1990,* 1990, The Society, pp 16-17.

Arbeter AM, Granowetter L, Starr SE, et al: Immunization of children with acute lymphoblastic leukemia with live attenuated varicella vaccine without complete suspension of chemotherapy, *Pediatrics* 85:338-344, 1990.

Armstrong B, Resnick MI and Richards F: Delayed cystitis due to cyclophosphamide, *N Engl J Med* 300:45, 1979.

Barson WJ and Brady MI: Management of infections in children with cancer, *Hematol Oncol Clin North Am* 1:801-839, 1987.

Blatt J and Bleyer WA: Late effects of childhood cancer and its treatment. In Pizzo PA and Poplack DG, eds: *Principles and practice of pediatric oncology,* Philadelphia, 1989, JB Lippincott, p 1005.

Bleyer WA: The impact of childhood cancer on the United States and the world, CA 40:355-367, 1990.

Bortin M and Buckner C: Major complications of marrow harvesting for transplantation, *Exp Hematol* 11:916-921, 1983.

Cameron GS: Central venous catheters for children with malignant disease: Surgical issues, *J Pediatr Surg* 22:702-704, 1987.

Chauvenet AR and Wofford MM: Cures in childhood cancer, *Pediatr Rev* 11:311-317, 1990.

Cohen MH and Martinson IM: Chronic uncertainty: Its effect on parental appraisal of a child's health, *J Pediatr Nurs* 3:89-96, 1988.

Cogliano-Shutta NA, Broda EJ, and Gress JS: Bone marrow transplantation: An overview and comparison of autologous, syngeneic and allogeneic treatment modalities, *Nurs Clin North Am* 20:49-66, 1985.

Committee on Infectious Disease: Report of the Committee on Infectious Diseases, ed 22, Elk Grove Village, Ill, 1991, American Academy of Pediatrics.

Deasy-Spinetta P and Tarr D: Public Law 94-142 and the student with cancer: An overview of the legal, organizational and practical aspects, *J Psychosoc Oncol* 3:97-105, 1985.

Evans WE, Petros WP, Relling MV, et al: Clinical pharmacology of cancer chemotherapy, *Pediatr Clin North Am* 36:1199-1230, 1989.

Feldman S and Lott L: Varicella in children with cancer: Impact of antiviral therapy and prophylaxis, *Pediatrics* 80:165-172, 1987.

Fochtman D, Fergusson J, Ford N, et al: The treatment of cancer in children. In Fochtman D and Foley GV, eds: *Nursing care of the child with cancer,* Boston, 1982, Little, Brown, pp 177-233.

Frick SB, DelPo E, Keith JA, et al: Chemotherapy-associated nausea and vomiting in pediatric oncology patients, *Cancer Nurs* 11:118-121, 1988.

Grose C and Giller RH: Varicella-zoster virus infection and immunization in the healthy and the immunocompromised host, *Crit Rev Oncol Hematol* 8:27-64, 1988.

Happ M: Life threatening hemorrhage in children with cancer. *J Assoc Oncol Nurses* 4:36-40, 1987.

Hartman GE and Shochat SJ: Management of septic complications associated with silastic catheters in childhood malignancy, *Pediatr Infect Dis J* 6:1042-1047, 1987.

Hathorn JW and Pizzo PA: Infectious complications in the pediatric cancer patient. In Pizzo PA and Poplack DG, eds: *Principles and practice of pediatric oncology,* Philadelphia, 1989, JB Lippincott, p 851.

Lawrence R, Gershon AA, Holzman R, et al: The risk of zoster after varicella vaccination in children with leukemia, *N Engl J Med* 318:543-548, 1988.

Lynam MJ: The parent network in pediatric oncology: Supportive or not? *Cancer Nurs* 10:207-216, 1987.

Marcoux C, Fisher S, and Wong D: Central venous access devices in children, *Pediatr Nurs* 16:123-133, 1990.

Mason CA: Septic shock, *J Assoc Oncol Nurses* 4:26-31, 1987.

McCalla JL: A multidisciplinary approach to identification and remedial intervention for adverse late effects of cancer therapy, *Nurs Clin North Am* 20:117-130, 1985.

Miser AW and Miser JS: The treatment of cancer pain in children, *Pediatr Clin North Am* 36:979-999, 1989.

Moore IM, Glasser ME and Albin AR: The late psychosocial consequences of childhood cancer, *J Pediatr Nurs* 3:150-158, 1988.

Neihaus CS, Meiller TF, Peterson DE, et al: The dental hygienist's role in a pediatric oncology center, *Dental Hygienist* 61:414-418, 1987.

Noyes NF: Chemotherapy. In Hockenberry MJ and Cody DK, eds: *Pediatric oncology and hematology,* St Louis, 1986, CV Mosby, p 326.

Ochs J and Mulhern RK: Late effects of antileukemic treatment, *Pediatr Clin North Am* 35:815-831, 1988.

Pack B and Maria BL: Neurological emergencies in pediatric oncology, *J Assoc Pediatr Oncol Nurses* 4:8-18, 1987.

Riley-Lawless K: School re-entry programs, *J Pediatr Oncol Nurses* 5:34-37, 1988.

Stevens MC, Kaye JT, Kenwood CP, et al: Facts for the teachers of children with cancer, *Arch Dis Child* 63:456-458, 1988.

Sutow WW, Fernbach DJ, and Vietti TJ: *Clinical pediatric oncology,* St Louis, 1984, CV Mosby.

Whaley L and Wong D: *Essentials of pediatric nursing,* St Louis, 1984, CV Mosby.

Wiley PM and House KU: Bone marrow transplant in children, *Semin Oncol Nurs* 4:31-40, 1988.

9 *Cerebral Palsy*

Shirley Steele

ETIOLOGY

Cerebral palsy is defined as a nonprogressive disorder of motion and posture caused by a brain insult or injury occurring during early periods of brain growth and involving a variety of distinct clinical entities such as spasticity, dyskinesia, and ataxia (Lord, 1984). It is classified according to the type of motor dysfunction and extremities involved. The major types of cerebral palsy are spasticity, dyskinesia (athetoid), ataxia, and mixed.

The child with *spastic* cerebral palsy has increased muscle tone, prolonged primitive reflexes, exaggerated deep tendon reflexes, clonus, rigidity of the extremities during flexion and extension, and a tendency to develop scoliosis and contractures. These findings most commonly occur in one of three characteristic patterns: (1) hemiplegia involving the arm and leg of one side of the body, (2) diplegia of the lower extremities with or without an associated interference with fine or gross (or both) motor function of the upper extremities (Fig. 9-1, *B*), and (3) quadriplegia with involvement of the trunk and all four extremities (Lord, 1984). The motor neuron involvement is associated with the extensive cerebral degeneration of the brain (spastic quadriplegia) or malformation of the cerebral hemisphere (spastic hemiplegia) (Fig. 9-1, *A*). These findings account for 70% to 75% of the cases of cerebral palsy.

The child with *dyskinetic* cerebral palsy has extreme difficulty in making purposeful movements; movements are abrupt, jerky, uncontrolled, and uncoordinated. Dyskinetic cerebral palsy is the result of a neurologic insult to the basal ganglia or extrapyramidal tracts and accounts for 15% to 20% of the cases.

The child with *ataxic* cerebral palsy has a wide-based gait and instability. In infancy, hypotonia or normal muscle tone may be found. Stiffness of the trunk, however, will become apparent at 8 to 10 months of age. This decreases the infant's ability to rotate. The stiffness eventually aggravates the child's ataxic movements and contributes to the unsteadiness. Righting and equilibrium reactions are frequently delayed in these children, resulting in increased falls and potential accidents. The ataxic characteristics become more apparent as the child tries to stand. Standing, if achieved, is delayed. If the child achieves walking, the knees are extended and a wide-based gait is used (Haynes, 1983). Ataxic cerebral palsy accounts for approximately 2% to 5% of the cases.

The child with *mixed* cerebral palsy displays characteristics of more than one type, usually a combination of spasticity and dyskinesia.

Research is essential to provide more information about cerebral palsy and its causes. At the present time it is not possible to reliably correlate a specific cause with a specific subtype of cerebral palsy. There are, however, some fairly predictable associations. For example, a combination of choreoathetosis and sensorineural deafness virtually always implies kernicteric brain damage attributable to bilirubin encephalopathy. In addition, pure congenital ataxia without associated diplegia is commonly familial in nature (Paneth, 1986). Children

148

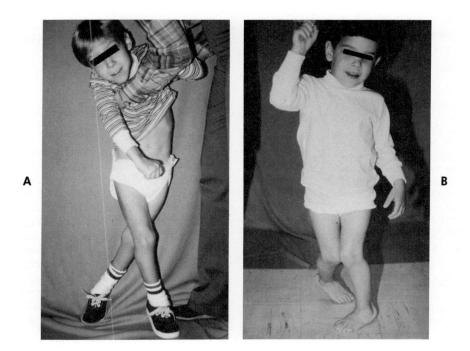

Fig. 9-1. Two children with adductor spasticity producing scissoring. **A,** Severe spasticity in nonambulatory child who has adduction deformity and severe scissoring. **B,** Ambulatory child with spastic diplegia whose legs scissor during walking. *From Canale, ST and Beaty, JH: Operative Pediatric Orthopaedics, St. Louis, 1991, Mosby–Year Book.*

with spastic diplegia frequently have a history of very low birth weight. Moreover, infants delivered in the breech position are at a higher risk of developing cerebral palsy than infants delivered vertex first.

The two most commonly cited risk factors for cerebral palsy are low birth weight and birth asphyxia (Hensleigh, Fainstat, and Spencer, 1986). Data from the National Collaborative Perinatal Project of the National Institute of Neurological and Communicative Disorders and Stroke (NCPP) indicate that children have a twentyfold incidence of having cerebral palsy when they weigh less than 1500 g at birth (Ellenberg and Nelson, 1979). In addition, children of normal weight who have Apgar scores of 3 or less have a 250-fold increased risk of having cerebral palsy. Seventy-five percent of all infants with cerebral palsy documented by the NCPP, however, had 5-minute Apgar scores of 7 or higher (Nelson and Ellenberg, 1981).

Stanley (1987) concluded that the majority of causes of cerebral palsy are unknown rather than the result of brain damage from birth asphyxia or other perinatal causes. The possibility of genetic, teratogenic, and early pregnancy influences on the development of cerebral palsy have yet to be thoroughly investigated. Fetal abnormalities, maternal mental retardation, and severe proteinuria late in pregnancy merit consideration in future studies, although these conditions would account for a very small proportion of cases (Nelson and Ellenberg, 1986). Growing evidence suggests that many of the risk factors historically cited as correlates of cerebral palsy account for only a small proportion of the actual cases. The box on p. 150 lists risk factors currently accepted as possible causes.

INCIDENCE

Prior to 1962, it was estimated that there were between 4.7 and 7.5 cases of cerebral palsy per

---

POTENTIAL RISK FACTORS FOR CEREBRAL PALSY

Prenatal

Hyperemesis gravidarum
Toxemia
Teratogenic drugs
Placenta previa
Placenta abruptio
Intrauterine viral or bacterial infection (toxoplasmosis, rubella, cytomegalovirus, herpes, and syphilis)
Chromosomal abnormality
Maternal malnutrition
Positive family history

Perinatal

Prematurity
Breech or face delivery
Intrauterine asphyxia
Asphyxia neonatorum
Low Apgar score, especially at 5, 10, and 20 minutes
Seizures
Respiratory distress syndrome
Hyaline membrane disease
Hyperbilirubinemia

Postnatal

Head trauma
Intracranial infections (encephalitis, meningitis)
Toxic encephalopathies (e.g., lead)
Cerebrovascular accident

From Taft LT and Matthew WS: Cerebral palsy. In Levine MD ed: *Developmental-behavioral pediatrics*, Philadelphia, 1983, WB Saunders, p 789.

1000 live births (Abroms and Panagakos, 1980). Currently estimates range from approximately 1.5 to 5 cases of cerebral palsy per 1000 live births (Lord, 1984; Paneth, 1986), and today approximately 400,000 children in the United States have cerebral palsy. Improved neonatal care and Rh immunization are probably responsible for the recent decline in incidence of cerebral palsy. Increased survival rates of very low birth weight infants, however, is contributing to an upward trend in incidence of all major types of cerebral palsy. To date, this has not contributed to an overall increase in the prevalence rate of cerebral palsy (Pharoah et al., 1987).

CLINICAL MANIFESTATIONS AT TIME OF DIAGNOSIS

The signs and symptoms of cerebral palsy are varied. Although the initial signs of cerebral palsy may be evident as early as the first few months of life, an official diagnosis is usually not made until 2 years of age unless a child is severely involved. Some children with early signs of neuromotor deficits can improve significantly with the maturation of the central nervous system (CNS), and early clinical signs can change or disappear entirely (Taft, 1987). This phenomenon is called "transient abnormal neurologic signs" and can occur in a large number of neonatal intensive care unit (NICU) graduates. Coolman and associates (1985) found the incidence of transient abnormal neurologic signs to occur in 43% of the post-NICU infants. A sizable number of these infants (21%) continued to

---

ASSESSMENT OF TONE IN INFANTS

Normal tone

Infant moves well against gravity and lacks high or low tone characteristics.

Low tone

Infant lacks tone to move against gravity; lacks resistance to passive movement; has low tone postures such as supine lying with arm abducted, legs abducted in a frogged position; or has decreased movement.

High tone

Infant becomes stiff when moving against gravity; the neck or extremities resist passive movement; infant has hypertonic head reactions such as hyperextension of the neck when rolling over, head pushing when supine or when pulled to sitting position; infant has high tone posturing such as increased extension of the head when supine lying, retracted shoulder girdle, and lordosis of the back of extended lower extremities.

Table 9-1. Normal values for dissolution and appearance (marked with*) of some neurological items, according to different authors (in months) (mainly averages and average ranges; only Paine gives full ranges)

Response	Taft-Cohen	DiLeo	Vassella	Mitchell	Dekaban	Milani-Comparetti	Illingworth	St. Anne-Dargassies	Paine et al.
Sucking	Persists				End 1st yr				
Rooting	3-4 mo	12 mo	4 mo		End 1st yr				
Palmar grasp	5-6 mo	4-5 mo	3-4 mo		3-4 mo	3.5 mo		3 mo	After 2 mo
Plantar grasp	9-12 mo	Walking age	End baby age			9 mo		12 mo	After 2 mo
Crossed extension	Persists						6 mo		
Asymmetric tonic neck	6-7 mo	4 mo	4-5 mo		3-6 mo	4 mo	4 mo		1-6 mo
Neck-righting	9-12 mo		4 mo		8 mo*→3.5 yr				1-10 mo*
Moro	4-6 mo	4-5 mo	4-5 mo	3-5 mo	3-6 mo	4 mo	6 mo		1-5 mo
Stepping	3-4 mo	1.5 mo	1 mo		2-6 mo				Early months
Tactile placing feet	1 yr				1 yr			3-6 mo	1 yr
Galant	2-3 mo		6 mo to walking						
Babinski	12-18 mo	During 2nd yr							
Positive supporting	Variable, 2-3 mo		3 mo		1-2 mo		2 mo	3-6 mo	1-9 mo
Landau	3 mo*→2nd yr		4 mo*	3 mo*→1 yr	10 mo*→28 mo	4 mo*		3 mo*→7 mo	1-2 mo*→7 mo
Parachute (prone)	7-9 mo*		5 mo*		6 mo*	4 mo*		7-9 mo*	7-12 mo*
Lateral supporting	5-7 mo*		7 mo*			6 mo*		7-9 mo*	

From Touwen BCL: The neurological development of the infant. In Davis JA and Dobbing J eds: *Scientific Foundations of Paediatrics*, Philadelphia, 1974, WB Saunders.

demonstrate subtle persistent non–cerebral palsy dysfunction until 1 or 2 years of age. Based on this study and previous work (Amiel-Tison, 1976; Drillien, 1972; Drillien, Thomson, and Burgoyne, 1980), infant neuromotor function should be classified only as normal or abnormal. After 2 years of age, persistent neuromotor dysfunction evidenced by the presence of primitive reflexes, delay in acquiring postural reflexes, hyperreflexia, or generalized hypertonia or hypotonia is indicative of cerebral palsy (see the box on p. 150 for an assessment guide for tone and Table 9-1 for normal values of reflexes).

Many infants with cerebral palsy have a history of opistonic posturing when crying, irritability, difficulty in feeding, and excessive drooling. The increased drooling can be caused by abnormal swallowing, abnormal posture of the lips, tongue, or jaws, or poor body posture (Weiss-Lambrou, Tetreault, and Dudley, 1989). Although any of these symptoms taken independently are not diagnostic of cerebral palsy, they should heighten awareness that a neuromotor problem may exist.

In the older infant and young toddler, another red flag is evidence of early hand preference. Preferential handedness before 1 year of age can signify hemiparesis associated with the other hand. Another suspicious sign is when one hand remains fisted while the other hand freely opens. Lower extremity hemiparesis may be observed in the child's crawl and walk. A child with hemiparesis uses the unaffected extremities and partially or competely drags the affected extremities, resulting in an asymmetric pattern. Other children may bunny-hop, crawling by first advancing both hands and then advancing both knees simultaneously. Persistent and consistent toe walking should raise the suspicion of spastic diplegia because the child so affected has tight heel cords, making it difficult to bring the feet into a neutral position (see Fig. 9-1, *B*).

TREATMENT

The therapy for each child is individualized and focuses on the particular symptoms and development of the child. The treatment aim is to minimize the effects of abnormal motor function and postural deficits. Often, children are referred to tertiary centers with interdisciplinary teams who focus on care of children with developmental disabilities. In addition, the family is enrolled in a home- or center-based early development program. This combination of services will optimize the child's growth and development and minimize deformities resulting from abnormal motor function.

The primary interventions focus on appropriate positioning and handling to promote maximum function and prevent contractures. Four basic positions are used in positioning: (1) side lying, (2) prone lying, (3) supported sitting, and (4) supported standing (Hanson and Harris, 1986). Positioning activities and alternating positions can help the children learn to engage in more normal activities. Children who have severe limitations in movement need to have their position changed on a definite schedule so that the chance of skin breakdown is minimized.

The focus on early and adequate positioning has improved the overall status of many children and has decreased the numbers of orthopedic surgeries that need to be performed. For example, the child who is supported in an appropriate position in a specialized wheelchair can maintain a more symmetric position, can decrease the effects of retained primitive reflexes, and can maintain extremities in a more relaxed, flexed position. Under these ideal conditions, the incidence and severity of contractures and scoliosis are decreased. Ankle, foot, knee, or spine orthoses are used to prevent, support, or correct a deformity, to improve function, and can also help to decrease the need for surgery.

Experimental treatments are often sought by parents. Some of these treatments may become future standard therapy, others will disappear with time, and others reappear periodically in the same or similar form. For example, nonsurgical drooling therapies have included radiotherapy (Smith and Goode, 1970), chin pressure devices (Harris and Dignam, 1980), oral musculature training (Harris and Dignam, 1980), and behavioral therapy (Garber, 1971). Surgical procedures have included salivary gland excision (Smith and Goode, 1970), translocation of salivary ducts (Crysdale, 1980), and chorda tympani neurectomy (Friedman, Swerdlow, and Pomarico, 1974). Biofeedback is sometimes used to eliminate temporomandibular (TMJ) pain, to improve muscle function, or to relieve muscular spasm (Kerr, 1984; Linkenhoker, 1983).

Orthopedic surgery provides correction of deformities but does not decrease the muscle spasticity. In selected children, selective posterior (dorsal) rhizotomy is being explored as one method of reducing spasticity and improving function (Shiminski-Maher, 1989). This surgery requires extensive postoperative therapy because the procedure renders the child's muscles flaccid. The child must be retaught to sit, stand, and walk (Brucker, 1990).

Therapy techniques by physical or occupational therapists are usually prescribed, although sound scientific research is not readily available to support their efficacy. Of the five most common neuromotor therapies being used, the Doman-Delacato approach (patterning) is the most controversial. The four other types and their chief proponents are Bobath's neurodevelopmental treatment, Rood's sensorimotor approach, Ayre's sensory integration approach, and Vojta's approach (Harris, Atwater, and Crowe, 1988; Tirosh and Rabino, 1989). Transcranial stimulation is also sometimes suggested to inhibit primitive reflexes (Malden and Charash, 1985).

ASSOCIATED PROBLEMS
Intellectual problems

One of the most serious associated problems is potential intellectual impairment. Fifty percent to 75% of all children with cerebral palsy are estimated to have intellectual disabilities ranging in degree from mild to severe mental retardation. Dyskinetic cerebral palsy results in few limitations in intellectual abilities. Many of the persons who have the most limiting physical symptoms are the ones who have the least cognitive impairment. Severe motor involvement interferes with speech production and the ability to exhibit intellectual capabilities unless the child has access to appropriate technology to help transmit intellectual ability.

Visual impairment

More than 50% of children with cerebral palsy are estimated to have vision problems (Rubin and Crocker, 1989). Refractive errors, strabismus, nystagmus, and amblyopia are common and often require surgery, lenses, or both for correction. Assessment, identification, and treatment are important to prevent amblyopia and other secondary problems.

Hearing impairment

Sensorineural hearing loss is not uncommon. It may occur in 5% to 15% of all children and in 67% of the children with postbilirubin dyskinetic cerebral palsy. Children with motor problems as infants may spend an inordinate amount of time in the recumbent position, predisposing them to increased episodes of acute and chronic serous otitis media resulting in temporary conductive hearing loss.

Mobility

Motor milestones are almost always delayed. Alterations in muscle tone and range of motion contribute to impairment in motor function (Shiminski-Maher, 1989). There is a persistence of primitive reflexes, now viewed as aberrant reflexes, as well as a delay in the acquisition of postural reactions. Scoliosis and contractures can further limit the level of motor function achieved.

Dental problems

Increased dental caries result from (1) improper dental hygiene, (2) congenital enamel defects (hypoplasia of primary teeth), (3) high carbohydrate intake and retention, (4) dietary imbalance with poor nutritional intake, (5) inadequate fluoride, and (6) difficulty in mouth closure and drooling. Spastic or clonic movements may interfere with the cleaning process. These movements can cause gagging or biting down on the toothbrush. Hypersensitivity around the mouth is also common, causing the child to resist dental hygiene. Malocclusion can occur in as many as 90% of the children. Gingivitis is secondary to inadequate dental hygiene and may be further complicated by the use of anticonvulsants. Bruxism and TMJ dysfunction are common findings (Pearlman, 1989). Fractured, avulsed, or devitalized anterior teeth secondary to trauma are seen, especially in the child with seizures.

Eating disabilities

It is not uncommon for an infant with cerebral palsy to have feeding problems. A poor sucking reflex and inability to chew or swallow are secondary to the involvement of oropharyngeal muscles, resulting in abnormal muscle tone and function of the tongue, lips, and cheeks (Rubin and Crocker, 1989). Abnormal posturing further contributes to difficulty in swallowing. Children with excessive extensor tone are especially prone to this problem (Haynes, 1983). In addition, respiratory status influences the child's eating abilities. Children who have abnormal, irregular, or inefficient breathing will have difficulty coordinating breathing and swallowing.

Drooling

Approximately 10% to 13% of children have drooling problems (Sochaniwskyj, 1982). Constant drooling causes excoriation of the chin, wet clothing, odor, discomfort, and social rejection. Both invasive and noninvasive techniques have been used to decrease or eliminate drooling. Referral to an occupational therapist or a surgeon may be indicated if the family desires further assessment.

Constipation

The increased incidence of constipation in various age groups can be the result of a variety of factors: chewing and swallowing difficulties, inadequate fluid intake, decreased intake of bulky foods, prolonged use of strained foods, decreased mobility, abnormality of muscle tone (including the muscles related to peristalsis), medications, lack of an established toileting pattern, fear of using the toilet, instability of the child while seated on the toilet, history of painful evacuations, inadequate positioning for evacuation, and behavior problems. Dioctyl sodium sulfosuccinate (Colace) or senna concentrate (Senokot) are often used with diet management to control and treat constipation.

Communication disorders

A large number of the children will have delayed communication and communication disorders. Poor quality of speech is the result of an inability to control muscles to provide oral-motor function, and language is affected by central processing difficulties. Technology has made a tremendous difference in helping these children to be able to communicate. Procurement of augmentative communication systems, including proper switching devices, is essential if they are to express themselves. This is especially relevant for children with dyskinetic cerebral palsy who often have intellectual capabilities that are underrecognized and utilized because they lack verbal skills and have decreased use of their hands to write.

Respiratory problems

Children with abnormal tone and muscle function are prone to respiratory problems. Weak respiratory muscles contribute to a decreased vital capacity. Decreased neuromuscular control makes it difficult to coordinate the activity of the respiratory muscles, often resulting in inadequate gas exchange (Haynes, 1983). The irregularity and reduced efficiency of the respiratory system predisposes the child to respiratory problems. Coughing or choking during feedings can result in aspiration. Aspiration can contribute to acute lower respiratory tract infections, and if they are a recurrent problem, chronic lung changes may occur (Jones, 1989).

Urinary tract infections

Children with cerebral palsy have an increased risk of developing urinary tract infections (UTIs) (Rubin and Crocker, 1989). Inadequate fluid intake, limited mobility, inadequate perineal hygiene, abnormal voiding patterns, and chronic constipation all are factors that predispose the child to UTIs. Girls also have a higher rate of vaginal infections that contribute to UTI predisposition. Poor perineal hygiene, often the result of tight hip adductors, makes it difficult for girls to be self-sufficient in toileting.

Seizures

Seizures of all types are common. It is estimated that 35% to 50% of all persons with cerebral palsy have seizures. Seizures occur in 69% of the children with hemiparesis, 39% of the children with quadriparesis, and 7% of the children with dyskinesia (Abroms and Panagakos, 1980). (For further discussion on seizure disorders, see Chapter 15.)

Hip dislocations, scoliosis, and contractures

Children with spasticity will have unbalanced muscle tone across one or both hip joints. This predisposes them to unilateral or bilateral dislocation, which can occur at any age (Fig. 9-2). Children who are nonambulatory are more prone to this condition (Lord, 1984). Because of abnormal muscle tone, scoliosis occurs more frequently in children with spasticity than in the general population. Uncorrected scoliosis can contribute to cardiorespiratory problems and decreases the child's functional ability. Joint contractures secondary to unbalanced musculature are also common. The most serious

Spasm　　　　　　Contracture　　　　　　Deformity

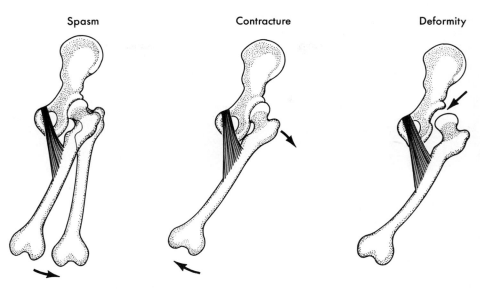

Fig. 9-2. Muscle spasm leading to contracture and eventual bony deformity.

ones are hip flexion and ankle plantar flexion deformities. Mild elbow flexion contractures, though common, cause less interference with function.

PRIMARY CARE MANAGEMENT
Growth and development

Growth retardation is anticipated in children with cerebral palsy. This retardation can be expressed as decreased height, weight, and weight for height, as well as skeletal immaturity. Children with oral-motor impairment are at greater risk for inadequate nutritional intake and subsequent growth retardation than children with cerebral palsy who do not have oral-motor impairments (Krick and Van Duyn, 1984). Growth retardation may also be influenced by increased energy requirements secondary to abnormal movements or seizures. Some improvement in growth has been demonstrated, however, when the child's nutritional status is improved through tube or gastrostomy feedings (Jones, 1989).

Obtaining accurate length and weight measurements of children with motor or posture disabilities is a challenge. If infants do not have seating balance, they are weighed supine on a balance scale. Older children are weighed in a chair scale or on a stretcher scale. Length is obtained by lying the child supine on a measuring board (Fig. 9-3). Children who have contractures or dyskinetic movements will need to be assisted to lie quietly and straight to get as accurate assessments as possible. Skinfold assessments are also obtained. Because of underdeveloped muscles and other associated problems, a thorough, combined analysis of all height, weight, and skinfold data will provide a more accurate picture of the child's growth.

Development. The child's development needs to be monitored in five domains: (1) self-help, (2) communication, (3) physical (fine-gross motor), (4) academic, and (5) personal-social. These areas can be assessed by parent interview using the Developmental Profile II, the Vineland Adaptive Behavior Scales, or the American Academy of Mental Deficiency Adaptive Behavior Scales (school version). Because children often have considerable "scatter" in their performance, assessing each developmental domain helps document the child's strengths and deficits. Adjustments for prematurity are indicated when the child less than 1 year of age is tested.

The Denver Development Screening Test (DDST), although widely used in screening, is re-

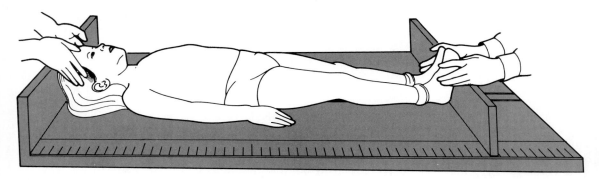

Fig. 9-3. Measuring length. Child with contractures or dyskinetic movements is helped to lie quietly and straight.

ported to underdetect infants with cerebral palsy when it is used during the first year of life (Campbell and Wilhelm, 1985; Sciarillo et al., 1986). A newer revision of the test may prove to be more sensitive, however. Moreover, the DDST is inappropriate to use in following the developmental progression of children already identified with cerebral palsy, particularly those with severe disabilities (Meisels, 1989). Tests that focus more specifically on motor development, such as the Bayley Scales of Infant Development (psychomotor development index) and the Milani-Comparetti Developmental Scale, Peabody Developmental Motor Scales, Movement Assessment of Infants, and the Infant Motor Screen are more sensitive for younger children than the DDST, and the Bruininks-Oseretsky Test of Motor Proficiency is more sensitive for children more than 4½ years of age if they do not have serious motor involvement.

Some of these instruments focus more specifically on the quantity than the quality of motor skills, so observation of motor performance must also be included in the assessment. For example, a child with ataxic cerebral palsy may be walking, but the gait is wide based and uncoordinated, causing swaying, or a child with hemiplegia may be walking but have foot and ankle equinus, producing instability.

Screening for language development is essential because deficits in language milestones are usually considered to be the best indicators of future cognitive performance (Pidcock, 1987). The sensitivity of the DDST is weak in this domain, failing to

identify more than half of the children who had expressive or articulation problems. The Denver Articulation Screening Examination is a quick assessment of articulation. The Clinical Linguistic and Auditory Scale (CLAMS) can be used to monitor the child's attainment of language milestones. Care should be taken to be certain that parents are not overestimating their child's expressive language by assuming that echolalia or grunting sounds are words or combinations of words. Pidcock (1987) suggests that children who fail the CLAMS can be given the second-step Emergent Language Milestone Scale for further evaluation.

Because many children with cerebral palsy have developmental delays, enrollment in a community-based or center-based interdisciplinary early developmental program is indicated. Special therapies, such as speech, language, physical, and occupational, are included in the programming.

Immunizations

Diphtheria, tetanus, and pertussis. Children with neurologic disorders, especially seizures, may have adverse reactions to pertussis vaccine. Therefore diphtheria, tetanus, and pertussis (DPT) immunization is sometimes deferred. The risk of diphtheria or tetanus is so low during the first year of life that it is not necessary to give DT vaccine if pertussis immunization is contraindicated. However, as early in the second year as possible, DT or DPT should be given. Charts of children where DPT immunization was deferred need to be flagged so that their condition is evaluated periodically and immunization given as soon as appropriate (Committee on Infectious Diseases, 1991). The risks and benefits of giving or withholding the immunization must be discussed with the parents and recorded in the child's record. Children with cerebral palsy without seizures are not at increased risk and may receive DPT as normally recommended.

Measles. Children with a history of previous seizures are at slightly increased risk, though minimal, of having a seizure after measle vaccination (see Chapter 15). The high risk of contracting measles with its known serious complications and the low incidence of reported seizure activity following vaccination warrant routine measles immunization (Committee on Infectious Diseases, 1991).

Haemophilus influenzae type b. The regular schedule for administering the *Haemophilus influenzae* type b (Hib) vaccine should be strictly followed. Because Hib bacteria are present in respiratory secretions and are easily transmitted from one child to another, children with cerebral palsy in group settings are at particular risk for infection because of their increased drooling.

Influenza vaccine. Although children with cerebral palsy are not targeted by the American Academy of Pediatrics as needing influenza vaccine (Committee on Infectious Diseases, 1991), those who are cared for in child care settings should be considered candidates. Influenza vaccine is administered in the fall before the beginning of the influenza season. It can be administered simultaneously with measles-mumps-rubella (MMR), Hib or oral polio vaccine.

Other immunizations. Immunizations for polio, mumps, and rubella are given as routinely scheduled. It is important to keep the child on schedule. Because these children have frequent respiratory tract infections, mild illness should not be a contraindication to vaccination otherwise completing the immunization schedule may be unnecessarily prolonged.

Screening

Vision. Because of the high incidence and variety of visual defects, many of these children are followed every 6 to 12 months by a pediatric opthalmologist. The primary care provider should also screen vision on a regular basis. The Hirschberg light reflex text, cover test, tracking, and fundo-

scopic examinations should be done at each visit.

Visual acuity screening can be done using a variety of instruments. The picture card test is used for children less than 3 years of age, the illiterate "E" test is used for children 3½ to 6 years of age, and older children may be able to use the Snellen chart or Titmus machine if their intelligence and communication skills are adequate (Holland, 1982). Children with motor deficits may have difficulty showing the direction of the E on the illiterate chart, and children with upper motor disabilities may have difficulty naming the letters or symbols. Practicing before the examination is essential.

Many children need glasses for correction. Young children may dislike keeping the glasses in place. Using a Velcro strap around the head helps secure the glasses. Correct positioning of glasses will increase visibility, improving sensory input. Eye patching, surgery, or both may be indicated to correct strabismus (Sprague, 1981).

Hearing. Because of the high incidence of hearing impairment, many children need to be followed by a pediatric audiologist or ear-nose-throat (ENT) physician. Infants and young children need to be referred for behavioral audiometry and an auditory evoked response under sedation to determine hearing activity. Older children should have periodic behavioral baseline hearing tests performed. Because of the increased susceptibility to ear infections, impedance audiometry should be done routinely to determine the patency of the eustachian tubes, the integrity of the ossicular chain, and the presence of perforation (Chow et al., 1984).

Children with hearing impairment are fitted with a hearing aid(s) as soon as the diagnosis is made. The family and child need to be taught the proper use and maintenance of these appliances as they can significantly increase the child's ability to learn and to interact effectively with others.

Dental. Dental care consisting of routine biannual pediatric dental appointments, daily dental hygiene of cleaning and flossing, attention to nutrition and fluoride, and early intervention to pathologic changes are essential. Dental sealants are often used to decrease the possibility of caries formation. Children who have seizures may be receiving phenytoin (Dilantin), a drug that causes gingival hyperplasia. A dentist needs to closely monitor this condition because it may eventually require surgical intervention.

Techniques that parents may be taught to improve dental hygiene include using a wash cloth instead of a toothbrush, cleaning the teeth while the child is lying down rather than sitting up, and omitting toothpaste if the child objects to it. Children who have severe deformities, are unable to cooperate, or who have extensive dental problems may need to be sedated to have an adequate dental examination and treatment. Assisting the parents in locating a dentist qualified and sensitive to these children's special needs is very important. Preparing the child for dental visits can help to decrease anxiety.

Blood pressure. Routine screening is recommended.

Urinalysis. Routine screening is recommended.

Hematocrit. Routine screening is recommended.

Tuberculosis. Routine screening is recommended.

Condition-specific screening

HIP DISLOCATION. Dislocation of the hips can occur at any age in the child with spastic cerebral palsy. Screening should occur at each well child visit. Because of the scissoring of the lower extremities, use of the Ortolani or Barlow test is often not possible. Screening must focus on a history of change in the joint. Suspected dislocation can be confirmed by radiographic testing.

SCOLIOSIS AND CONTRACTURES. Scoliosis and musculoskeletal contractures also can occur at any time and must be screened for at each well child visit. Measurement of spinal curvature and joint flexibility should be done. Changes in flexibility should be documented and reported to the appropriate team specialist. The primary provider plays an important role in prevention of these deformities by reinforcing the importance of physical therapy when counseling the child and family

Drug interactions

Medications, other than for seizure control, are not routinely prescribed for children with cerebral palsy. Tranquilizers and muscle relaxants have been found to result in quantitative relaxation of muscle tension but provide little functional improvement (Diamond, 1986).

DIFFERENTIAL DIAGNOSIS AND MANAGEMENT OF COMMON PEDIATRIC CONDITIONS
Fever

Young children with impaired neurologic systems are prone to fever. Temperature more than 38.6° C is often caused by an acute infectious process, usually of viral origin. About half of these infections are related to upper or lower respiratory tract infections and the other half to genitourinary or gastrointestinal (GI) tract infection. Infants less than 6 months of age, children having high fevers or fever for more than 72 hours without symptoms, children appearing acutely ill, or children who have seizures with fever need to be seen for physical assessment and laboratory studies (urinalysis, white blood cell and differential counts, and throat or blood culture consistent with physical findings).

If the fever persists beyond 1 week, the child is irritable, listless, or lethargic, or the condition seems to worsen, the child should be evaluated by the primary care provider. Children with severe cerebral palsy have a low baseline of homeostasis. A relatively minor illness can result in significant physiologic distress. Their condition must be closely monitored.

Respiratory tract infections

The most common location of infection in the upper respiratory tract are the middle ears, throat, and sinuses. Otitis media frequently occurs in children with cerebral palsy and must be high on the list of suspected diagnoses. Routine antibiotic and symptomatic treatment is indicated, with special emphasis on follow-up for evaluation of continued suppurative or serous effusion and loss of hearing. If recurrent otitis media develops, a referral to an ENT specialist is advised because myringotomy tubes are often recommended for this population.

Pain is one symptom of infection that may be difficult to assess in children with severe cerebral palsy. Signs of pain in an infant with upper respiratory tract infections may be rubbing or pulling on the ears or facial grimaces when swallowing. Drooling may also increase because of pain on swallowing. The older child may be able to respond to questions concerning pain by shaking his or her head. Children who use communication systems have facial symbols that can identify pain and may have pictures of body parts to which they can point.

School-aged children may be able to understand systems that ask for variations in degree of pain, such as: "If 1 is a little pain and 4 is the worst pain you've every had, what is this pain like?" Patience is needed when a child is not feeling well and has impaired verbal or motor skills to get an adequate assessment of the child's condition and health problem.

In children with moderate or severe cerebral palsy associated with limited mobility and compromised nutritional and respiratory status, lower respiratory tract infections are more common and are potentially life threatening. Aspiration pneumonia, as well as routine viral and bacterial pneumonia, must be high on the list of differential diagnosis whenever the child has respiratory symptoms. These children must be closely monitored. Excessive secretions and ineffective cough mechanisms may lead to respiratory difficulty and airway obstruction. Fever may rapidly result in dehydration and increased mucous viscosity.

If pneumonia is diagnosed on physical examination or by chest x-ray studies, the practitioner will need to determine if hospitalization is required. Home management of the mild to moderately ill child can be attempted if adequate follow-up can be arranged and the family is able and willing to care for the child. The practitioner will need to carefully educate the family on respiratory assessment and identify specific instructions for treatment and follow-up. Many parents become skilled at identifying subtle changes in their child's condition, but they must never feel it is their ultimate responsibility to make critical assessment decisions.

Urinary tract infections

Urinary tract infections are more common in children with cerebral palsy and, as with all children, are often difficult to diagnose by history and physical examination alone. The practitioner must have a high index of suspicion and order urinalysis or urine cultures whenever symptoms indicate the possibility of a UTI. Nonspecific symptoms include lethargy, irritability, anorexia, vomiting, diarrhea, and fever. More specific symptoms include abdominal or flank pain, frequent urination, burning, loss of previously obtained continence, and foul-smelling urine.

Standard antibacterial therapy is indicated for positive urine cultures. Additional comfort measures include increasing fluid intake, increased rest, increased attention to cleansing the perineal area after voiding, routine toileting schedule to encourage reestablishment of continence, and taking acetaminophen based on body weight for pain relief. Follow-up evaluations are imperative. Repeat urine culture should be sterile 48 to 72 hours after therapy is instituted. If not, the practitioner should consider the advisability of changing antibiotics. After 2 weeks another urine culture should be done. Long-term follow-up is required because recurrent UTIs are common. Recurrent infections require further diagnostic studies for exploration of urinary tract abnormalities, and a referral to a urologist is indicated.

Gastrointestinal problems

Diarrhea and vomiting are frequent symptoms during childhood. Children with cerebral palsy are often poorly nourished, and consequently diarrhea and vomiting can be a serious problem needing close evaluation. If only diarrhea is present, the parents are advised to provide adequate fluid intake to prevent dehydration and omit solid foods for 24 to 48 hours to rest the bowel. If vomiting is present, all solids foods are withheld. The child is given only sips of an oral electrolyte solution (e.g., Lytren or Pedialyte), flat cola, ginger ale, or lemon-lime soda for 24 to 48 hours. Fluids are gradually increased as vomiting decreases. If vomiting or diarrhea is severe or associated with pain, the child should be seen by the practitioner. Careful monitoring of fluid loss by examination and weight checks is advised because children can become dehydrated quickly.

The primary care provider must always remember that appendicitis, bowel obstruction, and mesentery artery syndrome are possible reasons for GI symptoms. In the child with severe cerebral palsy, many of the classic historical or physical findings may be absent or altered, making diagnosis difficult.

DEVELOPMENTAL ISSUES
Safety

Children with cerebral palsy, even those mildly affected, have balance and coordination problems. Bike riding, skiing, rock climbing, ice skating, or boating are examples of activities that require good balance and may be difficult for children with even mild cerebral palsy. These and similar activities are not contraindicated but should be initiated slowly, with adult supervision, and with recognition of the potential safety hazards.

Children who have seizures should wear a helmet when trying to ambulate or during play activities to prevent head injuries if a seizure should occur. Children who are prone to falls should be encouraged to ambulate or play in areas away from sharp-angled objects, steps, or uneven surfaces. Children with moderate to severe cerebral palsy create a different picture.

Seat belts are essential whenever the child is in the upright seated position to prevent falls. Generally the seat belt should come across the child's hips at a 45-degree angle and clasp over the pelvis. Car safety seats are required and can be manufactured individually for the child if standard car seats do not position the child correctly. Parents should be cautioned against attempting to modify standard car seats, such as altering strap positions, to avoid reducing the seat's effectiveness in an automobile accident (Bull, Stroup, and Gerhart, 1988). Infants and children without good head control should be positioned facing the rear of the car until adequate head control is attained.

For the child who spends a great deal of time in a wheelchair or travel chair, several other important safety factors must be taken into account. It is imperative to check for pressure areas and to relieve points of stress as soon as possible. Careful attention is paid to ensure that the chair's brakes are appropriately applied. Precautions need to be taken when the wheelchair is moved from one level to another, and the use of ramps is encouraged. The bedroom window of a child who uses a wheelchair should be marked with an emergency alert sticker and the local fire station personnel informed of the child's condition and whereabouts in case of an emergency.

Child care

Children requiring care outside the home can be serviced in preschool or day-care programs that are designed specifically for children with special health care needs or mainstreamed into programs serving nondisabled children. The family needs to assess and observe the child care program before

---

QUESTIONS ON CHILD CARE

1. Has the child care center ever had a child with similar problems?
2. Do the personnel seem to understand what the family identifies as special needs of their child?
3. What policies are in place regarding illness and infection control?
4. What provisions are made for serving children with minor illness?
5. What are the preentrance requirements for immunizations?
6. What is the adult/child ratio?
7. How does the staff respond when children cannot participate in a scheduled activity because of physical limitations?
8. Are the furniture, toys, and so forth appropriate to meet their child's needs?
9. Are they willing to adapt the environment to meet the child's special needs (e.g., using switches, applying Velcro, using built-up handles)?
10. Is the staff willing to teach the child self-help skills even if it takes more time?
11. What will the child do if he or she cannot engage in special activities that are planned?
12. What arrangements are made for transporting a child with a wheelchair (if appropriate) or seating instability?
13. What behavior management approaches are used to control negative behaviors?
14. If the child care personnel do not have experience with children with cerebral palsy, are they willing to have in-service education or technical assistance to learn skills that they need?

---

placing the child to be certain that the program is able to respond to the needs of children with cerebral palsy (see the box above). The practitioner can provide a valuable service to the family and day-care center by being available to answer questions concerning health care needs of the child.

Diet

Children with moderate or severe cerebral palsy may have dietary problems throughout their life.

The infant's inability to use his or her mouth and tongue effectively makes feeding difficult. Parents may need to thicken formula or put a larger hole in the nipple to aid in swallowing and to compensate for a weak suck. Parents are discouraged from putting the infant's head back and pouring the formula into the mouth because of the risk of aspiration. When fluids or food need to be wiped from the infant's chin, a gentle patting or blotting motion is indicated to minimize stimulation of the often hypersensitive oral area. To obtain adequate nutrition, infants with severe feeding problems are fed small feedings of highly concentrated foods at frequent intervals. Jaw control is achieved by placing the fingers in a V position over the child's chin. Because these children are often highly distractable, confusion and activities need to be minimized. A mirror can be placed in front of the child to focus attention on feeding.

When an infant feeds poorly, a cycle of frustration occurs because the parent feels inadequate in satisfying the infant and the infant does not obtain satisfaction from the feeding and becomes irritable and fussy. The parents may need assistance in reading the infant's cues so that the infant is fed when most alert (Snow and Frye, 1990). This is especially important when one is feeding an infant with hypotonia because this infant may sleep a great deal and not cry to alert the parent to provide a feeding.

Parents often delay introducing textured foods when feeding problems are present. They need to be encouraged to increase texture and to provide a variety of foods. Parents are discouraged from giving the child only foods that are readily accepted, such as high caloric foods, strained fruits, or sweetened liquids, to the exclusion of nutritious foods from the basic four food groups (Weigley, 1990). When a child has severe cerebral palsy, spoon feeding may be difficult and the assistance of an occupational therapist in teaching parents appropriate techniques is often very valuable.

As soon as it is developmentally appropriate, the child can begin finger feeding. Finger foods, such as raw fruits or crackers, will encourage chewing and strengthen the jaw muscles. The parents need to know that choking can occur and must be prepared to perform the Heimlich maneuver if necessary.

When it is necessary to provide feeding through either a nasogastric or gastrostomy tube, the child's normal sensory experiences are decreased. Even minor attempts to suck and swallow are important movements, and their loss can influence the child's future ability to be fed by mouth. Because the mouth area receives less normal stimulation, it can become hypersensitive to any touch sensation. In addition, if painful stimuli such as suctioning, intubation, and tube insertions take place, the hypersensitivity can be heightened. A referral for video fluoroscopy may be useful if feeding is not improved and growth is not taking place. An occupational therapist can also assist the child in developing or maintaining prefeeding skills through an oral-motor treatment program (Morris and Klein, 1987).

If a child is unable to maintain a normal growth pattern, a 3-day dietary intake can help in the assessment process. If nutritional intake is adequate or excessive, a child who has limited mobility may gain excessive weight. On the other hand, a child with seizures or dyskinesia may need additional calories to compensate for increased motor activity. The primary care provider should provide nutritional counseling or refer the parents to a nutritionist.

Discipline

All children need consistent discipline to develop. Because many children with cerebral palsy start life with serious threats to their viability, parents are often initially wary and tend to respond to their child's every demand. The parents may be uncertain about their ability to successfully parent. If the child has difficulties or frequent illnesses, the parents may be tempted not to discipline the child in any way or to be inconsistent with discipline. As the child gets older, lack of discipline can lead to behavior problems that will need strict behavior management programs to eradicate. Therefore, parents are encouraged to set reasonable limits for the child, to be consistent within the parameters they establish, and to use behavior management techniques that are appropriate, such as short time-out periods, to control aberrant behavior.

Toileting

Because of the motor delays and potential associated developmental delays, toileting is usually

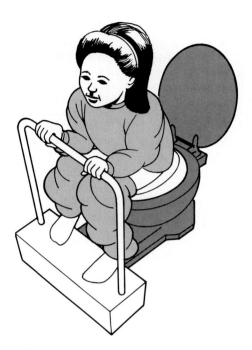

Fig. 9-4. Child uses adaptive equipment for toileting.

started later. The parents need to be apprised of readiness signs for toilet training, such as the child recognizing a wet diaper or exhibiting appropriate motor skills. It is very helpful to have the parent keep a record of the child's elimination for 1 week before a toileting routine is started to identify the child's normal pattern of elimination. When toileting is started, the child needs a steady seat such as a child potty chair or a seat attachment for the commode. The child's feet should be placed firmly on the floor or a box and a seat belt used (Fig. 9-4). An inverted long-leg stool can serve this purpose. A side support, such as rails, is also helpful so that the child does not fear falling.

If muscle tone is extremely poor, constipation can be a persistent problem. It may be necessary to increase roughage and fluids in the diet, to use stool softeners or suppositories, and even to resort to enemas or manual removal in extreme cases. Establishing a consistent toileting time can assist in developing periodic evacuations of the bowel. The time set aside for toileting is determined by the family's schedule. When a convenient time is established, the child should finish a meal and then be placed on the toilet. The child may need to have an adult close by for support during the time that the toilet is being used. A quiet time with encouragement will contribute to success. After 10 to 25 minutes the child should be removed from the toilet and praised for efforts regardless of whether evacuation takes place. Parents should be discouraged from scolding the child when evacuation does not occur.

Whether or not the child will achieve urinary and bowel continence and at what age it will occur are highly individualized. The practitioner needs to work closely with the family so that toileting is started at an appropriate time and maximum function is achieved.

Sleep patterns

A variety of sleep disturbances can be present. Keeping a weekly record of the child's sleep-wake pattern can assist the practitioner to plan appropriate interventions. The infant or young child who is hypotonic or has spasticity should not be allowed to sleep in the froglike position. A neutral alignment of the arms and legs should be attempted, and the head and trunk need to be slightly flexed. This positioning is obtained by using a firm mattress and placing the child in a side-lying position or by having the child sleep between two long bolsters (Haynes, 1983). In the early months it may be necessary to reposition the child frequently during the night. Practicing sleep positions during the day can facilitate the child's comfort level and encourage new positioning and development of independent sleep skills, such as the ability to turn over. The occupational therapist and physical therapist are most helpful in educating parents on body alignment and positioning techniques.

The infant or young child with hypotonia may also evidence stridor when placed in bed. Intrinsic or extrinsic blockage of the upper airway may cause a harsh respiratory sound. This blockage is usually relieved by altering the flexion of the head and neck. Intermittent respiratory stridor that does not respond to a change in position should be evaluated by the practitioner even though it is usually not a cause for concern. A continuous stridor requires immediate medical evaluation.

Children who drool excessively benefit from the side-lying position. Bibs that are often worn during daytime hours should be removed when the child is sleeping to avoid potential strangulation. The infant who is not satisfied with feeding will often be awake many more hours than anticipated. In this instance, focusing on improving the infant's nutritional status can also improve the infant's sleep pattern.

School issues

For the child with cerebral palsy who has attended a preschool program, an educational transition program should be planned so that there is a smooth transition from the preschool program to the elementary school program. The child may be mainstreamed into attending an elementary school program for children the same age or may be in the special education program. In either case, the child should receive educational and related services in the least restricted environment.

The school-aged child needs an individualized education plan (IEP) that clearly identifies all of the resources that need to be in place so that the child can achieve in school. Technology can often improve the child's ability to learn and communicate. An augmentative communication system should be chosen on the basis of the child's capabilities, such as an eye gaze system for the child with severe quadraplegia, communication board for the child with some upper extremity movement, or a computer with a keyboard voice synthesizer for those children with severe speech impairment.

The child will often need physical or occupational therapy services. The development of fine and gross motor skills can enhance learning and are incorporated with the child's school activities. Speech and language therapy can be done individually, can be done in small groups, or can be incorporated into classroom activities.

The school needs to know whether or not the child requires modifications in the school environment, such as a cut-out desk, special seating, or special adaptations for eating. Adapted physical education is often necessary. During physical education the child should be taken out of the wheelchair so that a change in position accompanies exercise. If a child has numerous needs, such as when the child is incontinent and requires clothing changes, the child is dependent on others for oral or gastrostomy feedings, or the child's seizures are uncontrolled, a personal assistant is required and should be provided by the school district.

Transportation issues need to be resolved well in advance of the school year so that the family knows how this will be accomplished. If the child is in a wheelchair, it is especially important to discuss this area to ascertain that the van or bus has a wheelchair lift and that the driver knows how to assist a child with a wheelchair.

Developmental disabilities, learning deficits, and the adaptation to the school environment and personnel all are potential road blocks to successful school performance. The practitioner should routinely assess the child's progress in school and offer support to the family in attaining additional needed services when indicated. School failure can be the first sign of emotional problems, so monitoring is essential.

A plan should be in place for actions to be taken in case of emergency. For the child in a wheelchair or with mobility problems, specific guidelines should be established for assisting the child in a fire drill or actual situation. In addition, if medications are required during the school program, the school personnel need written instructions from the primary caretaker. Ideally a school nurse is available for ongoing consultation with the school personnel and serves as a liaison with the family and the primary care providers.

As adolescence approaches, changes may occur. For example, younger adolescents may try to deny the permanence of their condition. As the reality of their limitations becomes evident, adolescents may become depressed as they begin to come to terms with the implications of their condition for their life script. Until resolution occurs, they may exhibit withdrawal from others, refuse to do school work, decline to participate in extracurricular activities, or express death wishes. In addition, if other nondisabled adolescents exhibit discomfort when in the presence of the adolescent with more severe cerebral palsy, the adolescent with a disability soon learns the stigma attached to being different (Taft and Matthews, 1983). Awareness of their own long-term condition and exclusion by peers combines to make this a potentially troublesome time.

Sexuality

The late adolescent years can find the person with cerebral palsy still being physically dependent on others. Often the more dependent and physically involved, the fewer opportunities there will be to engage in sexual-social interactions and explorations. When opportunities for sexual expressions occur, the person may have difficulty engaging in interactions that are mutually rewarding to each partner. Consideration needs to be focused on ways to make the social-sexual experience possible and positive. Intimacy needs will be influenced by their capabilities as well as their physical disabilities. However, having disabilities does not rule out the possibility for significant relationships to occur. A variety of resources to assist with intimate relationships are available, and a referral to a sexual counselor or therapist may be warranted. With the emphasis on normalization, social-sexual experiences will become more important as choices to date, marry, and bear children increase.

SPECIAL FAMILY CONCERNS

Having a child with mild cerebral palsy may have minimal affect on the family and family function, but the time spent providing care to the child with severe cerebral palsy can be extreme. Increased physical care needs and prolonged years of dependency may overwhelm the family. Families need assistance, from whatever sources are available, in the day-to-day care of their child so that the personal needs of all family members, including siblings, can be met. Respite care opportunities are essential for the overall health and well-being of the family.

SUMMARY OF PRIMARY CARE NEEDS FOR THE CHILD WITH CEREBRAL PALSY

Growth and development

Children with cerebral palsy usually have slow growth in weight and height and may become overweight because of decreased mobility.

Children with dyskinetic cerebral palsy often need extra calories to maintain growth and to compensate for increased movements or seizures.

Skinfold and height and weight should be assessed to monitor growth.

Eating and feeding problems contribute to poor growth patterns.

The validity of developmental tests for this population is questionable.

Quality and quantity of skills in various domains should be assessed.

Delayed development especially in physical and communication skills is common.

Intellectual abilities vary widely depending on the degree of involvement; more involved (dyskinesis) often have intellectual abilities that are not readily exhibited.

Technologic advances have increased the potential for these children.

Immunizations

During the first year of life the DPT vaccine is sometimes deferred if the infant has uncontrolled seizure activity. If it is deferred, DT or DPT vaccine is given as soon as possible in the second year.

Measles vaccine can cause seizures if children have a history of seizures, but a high incidence of measles makes the risk/benefit ratio favor administration.

Haemophilus influenzae type b is strongly recommended.

Influenza vaccine may be warranted in the fall if the child receives child care outside the home.

Other immunizations are given as recommended. Minor illness should not interfere with administration.

Screening
Vision

The Hirschberg test, cover test, ability to track, and fundoscopic examination should be done at each visit. The choice of tests for acuity is based on the child's age and capabilities. Because of the high incidence of visual defects, referral to an ophthalmologist is recommended during infancy.

Hearing

Routine office screening is done. Auditory brainstem evoked response may be indicated for younger children unable to participate in behavioral testing. The high incidence of hearing impairment and recurrent otitis media may require referral to an audiologist and ENT specialist.

Dental

Evaluation by a pediatric dentist is done biyearly. Parent counseling on dental care techniques is needed.

Hematocrit

Routine screening is recommended.

Tuberculosis

Routine screening is recommended.

Condition-specific screening

Hip dislocation, scoliosis, and musculoskeletal contracture may occur at any age. Screening for these deformities should be done at each well child visit.

Drug interactions

Except for medications for seizures, no medications are prescribed routinely.

Differential diagnosis
Fever

Respiratory tract, genitourinary, and GI tract infections should be ruled out. Management of fever symptoms is routine.

Respiratory tract infections

Upper respiratory tract, middle ears, throat, and sinuses are common locations. Lower respiratory tract infection should be ruled out. Adequate follow-up is essential.

Continued.

SUMMARY OF PRIMARY CARE NEEDS FOR
THE CHILD WITH CEREBRAL PALSY — cont'd

Urinary tract infections

Infections should be ruled out. If UTIs occur repeatedly, urinary tract abnormalities should be ruled out.

Gastrointestinal problems

Careful monitoring is required to prevent dehydration.

Developmental issues
Safety

Risk of injury is increased because of incoordination, instability, delayed motor skills, and potential seizures.

Child care

Appropriate special day-care or mainstreamed programs should be selected based on the child's assets and deficits and the family's needs. The potential for infection is increased.

Diet

The infant may have early feeding problems because of oromotor muscle problems and difficulty with swallowing and drooling. Regurgitation can be a problem. Feeding problems can be lifelong, and sometimes gastrostomy is indicated.

Discipline

Significant life-threatening health problems can contribute to a lack of discipline by parents. Limit setting should be encouraged so that behavior management techniques do not have to be instituted to correct protracted negative behavior.

Toileting

Bowel and bladder training may be delayed. Positioning is required when toileting is instituted.

Sleep patterns

Frequent sleep problems are sometimes associated with positioning and inadequate nutritional intake. Behavioral sleep problems respond to structured program.

School issues

Public Law 99-457 will make early development programs more common for preschool children with an individualized family service program. Public Law 94-142 requires IEPs for school-aged children. These children should receive specialized programming or mainstreaming in the LRE. Consideration of therapies and technology assistance is essential. Learning problems are common, and adolescence brings increased awareness of the disability and its consequences for lifetime planning.

Sexuality

Physical involvement may interfere with normal social-sexual interactions. Normalization in the community will lead to increased opportunities for dating, marriage, and childbearing.

Special family concerns

Lifelong attention to special needs can stress the family and requires respite opportunities for both the child and family.

RESOURCES

Organizations

United Cerebral Palsy Association, Inc.
1522 K St, NW
Washington, DC 20005

> *The United Cerebral Palsy Association, Inc. is a nationwide organization with local chapters that address the needs of families who have a member with cerebral palsy.*

REFERENCES

Abroms IF and Panagakos PG: The child with significant development motor disability (cerebral palsy). In Scheiner AP and Abroms IF, eds: *The practical management of the developmentally disabled child,* St Louis, 1980, CV Mosby, pp 145-166.

Amiel-Tison C: A method for neurologic evaluation within the first year of life, *Curr Probl Pediatr* 7:1-50, 1976.

Bull MJ, Stroup KB, and Gerhart S: Misuse of car safety seats, *Pediatrics* 81:98-101, 1988.

Campbell SK and Wilhelm IJ: Development for birth to 3 years of age 15 children at high risk for central nervous system dysfunction, *Phys Ther* 65:463-469, 1985.

Chow MP, Durand BA, Feldman MN, et al: *Handbook of pediatric primary care,* ed 2, New York, 1984, John Wiley & Sons, pp 933-977.

Committee on Infectious Diseases: *Report of the Committee on Infectious Diseases,* ed 22, Elk Grove Village, Ill, 1988, American Academy of Pediatrics.

Coolman RB, Bennett FC, Sells CJ et al: Neuromotor development of graduates of the neonatal intensive care unit: Patterns encountered in the first two years of life, *Dev Behav Pediatr* 6:327-333, 1985.

Crysdale WS: Drooling patient: Evaluation and current surgical options, *Laryngoscope* 90:775-783, 1980.

Diamond M: Rehabilitation strategies for the child with cerebral palsy, *Pediatr Ann* 15:230-236, 1986.

Drillien CM: Abnormal neurologic signs in the first year of life in low-birthweight infants: Possible prognostic significance, *Dev Med Child Neurol* 14:575-584, 1972.

Drillien CM, Thomson AJM and Burgoyne K: Low birthweight children at school age: A longitudinal study, *Dev Med Child Neurol* 22:26-47, 1980.

Ellenberg J and Nelson KB: Birthweight and gestational age in children with cerebral palsy or seizure disorders, *Am J Dis Child* 133:1044-1048, 1979.

Friedman WH, Swerdlow RS, and Pomarico JM: Tympanic neurectomy: Revise and additional indication for this procedure, *Laryngoscope* 84:568-577, 1974.

Garber NB: Operant procedures to eliminate drooling behavior in cerebral-palsied children, *Dev Med Child Neur* 13:641-644, 1971.

Hanson MJ and Harris SR: *Teaching the young child with motor delays,* Austin, Tex, 1986, Pro-Ed.

Harris MM and Dignam PF: Non-surgical method of reducing drooling in cerebral-palsied children, *Dev Med Child Neurol* 22:293-299, 1980.

Harris SR, Atwater SW, and Crowe TK: Accepted and controversial neuromotor therapies for infants at high risk for cerebral palsy, *J Perinatol* 8:3-13, 1988.

Haynes U: *Holistic health care for children with developmental disabilities,* Baltimore, 1983, University Park Press.

Hensleigh PA, Fainstat T, and Spencer R: Perinatal events and cerebral palsy, *Am J Obstet Gynecol* 154:978-981, 1986.

Holland SH: 20/20 vision screening, *Pediatr Nurs* 8:81-87, 1982.

Jones PM: Feeding disorders in children with multiple handicaps, *Dev Med Child Neur* 31:398-406, 1989.

Kerr AH: Help for the cerebral palsy patient. *Orthop Nurs* 3:44-46, 1984.

Krick J and Van Duyn MAA: The relationship between oral-motor involvement and growth: A pilot study in a pediatric population with cerebral palsy, *J Am Diet Assoc* 84:555-559, 1984.

Linkenhoker D: Tools of behavioral medicine: Application of biofeedback treatment for children and adolescents, *Dev Behav Pediatr* 4:16-20, 1983.

Lord J: Cerebral palsy: A clinical approach, *Arch Phy Med Rehabil* 65:542-548, 1984.

Malden JW and Charash LI: Transcranial stimulation for the inhibition of primitive reflexes in children with cerebral palsy, *Neurol Rep* 9:33-38, 1985.

Meisels SJ: Can developmental screening tests identify children who are developmentally at risk? *Pediatrics* 83:578-584, 1989.

Morris SE and Klein MD: *Pre-feeding skills,* Tucson, Ariz, 1987, Therapy Skill Builders.

Nelson KB and Ellenberg JH: Apgar scores as predictors of chronic neurologic disability, *Pediatrics* 68:36-44, 1981.

Oppenheim WL, Peacock WJ, Staudt LA, et al: Selective posterior rhizotomy for cerebral palsy. Presented in San Francisco, Oct 26, 1989. California

Paneth N: Etiologic factors in cerebral palsy, *Pediatr Ann* 15:191-201, 1986.

Pearlman J: Dental management. In Rubin IL and Crocker AC, eds: *Developmental disabilities: Delivery of medical care for children and adults,* Philadelphia, 1989, Lea & Febiger, pp 320-333.

Pharoah POD, Cooke T, Rosenbloom I, et al: Trends in birth prevalence of cerebral palsy, *Arch Dis Child* 62:379-384, 1987.

Pidcock FS: Developmental screening techniques for pediatricians, *Pediatr Basics* 50(5):8-12, 1987.

Rubin IL and Crocker AC: *Developmental disabilities: Delivery of medical care for children and adults,* Philadelphia, 1989, Lea & Febiger.

Sciarillo WG, Brown MM, Robinson NM, et al: Effectiveness of the Denver Developmental Screening Test with biologically vulnerable infants, *J Dev Behavior Pediatr* 7:77-83, 1986.

Shiminski-Maher T: Selective posterior rhizotomy in the pediatric cerebral palsy population: Implications for nursing practice, *J Neurosci Nurs* 21:308-312, 1989.

Snow LS and Frye ME: Formula feeding in the first year of life, *Pediatr Nurs* 16:442-446, 1990.

Sochaniwskyj AE: Drool quantification: Noninvasive technique. *Arch Phys Med* 63:605-607, 1982.

Smith RA and Goode RL: Sialorrhea, *N Engl J Med* 283:917-918, 1970.

Sprague J: Opthalmological evaluation. In Frankenburg WK, Thornton SM, Cohrs ME, eds: *Pediatric developmental diagnosis,* New York, 1981, Thieme-Stratton, pp 57-65.

Stanley FJ: The changing face of cerebral palsy? *Dev Med Child Neurol* 29:258-270, 1987.

Taft LT: Cerebral palsy. In Hoelkelman RA, Blatman S, Friedman SB, et al, eds: *Primary pediatric care.* St Louis, 1987, CV Mosby, pp 1183-1186.

Taft LT and Matthews WS: Cerebral palsy. In Levine MD, et al ed: *Developmental-behavioral pediatrics,* Philadelphia, 1983, WB Saunders, pp 789-797.

Tirosh E and Rabino S: Physiotherapy for children with cerebral palsy, *Am J Dis Child* 143:552-555, 1989.

Weigley EM: Changing patterns in offering solids to infants, *Pediatr Nurs* 16:439-441, 1990.

Weiss-Lambrou R, Tetreault; S, and Dudley J: The relationship between oral sensation and drooling in persons with cerebral palsy, *Am J Occup Ther* 43:155-161, 1989.

10 Congenital Adrenal Hyperplasia

Judith A. Ruble

ETIOLOGY

The adrenal glands are small triangular organs located on the top of each kidney. They are divided into two major components: the adrenal medulla, which is in the center of the gland, and the adrenal cortex, which surrounds the medulla.

The adrenal cortex synthesizes glucocorticoids (primarily cortisol), mineralocorticoids (mainly aldosterone) and androgens through complex metabolic pathways. A simplified diagram of these pathways is shown in Fig. 10-1. Cortisol, aldosterone, and adrenal androgens play a crucial role in maintaining homeostasis by helping to regulate the body's blood pressure, glucose, sodium, and water levels, sexual development, and other metabolic processes (Bacon et al., 1990; Miller and Levine, 1987).

Congenital adrenal hyperplasia (CAH) is caused by a deficiency of one of the enzymes used by the adrenal cortex to produce cortisol and aldosterone. Although there are six possible enzyme defects, approximately 90% to 95% of CAH is caused by 21-hydroxylase deficiency (Bacon et al., 1990; Miller and Levine, 1987). The other five enzyme defects are quite rare and are not discussed here. Each of the enzyme defects causing CAH is inherited as a separate autosomal recessive genetic trait. The gene responsible for CAH has been identified and is located on the short arm of chromosome 6, linked to the human leukocyte antigen gene B (HLA-B) (Miller and Levine, 1987).

The adrenal production of glucocorticoids is regulated by a feedback system to the hypothalamus and pituitary gland (Fig. 10-2). Normally the hypothalamus secretes corticotropin-releasing factor (CRF), which causes the pituitary gland to produce adrenocorticotropic hormone (ACTH). In turn, ACTH stimulates the adrenal glands to synthesize glucocorticoids (primarily cortisol). The "switch" that controls this feedback system is cortisol. When blood levels of cortisol are low, the system turns on; the hypothalamus releases CRF, which signals the pituitary to release ACTH, which stimulates the adrenal glands to synthesize cortisol. When blood levels of cortisol rise, the system turns off; the hypothalamus stops releasing CRF, the pituitary gland stops releasing ACTH, and the adrenal glands stop synthesizing cortisol (Bacon et al., 1990; Miller and Levine, 1987). Because cortisol production is blocked in CAH, the hypothalamic-pituitary-adrenal system is not turned off, resulting in high ACTH levels that continuously stimulate the adrenal glands (Bacon et al., 1990; Miller and Levine, 1987). The continual stimulation by ACTH leads to hypertrophy of the adrenal glands and a buildup of precursors to cortisol and an overproduction of adrenal androgens, as described in Fig. 10-1.

Aldosterone synthesis is regulated primarily by the renin-angiotensin system of the kidney, so that a block in aldosterone synthesis will cause very high plasma renin activity levels, just as a block

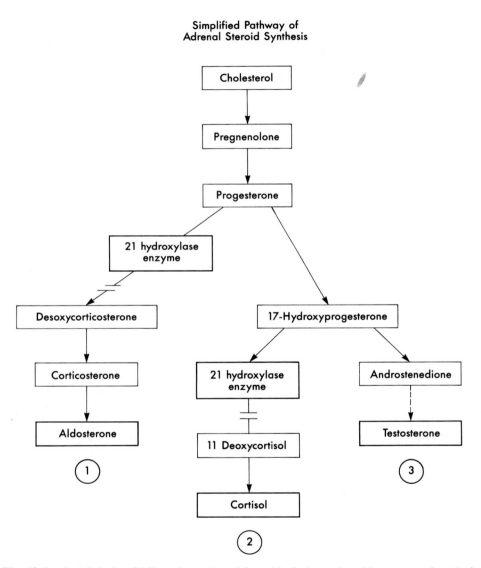

Fig. 10-1. In salt-losing CAH, pathways 1 and 2 are blocked, causing aldosterone and cortisol deficiencies. In non–salt-losing CAH, only pathway 2 is blocked, causing cortisol deficiency. In both forms of CAH there is a buildup of precursors and overproduction of adrenal androgens.

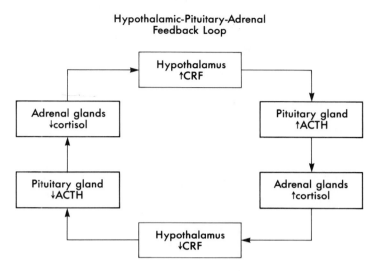

Fig. 10-2. Blood levels of cortisol turn the hypothalamic-pituitary-adrenal system "on" and "off": low cortisol levels cause the hypothalamus to make CRF; CRF causes the pituitary to release ACTH; ACTH stimulates the adrenal cortex to synthesize cortisol; high cortisol levels cause the hypothalamus to stop making CRF; without CRF, the pituitary stops producing ACTH; without ACTH, the adrenal cortex stops synthesizing cortisol; the cycle repeats.

in cortisol synthesis will cause high ACTH levels (Bacon et al., 1990; Levine and New, 1986).

There are two forms of "classical" 21-hydroxylase deficiency: salt-losing CAH and non-salt-losing (or simple virilizing) CAH. In the salt-losing form both cortisol and aldosterone production are blocked (see Fig. 10-1). The absence of aldosterone results in excessive sodium loss through the kidneys and the inability to maintain normal serum electrolyte balance. In the non-salt-losing form, only cortisol production is blocked and there is adequate aldosterone production to meet the body's normal needs. However, there may be a mild deficit, as indicated by elevated plasma renin activity levels or mild hyponatremia during stress (Bacon et al., 1990; Miller and Levine, 1987; Rosler et al., 1977).

The alterations in adrenal steroid metabolism caused by 21-hydroxylase deficiency lead to the buildup of precursors and overproduction of adrenal androgens, which do not require the 21-hydroxylase enzyme (see Fig. 10-1). Laboratory assays for these substances, such as serum 17-hydroxyprogesterone (17-OHP) or urine 17-ketosteroids and pregnanetriol, are used to monitor the adequacy of

cortisol replacement therapy for CAH. Laboratory assay of plasma renin activity is used to monitor the mineralocorticoid replacement in the salt-losing form.

There is another type of 21-hydroxylase deficiency commonly called the "nonclassic," "late-onset," or "cryptic" form, which is not apparent at birth by either physical findings or newborn screening tests. Its clinical features are similar to those of classical 21-hydroxylase deficiency but occur later in childhood and are much milder (many are asymptomatic) without salt losing and acute adrenal insufficiency (Drucker and New, 1987). Nonclassic 21-hydroxylase deficiency does not present the management difficulties and risks of the classical form.

INCIDENCE

A multinational neonatal screening study documented the overall incidence of classical 21-hydroxylase deficiency CAH in the United States, Italy, France, New Zealand, and Japan at approximately 1:5000 to 1:15,000 live births with males and females equally affected (Drucker and New,

1987; Pang et al., 1988). Some isolated populations have an extraordinarily high incidence of CAH, such as the Yu'pik-speaking Eskimos of Alaska (1:282) and the people of LaReunion, France (1:2141) (Pang et al., 1988). The incidence of CAH based on large-scale neonatal screening studies is significantly higher than that based on case reports, which suggests that many children with CAH go undiagnosed (Drucker and New, 1987; Pang et al., 1988).

The same neonatal screening study found that the salt-losing form of CAH is 2 to 3 times as frequent as the non-salt-losing form rather than the equal frequency previously described in case report studies (Pang et al., 1988). This discrepancy is believed to be the result of early deaths of infants with salt-losing CAH before the diagnosis was made. Methods for prenatal and neonatal screening of individuals known to have a blood relative with CAH are presently available. Screening could significantly reduce the number of deaths from undiagnosed CAH, as well as reduce the morbidity associated with nonfatal episodes of acute adrenal insufficiency and excessive virilization (Gueux et al., 1988; Hughes, Riad-Fahmy, and Griffiths, 1979; Pang et al., 1977, 1988; Strachan et al., 1987).

CLINICAL MANIFESTATIONS AT TIME OF DIAGNOSIS

Nearly all female infants with CAH will have virilization apparent on physical examination at birth (Fig. 10-3). The findings range from a mildly enlarged clitoris to complete fusion and rugation of the labia, with the urethra opening through a urogenital sinus at the base of the phallus or even on the phallus (Anon., 1980; Drucker and New, 1987; Levine and New, 1986; Pagon, 1987).

Female infants with a mildly enlarged clitoris often go undetected, but the alert primary care provider can identify these infants by paying close attention to clitoral size. When measured at the base with redundant skin retracted, the normal clitoral breadth (not length) in a female infant is 2 to 6 mm; this range applies to all gestational ages of newborns and for infants up to 1 year of age (Riley and Rosenbloom, 1980).

The middle range virilization of a female infant

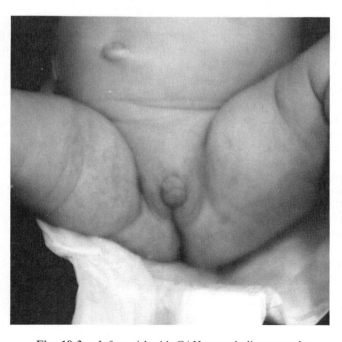

Fig. 10-3. Infant girl with CAH-caused clitoromegaly.

looks abnormal enough to prompt an immediate search for the cause. Unfortunately, the severely virilized female infants may go undiagnosed, being mistaken for cryptorchid males with hypospadias or micropenis.

The label "ambiguous genitalia" should be applied to any infant with either hypospadias and no palpable gonads or a micropenis and no palpable gonads. Since the most common cause of ambiguous genitalia is CAH, it should be high in the clinician's index of suspicion and part of the diagnostic work-up (Pagon, 1987).

Newborn boys with CAH look normal and cannot be reliably identified by physical examination, although there may be slight enlargement of the penis and mildly increased genital pigmentation (Anon., 1980; Bacon et al., 1990).

Newborns with salt-losing CAH will have elevated plasma renin activity levels at birth, although elevated serum potassium levels and decreased serum sodium levels may not be apparent for 1 week or more (Bacon et al., 1990). Newborns with either form of classical CAH will have significantly elevated 17-OHP levels by 24 to 36 hours of age (the infant's age should be noted on the specimen). However, there is a possibility of false positive results in premature infants or very sick term infants (Bacon et al., 1990; Hughes, Riad-Fahmy, and Griffiths, 1979; Pang, 1977).

If salt-losing CAH is not diagnosed and replacement therapy is not begun at birth, both male and female infants will have symptoms of acute adrenal insufficiency and a salt-losing crisis within the first few weeks of life. These symptoms include failure to thrive, weakness, vomiting, and dehydration. Unfortunately these symptoms are nonspecific and usually prompt a work-up for sepsis, pyloric stenosis, or severe malabsorption. Because the routine evaluation of infants with these symptoms normally includes serum electrolyte values, hyponatremia and hyperkalemia should signal the clinician to suspect acute adrenal insufficiency.

The lack of specific symptoms combined with a low index of suspicion on the part of medical personnel can lead to a high mortality rate for undiagnosed infants, especially boys. The difference in the frequency of salt-losing CAH based on early case reports versus newborn screening reinforces the belief that many of these infants die because

of a salt-losing crisis without being diagnosed (Fife and Rappaport, 1983; Pang et al., 1988).

Children with non-salt-losing CAH (who have only cortisol deficiency) may go undiagnosed for years. These children have impaired ability to withstand stress, so that minor illnesses such as acute otitis media, streptococcal pharyngitis, bronchitis, and febrile (temperature >38.4° C) illnesses may cause excessive weakness, pallor, hypotension, and prolonged convalescence (Burnett, 1980). Severe stress such as surgery or a fractured bone can trigger acute adrenal insufficiency with extreme weakness, abdominal pain, vomiting, dehydration, hypotension, and, if not adequately treated, vascular collapse and death (Levine and New, 1986).

TREATMENT

It was not until the 1950s that an understanding of the metabolic defect in CAH led to the current concept of replacement therapy, and it was another decade before adequate therapy was routinely employed (Bartter, 1977). It is not yet possible to correct the genetic defect that blocks the adrenal metabolic pathways, but the clinical consequences of the defect can be prevented by replacing the blocked glucocorticoid and mineralocorticoid end products of cortisol and aldosterone.

In both salt-losing and non–salt-losing CAH, hydrocortisone tablets or liquid (Cortef) are given as a replacement for the glucocorticoid cortisol; in salt-losing CAH, fludrocortisone acetate (Florinef) is added as a replacement for the mineralocorticoid aldosterone.

The basal nonstress dose of hydrocortisone is designed to simulate normal cortisol serum levels. A common regimen is 15 to 25 mg/m^2/day divided into three doses and given orally every 8 hours, but there is still considerable disagreement on the optimal dosage regimen (Anon., 1980; Bacon et al., 1990; Levine and New, 1986; Miller and Levine, 1987). Excessive hydrocortisone dosage can produce Cushing's syndrome, with stunted linear growth, truncal obesity, striae, bruising, hirsutism, muscle weakness, and hypertension (Levine and New, 1986; Stern and Tuck, 1986). Inadequate dosage puts the child at risk for acute adrenal insufficiency and allows excessive androgen production, which causes virilization and accelerates growth and bone age advancement.

GUIDELINES ON STRESS DOSES OF HYDROCORTISONE*

1. For temperature 38.4° to 38.9° C (orally) or for mild illness, give double the basal dose orally.
2. For temperature 38.9° C or higher (orally) or for moderate illness, give triple the basal dose orally.
3. For minor injury (e.g., sprain), give double the basal dose orally.
4. For vomiting only once and acting well, wait 20 minutes and give double the basal dose orally.
5. For vomiting only once but acting ill, vomiting more than once, or acting ill in spite of increased oral dose, give hydrocortisone intramuscularly.
6. For serious injury (e.g., fracture or concussion), give hydrocortisone intramuscularly.
7. If the child looks severely ill or has symptoms of acute adrenal insufficiency, give hydrocortisone intramuscularly and go to the emergency room.
8. If the child is unconscious for any reason, give injectable hydrocortisone intramuscularly and go to the emergency room.
9. In general, emotional stress does not require increased hydrocortisone doses; for severe, prolonged emotional upheaval, consult with the endocrinologist for advice.
10. Call the endocrinologist or primary care provider for all but mild illnesses.
11. Prior to all surgical procedures consult with endocrinologist.

NOTE: **When in doubt, give stress doses of hydrocortisone.** The stress dose should be reduced to basal levels after the acute phase of the illness, injury, or stress; it does not require a prolonged taper.
*From Children's Hospital, Oakland, California.

SIGNS AND SYMPTOMS OF ACUTE ADRENAL INSUFFICIENCY

1. Nausea or vomiting
2. Pallor
3. Cold, moist skin
4. Weakness
5. Dizziness or confusion
6. Rapid heart rate
7. Rapid breathing
8. Abdominal, back, or leg pain
9. Dehydration
10. Hypotension

The basal hydrocortisone dose is doubled or tripled during the acute phase of an illness (e.g., temperature >38.4° C, significant malaise, or pain) or mild to moderate stress. Stress doses do not require prolonged tapering and should be returned to basal levels as soon as the acute stress is resolved (Bacon et al., 1990; Stern and Tuck, 1986). Examples of stresses and dosage guidelines are provided in the box at left.

If the child vomits more than once, the stress is severe, or the child does not respond to oral treatment, injectable hydrocortisone (Solu-Cortef) must be given. The dose, typically 50 to 100 mg, is based on the size and usual replacement dose of the child and should be prescribed in conjunction with the endocrinologist (Bacon et al., 1990; Stern and Tuck, 1986). Parents should have injectable hydrocortisone on hand, know the indications for using it, and learn how to prepare and give an intramuscular (IM) injection. Parents who are unable to give injectable hydrocortisone must have rapid (5- to 10-minute) access to a hospital emergency room or health care provider who is equipped to administer hydrocortisone parenterally.

Whenever there is uncertainty about the necessity of giving emergency treatment, keep in mind that *there is no physical harm in treating for suspected acute adrenal insufficiency that is not present, and the consequence of not treating acute adrenal insufficiency can be the death of the child* (Stern and Tuck, 1986). In this type of situation it is always best to err on the side of prompt, aggressive treatment.

During acute adrenal insufficiency, injectable hydrocortisone (Solu-Cortef or hydrocortisone 21-phosphate) is given intravenously in 3 to 5 times the basal dose, along with appropriate intravenous (IV) therapy to restore intravascular volume and electrolyte balance (see the box above for symptoms of acute adrenal insufficiency) (Levine and New, 1986). If IV access is not available, the hydrocortisone should be given intramuscularly rather than delaying until IV therapy can be started (Stern and Tuck, 1986).

The usual dose of mineralocorticoid is 50 to 200 μg daily, given orally in a single dose. Newborns may temporarily need doses as high as 200 to 300 μg daily for stabilization, and adolescents may also require up to 250 to 300 μg daily during the rapid growth period (Levine and New, 1986). Excessive amounts of mineralocorticoid will result in hypokalemia, weight gain, edema, hypertension, and headache. Inadequate dosage will impair growth and put the child at risk for a salt-losing crisis (Rosler et al., 1977; Stern and Tuck, 1986).

The basal mineralocorticoid dose does not need to be increased during illnesses because the increased amount of hydrocortisone given during stress has enough mineralocorticoid activity to make additional fludrocortisone acetate unnecessary (Stern and Tuck, 1986).

In addition to treatment with cortisol and aldosterone replacement, the majority of girls with CAH have severe enough virilization of their external genitalia to require surgical correction. The corrective surgery frequently requires more than one procedure (e.g., clitoral reduction, separation of the fused labia, correction of a urogenital sinus, and vaginoplasty), with the initial correction done before 2 years of age (Engert, 1989; Jones et al., 1970; Whitaker, 1989). Although satisfactory cosmetic and functional results are usually achieved, additional surgery may be necessary during adolescence to enlarge the vagina to allow for intercourse and to avoid the need for repeated dilatation (Engert, 1989; Jones et al., 1970; Whitaker, 1989). All surgical procedures are a major stress to the child and require consultation with the endocrinologist for perioperative management.

PROGNOSIS

The major risk for these children is death from a misdiagnosed salt-losing crisis early in infancy or from inadequately treated acute adrenal insufficiency during stress. Screening of individuals with a family history of CAH for the carrier state, prenatal screening, and routine neonatal screening have the potential for greatly reducing the number of children who die of CAH (Gueux et al., 1988; Lejeune-Lenain et al., 1980; Pang et al., 1988;

Strachan et al., 1987). Efforts are being made to include CAH in routine newborn screening programs in this country.

Currently nearly all female infants with CAH have morbidity associated with prenatal virilization and the surgical procedures necessary to correct it. Preliminary work on prenatal treatment shows that virilization of a female fetus can be prevented by treating the mother with glucocorticoids. If this becomes available as a standard treatment, it should have a substantial effect on reducing the morbidity in girls with CAH (David and Forest, 1984).

ASSOCIATED PROBLEMS

In children who are receiving appropriate therapy, the problems associated with CAH will be limited. However, the primary care provider must be aware of the potential for acute adrenal insufficiency, growth disorders, virilization, and problems surrounding issues of sexuality.

Acute adrenal insufficiency

Children with CAH may develop acute adrenal insufficiency with any significant illness or injury because they lack the ability to produce increased amounts of cortisol as part of the body's normal stress response. (See the boxes on p. 174.)

Accelerated growth and bone age

In children with undiagnosed or inadequately treated CAH, excessive androgen production will cause accelerated linear growth and muscle development so that a 5-year-old child could have the height and build of an 8- or 10-year-old. Another consequence of excessive androgen production is rapidly advancing bone age with early closure of the growth plates. The 5-year-old with the height and build of a 10-year-old may have the bone age of a 15-year-old. This means that a child who was unusually large for his or her age during the early years will stop growing early because of early closure of the growth plates and end up as a significantly short adolescent and adult (Anon, 1980; Bacon et al., 1990; Duck, 1980).

Virilization

Virilization of the fetus begins at approximately the tenth week of gestation, so virtually all newborn girls with CAH have ambiguous genitalia that will require surgical correction (Bacon et al., 1990; Jones et al., 1970; Miller and Levine, 1987).

By early school age, untreated boys may have an adult-sized penis (the testes remain normal size for age), and untreated girls will be severely virilized with fused labia and a markedly enlarged clitoris. Both sexes will have adult-appearing pubic and axillary hair. By adolescence, if the condition remains untreated, changes from prolonged exposure to very high testosterone levels will no longer be reversible. Boys may have impaired testicular development or spermatogenesis, and girls will not have breast development or menarche (Anon., 1980).

Fertility

Menstrual irregularities are common in adolescent girls who are noncompliant with their replacement therapy, but the majority of girls who were diagnosed early and adequately treated can be expected to have normal puberty and fertility (Bacon et al., 1990; Miller and Levine, 1987).

Prolonged exposure to high levels of androgens in undiagnosed or inadequately treated children will eventually result in irreversible infertility and virilization in girls and may cause impaired fertility in boys (Miller and Levine, 1987; Mulaikal, 1987).

Congenital anomalies

The incidence of congenital anomalies associated with CAH is not believed to be significantly increased over the general population. Although there have been reports of an increased incidence of upper urinary tract abnormalities and testicular tumors, these have not been clearly established (Bacon et al., 1990).

PRIMARY CARE MANAGEMENT
Growth and development

Because abnormal linear growth is an indication of inappropriate treatment or noncompliance, careful monitoring of growth is an essential component of primary care. Linear growth should be measured every 1 to 4 months for infants and every 3 to 6 months for children more than 2 years of age. These measurements should be done carefully using an infantometer for lengths and a stadiometer for heights. The standard scale-mounted measuring device is not accurate enough to detect slight varia-

tions in growth. The measurements should be plotted on a standardized growth chart and assessed for changes in growth rate (e.g., increase or decrease in centile).

Poor growth. Linear growth is acutely sensitive to excessive levels of hydrocortisone; therefore, any decrease in height centile on the growth chart should prompt a reassessment of the hydrocortisone dosage. Occasionally a child's hydrocortisone therapy will be increased based on a high laboratory 17-OHP result, when the result was high because of an acute illness, stress caused by an unusually traumatic venipuncture, or frequently missed hydrocortisone doses before sampling.

To avoid unnecessary and possibly harmful increases in hydrocortisone dosage, the clinician must rule out these other causes of high 17-OHP values with a careful history and comparison of the prescribed dose of hydrocortisone with established dosage ranges before making medication increases. The primary care provider may be in a position to identify these other causes and should contact the endocrinologist with this information.

Another cause of poor linear growth in children with CAH is chronically inadequate mineralocorticoid levels (Duck, 1980). A plasma renin activity level that is abnormally high indicates that the child needs additional mineralocorticoid or dietary sodium. A careful history and comparison with established dosage ranges will determine if the problem is one of compliance or inadequately prescribed dosage.

A child with poorly controlled CAH or one who was not diagnosed until preschool or school age may have early cessation of growth because of premature closure of the epiphyses. Bone-age x-ray studies should be done to assess skeletal maturity if this is suspected.

Excessive growth. Inadequate hydrocortisone replacement will allow continued androgen synthesis by the adrenals and will result in accelerated linear growth. An elevated serum 17-OHP level or clinical findings of increased virilization (e.g., pubic and axillary hair, oily skin, acne, enlargement of the phallus) will confirm the cause of excessive growth. Again, the clinician must be careful to assess whether the inadequate hydrocortisone replacement is secondary to an inappropriately prescribed dose or poor adherence.

DEVELOPMENT. Children with CAH that was diagnosed in infancy or very early childhood and receive adequate, consistent treatment should develop normally.

If the diagnosis of CAH is not made until late childhood, the child will be much taller and more mature looking than his or her peers. Because of mature physical appearance, people may expect the child to have the emotional maturity and behavior of a much older child. This may lead to frustration for all concerned, inappropriate demands and punishment, and the possibility of creating or exacerbating behavior problems.

If these children stop growing early because of early epiphyseal closure, they will go from being the largest to the shortest child in their peer group. Short stature is known to have an impact on behavior and social relationships, and it very likely to have an even greater impact on someone who spent early childhood as the largest person in any group of peers (Holmes, Karlsson, and Thompson, 1986; Young-Hyman, 1986).

Parents, school personnel, child care workers, and others who regularly interact with the child should be given clear, frequently reinforced guidelines on age-appropriate expectations to avoid demanding too much of the large but immature child or asking too little of the small adolescent.

Immunizations

Children with CAH are not immunosuppressed and should receive all of the standard immunizations at the usual ages. At present there is no recommendation for or against giving additional immunizations (e.g., pneumococcal, influenza, or varicella when available); the benefits of immunity to these diseases must be weighed against the possibility of adverse reactions to the vaccine. In weighing these factors, many clinicians believe that giving additional immunizations is worthwhile to reduce the risk of acute adrenal insufficiency triggered by illness.

It is not necessary to increase the basal dose of hydrocortisone before immunizations are given unless there is a history of adverse reactions to previous immunizations with that vaccine. A common but discretionary recommendation is to give the child acetaminophen a few hours before giving an immunization that is likely to produce a rapid-onset febrile reaction (e.g., pertussis), and continue it for 24 to 48 hours afterward.

Stress doses of hydrocortisone should be given if the child develops a temperature of more than 38.4° C or is very fussy or lethargic after an immunization. (See the box on p. 174 for stress dose guidelines.) Any immunization reaction should be documented so that stress doses of hydrocortisone can be given before subsequent immunizations with the same vaccine.

Screening

Vision. Routine screening is recommended.

Hearing. Routine screening is recommended.

Dental. Routine screening is recommended.

Blood pressure. Blood pressure should be checked at each visit. This will require special equipment, such as a Dinamap, for infants. Every effort should be made to have the child relaxed and quiet so that the readings obtained are accurate.

Elevated blood pressure (in a quiet child) may indicate excessive mineralocorticoid or hydrocortisone dosage, whereas low blood pressure may indicate an inadequate mineralocorticoid or hydrocortisone dosage. Either situation should prompt an evaluation of the replacement therapy regimen and compliance.

Hematocrit. Routine screening is recommended.

Urinalysis. Routine screening is recommended.

Tuberculosis. Routine screening is recommended.

Condition-specific screening

SERUM 17-OPH. It may be desirable for the primary care provider to order additional screening tests to more closely monitor the adequacy of replacement therapy in children who have difficulty with compliance. The serum 17-OHP level has become widely accepted as a convenient measure of hydrocortisone therapy even though it has the disadvantage of being influenced by temporary stress (e.g., traumatic venipuncture), the length of time since the last hydrocortisone dose, and diurnal fluctuations. To help evaluate the significance of 17-OHP results, clinicians should note on the specimen the time of day (preferably morning) and the time of the last dose of hydrocortisone. Some clinicians continue to rely on 24-hour urinary 17-ketosteroid and pregnanetriol levels to monitor hydrocortisone therapy in spite of the difficulty in collecting a 24-hour specimen because of the lack of short-term fluctuations. Mineralocorticoid therapy is monitored by plasma renin activity level.

Serum 17-OHP levels should be no more than 3 times normal, preferably less than 200 ng/dl; urinary 17-ketosteroid and pregnanetriol levels should also be in the normal to near-normal range for age, as should plasma renin activity. Specimens ordered by the primary care provider should be coordinated with the endocrinologist and sent to the same laboratory to assure consistency.

BONE AGE. The frequency of bone-age x-ray studies depends on the clinical course. Bone ages in newborns are not helpful. Initial bone age should be determined early in childhood at 2 to 3 years of age (or at the time of diagnosis if the diagnosis is delayed) and can be used as a baseline for future studies. If the child is growing normally and has consistently acceptable 17-OHP and plasma renin activity levels, routine screening should not be necessary more often than every few years.

If the child has growth acceleration, physical findings of increased virilization, or consistently high laboratory results, bone age should be determined to further assess the degree of androgen excess. If the bone age has accelerated, it can be used to help impress on the family the serious and permanent consequences of poor compliance. Ideally, all bone-age studies should be read by the same person to avoid inconsistencies in interpretation.

Drug interactions

Families often are afraid of giving their child "steroids" because of negative publicity in the popular press. It is important to stress to families that the Cortef and Florinef medications their child takes for CAH are replacing substances that are normally produced by their bodies and that the dosages recommended are calculated to match normal blood levels as closely as possible. This is an entirely different situation than taking a foreign substance such as an antibiotic. It is also very different from taking high doses of glucocorticoids to treat diseases such as rheumatoid arthritis. Because the medications for CAH are replacements, concern about using other medications is limited to their effect on absorption or rate of metabolism.

Barbiturates (phenobarbital, butalbital [Fiorinal, Fioricet], pentobarbital [Nembutal, Donnatal], secobarbital [Seconal, Tuinal], phenytoin [Dilantin], rifampin [Rifadin, Rifamate, Rimactane] increase the rate of metabolism of glucocorticoids; therefore, children with CAH who are taking any of these medications for more than a few weeks may require a higher than usual dose of hydrocortisone for adequate cortisol replacement (Stern and Tuck, 1986).

A serum 17-OHP level done approximately 2 weeks after beginning the medications will show if an adjustment in the hydrocortisone dose is necessary. The short-term use of barbiturates perioperatively or the prophylactic use of rifampin for *Haemophilus influenzae* meningitis should not require a change in hydrocortisone dose.

Antibiotics, decongestants, antihistamines, cough preparations, analgesics, antipyretics, and topicals have no unusual adverse effects.

DIFFERENTIAL DIAGNOSIS AND MANAGEMENT OF COMMON PEDIATRIC CONDITIONS

Children with CAH are not immunosuppressed and are no different than their peers in their susceptibility to common childhood illnesses; it is their ability to withstand the stress of illness that is impaired. During periods of illness these children must be followed closely and consultation with the endocrinologist is necessary if the child shows any signs or symptoms of acute adrenal insufficiency.

The primary care provider should consider keeping injectable hydrocortisone in the office for emergencies. The most commonly used preparation is the 100-mg Solu-Cortef Mix-O-Vial because of its long shelf life and convenience. It does not require refrigeration. When reconstituted by rotating and depressing the plunger-stopper, it contains 100 mg of hydrocortisone in 2 ml and can be given intramuscularly or intravenously.

Upper respiratory tract infections and allergies

If the symptoms are mild and the child does not have fever or marked malaise, no specific treatment or increase in basal dose of hydrocortisone is necessary for upper respiratory tract infections or allergies. The parents should watch for worsening of the symptoms, fever, or unusual lethargy; a school-aged child should know to report these symptoms to the teacher and contact his or her parents.

If the symptoms worsen or complications develop, the child should be treated promptly with a stress dose of hydrocortisone and seen by the primary care provider for assessment and specific therapy for the illness.

Acute illnesses

Any known or suspected bacterial illness such as acute otitis media, urinary tract infection, streptococcal pharyngitis, and cellulitis should be treated aggressively with the appropriate antibiotic and stress doses of hydrocortisone during the acute phase of the illness if fever, pain, and malaise are present (see guidelines in the box on p. 174).

When the diagnosis is uncertain or has a significant risk of secondary infections or complications (e.g., a suspicious but not clearly inflamed tympanic membrane, viral pneumonia, or prolonged or marked nasal congestion in a child with a history of frequent acute otitis media or sinusitis), it is wise to treat with antibiotics rather than wait for the situation to worsen.

The child must be followed closely, with an initial office visit for diagnosis and assessment of the child's overall condition and daily telephone progress reports until the acute phase of the illness has passed. Follow-up office visits should be scheduled as for any other child.

Fever

Although fever is a physiologic response to illness, it is also a stress; for this reason fever in a child with CAH should be treated with acetaminophen in the usual recommended dose for age. Stress doses of hydrocortisone should be given using the guidelines in the box on p. 174. It is important to advise the family that reducing the fever does not cure the illness and that other treatments such as antibiotics and stress doses of hydrocortisone should continue to be given as directed.

The child must be followed closely, as described for bacterial and viral illnesses, until the illness has resolved.

Vomiting

If a child with CAH vomits once but appears well otherwise, wait about 20 minutes, give twice the usual oral dose of hydrocortisone, and observe the child closely. If the child appears weak or lethargic after vomiting only once or vomits more than once, the family should give injectable hydrocortisone intramuscularly and contact the endocrinologist immediately.

If family members are not able to give injectable hydrocortisone, they must immediately take the child to the nearest emergency room to receive hydrocortisone intravenously and appropriate fluid and electrolyte therapy. *This can be a life-threatening situation.* Emergency room personnel should contact the endocrinologist but should not delay hydrocortisone therapy while awaiting consultation.

Injury

The child with a significant injury such as a fracture or concussion or injury from automobile accident should immediately be given hydrocortisone intramuscularly and evaluated further for acute adrenal insufficiency at an emergency room. Emergency room personnel should contact the endocrinologist but should not delay hydrocortisone therapy while awaiting consultation.

Acute adrenal insufficiency

Acute adrenal insufficiency is a life-threatening situation. Symptoms of acute adrenal insufficiency include weakness, nausea, abdominal discomfort, vomiting, dehydration, and hypotension. Any of these signs or symptoms in a child with CAH should be presumed to indicate acute adrenal insufficiency and be treated with hydrocortisone intravenously or intramuscularly in 3 to 5 times the basal dose; this should be done at home (or in the primary care setting if the child is there) rather than delaying initial treatment until the child arrives at an emergency room.

The diagnosis of acute adrenal insufficiency can be confirmed by laboratory values showing hyponatremia and hyperkalemia in children with salt-losing CAH. Although consultation with an endocrinologist should be sought, treatment should not be delayed.

An IM injection of hydrocortisone or IV therapy in an emergency room are frightening experiences that no one wants to go through unnecessarily. However, as mentioned earlier, in this type of situation it is always best to err on the side of aggressive treatment.

DEVELOPMENTAL ISSUES
Safety

Children with CAH are not physically impaired and are not at increased risk for any of the usual physical hazards of childhood, but they are at risk for having their special needs ignored when they are away from home. Injuries such as a broken bone may not be recognized as a potentially life-threatening event.

Teachers, child care personnel, coaches, and others who are in regular contact with the child should have written information describing the condition and the need for prompt treatment in an emergency. The child should wear a Medic-Alert bracelet with similar information on it.

The decision of whether or not to keep injectable hydrocortisone at school or day care depends on the situation and must be made on a case by case basis. Factors to consider are: Can the primary care provider or emergency room be reached in 5 to 10 minutes? Is a parent always available at short notice? Are there personnel at the site who are trained and willing to give an IM injection? Does the child engage in activities with a high risk of serious injury?

If injectable hydrocortisone is kept at school or day care, the most convenient preparation is the 100-mg Solu-Cortef Mix-O-Vial, which is easy to use and store. Written indications for use and dosage should be provided by the endocrinologist.

Participation in sports is a normal part of childhood and should be encouraged; however, if at all possible the child with CAH should be directed toward activities with a low risk of serious injury, such as swimming, track, or tennis (bruises, mild or moderate sprains, abrasions, etc. are not cause for special concern). If the child is involved in high-risk sports such as football, the parents should meet with the coach to explain the child's special needs in an emergency and provide appropriate written materials, instructions, and authorization for treatment. Ideally someone such as a parent or team physician should be present and have hydrocortisone for IM injection on hand during competition. This should be mandatory if the activity takes place more than 15 minutes away from a source of emergency care.

Child care

Parents should meet with child care personnel before enrollment to explain their child's special needs. Child care personnel do not require detailed knowledge of CAH, but they should be given a clear explanation that the child has a metabolic disorder that requires simple but very important treatment. Written information for the child care center should include written authorization to give hydrocortisone in oral form with instructions on the dose, time, and purpose, instructions on when to call the parents and telephone numbers where they can be reached, what symptoms or events require emergency care, where to take the child for care, authorization for treatment, and the name and telephone number of the primary care provider and endocrinologist.

It is neither necessary nor desirable to have special rules or restrictions on activities at school or child care for children with CAH. The usual policies on safety and appropriate play are sufficient to avoid serious injury.

Since hydrocortisone is usually given every 8 hours, many children will need at least one dose while in day care. Mineralocorticoid for children with salt-losing CAH is given once daily and can be administered at home. Although most child care providers are conscientious, occasionally they miss or delay doses of hydrocortisone because they do not understand its importance and are distracted by other demands on their attention. A routine that ties medication time to a regular activity, such as rest period or story time, can be established, or the child can wear a watch programmed to beep at the desired time. A letter from the primary care provider or the endocrinologist is very helpful in making this invisible condition real to people who care for these children.

Diet

The only required modification to a regular diet is to allow for adequate sodium intake. Although an appropriate dose of mineralocorticoid will prevent significant sodium depletion in children with salt-losing CAH the children should be offered salty foods and allowed to salt their food to taste. This recommendation also applies to children with non–salt-losing CAH because they may have a mild salt deficit compared with unaffected children (Rosler et al., 1977). Some clinicians use a sodium chloride supplement of 3 to 5 mEq/kg/day for infants; this is divided into two to four parts and given crushed and dissolved in the formula (Bacon et al., 1990; Levine and New, 1986).

Discipline

Children with CAH should be expected to behave appropriately for their age. The only special consideration has to do with children who appear older than their actual age. Parents, teachers, and others must be given clear guidelines on appropriate expectations for the child's developmental stage if it differs from his or her appearance.

Another area that raises disciplinary issues is compliance with taking medication, especially during toddlerhood and adolescence when the child struggles with issues of dependency and autonomy. The parents should be advised from the beginning to use a matter-of-fact approach and avoid negotiating something that is not negotiable. During infancy and the early school years the parents have full responsibility for giving medications. As the child matures and is able to assume more responsibility, the parents should encourage more active participation by the child such as remembering when it is "pill time," marking off the calendar for each dose, or filling a pill box.

The adolescent should have the primary responsibility for taking the medication with the parents offering support. Using a watch with a beeper is helpful for adolescents, as is a pillbox, which coincidentally provides an unobtrusive way for a parent to see if the medication disappears on schedule.

Clinicians can help make older children and adolescents aware of the consequences of poor compliance by pointing out signs of virilization to the girls and slowed growth to both sexes and emphasizing that it is within their power to "get back to normal." The risks of acute adrenal insufficiency and impaired fertility associated with poor adherence should also be discussed with adolescents, again emphasizing that these things are avoidable.

Occasionally an adolescent will choose to make compliance with medications the focus of serious rebellion. Every effort should be made to explain the purpose and necessity of the medication, and counseling should be sought promptly if the problem is severe or chronic.

Toileting

Children who have obvious virilization of their external genitalia should be allowed privacy when using the toilet to avoid being teased. Usually the initial corrective surgery for virilized girls is done at an early age to avoid problems related to looking different. Although there may be some regression in the amount of pubic hair and penile size in boys when adequate treatment is established, those who have become excessively virilized will be noticeably different from their peers until adolescence when normal secondary sexual characteristics occur.

These children are otherwise no different in toileting readiness or skills than their age group and are not unusually prone to constipation, incontinence, enuresis, polyuria, or other disorders related to toileting.

Sleep patterns

Children with CAH do not differ from their peers in their sleep patterns or needs. Unusual fatigue may indicate an illness or inadequate cortisol replacement and should be evaluated.

School issues

Children with CAH do not have any learning disabilities or intellectual impairment related to their disorder and should not need special resources (Galatzer and Laron, 1989; Ehrhardt and Baker, 1977). If the child's appearance differs from his or her age, teachers may have inappropriate behavioral and academic expectations. This issue must be addressed in parent-teacher conferences and frequently reinforced.

The child with CAH may have more absences than usual because of the need for close observation at home during acute illnesses. Concerns about excessive absences should be brought to the attention of the primary care provider who can assess their appropriateness. Legitimate absences include any illness that would keep other children at home. In addition, symptoms such as a scratchy throat and malaise that might be ignored in other children should be initially observed at home.

Sexuality

Virilization is nearly always present at birth in infant girls. Since multiple surgeries usually are needed, these girls learn that there is something "wrong" with them and that it has to do with their genitals. It is very important to reassure these girls that they have all the normal female organs, hormones, and chromosomes and that the surgeries are simply to correct a cosmetic mistake that happened before they were born (Mazur, 1983).

Although some observers have noted "tomboyish" behavior in girls with CAH, special anticipatory guidance in this area is not justified given the lack of data on long-term outcomes for girls who have received early and consistently adequate treatment (Galatzer and Laron, 1989; Hochberg, Gardos, and Benderly, 1987; Money, Schwartz, and Lewis, 1984; Erhardt and Baker, 1977).

Some studies have shown a high incidence of delayed menarche and menstrual irregularities in girls with CAH, but inadequate treatment or poor adherence with medications during puberty contributes to this (Klingensmith et al., 1977; Mulaikal, Migeon, and Rock, 1987). Young women with CAH, particularly the salt-losing form, may have impaired fertility, and those who become pregnant may require Cesarean delivery because of a small birth canal (Klingensmith et al., 1977; Mulaikal, Migeon, and Rock, 1987). A significant number of women in one study had successful pregnancies in spite of late diagnosis, inadequate reconstruction of the introitus, which prevented or reduced the frequency of intercourse (35% of the subjects); and poor compliance with replacement therapy (25%), all of which contribute to reduced fertility (Mulaikal, Migeon, and Rock, 1987).

Prolonged androgen excess can eventually result in infertility in men, but the majority are fertile (Urban, Lee, and Migeon, 1978).

When these children reach adolescence, the primary care provider or endocrinologist should discuss with them the availability and purpose of genetic counseling, screening for carriers, and prenatal and neonatal diagnosis. Because CAH is an autosomal recessive trait, children must receive an abnormal gene from each parent to have the disorder; if one parent has CAH and the other is not a carrier, their children will not have CAH. All unaffected children with a parent with CAH will be carriers of the trait.

SPECIAL FAMILY CONCERNS

The parents of an infant girl with CAH must cope with the impact of ambiguous genitalia and possibly a delayed or even incorrect gender assignment. It is critical that the initial explanations and reassurances given to the family by health care personnel be both sensitive and accurate to prevent serious misperceptions of the child's condition and prognosis (Darland, 1986; Mazur, 1983). Discussions with parents should focus on listening to their concerns and reinforcing the normality of their daughter's internal female organs and chromosomes and explaining that the appearance of the external genitals is correctable and the underlying condition treatable (Darland, 1986). Even after the best explanations and reassurances, these families continue to have a great deal of anxiety about their child's normality and constant reinforcement and support are necessary.

The family must be taught to be assertive in communicating the urgency of their child's need for hydrocortisone to health care personnel who are not familiar with their child or with CAH. Unfortunately, it is common for treatment to be delayed because of lack of understanding of the implications of acute illness in a child with CAH. The primary care provider can help avoid delays in treatment by alerting other health care personnel (e.g., call group, emergency room staff) to the child's special needs. The endocrinologist should be consulted for any questions about treatment.

Parents initially have difficulty believing the seriousness of CAH unless the diagnosis was made during an episode of acute adrenal insufficiency. However, once they experience the rapidity with which their child can change from being robustly healthy to being deathly ill, they may become very fearful of future episodes. It is difficult for these parents to find a balance between protecting their child from serious harm and allowing them to have an active, normal life. This balance needs to be assessed at each visit by asking about the child's social and academic progress, outside interests and activities, and special concerns; any problem areas should be discussed.

The child with CAH may experience emotional disturbances related to the multiple factors involved in having this chronic condition, including being concerned about sexuality and fertility, being perceived and treated as different by others (including their parents), receiving mixed or confusing messages from health care personnel, being overprotected by their parents, and dealing with their own fears related to life-threatening crises they may have experienced. Psychotherapy is indicated for significant emotional disturbance and behavioral problems and has proved to be helpful (Jones et al., 1970).

Newborn siblings also should be screened for CAH. At birth their plasma renin activity and serum electrolyte levels should be evaluated, and at 24 to 36 hours of age their 17-OHP concentration should be checked (Hughes, Riad-Fahmy, Griffiths, 1979; Pang et al., 1977). All older male and female siblings with virilization or accelerated growth should also be screened. Testing for the carrier state is available (although costly) and should be explained to unaffected siblings and other first-degree relatives (Lejeune-Lenain et al., 1980).

Prenatal testing has been done successfully by radioimmunoassay for adrenal steroids in amniotic fluid as early as 10 to 12 weeks of gestation, and by DNA probe of chorionic villus samples at 9 to 11 weeks (Gueux et al., 1988; Strachan et al., 1987). Early attempts to prevent virilization of female fetuses with CAH by administering glucocorticoids to the mother during pregnancy have produced promising results (David and Forest, 1984). However, glucocorticoid therapy must be started before virilization begins at about 10 weeks of gestation. Because this may be before a prenatal diagnosis of CAH is available, a decision to treat will initially include nonaffected fetuses and their mothers.

Prenatal diagnosis and treatment for CAH are areas of intense interest and rapid progress; it is very likely that these procedures will be refined and become more readily available in the future, and they should be discussed with families who have a first-degree relative with CAH.

SUMMARY OF PRIMARY CARE NEEDS FOR THE CHILD WITH CONGENITAL ADRENAL HYPERPLASIA

Growth and development

If CAH is diagnosed in infancy and adequately and consistently treated, growth and development is normal.

Accelerated linear growth occurs if CAH is inadequately treated.

Accelerated bone age advancement and early closure of epiphyses with reduced final adult height will occur if CAH is inadequately treated.

Stunted linear growth will occur if CAH is overtreated with hydrocortisone.

Immunizations

Give all routine immunizations according to usual guidelines.

Giving additional vaccines (pneumococcal, influenza, varicella when available) is discretionary.

Increased "stress" doses of hydrocortisone are not necessary prophylactically unless there is a history of previous adverse reaction to the vaccine.

Give increased "stress" dose of hydrocortisone for immunization reactions involving fever, unusual malaise, and lethargy.

Giving acetaminophen prior to immunization with likelihood of febrile reaction (e.g., pertussis) is discretionary.

Routine screening
Vision

Routine screening is recommended.

Hearing

Routine screening is recommended.

Dental

Routine screening is recommended.

Blood pressure

Blood pressure should be checked at each visit (including infants). Children with abnormal findings should be referred to an endocrinologist.

Hematocrit

Routine screening is recommended.

Urinalysis

Routine screening is recommended.

Tuberculosis

Routine sceening is recommended.

Special screening

Screening serum 17-OHP levels or 24-hour urine pregnanetriol values may be indicated and should be coordinated with the endocrinologist.

Checking plasma renin activity levels may be indicated and should be coordinated with the endocrinologist.

Bone age should be checked every 2 to 3 years, more often if there are indications of androgen excess.

Drug interactions

Long-term use of barbiturates, phenytoin, or rifampin increase the rate of metabolism of glucocorticoids. Adjustments in dosage may be required.

Differential diagnosis

If the child has nausea or vomiting, pallor, cold moist skin, weakness, dizziness or confusion, rapid heart rate, rapid breathing, abdominal, back or leg pain, dehydration, or hypotension, acute adrenal insufficiency should be ruled out.

Temperature greater than 38.4° C, significant malaise, pain, lethargy, or persistent vomiting (regardless of cause) should be covered by stress doses of hydrocortisone in addition to appropriate specific therapy.

If the child has hypertension, excessive dietary sodium intake or overtreatment with mineralocorticoids or glucocorticoids should be ruled out.

If the child has hypotension, inadequate mineralocorticoid or glucocorticoid dosage should be ruled out.

Developmental issues
Safety

These children have no increased susceptibility to injury.

There is a risk of acute adrenal insufficiency with a serious injury (e.g., fracture, concussion).

A Medic-Alert bracelet or necklace should be worn.

Child care

Child care providers must be aware of special needs with illness and injury and the importance of routine and stress medication.

Diet

Children should be allowed to salt to taste and eat salty foods.

Discipline

Expectations are normal based on age and developmental level.

Physical appearance may differ from age and developmental level, leading to inappropriate expectations.

Toileting

There is no impairment in readiness or functioning. Children with obvious virilization should be allowed privacy.

Sleep patterns

Unusual fatigue or lethargy may indicate the need for increased doses of hydrocortisone.

School issues

There are no special educational needs.

School personnel should be aware of special needs regarding illness and injury.

Sexuality

Virilization of infant girls requires surgical correction.

Inadequate treatment results in continued virilization, menstrual irregularities, and infertility in girls and may impair fertility in boys.

Most will be fertile.

Special family concerns

Rapid onset of acute adrenal insufficiency is possible.

Appropriate emergency treatment may be delayed because of lack of awareness or knowledge of CAH by health care providers.

The normality of girls should be stressed.

Others in the family may possibly be affected (siblings, children of affected child).

RESOURCES

At present there is no national organization for CAH, but individual families can ask to be introduced to each other through their endocrinology clinic. Literature available on the subject of CAH is typically produced by individual medical centers and given to patients and health professionals who request it (usually for a small charge).

Informational materials

Burnett J: A boy with CAH. *Am J Nurs* 80:1306-1308, 1980.

This article is easy to read, and families will identify with the description of life with a child with CAH. This is also a good article to give to school and child care personnel because it gives a simple explanation of the disorder and its management without overwhelming the reader with technical information.

From the Department of Education, University of Wisconsin Hospital, 600 Highland Ave, Madison, WI 53792:

Guidelines for the Child Who is Cortisol Dependent, a leaflet for parents with information on cortisone replacement and illness management.

How to Mix and Inject Injectable Hydrocortisone, a small pamphlet for parents with a clear description of this procedure.

Congenital Adrenal Hyperplasia, an 8-page handout explaining CAH and its management. It is primarily for families but also is of interest to professionals unfamiliar with CAH.

From Patient/Parent Education Department, British Columbia's Children's Hospital, 4480 Oak St, Vancouver, British Columbia, V6H 3V4, Canada:

Congenital Adrenal Hyperplasia, a 28-page illustrated booklet describing the condition and treatment. It is primarily for families but also is of interest to professionals unfamiliar with CAH.

Hydrocortisone/Florinef Handout, a concise 2-page handout for parents that includes information on illness management.

From Pediatric Endocrinology, CB 7220, Burnett-Womack, University of North Carolina at Chapel Hill, Chapel Hill, NC 27599:

Medication Instructions for Patients with Congenital Adrenal Hyperplasia, instructions for families. It also describes dosages.

Organizations

Pediatric Endocrinology Nursing Society (PENS): This organization has members in many regions who are willing to speak to parent, school, professional, or other groups. For information, write to PENS, CB 7220, 509 Burnett-Womock, UNC-CH, Chapel Hill, NC 27599

Products

From Medic-Alert Foundation, PO Box 1009, Turlock, CA 95381-1009:

Medic-Alert bracelets and necklaces, which are recommended for all children with CAH.

REFERENCES

Anonymous: Congenital adrenocortical hyperplasia, the syndrome, *Am J Nurs* 80:1306-1308, 1980.

Bacon G, Spencer M, Hopwood N, et al: *A practical approach to pediatric endocrinology,* ed 3, Chicago, 1990, Year Book Medical Publishers, pp 157-182.

Bartter F: Adrenogenital syndromes from physiology to chemistry (1950-1975). In Lee P, Plotnick L, Kowarski A, Migeon C, eds: *Congenital adrenal hyperplasia,* Baltimore, 1977, University Park Press, pp 9-18.

Burnett J: A boy with CAH, *Am J Nurs* 80:1304-1305, 1980.

Darland N: Congenital adrenocortical hyperplasia: Supportive nursing interventions, *J Pediatr Nurs* 1:117-123, 1986.

David M and Forest M: Prenatal treatment of congenital adrenal hyperplasia resulting from 21-hydroxylase deficiency, *J Pediatr* 105:799-803, 1984.

Drucker S and New M: Nonclassic adrenal hyperplasia due to 21-hydroxylase deficiency. In Mahoney C, editor: *Pediatric clinics of North America: Pediatric and adolescent endocrinology,* Philadelphia, 1987, WB Saunders, pp 1069-1081.

Duck S: Acceptable linear growth in congenital adrenal hyperplasia, *J Pediatr* 97:93-96, 1980.

Ehrhardt A and Baker S: Males and females with congenital adrenal hyperplasia: A family study of intelligence and gender-related behavior. In Lee P, Plotnick L, Kowarski A, eds: *Congenital adrenal hyperplasia,* Baltimore, 1977, University Park Press, pp 447-461.

Engert J: Surgical correction of virilised female external genitalia, *Progr Pediatr Surg* 23:151-164, 1989.

Fife D and Rappaport EB: Prevalence of salt-losing among congenital adrenal hyperplasia patients, *Clin Endocrinol* 18:259-264, 1983.

Galatzer A and Laron Z: The effects of prenatal androgens on behavior and cognitive functions. In Forest M, ed: *Androgens in childhood,* 1989, Karger, Basel, pp 98-103.

Gueux B, et al: Prenatal diagnosis of 21-hydroxylase deficiency congenital adrenal hyperplasia by simultaneous radioimmunoassay of 21-deoxycortisol and 17-hydroxyprogesterone in amniotic fluid, *J Clin Endocrinol Metab* 66:534-537, 1988.

Hochberg Z, Gardos M, Benderly A: Psychosexual outcome of assigned females and males with 46,XX virilizing congenital adrenal hyperplasia, *Eur J Pediatr* 146:497-499, 1987.

Holmes C, Hayford J, and Thompson R: Parents' and teachers' differing views of short children's behaviour, *Child Care Health Dev* 8:327-336, 1982.

Holmes C, Karlsson J, and Thompson R: Longitudinal evaluation of behavior patterns in children with short stature. In Stabler B and Underwood L, eds: *Slow grows the child,* Hillsdale, NJ, 1986, Lawrence Erlbaum Assoc, pp 1-12.

Hughes IA, Riad-Fahmy D, Griffiths K: Plasma 17 OH-progesterone concentrations in newborn infants, *Arch Dis Child* 54:347-349, 1979.

Jones H, Verkauf B, Lewis V, et al: The relevance of surgical, psychologic, and endocrinologic factors to the long-term end result of patients with congenital adrenal hyperplasia: A study of eighty-nine patients, *Int J Gynaecol Obstet* 8:398-401, 1970.

Klingensmith G, Garcia S, Jones H, et al: Glucocorticoid treatment of girls with congenital adrenal hyperplasia: Effects on height, sexual maturation, and fertility, *J Pediatr* 90:996-1004, 1977.

Lejeune-Lenain C, Cantraine F, Dufrasnes M, et al: An improved method for the detection of heterozygosity of congenital virilizing adrenal hyperplasia. *Clin Endocrinol* 12:525-535, 1980.

Levine L and New M: Congenital adrenal hyperplasia. In Lavin N, ed: *Manual of endocrinology and metabolism,* Boston, 1986, Little, Brown, pp 143-162.

Mazur T: Ambiguous genitalia: Detection and counseling, *Pediatr Nurs* 9:417-422, 1983.

Miller W and Levine L: Molecular and clinical advances in congenital adrenal hyperplasia, *J Pediatr* 111:1-17, 1987.

Money J, Schwartz M, and Lewis V: Adult erotosexual status and fetal hormonal masculinization and demasculinization: 46,XX congenital virilizing adrenal hyperplasia and 46,XY androgen-insensitivity syndrome compared, *Psychoneuroendocrinology* 9:405-414, 1984.

Mulaikal R, Migeon C, Rock J: Fertility rates in female patients with congenital adrenal hyperplasia due to 21-hydroxylase deficiency, *N Engl J Med* 316:178-182, 1987.

Pagon R: Diagnostic approach to the newborn with ambiguous genitalia. In Mahoney C, ed: *Pediatric Clinics of North America,* Philadelphia, 1987, WB Saunders, pp 1019-1031.

Pang S, Hotchkiss J, Drash A, et al: Microfilter paper method for 17-hydroxyprogesterone radioimmunoassay: Its application for rapid screening for congenital adrenal hyperplasia, *J Clin Endocrinol Metab* 45:1003-1008, 1977.

Pang S, Wallace M, Hofman L, et al: Worldwide experience in newborn screening for classical congenital adrenal hyperplasia due to 21-hydroxylase deficiency, *Pediatrics* 81:866-874, 1988.

Riley W and Rosenbloom A: Clitoral size in infancy, *J Pediatr* 96:918-919, 1980.

Rosler A, Levine L, Schneider B, et al: The interrelationship of sodium balance, plasma renin activity and ACTH in congenital adrenal hyperplasia, *J Clin Endocrinol Metab* 45:500-512, 1977.

Stern N and Tuck M: The adrenal cortex and mineralocorticoid hypertension. In Lavin N, ed: *Manual of endocrinology and metabolism,* Boston, 1986, Little, Brown, pp 107-130.

Strachan T, Sinnott P, Smeaton I, et al: Prenatal diagnosis of congenital adrenal hyperplasia, *Lancet* 2:1272-1273, 1987.

Urban M, Lee P, and Migeon C: Adult height and fertility in men with congenital virilizing adrenal hyperplasia, *N Engl J Med* 299:1392-1396, 1978.

Whitaker RH: Genitoplasty for congenital adrenal hyperplasia: anatomy and technical review, *Prog Pediatr Surg* 23:144-150, 1989.

Young-Hyman D: Effects of short stature on social competence. In Stabler B and Underwood L, eds: *Slow grows the child,* Hillsdale, NJ, 1986, Lawrence Erlbaum Assoc, pp 27-45.

11 *Congenital Heart Disease*

···

Elizabeth Cook and *Sarah S. Higgins*

ETIOLOGY

Congenital heart disease (CHD) is commonly categorized by two hemodynamic changes that occur as a result of the specific heart anomaly: (1) acyanotic heart disease, in which the systemic circulation is not compromised by oxygenated blood; and (2) cyanotic heart disease, characterized by unoxygenated blood mixing in the systemic circulation (Fig. 11-1) (see also the box on p. 191).

Most heart defects occur within the first 8 weeks of gestation (Nora, 1989). Approximately 90% of congenital heart defects have a multifactorial cause in which there is an interplay of a genetic predisposition for cardiac maldevelopment with an environmental trigger (e.g., a virus, toxin, or maternal ingestion of certain drugs) at a vulnerable time of cardiac development (Nora, 1989).

Genetic factors acccount for about 8% of CHD and are usually associated with a syndrome in which other systems are also affected (Table 11-1). One of the most common genetic associations of CHD is with Down syndrome; approximately 40% of these children have a heart defect (Ferencz et al., 1989) (see Chapter 14). Other syndromes, such as asplenia syndrome, DiGeorge syndrome, and VACTERL syndrome,* which do not have an iden-

tified chromosomal defect, frequently have CHD as one of many anomalies.

Maternal exposure to environmental factors during cardiac development of the fetus may also result in heart defects (see Table 11-1). Purely environmental causes for the development of CHD are estimated at 2% to 3% (Nora, 1989). The vulnerable period for exposure to a cardiac teratogen is during the first 8 weeks of gestation.

INCIDENCE

Congenital heart disease generally occurs in .8% to 1% of live births (Hoffman, 1987). Some authorities cite 2% as the incidence of CHD; this percentage usually includes bicuspid aortic valve and mitral valve prolapse (Moller, 1982). The incidence of specific heart defects is presented in Table 11-2. Boys tend to have a higher overall incidence of CHD, although certain defects exhibit some sex preference. Defects more common among girls are PDA and ASD; among boys valvular aortic anomalies, coarctation of the aorta (COTA), and transposition of the great arteries (TGA) are more common (Fyler et al., 1980).

The recurrence risk of CHD in the same family depends on several factors (Nora, 1989). If one child has a heart defect, the recurrence risk is about 1% to 4%, with the risk being higher in more common heart defects than in a defect with a lower

---

*VACTERL syndrome refers to abnormalities of vertebral, anus, cardiovascular tree, trachea, esophagus, renal system, and limb buds.

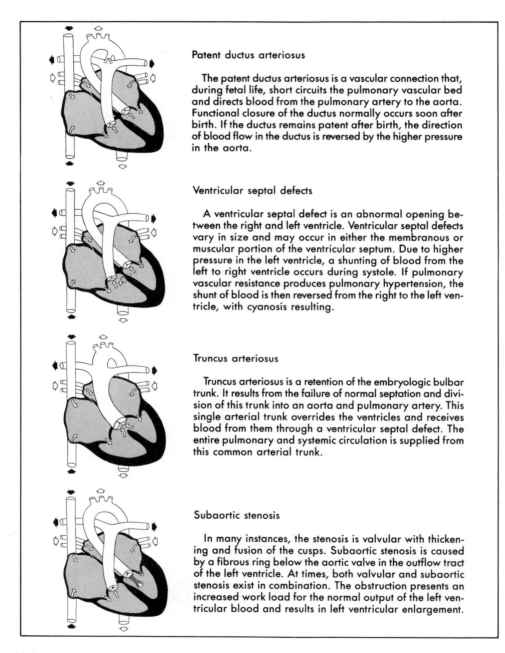

Patent ductus arteriosus

The patent ductus arteriosus is a vascular connection that, during fetal life, short circuits the pulmonary vascular bed and directs blood from the pulmonary artery to the aorta. Functional closure of the ductus normally occurs soon after birth. If the ductus remains patent after birth, the direction of blood flow in the ductus is reversed by the higher pressure in the aorta.

Ventricular septal defects

A ventricular septal defect is an abnormal opening between the right and left ventricle. Ventricular septal defects vary in size and may occur in either the membranous or muscular portion of the ventricular septum. Due to higher pressure in the left ventricle, a shunting of blood from the left to right ventricle occurs during systole. If pulmonary vascular resistance produces pulmonary hypertension, the shunt of blood is then reversed from the right to the left ventricle, with cyanosis resulting.

Truncus arteriosus

Truncus arteriosus is a retention of the embryologic bulbar trunk. It results from the failure of normal septation and division of this trunk into an aorta and pulmonary artery. This single arterial trunk overrides the ventricles and receives blood from them through a ventricular septal defect. The entire pulmonary and systemic circulation is supplied from this common arterial trunk.

Subaortic stenosis

In many instances, the stenosis is valvular with thickening and fusion of the cusps. Subaortic stenosis is caused by a fibrous ring below the aortic valve in the outflow tract of the left ventricle. At times, both valvular and subaortic stenosis exist in combination. The obstruction presents an increased work load for the normal output of the left ventricular blood and results in left ventricular enlargement.

Fig. 11-1. Congenital heart abnormalities. *Reprinted with permission of Ross Laboratories, Columbus, Ohio 43216, from Clinical Education Aid No. 7, Copyright 1970 Ross Laboratories.*

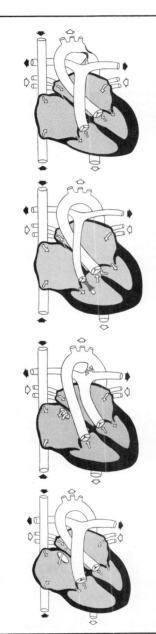

Coarctation of the aorta

Coarctation of the aorta is characterized by a narrowed aortic lumen. It exists as a preductal or postductal obstruction, depending on the position of the obstruction in relation to the ductus arteriosus. Coarctations exist with great variation in anatomic features. The lesion produces an obstruction to the flow of blood through the aorta causing an increased left ventricular pressure and work load.

Tetralogy of Fallot

Tetralogy of Fallot is characterized by the combination of four defects: (1) pulmonary stenosis, (2) ventricular septal defect, (3) overriding aorta, (4) hypertrophy of right ventricle. It is the most common defect causing cyanosis in patients surviving beyond two years of age. The severity of symptoms depends on the degree of pulmonary stenosis, the size of the ventricular septal defect, and the degree to which the aorta overrides the septal defect.

Complete transposition of great vessels

The anomaly is an embryologic defect caused by a straight division of the bulbar trunk without normal spiraling. As a result, the aorta originates from the right ventricle, and the pulmonary artery from the left ventricle. An abnormal communication between the two circulations must be present to sustain life.

Atrial septal defects

An atrial septal defect is an abnormal opening between the right and left atria. Basically, three types of abnormalities result from incorrect development of the atrial septum. An incompetent foramen ovale is the most common defect. The high ostium secundum defect results from abnormal development of the septum secundum. Improper development of the septum primum produces a basal opening known as an ostium primum defect, frequently involving the atrio-ventricular valves. In general, left to right shunting of blood occurs in all atrial septal defects.

Fig. 11-1, cont'd.   Congenital heart abnormalities.   *Continued.*

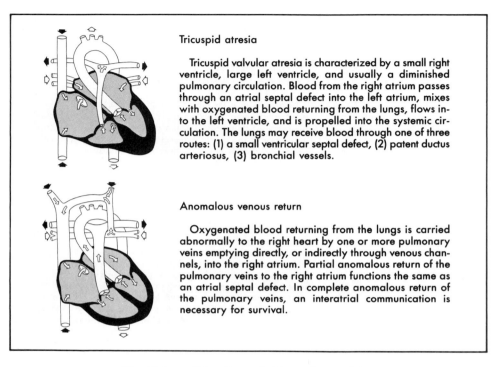

Tricuspid atresia

Tricuspid valvular atresia is characterized by a small right ventricle, large left ventricle, and usually a diminished pulmonary circulation. Blood from the right atrium passes through an atrial septal defect into the left atrium, mixes with oxygenated blood returning from the lungs, flows into the left ventricle, and is propelled into the systemic circulation. The lungs may receive blood through one of three routes: (1) a small ventricular septal defect, (2) patent ductus arteriosus, (3) bronchial vessels.

Anomalous venous return

Oxygenated blood returning from the lungs is carried abnormally to the right heart by one or more pulmonary veins emptying directly, or indirectly through venous channels, into the right atrium. Partial anomalous return of the pulmonary veins to the right atrium functions the same as an atrial septal defect. In complete anomalous return of the pulmonary veins, an interatrial communication is necessary for survival.

Fig. 11-1, cont'd. Congenital heart abnormalities.

incidence. If two first-degree relatives are affected, the recurrence risk is tripled. If the defect is part of a syndrome or chromosomal abnormality, the recurrence risk of the heart lesion is related to the recurrence risk of the syndrome. The recurrence risk if a mother has CHD may be as high as 16%, whereas the risk to offspring if the father is affected is approximately 1% to 4% (Nora and Nora, 1987; Whittemore, Hobbins, and Engle, 1982). Additional information indicates that certain left-sided cardiac lesions, most notably hypoplastic left heart syndrome (HLHS), have a very high recurrence rate (Boughman et al., 1987).

CLINICAL MANIFESTATIONS AT TIME OF DIAGNOSIS

The clinical presentation of a child with CHD will vary depending on the specific defect. Symptoms usually relate to the degree of congestive heart failure (CHF) or cyanosis.

Congestive heart failure

The majority of cases of CHF result from CHD, and most of these cases occur within the first year of life. Congestive heart failure occurs when there is a strain on the myocardium, usually because of pressure or volume overload, severe enough to reduce cardiac output to a level insufficient to meet the body's metabolic demands (Engle, 1987). Symptoms of CHF result from the decreased cardiac output and the body's compensatory mechanisms. These include cardiac hypertrophy, cardiac dilatation, and stimulation of the sympathetic nervous system. The infant with CHF will be tachypneic, dyspneic, tachycardic, pale, cool, diaphoretic, and easily fatigued. Additional symptoms include periorbital edema, hepatomegaly, and a persistent cough. A history of difficult feeding and decreased food intake are classic signs of CHF. Failure to thrive is therefore common in the infant with CHF.

CLASSIFICATION OF CONGENITAL HEART DEFECTS

Acyanotic heart defects

Increased pulmonary blood flow	Normal pulmonary blood flow
Atrial septal defect (ASD) Ventricular septal defect (VSD) Patent ductus arteriosus (PDA) Atrioventricular (AV) canal	Aortic stenosis (AS) Coarctation of the aorta (COTA) Pulmonary stenosis (PS)

Since the pressure in the left side of the heart is greater than that in the right side, an abnormal opening between the two sides will result in blood flow from the left (oxygenated) to the right (unoxygenated) side of the heart. This "left to right shunting" commonly causes overcirculation of the lungs and may result in congestive heart failure

Cyanotic heart defects

Increased pulmonary blood flow	Normal pulmonary blood flow	Decreased pulmonary blood flow
Truncus arteriosus type I Total anomalous pulmonary venous return (TAPVR) Transposition of the great arteries (TGA) Single ventricle Hypoplastic left heart syndrome (HLHS)	Truncus arteriosus type II, III Single ventricle with pulmonary stenosis (PS)	Tetralogy of Fallot (TOF) Pulmonary atresia (PA) Tricuspid atresia (TA) Ebstein's anomaly Truncus arteriosus type IV

Cyanotic heart defects are generally a result of blood flow obstruction on the right side of the heart and an abnormal intracardiac communication causing deoxygenated blood on the right side of the heart to mix with oxygenated blood on the left side of the heart. Undercirculation to the lungs, accompanied by right to left shunting, results in cyanosis.

Congestive heart failure is manifested in the neonate in the presence of a severe cardiac defect. Infants with defects causing large left to right shunts, such as PDA, AV canal defect, or VSD, usually do not develop symptoms until 4 to 8 weeks of age when the high pulmonary vascular resistance of the fetal period becomes low enough to cause increased pulmonary blood flow. The onset of symptoms is usually gradual, with tachypnea, changes in feeding patterns, and poor weight gain often being early clues. Premature infants with a left to right shunt may develop symptoms of CHF earlier than a term infant because pulmonary vascular resistance in the premature infant drops faster than in the term infant (Neal and Morgan, 1981).

Hypoxemia and cyanosis

Hypoxemia is defined as the presence of arterial oxygen saturation that is less than normal. Cyanosis is the blue coloration of the skin and mucous membranes caused by hypoxemia. The coloration is usually seen in the lips, gums, and nailbeds and around the eyes. Cyanosis is more difficult to detect in children with dark pigmentation; it will be perceived best by observing the mucous membranes and nailbeds in natural light. The child with cyanosis often has slowed growth, though is not usually a poor feeder. Polycythemia occurs in the chronically hypoxemic child as the body attempts to increase its oxygen-carrying capacity. Cyanotic toddlers usually limit themselves in their activity but

Table 11-1. Conditions commonly associated with cardiac malformations

Condition	Associated defect
INFANT SYNDROME	
Trisomy 13 syndrome	VSD, PDA, dextrocardia
Trisomy 18 syndrome	VSD, PDA, PS
Trisomy 21 syndrome	AV canal, VSD, ASD
Turner's syndrome	COTA, ASD, AS
Marfan syndrome	Great artery aneurysms, aortic insufficiency (AI), mitral regurgitation (MR)
Noonan's syndrome	PS, ASD, idiopathic hypertrophic subaortic stenosis (IHSS)
Cri du chat syndrome	VSD, PDA, ASD
Ellis–van Creveld syndrome	ASD, single atrium
Osteogenesis imperfecta	Aortic valve disease
DiGeorge syndrome	Interrupted aortic arch, TOF, truncus arteriosus, ASD
Holt-Oram syndrome	ASD, VSD, single atrium
Treacher Collins syndrome	VSD, PDA, ASD
Asplenia syndrome	VSD, single ventricle, common AV valve, TGA
VACTERL syndrome	TOF
MATERNAL CONDITION	
Rubella	PDA, ASD, VSD, peripheral pulmonary stenosis
Diabetes	TGA, VSD, COTA, cardiomegaly
Lupus erythematosis	Heart block
Phenylketonuria	TOF, VSD, ASD
MATERNAL INGESTION	
Alcohol	VSD, PDA, ASD
Trimethadione	TGA, TOF, HLHS
Lithium	Ebstein's anomaly, ASD, TA
Retinoic acid	VSD
Amphetamines	VSD, PDA, ASD, TGA
Hydantoin	PS, AS, COTA, PDA
Sex hormones	VSD, TGA, TOF
Thalidomide	TOF, truncus arteriosus, VSD, ASD

Adapted from Nora JJ: Etiologic aspects of heart disease. In Adams FH and Emmanouilides GC, eds: *Moss's Heart Disease in Infants, Children and Adolescents,* ed 4, Baltimore, 1989, Williams and Wilkins, pp 15-23.

will become easily fatigued and breathless if running, climbing stairs, or playing for long periods of time. The child with a symptomatic cyanotic defect, most commonly tetralogy of Fallot (TOF), may assume a squatting position for relief of exertional dyspnea and fatigue. Increasing cyanosis may be subtle and difficult to discern; monitoring an increasing hemoglobin level may help in the determination of progressive hypoxemia.

TREATMENT

Medical management of the child with CHD is aimed at allowing the infant to grow and the organs to mature so that surgery can be performed at the optimal time. One goal of primary care management is to control CHF, which is usually achieved with the use of digitalis and diuretics. Since failure to thrive is a common complication of CHF, support with feeding also becomes a priority in manage-

Table 11-2. Incidence of specific heart defects

Defect	CHD (%)
Ventricular septal defect (VSD)	20-25
Patent ductus arteriosus (PDA)	10 (excluding premature)
Tetralogy of Fallot (TOF)	10
Coarctation of the aorta (COTA)	8
Atrial septal defect (ASD)	5-10
Pulmonary stenosis (PS)	5-8
Transposition of the great arteries (TGA)	5
Aortic stenosis (AS)	5
Atrioventricular (AV) canal	3-4
Hydroplastic left heart syndrome (HLHS) 1 - 2	1-2
Tricuspid atresia (TA)	1-2
Total anomalous pulmonary venous return (TAPVR)	1
Pulmonary atresia (PA)	<1
Ebstein's anomaly	<1
Truncus arteriosus	<1
Single ventricle	<1

From Park MK: *Pediatric cardiology for practitioners,* ed 2, Chicago, 1988, Year Book Publishers.

ment. This may include methods of decreasing fatigue during the feeding, increasing the caloric concentration of formula, and occasionally providing gavage feeding.

The cyanotic infant additionally requires monitoring for progressive cyanosis, anemia, and dehydration. The parents of the cyanotic child need to be taught to identify increasing blueness and cyanotic spells. They can be taught to place the child in the knee-chest position to alleviate cyanotic spells (Higgins and Kashani, 1986).

The decision for surgery depends on the severity of the lesion, associated defects, the child's age and size, concurrent medical or surgical problems, and family and cultural factors. A cardiac catheterization is usually performed within the first 6 months of the child's life to identify the exact anatomy and physiology of the child's heart defect. The natural history of some defects (e.g., ventricular septal defect (VSD), PDA, and ASD) is such that spontaneous improvement may occur, thus avoiding surgery. Most lesions, however, require surgery. The timing of surgical intervention varies among cardiac centers. As surgical techniques improve, the trend nationwide is toward earlier corrective surgery, often by midinfancy.

Some complex defects require an initial palliative surgery at birth with definitive surgery occurring later (Graham, 1984) (see the box on p. 194). Crucial in determining the timing of surgery is the prevention of irreversible pulmonary hypertension. Large left to right shunts rarely cause irreversible changes in the pulmonary vasculature before 12 to 18 months of age. However, once these irreversible changes occur, surgery is contraindicated and the child will become progressively cyanotic.

Neonates who need palliative surgery are those with inadequate pulmonary blood flow and those with uncontrolled CHF (Graham, 1984). These infants need close follow-up after surgery to ensure that pulmonary blood flow is maintained in cyanotic children and that excessive pulmonary blood flow is restricted in children with CHF.

Infants who need surgery are followed closely by the cardiologist to manage CHF or cyanosis and time surgery. Communication between the primary care provider and cardiologist is important. Symptoms of increasing tachypnea, decreasing feeding, slowed weight gain, or increased cyanosis should be reported to the cardiologist.

Children whose cardiac defects warrant delaying surgery for several years include those who

---

TIMING OF CARDIAC SURGERY

I. Patent ductus arteriosus
   A. Large with CHF; urgent operation
   B. Small to moderate with few or no symptoms; elective surgery, late infancy to school age

II. Ventricular septal defect
   A. Large with CHF; repair at any age, usually not necessary before 3 to 6 months
   B. Moderate to large shunt with CHF-controlled repair at 6 to 18 months
   C. Small defect with small shunt; surgery not indicated

III. Atrial septal defect
   A. Elective repair at 4 to 5 years in most patients
   B. Small defects; repair not required

IV. Atrioventricular canal defect
   A. Incomplete AV canal; usually repair at 4 to 5 years
   B. Complete AV canal; repair in infancy

V. Coarctation of the aorta
   A. Symptomatic; repair at manifestation
   B. Asymptomatic; repair at school age or older

VI. Aortic stenosis
   A. Symptomatic infant or child; urgent operation
   B. Asymptomatic; usually valvulotomy if LV-Ao gradient is more than 80 mm Hg

VII. Pulmonary stenosis
   A. Symptomatic infant with critical PS; urgent valvulotomy
   B. Asymptomatic; elective balloon dilatation or surgery if RV pressure is more than systemic pressure

VIII. Tetralogy of Fallot
   A. Asymptomatic; elective repair at 18 to 36 months
   B. Minimal cyanosis; repair at 12 to 24 months
   C. Significant cyanosis
      1. Less than 6 months; palliative shunt; repair at 18 to 36 months
      2. More than 6 months; repair when symptomatic

IX. Transposition of the great arteries
   A. Arterial switch procedure as neonate
   B. With PS; shunt in infancy; Rastelli repair as toddler

X. Tricuspid atresia
   A. Shunt in infancy; Fontan procedure at 4 to 6 years or older

XI. Single ventricle
   A. With PS; shunt in infancy; Fontan at 4 to 6 years or older
   B. Without PS; PA band in infancy; subsequent shunts

XII. Pulmonary atresia
   A. Emergency shunt as neonate; possible repair at 3 to 6 years

XIII. Truncus arteriosus
   A. Repair in infancy; conduit replacements with growth

XIV. Hypoplastic left heart syndrome
   A. Palliation as neonate; Fontan as toddler

Adapted from Graham TP Jr: When to operate on the child with congenital heart disease, *Pediatr Clin North Am* 31:1275-1291, 1984.

---

rarely develop early pulmonary hypertension or myocardial strain, such as small PDAs, ASDs, VSDs, and mild coarctation of the aorta. These children are usually asymptomatic. They may have more contact with their primary care provider than their cardiologist after initial diagnosis, so communication with the cardiologist is again important.

For certain defects, interventional cardiac catheterization can replace surgery. Some forms of pulmonary and aortic stenosis can be repaired through balloon valvuloplasty. Closure of PDAs, ASDs, VSDs, and unnecessary collateral blood vessels is being performed on a limited basis via cardiac catheterization and placement of various occlusion devices within the defect (Radtke & Lock, 1990). In addition, electrophysiologic studies in conjunction with cardiac catheterization are used to identify cardiac dysrhythmias, induce rhythm disturbances, and then evaluate the effectiveness of certain drugs under controlled circumstances. This field is still in the early stages of development, but it is becoming a valuable therapy in managing some children with CHD.

PROGNOSIS

The prognosis for children with CHD is good for the majority of lesions. Only the most complex defects require multiple surgeries. Many children, therefore, have had a definitive repair by their first or second year. The surgical mortality for the less complex defects is generally less than 5% (Park, 1988). Children with these defects usually are symptom free postoperatively and do not require further surgery. The operative risk for some complex lesions may be as low as 5% to 10% but can rise to 20% to 25% for the series of surgical procedures required with severe lesions (Park, 1988). Long-term postoperative follow-up by the cardiologist is required to evaluate the child for problems such as scarring or stenosis at suture sites, heart rhythm disturbances, and valve malfunctioning.

ASSOCIATED PROBLEMS
Hematologic problems

Children with cyanotic heart disease develop polycythemia to increase the oxygen-carrying capacity of the blood (Park, 1988). If the hematocrit value reaches 60% or higher, there is a marked increase in the viscosity of the blood and an increased tendency for thrombus formation (Hoffman, 1987). Bleeding disorders are also seen in the polycythemic child, most commonly thrombocytopenia and defective platelet aggregation. These children may bruise easily or develop petechiae, gingival bleeding, or epistaxes (Park, 1988).

Anemia can be a special problem in the child with CHD. In the child with existing CHF, a decreased hemoglobin level may exacerbate failure (Lister et al., 1982). In the cyanotic infant, iron deficiency anemia has been associated with cerebral vascular accidents and slowed growth (Hoffman, 1987). Cyanosis will not be as obvious in the anemic child as in the child with a normal or elevated hemoglobin level. Because of these problems associated with anemia, the child with a cyanotic

heart defect should have a hemoglobin value of at least 16 g/dl (Gidding and Rosenthal, 1984); the child with an acyanotic heart defect should have a hemoglobin value within normal range for their age.

Infectious processes

Children with significant heart defects are at high risk for developing a variety of infections. Recurrent respiratory tract infections are especially common in children with lesions causing increased pulmonary blood flow. Other systemic infections, such as sinusitis, are common nonspecific infections seen in the older cyanotic child. Infections can have a significant impact on the child's health. For example: (1) severe respiratory tract infections can exacerbate hypoxemia in the cyanotic child; (2) fever can increase oxygen demands and precipitate myocardial decompensation; (3) dehydration in a child with polycythemia can lead to thrombus formation; and (4) electrolyte imbalances from vomiting, diarrhea, or fever in a child receiving digoxin can lead to digoxin toxicity (Gidding and Rosenthal, 1984).

The child with asplenia syndrome (a condition that includes absence of the spleen and complex cardiac defects) is extremely susceptible to bacteremia; *Streptococcus pneumoniae* and *Haemophilus influenzae* type b are the most common pathogens. Daily antimicrobial prophylaxis is required for 5 years and strongly recommended thereafter. Experts advise 125 mg of penicillin G or V twice daily or 20 mg of amoxicillin/kg/day or 4 mg/kg/day of trimethoprim and 20 mg/kg/day mg of sulfamethaxozole (Septra) for children less than 5 years. For children more than 5 years of age, 250 mg of penicillin twice daily is recommended (Committee on Infectious Diseases, 1991).

Infective endocarditis

Endocarditis may occur because of blood-borne bacteria lodging on damaged or abnormal heart valves, prosthetic material, or the endocardium near congenital anatomic defects. This may occur if prophylaxis precautions are not followed during all dental procedures, incision and drainage of infected tissue, and surgical or invasive procedures involving mucosal surfaces or contaminated tissues (Dajani et al., 1990) (see the box on p. 196). The

---

INFECTIVE ENDOCARDITIS PROPHYLAXIS*

Cardiac conditions

Endocarditis prophylaxis recommended

Prosthetic cardiac valves

Most congenital cardiac malformations

Rheumatic and other acquired valvular dysfunction

Previous history of bacterial endocarditis

Mitral valve prolapse with valvular regurgitation

Hypertrophic cardiomyopathy

Endocarditis prophylaxis not recommended

Isolated secundum atrial septal defect

Surgical repair without residua beyond 6 months of secundum ASD, VSD, or PDA

Physiologic, functional, or innocent heart murmurs

Mitral valve prolapse without valvular regurgitation

Previous Kawasaki disease without valvular dysfunction

Previous rheumatic fever without valvular dysfunction

Indwelling cardiac pacemakers

Procedures for which endocarditis prophylaxis is recommended

Dental procedures known to induce gingival or mucosal bleeding, including professional cleaning

From Dajani, AS et al.: Prevention of bacterial endocarditis, JAMA 264:2919-2922. Copyright 1990 by American Medical Association. Adapted by permission.

*This table lists common pediatric conditions and procedures but is not meant to be all inclusive

Tonsillectomy and/or adenoidectomy

Surgical procedures that involve intestinal or respiratory mucosa

Bronchoscopy with rigid bronchoscope, or with biopsy

Cystoscopy

Urethral dilatation

Urethral catheterization if urinary tract infection is present

Urinary tract surgery if urinary tract infection is present

Incision and drainage of infected tissue

Vaginal delivery in the presence of infection

Procedures for which endocarditis prophylaxis is not recommended

Dental procedures not likely to cause gingival bleeding, such as simple adjustment of orthodontic appliances or fillings above the gum line

Shedding of deciduous teeth

Insertion of tympanostomy tubes

Bronchoscopy with flexible bronchoscope, or without biopsy

Endotracheal intubation

Cardiac catheterization

Endoscopy with or without gastrointestinal biopsy

Cesarean section

In the absence of infection for urethral catheterization, dilatation and curettage, uncomplicated vaginal delivery, therapeutic abortion, sterilization procedures, or insertion or removal of intrauterine devices

---

most common organisms are streptococci and staphylococci, which account for 80% to 90% of the cases (Hoffman, 1987; Park, 1988).

Central nervous system complications

In cyanotic children bacteria normally filtered out of the blood in the pulmonary circulation may be shunted directly to the systemic circulation. As a result they are at an increased risk for brain abscess, most commonly after 2 years of age (Hoffman, 1987). Cyanotic infants with iron deficiency anemia are prone to develop cerebral vascular accidents. A possible explanation for this finding is that hyperviscosity caused by polycythemia may be aggravated by microcytosis of iron deficiency anemia, thus increasing the risk of cerebral thrombus formation (Park, 1988).

Dysrhythmias

Rhythm disturbances can occur in the child with CHD as a direct result of the cardiac defect or from the surgical repair. Atrial dysrhythmias are more common than ventricular rhythm disturbances in children. Infants with Ebstein's anomaly are predisposed to develop supraventricular tachycardia (SVT). Congenitally corrected transposition of the great arteries (L-TGA) may also lead to SVT or varying degrees of heart block.

Postoperatively, disturbances in atrial rhythms may be seen in children after a Mustard procedure for TGA, repair of ASD, Fontan procedure, and total anomalous pulmonary venous return (TAPVR) (Park, 1988). Postoperative second- or third-degree heart block is an uncommon occurrence in VSD repair, atrioventricular (AV) canal repair, and TOF repair. In addition, children who have had total repair of TOF can develop ventricular dysrhythmias, which rarely leads to sudden death (Denfield and Garson, 1990).

Digoxin toxicity can cause a wide variety of dysrhythmias, including profound bradycardia, SVT, and varying degrees of heart block (Park, 1988). A low serum potassium concentration potentiates the effects of digoxin. A child receiving a non–potassium-sparing diuretic, such as furosemide (Lasix), without potassium replacement may be at particular risk of digoxin toxicity. A therapeutic digoxin level is generally 1 to 2 ng/dl, although toxicity has been seen at lower levels, and higher levels may not be toxic for some infants (Schneeweiss, 1986). A sound rule is to assume that a dysrhythmia noted in a child on digoxin therapy is caused by digoxin until proved otherwise. If extra beats or an abnormal rhythm, including bradycardia and tachycardia, is identified by the practitioner, the child should be referred to the cardiologist for further evaluation as soon as possible.

Failure to thrive

Growth failure has been frequently observed in children with CHD (Nadas, Rosenthal, and Crigler, 1981; Salzer et al., 1989). The decreased growth is usually more pronounced in weight than height. Congestive heart failure is one of the most potent factors in the development of failure to thrive because of both inadequate caloric intake secondary to tachypnea and the relative hypermetabolism associated with CHF (Bougle et al., 1986; Nadas, Rosenthal, and Crigler, 1981; Salzer et al., 1989). Growth failure is particularly important to recog-

nize because it may suggest significant hemodynamic compromise necessitating an alteration in the drug regimen or surgery. Corrective surgery, particularly in infancy, generally restores a normal growth pattern. Weight usually improves more quickly than height (Nadas, Rosenthal, and Crigler, 1981). Palliative surgery generally improves growth, though not to the same degree as corrective surgery (Gidding and Rosenthal, 1984).

Development

The majority of children with CHD show development within the normal range (Gidding and Rosenthal, 1984). However, studies of the effects of cyanosis on IQ have suggested that cyanotic children may have a lag in intellectual development (Linde, Rasof, and Dunn, 1970). Generally early correction of cyanotic lesions results in improved intellectual functioning (Newberger et al., 1984). Congestive heart failure has also been implicated as a factor in delayed mental and motor function (Aisenberg et al., 1982). Parental overprotection and lack of activity may also contribute to delayed development (Linde et al., 1966). Though delayed development has been identified, researchers have emphasized that children with cyanotic and acyanotic defects have IQs well within the normal range, and the practical importance of the difference in IQ may be insignificant (Aram et al., 1985).

Vulnerable child syndrome

Although overprotection is a problem for the child with a chronic condition in general, the child with a heart defect is at high risk for overprotection (Bergman and Stamm, 1967). Parental anxiety can relate to the disturbing array of clinical symptoms of a child with CHF or cyanosis, as well as the fear of a sudden catastrophic event (Glaser, Harrison, and Lynn, 1964; Higgins and Kashani, 1984). In addition, feeding problems have been identified as a primary source of anxiety for parents (D'Antonio, 1976). However, the mere presence of the defect unrelated to its severity can produce severe anxiety leading to overprotection (Linde et al., 1966). Because overprotection may delay the development in a child with existing physical impediments, the practitioner should be aware of feelings of vulnerability in the parents and child and reinforce the importance of treating the child normally.

PRIMARY CARE MANAGEMENT
Growth and development

Significant delays in both height and weight are seen in children with symptomatic CHD (Nadas, Rosenthal, and Crigler, 1981; Salzer et al., 1989). Generally height is not affected as much as weight, and head circumference is not affected by CHD. If growth is slowed to a point of the child's growth curve flattening, the child should be referred to the cardiologist for an evaluation of worsening CHF. A weight gain of approximately 1 lb/month is acceptable for the infant with controlled CHF (Higgins, 1987). Because the growth of a child whose CHF is well controlled may still be slow, it is important to look at trends of weight gain in addition to comparison with the norms.

In assessing the developmental and emotional status of the child with CHD, the practitioner needs to take into account factors such as hypoxemia, CHF, parental overprotection, and physical incapacity. Preoperatively the infant in CHF is often too exhausted to pass all of the developmental tasks in screening tests. If a child is developing at a slower but progressive rate, referral for additional developmental testing is not immediately warranted. If there appear to be significant alterations in the level of alertness or if there is no progress in mastering developmental tasks, further screening is advised. If CHD is part of a syndrome that involves developmental delay, referral and enrollment in an infant stimulation program would be important.

Crying is a major developmental concern of most parents of children with CHD. They worry that crying will hurt the heart or precipitate a medical crisis. Parents need to be informed that short periods of crying will not harm the infant. They should treat crying as if the child did not have a heart defect. Parents can be counseled that prompt attention to crying will usually console the infant faster (Barnard, 1978) and reduce crying and irritability in subsequent months (Bell and Ainsworth, 1970). Parents should attend to the crying child for these reasons, not because crying is dangerous for the child. It is important to discuss crying issues with both parents because there frequently are differences in philosophies and subsequent conflicts between parents regarding crying in children.

When developmental concerns are discussed with parents, it is critical to help parents normalize their reactions to their child. The practitioner can guide the parents in treating the child normally, reinforcing that symptomatic children will limit themselves naturally.

Immunizations

The standard immunization protocol is recommended for children with CHD. However, a significant percentage of infants with CHD either never receive immunizations or receive them well after the recommended dates (Gidding and Rosenthal, 1984; Uzark et al., 1983). Immunizations should not be given before cardiac catheterization or surgery because a fever would delay the procedure. Also, measles, mumps, and rubella (MMR) vaccine should be delayed for 3 months after a child has received blood products because passively acquired antibodies might interfere with the response to the immunization (Committee on Infectious Diseases, 1991). After surgery, immunizations should be delayed approximately 6 weeks so that a fever from an immunization is not confused with a postoperative infection.

Children with hemodynamically significant CHD may be more susceptible to complications of influenza and should receive the influenza vaccine yearly beginning at 6 months of age (Committee on Infectious Diseases, 1991). Polyvalent pneumococcal vaccine is recommended for all asplenic children 2 years old and older as a single intramuscular or subcutaneous 0.5-ml dose (Committee on Infectious Diseases, 1991).

Screening

Vision. Routine screening is recommended.
Hearing. Routine screening is recommended.
Dental. Routine dental care should be meticulously followed to prevent caries that may predispose the child to bacteremia if left untreated. Endocarditis prophylaxis is recommended during all dental procedures except simple adjustment of braces and shedding of deciduous teeth (Dajani, et al., 1990) (see the box on p. 199). Nearly all children with CHD need antibiotic prophylaxis both preoperatively and postoperatively. The specific regimen depends on the type of defect, procedure being performed, and the child's sensitivity to pen-

ENDOCARDITIS PROPHYLAXIS RECOMMENDATIONS*

For dental procedures and surgery of the upper respiratory tract

1. For most patients: Amoxicillin 50 mg/kg (maximum 3.0 g) orally 1 hour before procedure; then half the dose 6 hours after the initial dose.
2. For patients allergic to Amoxicillin or Penicillin: Erythromycin ethylsuccinate 20 mg/kg (maximum 800 mg) or erythromycin stearate 20 mg/kg (maximum 1.0 g) orally 2 hours before procedure; then half the dose 6 hours after the initial dose;

or

 Clindamycin 10 mg/kg (maximum 300 mg) orally 1 hour before procedure; then half the dose 6 hours after the initial dose.
3. For patients unable to take oral medications: Ampicillin 50 mg/kg (maximum 2.0 g) IM or IV 30 minutes before the procedure; then half the dose 6 hours after the initial dose.
4. For patients allergic to Penicillin who are unable to take oral medications: Clindamycin 10 mg/kg (maximum 300 mg) IV 30 minutes before the procedure; then half the dose 5 hours after the initial dose.

From Dajani, AS et al.: Prevention of bacterial endocarditis, JAMA, 264:2919-2922. Copyright 1990 by American Medical Association. Adapted by permission.

*The American Heart Association recommends the standard oral prophylactic regimen to patients who have prosthetic heart valves and in other high-risk groups. Some practitioners may prefer to use parenteral prophylaxis in these high-risk group patients.

5. For high-risk patients no candidates for standard regimen: Ampicillin 50 mg/kg (maximum 2.0 g) IV, plus Gentamicin 2.0 mg/kg (maximum 80 mg) IV, 30 minutes before procedure; then Amoxicillin 25 mg/kg (maximum 1.5 g) orally 6 hours after initial dose; alternatively, the IV dose may be repeated 8 hours after initial dose.
6. For high-risk patients allergic to Penicillin: Vancomycin 20 mg/kg (maximum 1.0 g) IV starting 1 hour before procedure; no repeat dose necessary.

For gastrointestinal and genitourinary tract procedures and surgery

1. For most patients: Ampicillin, Gentamicin and Amoxicillin. Ampicillin 50 mg/kg (maximum 2.0 g) IM or IV, plus Gentamicin 2.0 mg/kg (maximum 80 mg) IM or IV 30 minutes before procedure; then Amoxicillin 50 mg/kg (maximum 1.5 g) orally 6 hours after the initial dose; alternatively, the IV regimen may be repeated once 8 hours after initial dose.
2. For patients allergic to Penicillin: Vancomycin and Gentamicin. Vancomycin 20 mg/kg (maximum 1.0 g) IV, over 1 hour + Gentamicin 2.0 mg/kg (maximum 80 mg) IV, 1 hour before procedure; may be repeated once 8 hours after initial dose.
3. For low-risk patients: Amoxicillin 50 mg/kg (maximum 3.0 g) orally 1 hour before procedure; then half the dose 6 hours after initial dose.

icillin. This information should be communicated to the practitioner by the child's cardiologist. Wallet-size cards for parents that outline specific prophylaxis regimens are available from the American Heart Association.

Blood pressure. Blood pressure should be obtained in upper and lower extremities for children with preoperative or postoperative coarctation of the aorta to identify discrepancies in pressure readings. A child who has had a Blalock-Taussig shunt procedure to increase blood flow to the lungs will have a diminished or absent pulse in the upper extremity on the side of the surgical scar.

Hematocrit. A rise in hemoglobin and hematocrit values may indicate progressive hypoxemia in the child with a cyanotic heart defect. Furthermore, because of the problems associated with anemia in the child with cyanosis or CHF, hemoglobin and hematocrit values should be checked regularly. Iron supplementation should be prescribed if the hemoglobin level is low for the child's specific condition. Because the child's cardiologist will be checking these values periodically, communication with the cardiologist concerning laboratory results may save the child the pain and expense of repeated laboratory tests.

Urinalysis. Routine screening is recommended.

Tuberculin. Routine screening is recommended.

Drug interactions

Children with CHF or heart rhythm problems often receive digoxin, diuretics, and other antidysrhythmic medications. Coadministration of digoxin and quinidine, verapamil (Calan), or amiodarone (Cordarone) may elevate digoxin plasma concentrations (Schneeweiss, 1986).

Decongestants should be avoided in a child with a rapid heart dysrhythmia (e.g., supraventricular tachycardia or atrial fibrillation) or hypertension because they may exacerbate tachydysrhythmias or increase blood pressure (Hoffman and Bigger, 1985). Aspirin should be avoided for 3 weeks before surgery because of its anticoagulant properties. Aminoglycosides can affect renal function and alter excretion of digoxin (Hoffman and Bigger, 1985). Also, phenobarbital speeds hepatic metabolism and can alter drug metabolism and efficacy (Gidding and Rosenthal, 1984), resulting in increased medication requirements. The practitioner may be monitoring certain drug levels (digoxin, antidysrhythmics) or response to drugs (prothrombin time in the child taking anticoagulants) in close association with the cardiologist.

DIFFERENTIAL DIAGNOSIS AND MANAGEMENT OF COMMON PEDIATRIC CONDITIONS

Children with CHD may be susceptible to certain common pediatric problems that can be more severe than in the child with a structurally normal heart. It is important for the practitioner to know these common problems that can lead to serious complications. It is equally important, however, to treat these children normally and look for the simple, uncomplicated problems. Families need reinforcement that their children are normal with special medical needs. Children who have had heart surgery are often scared or hesitant to allow an examination, particularly of their chest. Taking the time to gain the trust of the child before the ex-

amination will make visits less stressful for the child and more productive for the practitioner.

Fever

Though febrile illnesses can have serious implications for the child with CHD, an acute fever may also be caused by a common, uncomplicated childhood illness. Practitioners should investigate and treat a fever the same way they would for any child the same age, keeping in mind the more serious possibilities. The chronic use of antibiotics without a diagnosis just because the child has CHD is not warranted and will put the child at risk of developing infections from resistant organisms (Gidding and Rosenthal, 1984).

A fever within a few weeks after heart surgery may be a sign of an operative infection or the postpericardiotomy syndrome (a reaction of the pericardial sac after heart surgery). A careful and complete examination is necessary to identify a source of infection. If no focus of infections such as otitis media or pharyngitis is found, the practitioner should obtain a complete blood cell (CBC) count with differential and a blood culture and should consult with or refer the child to the cardiologist or surgeon. In addition, if there are any signs of a superficial wound infection, the child should be referred to the cardiologist or surgeon. The postpericardiotomy syndrome should be suspected by the presence of a fever with a pericardial friction rub, chest pain, or enlargement of the cardiac silhouette on chest x-ray film (Park, 1988). It is rarely seen in children less than 2 years of age. Referral to the cardiologist is necessary.

A fever will increase the metabolic demands and thus the work of the heart. It is therefore important to evaluate the febrile child with CHD for developing or worsening CHF.

The infant or child with asplenia is at particular risk for infection. These children need to be seen by the practitioner immediately on developing a fever for a complete septic work-up to identify the cause and initiate antibiotic therapy.

Infective endocarditis

The practitioner should be alert to signs of endocarditis in a child with CHD who has a sustained, unexplained fever, because symptoms may be nonspecific and insidious. Fever may be associated with decreased activity, anorexia, malaise, night sweats, petechiae, splenomegaly, or a new murmur (Hoffman, 1987). Children with an unexplained fever and these symptoms should be referred to their cardiologist for evaluation, including an echocardiogram, to look for vegetations within the heart. Blood cultures should be drawn before antibiotics are begun. Infective endocarditis rarely is seen in children less than 2 years of age. Children at high risk are those who are cyanotic, have had palliative systemic to pulmonary shunts, have prosthetic valves, and those with obstructive defects.

Upper respiratory tract infection

The child with CHD, particularly the child with a defect causing left to right shunting, may have frequent or significant upper and lower respiratory tract infections (Hoffman, 1987). It is important to evaluate the degree of respiratory compromise compared with the child's baseline respiratory status. If there is an increase in respiratory effort or the presence of adventitious breath sounds, a chest x-ray film should be obtained to rule out pneumonia or worsening CHF. Infiltrates on x-ray film, fever, and productive cough indicate a lower respiratory tract infection; cardiomegaly, poor feeding, sweating, and a dry cough would signal CHF. The practitioner should have follow-up contact with the family 24 hours after initial contact to evaluate the child's progress.

Gastrointestinal symptoms

Vomiting or anorexia may occur secondary to gastroenteritis, worsening CHF, or digoxin toxicity. The child must be evaluated for other symptoms of CHF and a serum digoxin level obtained if the history and physical findings are not compatible with more common causes of gastrointestinal (GI) symptoms.

Excessive fluid losses from vomiting, diarrhea, or anorexia can lead to dehydration and thrombus formation in the cyanotic, polycythemic child. Replacement fluids or consultation with the cardiologist to hold diuretic therapy may be necessary until the GI disturbance is resolved.

Neurologic symptoms

The child with unexplained fever, headache, focal neurologic signs, or seizures requires immediate referral to a medical center because of the risk of a brain abscess or cerebrovascular accident (CVA).

DEVELOPMENTAL ISSUES
Safety

In addition to standard safety precautions, the child with CHD has unique safety needs. For example, digoxin elixir has a pleasant taste and attractive color, which increases the potential for accidental ingestion by the child or siblings. Therefore, safe storage and administration of medications is essential. A surprising number of parents had inadequate knowledge to safely and wisely administer digoxin to their children (Jackson, 1979). Marking a syringe at the correct dose, giving written instructions on digoxin administration, and allowing the parent to practice drawing up the digoxin will help ensure the safe use of this valuable but potentially dangerous medication. It is important for the family to find a schedule that not only maintains the correct timing of medications but also fits into their life to prevent a missed or repeated dose.

Electrical safety is critical for the child with a permanent pacemaker. An electric shock may irreparably damage the pacemaker, requiring immediate surgical replacement. There is no risk of electromagnetic interference between a permanent pacemaker and common household items such as electrical appliances, radios, or electronic equipment. Microwave ovens and the pacemaker itself have filtering systems that prevent interference with the pacemaker's function. Large magnets placed directly over the pacemaker will temporarily change its function. Magnetic resonance imaging is therefore not recommended for a child with a permanent pacemaker (Moses et al., 1987). Metal detectors should also be avoided, because they have an electromagnetic field that may alter the pacemaker's function temporarily as well as set off the alarm because of the metal in the pacemaker. Small magnet toys, however, will not alter the pacemaker's function. A pacemaker identification card or letter from the practitioner should be sufficient to avoid the metal detector. Older children with pacemakers and children receiving anticoagulants should wear Medic-Alert bracelets for emergencies.

Children with permanent pacemakers or on anticoagulant therapy for prosthetic valves can maintain most normal activities. They should be counseled to avoid contact sports such as football, boxing, or karate that could damage the pacemaker or cause excessive bleeding (Shannon, 1986).

Travel may need to be altered for the child with CHD. Altitudes of 5000 feet or more are not recommended for children with moderate to severe pulmonary hypertension, severe CHF, or significant hypoxemia (partial pressure of oxygen [PO_2] < 50 mm Hg) (Canobbio, 1987; Gidding and Rosenthal, 1984). Flying for these children may require precautions because cabin pressure is usually equivalent to an altitude of 5000 to 7500 feet. Supplemental oxygen can be supplied by the airlines to increase the inspired oxygen to 20%.

It has been reported that cardiopulmonary resuscitation (CPR) training for parents of children with CHD is effective and particularly warranted for certain problems (Higgins, Hardy, and Higashino, 1989). Suggesting CPR training to parents as a skill that is worthwhile to know can allay potential concerns about the importance of learning CPR. The Red Cross and American Heart Association offer CPR training to families.

Child care

Some parents choose to stop work when they have a child with a chronic condition, but many do not have that option. Child care is necessary for most families. Several factors need to be balanced when parents are deciding to return to work: (1) the financial and emotional need to return to work; (2) parents' anxiety about leaving the child; (3) the increased incidence of infection for children in child care and the impact of infection on the child's cardiovascular status; and (4) parents' confidence in the child care provider's ability to recognize symptoms, give medications properly, and respond to emergencies appropriately.

Before surgery or cardiac catheterization, parents may be counseled to take their child out of child care to avoid exposure to infections that would cancel surgery. Children with asplenia or DiGeorge syndrome are at the highest risk of infection. For these infection-prone children, home day care or small group day care would be advised. For 6 weeks after surgery, parents should limit the activities that stress the child's sternum, such as climbing, pulling, heavy lifting, rough playing, or lifting the child under the arms. The parents need to communicate these restrictions to the child care provider to determine if it is realistic or safe to return the child to day care before normal activity is allowed. The practitioner can play a key role in educating child care providers about the child's condition and reinforcing activity limits, as well as lack of limits.

Diet

Feeding is often a major problem for children with CHD, particularly if they are in CHF. The infant in CHF often has difficulty coordinating the suck, swallow, and breath of feeding. The distribution of calories in these infants is similar to the recommended dietary allowances (Gervasio and Buchanan, 1985). However, if the infant is not gaining weight adequately, the caloric intake may need to be increased by concentrating formula. Concentrating the formula to 24 to 30 calories/oz will improve total calories without increasing total volume. If formula is concentrated by decreasing the amount of water added to powder or concentrate, it is important to consider the increased renal solute load the infant receives. An alternative is to add low-osmolarity glucose polymers or oils to standard formulas to increase the caloric density. A diet providing increased carbohydrates and fats may lead to increased retention of nitrogen for growth (Gervasio and Buchanan, 1985). Two common preparations used are Polycose, which delivers 23 calories/15 ml, and medium-chain triglycerides (or MCT oil), which delivers 120 calories/15 ml. Consulting with a nutritionist and the cardiologist would be advised if nutritional manipulations are used.

Breast-feeding the child with even significant hemodynamic changes is not contraindicated if growth is adequate. Breast milk is the best source of nutrition for the child with CHD (Committee on Nutrition, 1985; Gidding and Rosenthal, 1984). The physiologic stress of breast-feeding may actually be less than the stress related to bottle-feeding (Meier and Anderson, 1987). Methods to decrease the work of feeding during breast- or bottle-feeding include holding the infant at a 45-degree angle to minimize tachypnea, feeding for no more than 40 minutes at a time to minimize fatigue, allowing the infant to develop his or her own rhythm of feeding and resting, and following the infant's cues for hunger, satiety, and tiring (Higgins and Kashani, 1984).

Rarely a child will not gain weight despite aggressive feeding and formula concentration. This child may need gavage feeding to minimize calories used with feeding. Using a pacifier during gavage feeding will help the infant develop a strong suck, facilitate the transition to oral feeding after surgery, and promote future language development (Bernbaum et al., 1983).

Parents often need tremendous support around feeding the child with CHD. The child with CHF and tachypnea has difficulty consuming adequate calories to satisfy hunger and may be irritable. Feeding may take a great deal of time because the child's cues are difficult to read. Parents may feel pressured to have the child gain weight for surgery. In addition, a parent's self-esteem may be tied to feeding and growth of the child (D'Antonio, 1976). The practitioner should stress to the parents that feeding can be a positive time for bonding and nurturing. Ongoing support includes teaching the parents to be sensitive to the infant's cues for hunger, satiety, and distress; pointing out the positive aspects of the child; and reinforcing their feeding skills. Through feeding the parent and child are developing their relationship (Satter, 1986). The practitioner who understands the potential problems with feeding can be instrumental in fostering a positive feeding relationship by providing support and counseling.

Discipline

Behavioral expectations of a child with CHD should be similar to those for a child without a heart defect. It is not uncommon for parents to overprotect and pamper children with CHD. Linde and associates (1966) observed that "the mere label of 'congenital heart disease' sets into motion complex changes in the family's approach and attitudes not only to the cardiac child but necessarily to his normal siblings." The practitioner can play a key role in reinforcing the importance of setting limits and disciplining the child as if there were no heart disease and helping to normalize the family dynamics in light of the risk of overprotection.

On the other hand, the infant with CHF who is irritable, hard to console, and difficult to feed may present a very stressful situation for the parents. The practitioner must be aware of the family stressors and infant characteristics that may lead to child abuse in the child with a chronic condition.

Toileting

The child on diuretic therapy may have difficulty with toilet training. If the child is receiving diuretics for a short period of time, the parents may want to delay toilet training until the medication has been discontinued.

Sleep patterns

Tachypneic infants with CHF may be unable to satisfy their hunger and have a difficult time sleeping through the night. Referral to the cardiologist is advised if the child's respiratory status is deteriorating to the point of interfering with feeding and sleeping. When discussing sleep with parents, the practitioner should ask them where the child sleeps. Because of the problem of parental anxiety and overprotection, some parents sleep with the child in their bed for up to 2 years. The practitioner should reinforce the stability of the child to help the parents deal with their anxiety. The transition to the child's bed should not occur when there has been a disruption in the child's routine or security, such as around surgery.

School issues

Most school-aged children with CHD are able to attend school with their peers. Missed school is often related to hospitalizations, recuperation from surgery, and cardiology visits. The practitioner can play an important role in assessing the need for home or in-hospital schooling for prolonged absences and facilitating services. Absenteeism may also be associated with the parent's perception of the child's vulnerability and lack of control over improving their child's health status (Fowler et al., 1987).

As children enter junior high and high school, they may have body image concerns related to their scar, small stature, and ability to keep up with peers. In general, children should be encouraged to participate in physical activity to their tolerance based on discussions that include the child, practitioner, cardiologist, parents, and school professionals (Freed, 1984). The American Heart Association (AHA) has developed guidelines for activity for young children with heart disease based on the particular defect and hemodynamic consequences (Gutgesell et al., 1986). Stress testing is often performed by the cardiologist to develop an individualized activity plan. This information should be relayed to the practitioner; an ongoing discussion with the parent and child will reinforce the realistic goals for activity and help to prevent overprotection.

Sexuality

The issues of contraception and the safety of pregnancy need to be discussed with the parents before the child's adolescence and with the child in early adolescence (Uzark, VonBargen-Mazza, and Messiter, 1989). Communication with the cardiologist will give the practitioner critical information about the child's risk factors for contraception and pregnancy given her particular physical status.

Oral contraceptives are not advised for women with pulmonary hypertension, cyanotic CHD, prosthetic valves, or for those who smoke cigarettes because of the risks associated with increased coagulation and thrombus formation (Gleicher and Elkayam, 1990). Because of the potential for cervicitis and subsequent bacteremia, the intrauterine device (IUD) is contraindicated in adolescents at risk for developing infective endocarditis (Canobbio, 1987; Gleicher and Elkayam, 1990). Barrier methods such as condoms and diaphragms with spermicidal cream are safe methods of birth control from a cardiac standpoint but are not as effective in preventing pregnancy. Certainly the condom represents the best method for preventing sexually transmitted diseases; with reliable use by her partner it is an acceptable form of contraception for the young woman with CHD (Gleicher and Elkayam, 1990).

For females at very high risk for cardiac compromise during pregnancy, surgical sterilization should be discussed. Tubal ligation in adolescents with long-standing pulmonary hypertension leading to Eisenmenger's syndrome carries with it a high surgical risk and should not be performed unless absolutely necessary (Gleicher and Elkayam, 1990). The preferred method of sterilization may therefore be vasectomy if there is one sexual partner.

Experts often look at the woman's cardiovascular status based on the New York Heart Association (NYHA) functional classification to determine the relative risk of pregnancy. Individuals with mild, unoperated heart disease or with well-repaired cardiac defects (NYHA class I or II) are at no higher risk from pregnancy than the general population (Canobbio, 1987; Elkayam, Cobb, and Gleicher, 1990; Whittemore, Hobbins, and Engle, 1982). The adolescent in class III will need special attention during pregnancy. The adolescent with pulmonary vascular disease or in CHF would be in NYHA functional class IV. She may not be able to safely carry a pregnancy to term, and the pregnancy may need to be terminated for safety of the mother (Gleicher and Elkayam, 1990). It is important for the practitioner to discuss the risks of pregnancy with the cardiologist so the recommendation can be reinforced to the adolescent. A multidisciplinary approach involving the cardiologist, obstetrician, and practitioner should be used for the pregnant adolescent with CHD.

SPECIAL FAMILY CONCERNS

The family of the child with CHD may have ongoing concerns about symptoms, feeding problems, sudden death, finances, and the long-term physical and emotional effects of multiple surgeries (Donovan, 1989; Garson et al., 1978). When parents are counseled about symptoms, it is important for the practitioner to convey that they will be watching for trends over time rather than minute by minute. Reinforcing to the parents that they become the expert in observing their child for changes decreases their feelings that only health care providers can adequately monitor their child.

The insurability of a child with heart disease depends on the particular defect and repair (Truesdell, Skorton, and Lauer, 1986). As children become older they often lose their parent's coverage and have difficulty obtaining insurance as an adult (Canobbio, 1987; Truesdell, Skorton, and Lauer, 1986). It is important for parents to investigate the options for extended coverage of the child on their health insurance plan well in advance of the policy expiring for the child. Children with CHD may qualify for the supplemental insurance of Crippled Children's Services depending on their parent's income.

Parents may also be concerned about the recurrence of CHD in subsequent children. Counseling a family about specific risk to future children should be performed by the cardiologist or genetic counselor; the practitioner should then reinforce the information and support the family in their decision making. Early prenatal diagnosis of CHD is possible using high-resolution ultrasound techniques.

---◆ ▬▬▬▬▬▬▬ ◆---

SUMMARY OF PRIMARY CARE NEEDS FOR THE CHILD WITH CONGENITAL HEART DISEASE

Growth and development

Significant delays in weight and height are common in children with symptomatic CHD preoperatively; corrective surgery improves growth.

Intellectual development is not significantly impaired by CHD; cyanosis, parental overprotection, and CHF may contribute to delayed development.

Infant crying is a major but unnecessary concern for parents.

Immunizations

Standard immunization protocol is recommended; delay should occur only around cardiac catheterization or surgery.

Delay MMR vaccine for 3 months after blood products are received.

With significant CHD, influenza vaccine is recommended.

With asplenia syndrome, daily antimicrobial prophylaxis and pneumococcal vaccine for children 2 years or older is recommended.

Screening
Vision

Routine screening is recommended.

Hearing

Routine screening is recommended.

Dental

Dental care is important to prevent caries, which predispose child to bacteremia and endocarditis. Endocarditis prophylaxis is recommended for all dental procedures except routine adjustment of braces and shedding of deciduous teeth (see the boxes on pp. 196 and 199).

Blood pressure

Check blood pressure in all four extremities for children with coarctation of the aorta preoperatively and postoperatively. Child with Blalock-Taussig shunt will have low or absent blood pressure values in the arm on the side of the shunt.

Hematocrit

A rise in hematocrit may indicate worsening cyanosis. Anemia is problematic in the child with CHF or cyanosis. Monitor hemoglobin levels closely in coordination with cardiologist.

Urinalysis

Routine screening is recommended.

Tuberculin

Routine screening is recommended.
Drug interactions

Accurate administration of digoxin is critical.

Phenobarbital may lower the plasma level of digoxin.

Aminoglycosides may decrease renal function and increase the digoxin level.

Decongestants are not recommended for the child with rapid heart dysrhythmias or hypertension.

Digoxin or anticoagulant dosages may need to be monitored.

Differential diagnosis
Fever

Postoperatively rule out (1) wound infection and (2) postpericardiotomy syndrome. If no focus is found, obtain CBC and blood culture. The child with asplenia with fever must be seen immediately.

Infective endocarditis

Symptoms are often vague; a high level of suspicion is needed to diagnose. It is rarely seen in children less than 2 years of age. Refer to the cardiologist if fever, malaise, anorexia, splenomegaly, or night sweats are present.

Respiratory tract infection

Frequent or significant upper and lower respiratory tract infections may occur; rule out CHF or pneumonia.

Continued.

SUMMARY OF PRIMARY CARE NEEDS FOR THE CHILD WITH CONGENITAL HEART DISEASE — cont'd

---

Gastrointestinal symptoms

Rule out digoxin toxicity and CHF; excessive fluid losses are dangerous in the child who is cyanotic or who is taking diuretics and digoxin.

Neurologic symptoms

Cyanotic children are at increased risk of brain abscess (if >2 years) or CVA (if <2 years); unexplained fever, headaches, seizures, or focal neurologic signs need immediate referral to a medical center.

Developmental issues
Safety

Safe storage of digoxin is critical.

For the child with a pacemaker, electrical safety is critical. There is no risk of damage with usual household appliances, including the microwave. Those with pacemakers should not have MRIs, should avoid metal detectors, and should wear a Medic-Alert bracelet.

Air travel and altitude may need to be limited depending on the defect.

Cardiopulmonary resuscitation training for parents is warranted for certain defects.

Child care

The provider must understand medications, must be able to recognize symptoms, and must know emergency procedures.

Infants with DiGeorge syndrome or asplenia syndrome are prone to infection; thus home day care or small group day care is recommended.

Vigorous activity is limited for 6 weeks after surgery.

Diet

Feeding is a major problem for the child with CHD, especially for the child in CHF; required daily allowances are normal, but formula may need to be concentrated for adequate caloric intake.

Breast-feeding is encouraged if growth is adequate.

Teach methods to decrease work of breathing.

Feeding is a major source of stress for parents, who will need much support.

Discipline

Normal behavior should be expected from children regardless of their CHD. Parents often overprotect and pamper children with CHD.

Toileting

Toilet training of the child receiving diuretics may be difficult.

Sleep patterns

Children may have difficulty sleeping through the night if they are tachypneic and unable to satisfy their hunger.

School issues

Children may need home tutoring around hospitalization and surgery time.

Self-image concerns about scar, keeping up with peers, and small stature may develop.

AHA publishes guidelines for activity limits based on each defect. Generally children limit themselves; the child who has a pacemaker or is taking anticoagulants should avoid rough contact sports.

Sexuality

Oral contraceptives are not recommended for individuals with pulmonary hypertension, cyanotic CHD, or prosthetic valves.

An IUD is not recommended for individuals at risk for developing endocarditis.

Risks associated with pregnancy are determined by the individual's heart defect and functional ability as assessed by the cardiologist; teens need early and thorough counseling.

Special family concerns

The family has ongoing concern about symptoms, multiple surgeries, and sudden death.

Insurability of the child is difficult.

Occurrence of CHD in subsequent children may be a concern; parents may want genetic counseling; prenatal diagnosis of CHD is possible through fetal echocardiography.

RESOURCES

Parent support groups are valuable resources and provide an important network for families coping with anxieties related to taking care of the child with CHD. Newsletters and special interest groups often develop from parent networking (see section on organizations). The practitioner should contact the local AHA or pediatric cardiology department to see if such groups exist. Written information covering many aspects of CHD is also available through the AHA. Public health or home health nursing may be an additional source of support, especially for the family learning to identify symptoms, give multiple medications, and provide adequate nutrition to the newly diagnosed infant with CHD.

Informational materials

The following resource booklets and pamphlets are available for families through the local or national chapter of the AHA (this is not a complete listing of resources):

If Your Child Has a Heart Defect — A Guide for Parents
Feeding Infants with Heart Disease — A Guide for Parents
Dental Care for Children with Heart Disease
Abnormalities of Heart Rhythm — A Guide for Parents
Caring for a Child with a Heart Condition — A Guide for Parents [San Francisco Chapter]
Caring for an Infant with Congestive Heart Failure — A Guide for Parents [San Francisco Chapter]
Marfan's Syndrome
Kawasaki's Disease

Organizations

American Heart Association
  National Center
  7320 Greenville Ave
  Dallas, TX 75231

The Heartline Group, Inc.
  10500 Noland Rd
  Overland Park, KS 66215
  (913) 492-6317

This is a national newsletter for parents of children with complex CHD.

The Heart Connection
(415) 970-7091

  This is a San Francisco Bay Area–based organization with monthly meetings for young adults with CHD.

Parents for Heart Support Group

  Check with the local AHA for listings.

REFERENCES

Aisenberg RB, Rosenthal A, Nadas AS, et al: Developmental delay in infants with congenital heart disease: Correlation with hypoxemia and congestive heart failure, *Pediatr Cardiol* 3:133-137, 1982.

Aram DM, Ekelman BL, Ben-Shachar G, et al: Intelligence and hypoxemia in children with congenital heart disease: Fact or artifact? *J Am Coll Cardiol* 6:889-893, 1985.

Barnard K: The nursing child assessment satellite training series. In *Learning resources manual,* Seattle, 1978, University of Washington School of Nursing Publications.

Bell SM and Ainsworth MDS: Infant crying and maternal responsiveness, *Child Dev* 43:1171-1190, 1970.

Bergman AB and Stamm SJ: The morbidity of cardiac nondisease in schoolchildren, *N Engl J Med* 276:1008-1013, 1967.

Bernbaum JC, Pereira GR, Watkins JB, et al: Nonnutritive sucking during gavage feeding enhances growth and maturation in premature infants, *Pediatrics* 71:41-45, 1983.

Boughman JA, Berg KA, Astemborski JA, et al: Familial risks of congenital heart defect assessed in a population-based epidemiologic study, *Am J Med Genet* 26:839-849, 1987.

Bougle D, Iselin M, Kahyat A, et al: Nutritional treatment of congenital heart disease, *Arch Dis Child* 61:799-801, 1986.

Canobbio MM: Counseling the adult with congenital heart disease. In Roberts WC, ed: *Adult congenital heart disease,* Philadelphia, 1987, FA Davis.

Committee on Infectious Diseases: *Report of the committee on infectious diseases,* ed 22, Elk Grove Village, Ill, 1991, The American Academy of Pediatrics, pp 52-53, 274-281, 373-378.

Committee on Nutrition: The American Academy of Pediatrics: *Pediatric nutrition handbook,* ed 2, Elk Grove Village, Ill, 1985, The American Academy of Pediatrics, pp 1-15.

Dajani AS, Bisno AL, Chung KJ, et al: Prevention of bacterial endocarditis: recommendations by the American Heart Association; *JAMA* 264:2919-2922, 1990.

D'Antonio IJ: Mothers' responses to the functioning and behavior of cardiac children in child-rearing situations, *Matern Child Nurs J* 5:207-256, 1976.

Denfield SW and Garson A Jr: Sudden death in children and young adults, *Pediatr Clin North Am* 37:215-231, 1990.

Donovan, EF: Psychosocial considerations in congenital heart disease. In Adams FH, Emmanouilides GC, eds: *Moss' heart disease in infants, children, and adolescents,* ed 4, Baltimore, 1989, Williams & Wilkins, pp 984-991.

Elkayam U, Cobb T, and Gleicher N: Congenital heart disease and pregnancy. In Elkayam U and Gleicher N, eds: *Cardiac problems in pregnancy: Diagnosis and management of maternal and fetal disease,* ed 2, New York, 1990, Alan R Liss, pp 73-98.

Engle MA: Cardiac failure. In Hoekelman RA, ed: *Primary pediatric care,* St Louis, 1987, CV Mosby, pp 1555-1558.

Ferencz C, Neill CA, Boughman JA, et al: Congenital cardiovascular malformations associated with chromosomal abnormalities: An epidemiologic study, *J Pediatri* 114:79-86, 1989.

Fowler MG, Johnson MP, Welshimer KJ, et al: Factors related to school absence among children with cardiac conditions, *Am J Dis Child* 141:1317-1320, 1987.

Freed MD: Recreational and sports recommendations for the child with heart disease, *Pediatr Clin North Am* 31:1307-1320, 1984.

Fyler DC, Buchley LP, Hellenbrand, WE, et al: Report of the New England regional infant cardiac program, *Pediatrics* 65(suppl):375-461, 1980.

Garson A, Benson RS, Ivler L, et al: Parental reactions to children with congenital heart disease, *Child Psychiatry Hum Dev* 9:86-94, 1978.

Gervasio MR and Buchanan CN: Malnutrition in the pediatric cardiology patient, *Crit Care Q* 8(3):49-56, 1985.

Gidding SS and Rosenthal A: The interface between primary care and pediatric cardiology, *Pediatr Clin North Am* 31:1367-1388, 1984.

Glaser HH, Harrison GS, and Lynn DB: Emotional implications of congenital heart disease in children, *Pediatrics* 3:367-379, 1964.

Gleicher N and Elkayam U: Fertility control in the cardiac patient. In Elkayam U and Gleicher N, eds: *Cardiac problems in pregnancy: Diagnosis and management of maternal and fetal disease,* ed 2, New York, 1990, Alan R Liss, pp 453-460.

Graham TP Jr: When to operate on the child with congenital heart disease, *Pediatr Clin North Am* 31:1275-1291, 1984.

Gutgesell, HP, Gessner IH, Vetter VL, et al: Recreational and occupational recommendations for young patients with heart disease, *Circulation* 74:1195A-1198A, 1986.

Higgins SS: Patterns of impairment: Congenital heart defects. In Rose MH and Thomas RB, eds: *Children with chronic conditions: Nursing in a family and community context,* Orlando, Fla, 1987, Grune & Stratton, pp 165-185.

Higgins SS, Hardy CE, and Higashino SM: Should parents of children with congenital heart disease and life-threatening dysrhythmias be taught cardiopulmonary resuscitation? *Pediatrics* 84:1102-1104, 1989.

Higgins SS and Kashani IA: Congestive heart failure: Parent support and teaching, *Crit Care Nurse* 4(4):21-24, 1984.

Higgins SS and Kashani IA: The cyanotic child: Heart defects and parental learning needs, *MCN* 11:259-262, 1986.

Hoffman BF and Bigger JT: Digitalis and allied cardiac glycosides. In Gillman AG, Goodman LS, Rall TW, et al, eds: *The pharmacologic basis of therapeutics,* ed 7, New York, 1985, MacMillan pp 16-47.

Hoffman JIE: The circulatory system. In Rudolph AM, ed: *Pediatrics,* Norwalk, Conn, 1987, Appleton & Lange, pp 1219-1358.

Jackson PL: Digoxin therapy at home: Keeping the child safe, *MCN* 4:106-109, 1979.

Linde LM, Rasof B, and Dunn OJ: Longitudinal studies of intellectual and behavioral development in children with congenital heart disease, *Acta Paediatr Scand* 59:169-176, 1970.

Linde LM, Rasof B, Dunn OJ, et al: Attitudinal factors in congenital heart disease, *Pediatrics* 38:92-101, 1966.

Lister G, Hellenbrand WE, Kleinman CS, et al: Physiologic effects of increasing hemoglobin concentration in left-to-right shunting in infants with ventricular septal defects, *N Engl J Med* 306:502-506, 1982.

Meier P and Anderson GC: Responses of small preterm infants to bottle- and breast-feeding, *MCN* 12:97-105, 1987.

Moller JH: Incidence of cardiac malformation. In Moller JH and Neal WA, eds: *Heart disease in infancy,* New York, 1981, Appleton-Century-Crofts, 1-14.

Moses, HW, Taylor GJ, Schneider JA, et al: *A practical guide to cardiac pacing,* ed 2, Boston, 1987, Little, Brown.

Nadas, AS, Rosenthal A, and Crigler JF: Nutritional considerations in the prognosis and treatment of children with congenital heart disease. In Suskind RM, ed: *Textbook of pediatric nutrition,* New York, 1981, Raven Press, pp 537-544.

Neal WA and Morgan MF: Care of the critically ill neonate with heart disease, *Crit Care Q* 4(1):47-58, 1981.

Newberger JW, Silbert AR, Buckley LP, et al: Cognitive function and age at repair of transposition of the great arteries in children, *N Engl J Med* 310:1495-1499, 1984.

Nora, JJ: Etiologic aspects of heart disease. In Adams FH, and Emmanouilides GC, eds: *Moss's heart disease in infants, children, and adolescents,* ed 4, Baltimore, 1989, Williams & Wilkins, pp 15-23.

Nora JJ and Nora AH: Maternal transmission of congenital heart diseases: New recurrence risk figures and questions of cytoplasmic inheritance and vulnerability to teratogens, *Am J Cardiol* 59:459-463, 1987.

Park MK: *Pediatric cardiology for practitioners,* ed 2, Chicago, 1988, Year Book Publishers.

Radke, W and Lock J: Balloon dilation, *Pediatr Clin North Am* 37:193-213, 1990.

Salzer HR, Haschke F, Wimmer M, et al: Growth and nutritional intake of infants with congenital heart disease, *Pediatr Cardiol* 10:17-23, 1989.

Satter EM: The feeding relationship, *J Am Diet Assoc* 86:352-356, 1986.

Schneeweiss A: *Drug therapy in infants and children with cardiovascular diseases,* Philadelphia, 1986, Lea & Febiger.

Shannon C: Care of the pediatric pacemaker patient. In Riegel B, ed: *Dreifus' pacemaker therapy: An interprofessional approach,* ed 2, Philadelphia, 1986, FA Davis, pp 219-240.

Truesdell SC, Skorton DJ, and Lauer RM: Life insurance for children with cardiovascular disease, *Pediatrics* 77:687-691, 1986.

Uzark K, Collins J, Meisenhelder K, et al: Primary preventive health care in children with heart disease, *Pediatr Cardiol* 4:259-264, 1983.

Uzark K, VonBargen-Mazza P, and Messiter E: Health education needs of adolescents with congenital heart disease, *J Pediatr Health Care* 3:137-143, 1989.

Whittemore R, Hobbins JC, and Engle MA: Pregnancy and its outcome in women with and without surgical treatment of congenital heart disease, *Am J Cardiol* 50:641-651, 1982.

12 Cystic Fibrosis

••

Ann Hix McMullen

ETIOLOGY

Cystic fibrosis (CF), a condition characterized by multisystem involvement, is the most common lethal genetic illness among white children, adolescents, and young adults. Significant advances in genetic and biomedical research over the past 10 years have increased our understanding of the condition, its etiology, clinical management, and approaches to detection.

In 1989, following a succession of scientific breakthroughs in genetics, the CF gene was isolated on the long arm of chromosome 7 and its protein product, cystic fibrosis transmembrane regulator (CFTR) protein, was identified (Rommens et al., 1989). To date, a number of mutations in the CFTR gene have been identified; these mutations account for approximately 85% of CF chromosomes. The remainder of the mutations have not been elucidated (Beaudet, et al., 1990; Fenwick, Fernbach, and O'Brien, 1990).

These breakthroughs in genetics have been accompanied by advances in biomedical research, which are leading to improved understanding of the etiology of CF. Although the fundamental cellular defect is not completely understood, progress has been made in understanding certain physiologic abnormalities present in CF epithelial cells. Scientists have demonstrated defective ion transport across these cells. Although both sodium and chloride are affected, the defect appears to be primarily a result of abnormal chloride movement (Quinton, 1989). It is hypothesized that the pathologic sequelae in

CF are a direct result of a chloride channel defect related to the abnormal CFTR protein. Most recently, molecular geneticists have inserted normal copies of the CFTR gene into CF respiratory epithelial cells in vitro, correcting the chloride channel defect (Rich, et al., 1990; Drum, et al., 1990). These and pioneering studies in other inherited diseases increase the possibility of gene therapy in CF patients in the future.

The pathology of CF is based on mucus-obstructing ducts in various body organs. Pathologic changes are produced in nearly every organ of the body. The most consistent changes occur in the exocrine glands, such as pancreatic acini, bile ducts and gallbladder, prostatic glands, salivary and lacrimal glands, mucous glands of the tracheo-bronchial tree, upper respiratory tract and intestinal wall, and the sweat glands (Lloyd-Still, 1983). Table 12-1 gives an overview of CF, delineating organ system pathogenesis, clinical manifestations, and treatment.

The impact of genetic discoveries on understanding etiology and treatment is only beginning to unfold. At the same time, approaches to detection are changing and reflect the new technologic advances. Carrier screening is available and reliable for siblings and family members of a child with CF (Beaudet et al., 1989). Appropriate DNA deletion and linkage analysis studies are highly complex, and any family member contemplating such screening should be referred to a regional CF center or pediatric genetics center for counseling.

Table 12-1. Overview of cystic fibrosis

System	Pathogenesis	Clinical manifestations	Complications	Management
Sweat glands	Abnormal electrolytes	High rate of salt loss; salt depletion	Heat prostration	Dietary salt replacement, Sweat test (see p. 214-215)
Lungs	Thick, tenacious mucus	Cough, decreased exercise tolerance	Infection	Chest physiotherapy: postural drainage, and cupping/vibration
	Mucus plugging	Air trapping: increased anteroposterior chest diameter	Fibrosis, bronchiectasis	Antibiotics: oral, intravenous (IV), aerosolized
	Obstruction	Hyperresonance	Atelectasis	Bronchodilators
	Decreased mucociliary clearance	Wheezing, fine and coarse crackles, clubbing	Hypoxia, respiratory failure	Cromolyn sodium
			Pneumothorax, hemoptysis	
			Cor pulmonale	
			Allergic bronchopulmonary aspergillosus	
			Failure to thrive (increased energy expenditure)	
			Hypertrophic osteoarthropathy	
Upper airway	Viscous mucus	Chronic sinusitis	Obstruction, mouth breathing	Decongestants; intermittent use
		Nasal polyposis		Nasal cromolyn sodium or corticosteroids
				Antibiotics
				Surgery
Gastrointestinal (GI) tract	Inspissated tenacious meconium	No passage of meconium	Obstruction: meconium ileus	Enema; surgery
		Abdominal distension	Meconium ileus equivalent	Pancreatic enzyme replacement
		Crampy abdominal pain		Dietary changes to avoid constipation
		Fecal mass in colon	Volvulus, intussusception	Laxatives
			Pancreatitis	Gastrografin enema or Go-LYTELY
			Fibrosis	Enzyme replacement
			Failure to thrive	Antacids
			Delayed maturation	H$_2$ antagonists
Pancreas	Viscous secretions obstruction, fibrosis	Maldigestion; bulky, greasy, foul-smelling stools		High-energy diet; normal fat intake
	Abnormal electrolytes	Fat malabsorption, including fat-soluble vitamins	Vitamin deficiency	Concentrated dietary supplements
	Suboptimal enzyme function		Rectal prolapse	Vitamin supplements
			Glucose intolerance	Aggressive nutritional supplementation

Continued.

Table 12-1. Overview of cystic fibrosis—cont'd

System	Pathogenesis	Clinical manifestations	Complications	Management
Biliary	Obstruction Fibrosis	Subclinical cirrhosis	Portal hypertension Cholelithiasis	
Salivary glands	Abnormal electrolyte concentrations	Probably not clinically significant		
Reproductive tract	Abnormally viscous secretions Obstruction	Male: obliteration of vas deferens Sterility Female: thick vaginal and cervical secretions, decreased fertility		Counseling Genetic and birth control counseling

Heterozygote (carrier) detection of the general population is at present technically possible but would allow identification of only about 70% of at-risk couples (Beaudet, Fenwick, Fernbach, and O'Brien, 1990). In addition, a number of mass population screening issues remain unstudied, such as public and professional education, human resource needs, and effects of information on legislative and health insurance systems. Before mass screening can be a feasible and responsible endeavor, pilot screening programs are needed to determine the impact of these issues and a larger percentage (90%-95%) of the mutations must be identified (Wilfond & Fost, 1990).

Prenatal diagnosis is also available to at-risk families (those who have had a child with CF) and has a test accuracy of 98% to 99% (Beaudet & Buffone, 1989; Beaudet et al., 1989). As a result increasing numbers of at-risk families are using these diagnostic resources and confronting the ethical dilemmas of therapeutic abortion versus continuation of the pregnancy. At present their decision making occurs in a milieu of rapidly advancing treatment and the variability of phenotypic expression of CF illness severity in an individual child.

INCIDENCE

The transmission of CF follows an autosomal recessive mode of inheritance and occurs in approximately 1 in 2000 to 2500 live births. The incidence in blacks is lower, about 1 in 17,000; Asians and American Indians are rarely affected, though its occurrence in any race is possible. With a gene frequency of 1 in 23 in the white population, it is estimated that 1 in 400 to 500 couples are both carriers of this recessive trait, with a subsequent 1 in 4 risk with each pregnancy of bearing an affected child (Schwartz, 1987; Stern, 1986).

CLINICAL MANIFESTATIONS AT TIME OF DIAGNOSIS

The pathophysiologic hallmarks of CF are (1) pancreatic enzyme deficiency from duct blockage by viscous mucus, (2) progressive chronic obstructive lung disease associated with viscous infected mucus and subsequent interstitial destruction, and (3) sweat gland dysfunction resulting in abnormally high sodium and chloride concentrations in the sweat (Schwartz, 1987).

There are three common clinical manifestations. The first is *meconium ileus in the neonate,* occurring in 7% to 10% of newly diagnosed infants. Occurrence of meconium ileus should be presumed to be CF until testing confirms or rules out the diagnosis. Meconium plug syndrome, although less frequently associated with the diagnosis of CF, should also raise the primary provider's suspicion.

Second is *malabsorption with failure to thrive* because of loss of or diminished exocrine pancreatic function; it occurs in 80% to 85% of children with CF. These children exhibit varying degrees of weight loss or poor growth patterns, usually in the presence of a normal to voracious appetite; frequent foul-smelling, greasy, bulky stools; rectal prolapse (seen in 25% of children), and a protuberant belly with decreased subcutaneous tissue of the extremities.

Third, *chronic or recurrent upper and lower respiratory tract infections* occur. Manifestations include nasal polyps, chronic sinusitis, recurrent pneumonia and bronchitis, bronchiectasis, or atelectasis. These children have a chronic cough that persists after an upper respiratory tract infection and may become paroxysmal and productive, provoking choking and vomiting. Auscultatory findings often include fine crackles and expiratory wheezes, particularly in the upper lobes and right middle lobe. Infants may have recurrent episodes of wheezing and tachypnea. *Staphylococcus aureus* and *Pseudomonas aeruginosa* are frequent isolates in a respiratory tract culture. Early roentgenographic changes include air trapping and peribronchial thickening, followed by atelectasis, infiltrates, and hilar adenopathy (Rosenstein and Langbaum, 1984; Schwartz, 1987). Without treatment, these early signs and symptoms progress and complications occur. The box below and Fig. 12-1 summarize the progressive changes in the clinical picture of CF lung disease.

PROGRESSIVE CHANGES IN THE CLINICAL PICTURE OF CYSTIC FIBROSIS

I. Early
   A. Dry, hacking, nonproductive cough
   B. Increased respiratory rate
   C. Decreased activity
II. Moderate
   A. Increased cough, increased sputum production
   B. Rales, musical rhonchi, scattered or localized wheezes
   C. Repeated episodes of respiratory tract infection
   D. Signs of obstructive lung disease
      1. Increased anteroposterior diameter
      2. Depressed diaphragm
      3. Palpable liver border
   E. Decreased appetite
   F. Failure to gain weight or grow, or weight loss
   G. Decreased exercise tolerance
III. Advanced
   A. Chronic, paroxysmal, productive cough
   B. Increased respiratory rate, shortness of breath on exertion, orthopnea, dyspnea
   C. Diffuse and localized fine and coarse crackles

   D. Signs of severe obstructive lung disease
      1. Marked increase in anteroposterior diameter (barrel chest, pigeon breast)
      2. Limited respiratory excursion of thoracic cage
      3. Depressed diaphragm
      4. Hyperresonance over entire chest
      5. Decreased ventilation, persistent hypoxemia
   E. Noisy respirations
   F. Marked decrease in appetite
   G. Muscular weakness
   H. Cyanosis
   I. Digital clubbing
   J. Rounded shoulders
   K. Fever, tachycardia, toxicity
   L. Hemoptysis
   M. Pneumothorax
   N. Lung abscess
   O. Signs of cardiac failure (cor pulmonale, edema, enlarged tender liver)
   P. Bone pain and osteoarthropathy

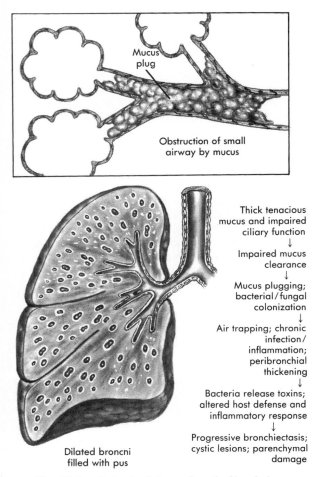

Mucus plug

Obstruction of small airway by mucus

Thick tenacious mucus and impaired ciliary function
↓
Impaired mucus clearance
↓
Mucus plugging; bacterial / fungal colonization
↓
Air trapping; chronic infection / inflammation; peribronchial thickening
↓
Bacteria release toxins; altered host defense and inflammatory response
↓
Progressive bronchiectasis; cystic lesions; parenchymal damage

Dilated broncni filled with pus

Fig. 12-1. Pathophysiology of cystic fibrosis lung disease.

INDICATIONS FOR SWEAT TESTING

Pulmonary

Chronic cough
Recurrent or chronic pneumonia
Staphylococcal pneumonia
Recurrent bronchiolitis
Atelectasis
Hemoptysis
Mucoid *Pseudomonas* infection

Gastrointestinal

Meconium ileus, steatorrhea, malabsorption
Rectal prolapse
Childhood cirrhosis (portal hypertension or bleeding esophageal varices)
Hypoprothrombinemia beyond newborn period

Other

Family history of CF
Failure to thrive
Salty sweat, salty taste when kissed, salt frosting of skin
Nasal polyps
Heat prostration, hyponatremia, and hypochloremia, especially in infants
Pansinusitis
Aspermatism
Digital clubbing

From Schwartz RH: Cystic fibrosis. In Hoekelman RH, ed: *Primary pediatric care*, 1205, St Louis, 1987, CV Mosby Co.

Although these manifestations are most common, the signs and symptoms of CF may be subtle, leading to diagnostic delays and creating an anxious and difficult period for both family and primary provider. Manifestations may be minimal or absent during childhood. Eight percent to 10% of children with CF are not diagnosed until adolescence (Fitzpatrick, Rosenstein, and Langbaum, 1986). Diagnostic delays may be decreased if the provider maintains a high level of suspicion of the wide variety of symptoms associated with CF. The box

above lists indications for sweat testing, the gold standard laboratory test for diagnosing CF.

Diagnosis of CF requires a positive sweat test result in the presence of either (1) clinical symptoms consistent with CF or (2) a family history of CF. Sweat testing is done by pilocarpine iontophoresis with quantitative analysis of sweat sodium and chloride. Collection and assay of sweat should be done only by a qualified laboratory. All of the 127 regional CF centers certified by the CF Foundation have clinical chemistry laboratories that meet specifications for accuracy and reliability of sweat tests. Sweat sodium and chloride concentrations greater than 60 mEq/L are consistent with the diagnosis of CF. A value of 40 to 60 mEq/L is considered borderline and should be repeated. These values should be considered reliable only if an adequate quantity of sweat (usually 50 mg) has been collected (National Academy of Sciences, 1976). Adequate quantities of sweat may be difficult to obtain on infants less than 4 weeks of age. Once the diagnosis has been established in a child, all siblings should also be tested.

TREATMENT
Pancreatic enzyme deficiency

The principal treatment for the resulting malabsorption in CF is oral pancreatic enzyme replacement. Recently enteric coating of enzyme preparations has decreased the likelihood of inactivation by gastric acid. Neutralization of gastric acid with antacids or inhibition of its production with H_2 antagonists may also improve the efficacy of the enzyme preparation. Because fat malabsorption is particularly problematic in CF and deficiencies in fat-soluble vitamins have been reported, many CF centers recommend doubling the recommended daily allowance of multivitamins and adding a water-miscible form of vitamin E. Vitamin K may also be supplemented during infancy, in the presence of hemoptysis, or when clotting studies are prolonged (Hubbard, 1985).

Caloric and protein requirements may be increased in CF because of malabsorption related to inadequate enzyme supplementation and because of progressive pulmonary disease. Most authorities agree that these children have a basal energy requirement 25% to 50% greater than the usual recommended daily allowance for energy intake (Hubbard, 1985). With pulmonary disease progression, children usually have chronic weight and nutrition problems as a result of their increased pulmonary energy requirements.

Calories are encouraged in both complex carbohydrates and fats. Because fats are a more concentrated source of calories, low-fat diets are discouraged because they may create essential fatty acid deficiencies. An individual may have difficulty with certain high-fat foods, and these may be limited; however, generally children should be encouraged to cover high-fat intake with additional enzymes. Aggressive nutritional supplementation (oral, enteral, and parenteral) has been used for children with weight loss and growth delay despite a reasonable intake. In the short term, improved weight gain and stabilization of pulmonary function have been achieved with this approach; long-term efficacy is under study (Soutter et al., 1986).

Pulmonary disease

Progressive lung disease is the major cause of morbidity and mortality in CF. The pathophysiologic basis of CF lung disease is bronchial mucoid infection. Children with CF are chronically colonized with gram-negative organisms that may quantitatively decrease with antimicrobial therapy but are not eradicated. The child's susceptibility to this bacterial growth is not fully understood, and controversies are widespread concerning the optimal approach to its long-term treatment. There is general agreement, however, that bacterial infection, its by-products, and the body's response to infection contribute to progressive damage in the lungs and that antimicrobial therapy plays a significant role in decreasing the rate of this deterioration (Marks, 1981).

Pulmonary exacerbations often follow mild viral illnesses, particularly upper respiratory tract infections; it has been hypothesized that viruses may cause suppression of host defenses (Mischler, 1985; Wang et al., 1984). Early use of oral antibiotic therapy with viral illness symptoms can be argued on the basis of its use to prevent exacerbation of the bacterial pulmonary infection during the viral illness. Traditional concerns regarding development of resistant organisms with overuse of antibiotics must be balanced against the greater concern for progressive deteriorative bronchiectasis (Stern, 1989). Initial choice of an antibiotic and its dosage should include consideration for broad-spectrum coverage, specifically for *S. aureus, S. pneumoniae,* and *Haemophilus influenzae.* Further considerations in children whose pulmonary infections have not responded to initial therapy include antibiotic susceptibility or resistance, lack of compliance, or abnormal pharmacokinetics (Taussig, Landau & Marks, 1984).

Other ongoing pulmonary therapeutic interventions are aimed at relief of bronchial obstruction.

Chest physical therapy (postural drainage and cupping, clapping, and vibration done 2 to 4 times daily) is standard therapy. Although evaluation of chest physical therapy remains difficult, its efficacy has been demonstrated and most CF centers believe that its routine use is beneficial in children with pulmonary involvement (Desmond et al., 1983). Exercise, particularly aerobic conditioning programs, is also encouraged because it positively influences general health, cardiopulmonary and musculoskeletal function, and airway clearance (Orenstein, Henke, and Cerney, 1983). Reactive airway disease (RAD) may result from chronic inflammation and infection; bronchodilators are often used if a clinical response can be observed or if a beneficial response can be demonstrated by pulmonary function testing (PFT) (Rosenstein, 1990). Many children with CF use an aerosolized bronchodilator before chest physical therapy, and some may also benefit from a theophylline preparation. Cromolyn sodium (Intal) may be used in tandem with this regimen.

Clinicians have long recognized the clinical efficacy of short courses of oral and inhaled corticosteroids in reactive airway disease associated with CF. Because immune-mediated inflammation may contribute to the progressive pulmonary damage in CF, the long-term use of corticosteroids and other antiinflammatory agents is being studied. In a large multicenter study, interim data on high dose alternate day prednisone (2 mg/kg) over a period of 1 to 4 years have shown increased frequencies of cataracts, growth retardation, and glucose abnormalities, with discontinuation of study protocol in the high-dose group of patients. This study continues comparing the low-dose prednisone (1 mg/kg) and placebo groups (Rosenstein and Eigen, 1991).

Aerosolized antibiotics may also be used in treating CF lung disease; the specific indications for their use are not fully documented, and they should be used in consultation with CF center providers. Mucolytic agents such as acetylcysteine (Mucomist) and expectorants have no clear efficacy; acetylcysteine may irritate the respiratory tract (Rosenstein, 1990). Current research in the treatment arena focuses on such efforts as development and testing of a new mucolytic agent, recombinant human deoxyribonuclease (DNase), use of aerosolized amiloride to change transmembrane chloride transport in respiratory epithelia, aerosolization of agents such as α1-antitrypsin to inhibit neutrophil elastase, a powerful enzyme that causes inflammation, and use of heart/lung and double lung transplantation in end-stage disease.

When pulmonary exacerbations are not controlled by outpatient management, hospitalization for a pulmonary and nutritional "tune-up" or "cleanout" may be necessary. These 2-week or longer hospital stays allow the CF center team to employ more aggressive strategies to contain infection and supplement nutrition. They include giving antibiotics intravenously, often an aminoglycoside with either a synthetic penicillin or third-generation cephalosporin, increasing pulmonary toilet, and offering nutritional support measures. Antibiotics are given intravenously because of their efficacy in treating *P. aeruginosa,* which is less responsive to oral therapy. A quinolone antibiotic, ciprofloxacin (Cipro), is currently the only oral preparation that effectively treats *Pseudomonas* species; it has not been approved by the Food and Drug Administration for use in individuals less than 18 years of age.

PROGNOSIS

Despite 40 years of remarkable progress in treatment and a recent surge of new approaches to treatment, CF remains a progressive disease without cure. The median survival age is 27 years, which has markedly increased over the past 20 years (Fig. 12-2). This change is likely the result of both improved treatment and appreciation and detection of the milder phenotypic expressions of the disease (Schwartz, 1987). With continued improvement in survival, CF has become an illness of children, adolescents, and young adults. Today adolescents whose parents were given a less optimistic picture on survival at diagnosis are being challenged to set goals for a future that may include college and vocational education, a career, and social relationships, including marriage. At the same time they struggle with increasing morbidity and higher rates of CF complications as they grow older.

Providers, as well, are faced with meeting the needs of a growing population of young adults. In most regional CF centers about 35% of the client population is more than 18 years of age. Transition programs that move the adolescent into care by

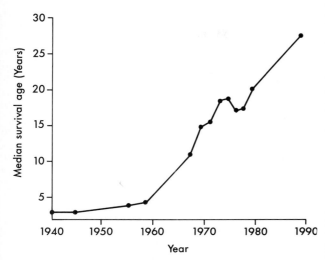

Fig. 12-2. Survival of individuals with cystic fibrosis. *Figures prior to 1970 are from estimates, and figures after 1970 are from Cystic Fibrosis Foundation Patient Registry data.*

adult providers have been developed in a number of these centers. They feature a committed team of adult providers who have developed CF care expertise and who become jointly involved with pediatric providers in care delivery during adolescence. Implementation of these programs has not been without problems, but they have innovatively addressed clients' developmental needs for independence and identity (Cappelli, MacDonald, & McGrath, 1989).

ASSOCIATED PROBLEMS
Salt depletion: hyponatremia and dehydration

Children with CF have abnormal sodium and chloride loss in their sweat and therefore are at risk for dehydration secondary to electrolyte imbalance. Risk factors include hot weather, febrile illnesses with or without vomiting and diarrhea, and strenuous physical activity. Excessive salt loss may lead to listlessness, vomiting, heat prostration, and dehydration. Infants are at particular risk because of the low salt content of breast milk, commercial infant formulas, and infant foods. Prevention includes supplementation of salt in infant formulas (¼ tsp/day) and adding salt to the older child's diet (Adams, 1988).

Rectal prolapse

Rectal prolapse occurs in about 25% of children with CF, usually in the first 3 years of life. It may be the presenting symptom and may occur only once or be a recurrent problem. Often, initiation of appropriate enzyme replacement or adjustment of enzyme dosage prevents its recurrence. Rarely, persistent or recurrent prolapse requires surgical intervention (deSant'Agnese and Hubbard, 1984). The first episode of rectal prolapse is frightening to both parents and child, and its reduction usually requires immediate telephone guidance and then assistance in the provider's office or an emergency room.

If a child experiences an episode of rectal prolapse, parents may learn to manually reduce a prolapse. With the child lying on his side and using a glove and KY-jelly, the parent is usually able to gently invert the mucosa through the rectal opening.

Nasal polyps and pansinusitis

Nasal polyps occur in 10% of children with CF, and their finding on physical examination should raise the suspicion of CF if it has not already been diagnosed. The upper respiratory tract, including sinuses, is lined with respiratory epithelial cells similar to that in the lungs and is also affected by CF pathologic conditions. Sinuses are frequently chronically infected, producing symptoms of frontal headaches, tenderness on palpation, purulent nasal discharge, and postnasal discharge, which further contributes to the chronic cough. Treatment includes extended use of antibiotics, nasal cromolyn sodium, corticosteroids, and intermittent use of nasal decongestants. Children may also find warm mist and saline nasal rinses to be helpful comfort measures. Surgical interventions for polyposis and sinusitis are occasionally necessary but have had variable degrees of success, with frequent recurrence of the problems over time (Davis, 1984).

Meconium ileus equivalent and constipation

Although the prevalence of meconium ileus equivalent (MIE) is higher in adolescents and young adults, even young children with CF are at risk for developing total or partial intestinal obstruction. Constipation is often the result of a combination of malabsorption, either from inadequate pancreatic enzyme dosage or a failure to take enzymes, decreased intestinal motility, and abnormally viscous intestinal secretions. Abdominal cramping with either diarrhea or absence of stool occurs, and stool masses may be palpable on examination, particularly in the right lower quadrant. These problems do not usually require surgical intervention and should be evaluated and managed by or in consultation with the CF center team. Treatment usually includes either Go-LYTELY or Colyte, osmotic solutions given orally or by nasogastric tube, or large-volume enemas of Gastrografin and Tween 80 which are monitored radiographically. Follow-up should include long-term use of some combination of a stool softener, mild stimulant, and bulk laxative, as well as the addition of bulk to the diet, consistent enzyme use, and exercise (Rubinstein, Moss, and Lewiston, 1986).

Hemoptysis

The appearance of blood-streaked mucus and small quantities of bright red blood is not uncommon in CF. Though initially alarming to the child and family, the bleeding is usually self-limiting. It reflects increased bronchial infection, inflammation, and irritation, requiring more aggressive treatment. In addition to an increase in routine pulmonary toilet, initiation or change of antibiotic therapy should be considered. Massive hemoptysis, on the other hand, requires immediate referral to the CF center team for management.

Other complications

Cystic fibrosis is a multisystem condition with an increased rate of complications and morbidity with

---

SERIOUS COMPLICATIONS OF CYSTIC FIBROSIS

Cor pulmonale
Massive hemoptysis
Pneumothorax
Hypertrophic pulmonary osteoarthropathy
Liver disease, including portal hypertension
Gallbladder disease
Glucose intolerance
Allergic bronchopulmonary aspergillosis

---

disease progression. Complications listed in the box below are more serious and usually require the expertise of the CF center team in their management. The primary provider must recognize early signs and symptoms of these complications so that timely referral for evaluation and treatment can be implemented.

PRIMARY CARE MANAGEMENT
Growth and development

Growth delay and difficulty maintaining adequate weight for height are common problems in CF. Weight loss and linear growth retardation may be presenting clinical signs both in infancy and in early adolescence. Following diagnosis and initiation of pulmonary and nutritional therapy, catch-up growth is frequently observed.

Growth and developmental failure have been observed in children with CF most commonly in the second and third decade of life. These delays involve not only height and weight but also skeletal, dental, and sexual maturation; they have been explained by a complex interrelationship of degree of severity of pulmonary disease, caloric intake and postulated endocrine mediated delays (Mitchell-Heggs, Mearns and Batten, 1976; Mearns, 1980; Shepherd, Cooksley, and Cooke, 1980; Mahaney and McCoy, 1986). Aggressive nutritional supplementation has been associated with short-term improvement in growth velocity and well-being and in slowed decline in pulmonary function (Levy et al., 1985; Shepherd et al., 1986). The primary provider should be alert to weight loss or a flattened growth curve associated with loss of appetite because these may be indicators of a pulmonary exacerbation; their presence should prompt further investigation with the child and family about an increase in pulmonary symptoms.

Growth retardation should also prompt review of GI status, specifically stool pattern and consistency, and symptoms of abdominal cramping or gastric "burning." The provider may adjust the enzyme dosage if stools are frequent and greasy; however, consultation with the CF center team regarding further interventions may become necessary.

The mean age of onset of puberty in CF is 14.5 years (Moshang and Holsclaw, 1980); this delay may be an acute source of concern for adolescents. The primary provider may be able to help the teen to understand that this delay is not unusual or unexpected and that sexual development, though delayed, will occur. Menarchal age has been associated with severity of illness, and adolescent girls who are underweight because of advancing disease and despite rigorous efforts in nutritional supplementation need support and reassurance.

Cystic fibrosis is not associated with intellectual deficits or delays in cognitive development. Problems in school performance are more likely to be related to either absenteeism because of physical illness or fatigue at school due to an impending exacerbation.

Immunizations

Infants and children with CF should receive all routine immunizations at the ages recommended by the American Academy of Pediatrics. In a few instances the CF team may recommend a brief delay to stabilize an acute pulmonary or nutritional problem; however, there is no evidence to support delay of routine immunizations.

Annual influenza vaccine is also recommended, following Centers for Disease Control (CDC) guidelines, which include use of split virus vaccine in children less than 13 years of age (Immunization Practices Advisory Committee, 1989). Pneumococcal vaccine is not routinely recommended because pneumococcal infections are rarely reported in children with CF (Stern, 1989; Committee on Infectious Diseases, 1991).

Screening

Vision. Routine visual screening is recommended. If corticosteroid dependent, the child should be annually monitored by a pediatric ophthalmologist for early detection of cataracts or glaucoma.

Hearing. In addition to routine hearing screening, any child treated with IV aminoglycoside therapy should be monitored by an audiologist for occurrence of high-frequency hearing loss.

Dental. Routine screening is recommended. Precautions regarding the use of tetracyclines before permanent tooth formation has occurred also apply for children with CF.

Blood pressure. Routine screening is recommended unless the child is corticosteroid dependent.

Hematocrit. Routine screening is recommended. The role of pancreatic insufficiency and pancreatic enzyme replacement therapy in iron absorption in CF is unclear; iron status should be evaluated periodically and appropriate supplementation provided if anemia is present (deSant'Agnese and Hubbard, 1984).

Urinalysis. Routine screening is recommended. Careful attention should be paid to the presence of glucose because this may indicate the onset of glucose intolerance.

Tuberculosis. Routine screening is recommended.

Condition-specific screening

PULMONARY FUNCTION TESTING. Pulmonary function testing (PFT) is performed routinely in children more than 6 years of age during CF center visits at least annually and more often as indicated. Chest roentgenography and PFT monitor pulmonary disease progression and identify acute problems.

MULTISYSTEM SCREENS. Other screening routinely performed at CF center visits includes blood and urine assays of liver and renal function cell counts and differential, and glucose levels.

Drug interactions

Primary providers routinely include anticipatory guidance about substance abuse with children, adolescents, and parents. Tobacco smoke, both active and passive, is an obvious detriment to children with CF. The growing evidence of an increased incidence of viral respiratory illness in all children exposed to passive smoke makes care giver smoking an added risk to the child with CF (Wall, 1987). Smoke is also known to increase airway reactivity (Stern et al., 1987). In a study comparing children with CF who had significant exposure to tobacco smoke with those who did not, Rubin (1990) suggests that passive exposure to smoke adversely affects the growth and lung function of children with CF.

In addition to the overall impact of alcohol, smoke, and psychoactive drugs on organ systems of the child and adolescent with CF, specific interactions have been reported. Alcohol use in individuals taking chloramphenicol (Chloromycetin) or cephalosporins has been associated with episodes of nausea, vomiting, and headache. Alcohol has also been reported to be associated with increased pulmonary symptoms, perhaps from suppression of the cough reflex, and with episodes of hemoptysis.

The provider should also be cognizant of certain interactions of drugs commonly used in the management of CF lung disease. Both erythromycin and ciprofloxacin alter the metabolism and excretion of theophylline, requiring a reduction in the theophylline dose during their use. With use of these antibiotics the provider should review signs of theophylline toxicity with clients and parents and discuss a plan for dosage reduction if they arise. Increased ultraviolet light sensitivity may occur in some children on tetracycline and sulfanomide therapy, and their use should be avoided when sun exposure is anticipated.

DIFFERENTIAL DIAGNOSIS AND MANAGEMENT OF COMMON PEDIATRIC CONDITIONS IN CHILDREN WITH CYSTIC FIBROSIS

Symptoms associated with common pediatric illnesses may also be symptoms specific to CF, and questions often arise regarding their etiology and management. Parents may need to hear often that their child will develop common minor childhood illnesses and will usually respond to routine management. They may be reassured to know that the CF center team is readily available to the primary provider whenever questions arise regarding etiology and treatment of an acute illness. Thorough history taking and examination are not only essential to the provider in making a differential diagnosis but also reassuring to parents and the child.

Gastrointestinal symptoms

Diarrhea, constipation, and abdominal cramping may be presenting complaints of a partial or complete intestinal obstruction. A history of cramping pain and changes in stool pattern in the absence of other acute GI and systemic symptoms is suggestive of MIE.

Fever and viral illness

Fever associated with a CF pulmonary exacerbation is a relatively uncommon manifestation, and evaluation of fever in children with CF should elicit the same broad-based approach used with other children. A brief initial febrile period with a viral illness should be anticipated in children with CF and symptomatically treated per usual practice protocols. When a viral illness exacerbates lower respiratory tract symptoms, as frequently occurs with upper respiratory tract infections, an increase in chest physical therapy and prompt and sustained (2-3 weeks) oral antibiotic coverage are usually recommended. Prevention of hyponatremia and dehydration during febrile illness includes use of electrolyte-balanced clear liquids such as Pedialyte, addition of salt to the child's intake, and review of warning signs of dehydration with the parent.

Chest pain

Children with CF frequently have complaints of chest pain. These should always be evaluated because of the potential occurrence of pneumothorax. Complaints associated with pneumothorax typically include sudden onset of sharp pain unilaterally, followed by dull aching and accompanied by profound shortness of breath and activity intolerance. This complication, confirmed by physical examination and chest roentgenogram, is best managed at the regional CF center following local emergency stabilization as indicated.

Bilateral musculoskeletal pain from coughing paroxysms is usually diffuse and occurs with a pulmonary exacerbation. It may also be localized, and the child will have pain on palpation at the site. Both usually respond to nonnarcotic pain relief. Some children and adolescents with CF experience midline chest and epigastric burning related to gastroesophageal reflux and esophagitis (Bendig et al., 1982). If antacids are not effective, the CF center team should be consulted, specifically regarding the use of H_2 antagonists.

Varicella

There has been no report in the CF literature of higher rates of complications from chickenpox in children with CF; however, there have been reports of exacerbation of pulmonary symptoms (MacDonald, Morris, and Beaudry, 1987). Management of coryzal symptoms is no different from other children. The same approach to antibiotic use with increased pulmonary symptoms should also apply to this viral illness. Use of antipruritic medications is not contraindicated; however, the child's cough may be suppressed by their use, and parents should increase chest physical therapy as soon as lesions permit.

Cough

A variably severe chronic cough is a hallmark of CF lung disease. At baseline it may be present in the early morning and with exercise. An increase in cough is alway of significance and requires intervention. Nighttime coughing may develop and may be associated with reactive airway disease, increased pulmonary infection and inflammation, or postnasal discharge from sinusitis or rhinitis. Delineating a clear cause may be difficult. Both antibiotic therapy and initiation of an increase in the use of aerosolized bronchodilators may be helpful. Cough suppressants are generally contraindicated and should be used only after consultation with the CF center team. A trial of decongestants may be useful. Antihistamines should be used with caution and in consultation with the CF center team because they may increase the viscosity of mucus and inhibit its mobilization.

Wheezing

Wheezing is a common manifestation of CF, particularly in infancy. It is most often attributed to heightened bronchial reactivity from chronic infection and inflammation (Mellis and Levison, 1978). Aerosolized bronchodilators and a course of an antibiotic often are effective; however, in addition a short burst of an oral corticosteroid may also be beneficial. Wheezing in infancy may be difficult to alleviate, but this problem often diminishes with age (Stern, 1989).

DEVELOPMENTAL ISSUES
Safety

In addition to routine anticipatory guidance about safety issues, the primary provider should emphasize safe storage and handling of the large quantities of medications frequently used by children with CF. Issues of accidental ingestion of pancreatic enzymes by another child may arise because these are routinely in ample supply at mealtimes in the home and carried by the child for use. They are not likely to be harmful if small quantities are ingested; they are activated in the small intestine and excreted in stool without major absorption in the bloodstream.

Child care

Parents of children with CF often struggle with day-care issues. They need reassurance that a child with CF is not immunocompromised and will mount an adequate response to communicable diseases. Day-care settings with few children, and therefore potentially lower viral illness exposure, may be a more appropriate environment for infants and toddlers. When a day-care program has been selected, day-care providers will need specific education regarding issues of (1) the child's individual nutritional and pulmonary treatment program, (2) the child's chronic cough and lack of contagion, and (3) how to prevent the spread of viral illness in the setting. (See the listing of available educational material on p. 226.)

Diet

Children with CF require high-calorie, high-protein diets. In infancy, breast-feeding should be continued whenever possible with enzyme supplementation and, when necessary, supplementation of higher calorie per ounce formula. Formula-fed infants are usually given a hydrolysate formula with medium-chain triglycerides (e.g., Pregestimil, Alimentum). Even though these formulas are predigested, some enzyme supplementation may also be necessary. Enzymes are given to infants by mixing the beads contained in the capsule in pureed fruit, usually applesauce, and feeding these by mouth.

Parents often have questions about enzyme supplementation dosage. Requirements depend on the degree of pancreatic insufficiency, the fat and protein content of the food ingested, the quantity eaten, and the type of enzymes used. Dosage is adjusted by trial until the stool pattern is acceptable (e.g., one to two stools daily in older children and more in infancy) and the child demonstrates reasonable growth. Enzymes should be taken within 30 minutes of eating, and the beads should not be chewed or crushed because destroying the enteric coating causes inactivation of the enzymes and excoriation of oral mucosa. Children should be encouraged to add extra enzymes when high-fat foods are eaten.

Parents of toddlers and preschoolers are often anxious about providing adequate food intake to maintain their child's well-being and growth. They need to understand the developmental stages of

TIPS TO BOOST ENERGY INTAKE

- Include snacks regularly, especially before bedtime. Serve snacks at least 2 hours before the next meal.
- Serve vegetables with cheese or cream sauces.
- Serve meats, potatoes, and other foods with sauces and gravies.
- When preparing fruit juice from concentrate, reduce water added by one fourth.
- Use whole milk fortified with powdered milk as a beverage, in cooking, and on food such as cereal.

Make the following additions to foods served:

Amount	Food	Adds (calories)	Use in or on
1 tsp	Butter or margarine	40	On hot cereal, vegetables, sandwiches, soups, casseroles, breads
1 T	Sour cream	26	Add to vegetables, salads
1 T	Mayonnaise	100	Use in salads, sandwiches, vegetables, deviled eggs
1 oz	Light cream	60	Cereal, hot chocolate, in cooking
1 oz	Evaporated milk*	50	Substitute for water or milk in cooking; add to hot cereal, hot chocolate
1 T	Powdered milk*	23	Add to whole milk, milkshakes, mashed potatoes, scrambled eggs, meatloaf, or hamburgers
1	Hard boiled egg*	80	Add to casseroles, meatloaf
1	Egg yolk, chopped*	60	Sandwich spreads
1 T	Peanut butter*	100	On bread, crackers, toast, apples or celery, in hot cereal, baked goods, milk shakes
1 oz	Cheese*	100	On vegetables, casseroles, meats, in sandwiches, salads, pasta, soup, dips
1 oz	Cream cheese	100	On toast, sandwiches, raw vegetables; add to scrambled eggs, jello salads
1 T	Chopped nuts*	49	Top puddings, ice cream; add to salads, casseroles, cereal, baked goods, fruit cup

From Adams EA: Nutrition care in cystic fibrosis. *Nutrition news,* Seattle, WA 1988, University of Washington Child Development and Mental Retardation Center.

*These foods add protein as well as calories.

toddlers and preschool children. Abnormal emphasis on food, force feeding, and mealtime battles should be avoided. Instead, parents should provide appropriate foods, set limits for mealtimes, and suggest trying some of each food offered. Small serving portions and nutritious snacks may also boost intake.

In preschool and older children, oral high-calorie, high-protein supplementation may be achieved using commonly purchased foods (see box above). The CF center nutritionist can provide many suggestions for fortifying the diet, and printed educational material is also available to families (see p. 226).

Taking enzymes in front of classmates may be difficult for school-aged children. Parents, the teacher, the school nurse, and the child can devise the best plan for their administration. As children grow older and have more control in selecting their diets, parents need to pay particular attention to the quality of snack foods available in the home. Parents often find that the adolescent's intake is better if a structured mealtime is maintained despite individual schedules.

Discipline

From the time of diagnosis parents of children with CF not only grieve their loss of a healthy child but also experience feelings of guilt associated with their genetic contribution, and they struggle to redefine a future for their child and family. The primary provider can provide ongoing support and counseling during this difficult adjustment period. Setting limits and encouraging similar responsibilities for the child with CF and siblings will help maintain consistency in family life.

The time commitment of daily therapy may not only create periodic conflict between parent and child but may also be seen by siblings as an inequity in parental attention. Conscious efforts by parents to give individual attention to each child may prevent feelings of jealousy and guilt. Extended family and community support are important ingredients in daily therapy, because parents need respite and the opportunity to develop individual interests (Venters, 1981).

Parents of adolescents with CF are frequently frustrated and anxious about disease progression when they experience difficulty in maintaining their child's adherence to the treatment program. Factors influencing compliance with chronic illness regimens are numerous and complex (Pidgeon, 1989). Normal adolescent behavior of limit testing, perceived invincibility, and risk taking is complicated by the chronicity and morbidity of CF. Experimentation with medications, both overuse and underuse, and refusal of chest physical therapy frequently occur. Teens with CF often experience no immediate consequences of these experimentations, further reinforcing their behaviors. Although the relative risk of not doing therapy is difficult to quantify, documentation of the efficacy of chest physical therapy cannot be ignored.

Parents who begin during early school years to transfer responsibility for illness management to their child often report fewer problems in adolescence. Even children age 5 to 6 years are old enough to understand the need for such treatments as enzymes and vitamins. Adolescents with CF may also be more adherent if allowed to take control of parts of their illness management, such as using a mechanical percussor for independence in therapy or substituting an exercise program for a therapy session. Encouraging school-aged children and adolescents to actively participate in clinic visits and involving them in decision making is essential to their development of autonomy. Behavioral contracts may be useful tools for families experiencing more problems with the adolescent.

Toileting

As with other children, toilet training should proceed as cues of developmental readiness are noted in the child. However, many children with CF continue to have stools more frequently than once daily and may have some abdominal cramping before stooling even on adequate enzyme therapy. These problems may impede the child's interest in toileting, and allowances should be made by parents for this delay.

Even though enzymes improve digestion of nutrients, some maldigested food often passes through the intestine. As a result, stools may be malodorous and an embarrassment to children and adolescents. Parents, teachers, and friend's parents should be aware of the need for privacy during toileting and assist the child with managing bathroom odor.

Sleep

Children with CF have a busy early morning routine, requiring early rising for school-aged children and adolescents. At the same time they are often more vulnerable to fatigue because of their increased basal metabolic rate. Sleep requirements, though not necessarily greater, should not be shortened.

Onset of nighttime coughing may also interfere with rest and contribute to general fatigue; prompt attention to these symptoms is important to overall well-being.

School issues

A number of issues may surface for the child with CF in the school environment, and it may be helpful for a CF center provider to make a school visit, meeting with the school nurse, classroom teacher or teachers, physical education teacher, principal, and, when appropriate, the director of special education. Commonly, school personnel have questions about the child's cough, bowel and pulmonary toilet needs, exercise tolerance, nutrition and medication needs during the school day, and school absenteeism for illness or hospitalization. Advice in handling these issues is greatly dependent on the individual child's severity of illness. Specific educational materials for school personnel are also available (see p. 226).

The degree to which short stature, difficulty in gaining and maintaining weight, and delayed pubertal development are present is variable. When significant, they affect the development of a positive body image and associated self-esteem, particularly in adolescence. These delays are often associated with increasing pulmonary involvement and alter the child's ability to fully participate in academics, social life, and sports and exercise programs. The primary provider may be able to suggest choices of recreational activities and skills that are more likely to be tolerated and in which the child may have an opportunity to excel, such as swimming, diving, baseball, archery, gymnastics, certain track and field events, playing a musical instrument, and art.

Sexuality

Ninety-eight percent of men with CF are sterile because of blockage of the vas deferens; a sperm count is recommended to confirm the expected aspermia (Rosenstein, 1990). Male adolescents need reassurance that this condition does not mean that they are impotent, and it will not diminish their ability to have normal sexual relations. Women with CF may have more difficulty becoming pregnant because of thick cervical mucus. They should also be carefully evaluated and counseled about the relative risk of pregnancy in their individual condition. This counseling is complex and includes such considerations as their level of pulmonary function and overall health status, the statistical genetic risk of having a child with CF, and their shortened life expectancy.

Contraception alternatives for adolescent and young adult women with CF have been controversial. Oral contraceptives have been reported to increase the viscosity of cervical mucus; they therefore carry the theoretical increased risk of having a similar effect on pulmonary mucous viscosity, although this has not been documented. Because of the comparative risk of pregnancy, many CF center providers recommend oral contraceptives after full discussion of these issues with the young woman. Reproductive issues in CF should be managed in consultation with the CF center team and an obstetrician or gynecologist.

SPECIAL FAMILY CONCERNS

Families who deal with CF have a myriad of special concerns, including coping with the stress of its prognosis, handling the added financial burden of medical care, and maintaining family life despite the uncertainty of exacerbations, hospitalizations, and disease progression. It has been demonstrated that families, though stressed, generally cope successfully (Phillips et al., 1985; Tavormina et al., 1976). McCubbin (1984) has identified circumstances that place a family dealing with CF at high risk for dysfunction and maladaptation: single-parent families, families with an older member who has CF, and families with limited income.

Parents often need guidance in presenting information and answering questions about CF with their child and with other family members. In addition to the CF center team's help, written material is available, including books for school-aged children (see p. 226). By age 10 to 12 years, most children's cognitive development is reaching formal operational thinking. Information regarding morbidity and mortality should be presented honestly and within a framework of hope for continued breakthroughs in treatment research.

The financial burden of this illness is formidable, and families often need additional assistance with health care costs. Cystic fibrosis is a diagnosis covered by programs for physically handicapped children or children with special needs in most states. Eligibility requirements are highly variable; the CF center staff can be helpful in coordinating these efforts for a family.

SUMMARY OF PRIMARY CARE NEEDS FOR THE CHILD WITH CYSTIC FIBROSIS

Growth and development

Growth and developmental delays vary; they are associated with pulmonary disease severity, maturational delay, and malabsorption.

Pubertal delay may be anticipated in most adolescents.

Immunizations

All routine immunizations should be given on schedule.

Influenza vaccine should be given annually per CDC guidelines.

Pneumococcal vaccine is not currently recommended.

Screening
Vision

A routine office examination is sufficient unless the child is receiving corticosteroids, then an annual examination by an opthalmalogist is recommended.

Hearing

Routine screening is recommended; a child on aminoglycoside therapy should have an audiology screen for high-frequency hearing loss.

Dental

Routine screening is recommended.

Blood pressure

Routine screening is recommended unless the child is corticosteroid dependent.

Hematocrit

Routine screening is recommended, along with full review of iron status as indicated, is recommended.

Urinalysis

Routine screening is recommended, but urine should be checked for glucose.

Tuberculosis

Routine screening is recommended.

Condition-specific screening

Chest roentgenogram, PFT results, and blood or urine assays (or both) of liver function, renal function, cell counts and differential, and glucose levels are usually monitored at routine CF center visits.

Drug interactions

Alcohol use with cephalosporins or chloramphenicol may cause headaches, nausea, and vomiting.

Erythromycin and ciprofloxacin may increase serum theophylline levels.

Differential diagnosis
Chest pain

Rule out pneumothorax.

Constipation or diarrhea

Rule out MIE.

Cough

Further differentiation of components of RAD, lower respiratory tract infection and inflammation, and rhinitis and sinusitis may be helpful in the selection of treatment choices.

Developmental issues
Safety

Safe storage of multiple medications should be emphasized.

Child care

Home care and small day-care programs are recommended during the first year of life to reduce viral exposure; day-care workers need information on CF.

Diet

High-calorie, high-protein diets are recommended. Fat intake is not restricted; target of 35% to 40% of daily intake in fat sources.

Pancreatic enzyme replacement and vitamin supplementation is necessary for children with malabsorption.

Discipline

Expectations are normal, with allowances during periods of illness exacerbation.

Lack of compliance with treatment programs may impact disease progression in adolescence.

Toileting

Delayed bowel training may occur secondary to increased frequency of stools and associated abdominal cramping.

Continued.

SUMMARY OF PRIMARY CARE NEEDS FOR THE CHILD WITH CYSTIC FIBROSIS — cont'd

Sleep patterns

Early morning routines require adjustment of bedtime. Nighttime cough may interfere with rest and requires prompt attention.

School issues

Multiple school questions may be best addressed in a school visit.

Adjustment problems related to altered body image and self-esteem may occur during adolescence.

School performance may be affected by fatigue and lethargy with an impending pulmonary exacerbation.

School absenteeism for hospitalizations requires coordination for ongoing academic services.

Sexuality

Male sterility should be confirmed.

Female reproductive issues are complex and require specialty consultation and counseling.

Special family concerns

Special family concerns include the uncertainty of illness progression and predicted lethality; family functioning during illness exacerbations requiring hospitalizations; and the impact of the treatment program on family life.

RESOURCES

The Cystic Fibrosis Foundation is a national organization committed to supporting research for the treatment and cure of CF. Local chapters are found in many of the larger cities in the United States. The Cystic Fibrosis Foundation also develops and distributes excellent informational material for the lay public and the professional community (see the list of informational materials). The 127 regional CF care centers in the United States offer expertise in the care and management of CF-related issues. Parents should be encouraged to keep in regular contact with the center; this ongoing and regular specialist care has been demonstrated to correlate with improved survival statistics (Wood, 1984). The CF center also offers a specialty team approach with a family focus in programming that often includes parent support groups, education programs, education and support for newly diagnosed families, and genetic counseling and testing services.

Informational materials

Farmer G and Willcox S: *Fat and loving it,* 1990.

This is a book on nutrition written for individuals with CF and is available from Gail Farmer, PO Box 5127, Belmont, CA 94002.

Luder E: *Living with cystic fibrosis: Family guide to nutrition,* Spring House, Pa, 1987, McNeil Pharmaceuticals.

Mandolfo A: *Cystic fibrosis,* Marietta, Ga, 1988, Reid Rowell Pharmaceuticals.

This is a booklet for young children.

Nakielna B, O'Loane M, and Durbach E: *For adults with cystic fibrosis,* Vancouver, BC, 1986, Shaughnessy Hospital CF Clinic.

Orenstein DM: *Cystic fibrosis: A guide for patient and family,* New York, 1989, Raven Press.

Ribando C and Langbaum T: *I have cystic fibrosis,* Baltimore, Md, 1985, The Johns Hopkins Medical Institutes.

This is a story for school-aged children.

Sondel S and Hartman L: *A way of life: Cystic fibrosis nutrition handbook and cookbook,* 1988.

This book is available from Karen Luther, F4/120 Food and Nutrition Services, University of Wisconsin Hospital and Clinics, Madison, WI 53792.

Stanzone A and Godwin SL: *Let's look at me,* Marietta, Ga, 1989, Reid Rowell Pharmaceuticals.

This is a workbook for young children.

Storey M and Adams E: *Snacks and more,* Rochester, NY, 1988, Pediatric Pulmonary Center, University of Rochester Medical Center.

Organizations

Cystic Fibrosis Foundation
6931 Arlington Rd
Bethesda, MD 20814
1-800-FIGHT CF
The following publications are available from the Cystic Fibrosis
   Foundation:
   A Guide to Cystic Fibrosis for Parents and Children
   Chest Physical Therapy: Segmental Bronchial Drainage
   An Introduction to Cystic Fibrosis
   The Genetics of Cystic Fibrosis
   A Teacher's Guide to CF
   Living with Cystic Fibrosis: A Guide for Adolescents

REFERENCES

Adams EA: Nutrition care in cystic fibrosis. In *Nutrition news,*
   Seattle, 1988, University of Washington Child Development
   and Mental Retardation Center.

Beaudet AL, Fenwick RG, Fernbach SD, and O'Brien WE:
   Genetic diagnosis using mutation analysis. In G Polgar, ed:
   *Pediatric pulmonology: Program and papers of Fourth An-
   nual North American and 1990 International Cystic Fibrosis
   Conference,* Suppl 5, 116-117, 1990.

Beaudet AL and Buffone GJ: Prenatal diagnosis of cystic fibrosis, *J Pediatr* 111:630-633, 1989.

Beaudet AL, Feldman GL, Fernbach SD, et al: Linkage disequilibrium, cystic fibrosis, and genetic counseling, *Am J
   Hum Genet* 44:319-326, 1989.

Bendig DW, Seilheimer MD, Wagner ML, et al: Complications
   of gastroesophageal reflux in patients with cystic fibrosis, *J
   Pediatr* 100:536-540, 1982.

Cappelli M, MacDonald N, and McGrath P: Assessment of
   readiness to transfer to adult care for adolescents with cystic
   fibrosis, Child Health Care 18:218-224, 1989.

Committee on Infectious Diseases: *Report of the Committee on
   Infectious Diseases,* ed 22, Elk Grove Village, IL, 1991,
   The American Academy of Pediatrics.

Cystic Fibrosis Foundation: *Discovery of cystic fibrosis gene,*
   Bethesda, MD, memorandum to the Cystic Fibrosis Center
   Directors, Aug 23, 1989.

Davis PB: Cystic fibrosis in adults. In Taussig LM, ed: *Cystic
   fibrosis,* New York, 1984, Thieme-Stratton, pp 408-433.

deSant'Agnese PA and Hubbard VS: The pancreas. In Taussig
   LM, ed: *Cystic fibrosis,* New York, 1984, Thieme-Stratton,
   pp 230-295.

Desmond KJ, Schwenk W, Thomas E, et al: Immediate and
   long term effects of chest physiotherapy in patients with
   cystic fibrosis, *J Pediatr* 103:538-542, 1983.

Drum ML et al: Correction of the cystic fibrosis defect in vitro
   by retrovirus-mediated gene transfer, *Cell,* 62:1227-1233,
   1990.

Fitzpatrick SB, Rosenstein BJ, and Langbaum TS: Diagnosis
   of cystic fibrosis during adolescence, *J Adolesc Health Care*
   7:38-43, 1986.

Hubbard VS: Nutritional considerations in cystic fibrosis, *Semin
   Respir Med* 6:308-313, 1985.

Immunization Practices Advisory Committee: Prevention and
   control of influenza: Part I, Vaccines, *MMWR* 38:297-311,
   1989.

Levy LD, Durie PR, Pencharz PB, et al: Effects of long-term
   nutritional rehabilitation on body composition and clinical
   status in malnourished children and adolescents with cystic
   fibrosis, *J Pediatr* 107:225-230, 1985.

Lloyd-Still JD: Pathology. In Lloyd-Still JD, ed: *Textbook of
   cystic fibrosis,* Boston, 1983, John Wright-PSG, pp 19-31.

MacDonald N, Morris R, and Beaudry P: Varicella in children
   with cystic fibrosis, *Pediatr Infect Dis J* 6:414-416, 1987.

Mahaney MC and McCoy KS: Developmental delays and pulmonary disease severity in cystic fibrosis, *Hum Biol* 58:445-
   460, 1986.

Marks MI: The pathogenesis and treatment of pulmonary infections in patients with cystic fibrosis, *J Pediatr* 98:173-
   179, 1981.

McCubbin M: Nursing assessment of parental coping with cystic
   fibrosis, *West J Nurs Res* 6:407-418, 1984.

Mearns MB: The heights of cystic fibrosis patients aged 2-9
   years allowing for parental height and severity of pulmonary
   episodes from birth. In Sturgess JM, ed: *Perspectives in
   cystic fibrosis,* Toronto, 1980, Cystic Fibrosis Foundation,
   pp 262-265.

Mellis C and Levison H: Bronchial reactivity in cystic fibrosis,
   Pediatrics 61:446-450, 1978.

Mischler EH: Treatment of pulmonary disease in cystic fibrosis,
   Semin Respir Med 6:271-284, 1985.

Mitchell-Heggs P, Mearns MB, and Batten JC: Cystic fibrosis
   in adolescents and adults, *Q J Med* 45:479-504, 1976.

Moshang T and Holsclaw DS: Menarchal determinants in cystic
   fibrosis, *Am J Dis Child* 134:1139-1142, 1980.

National Academy of Sciences: Report of the committee for a
   study for evaluation of testing for cystic fibrosis, *J Pediatr*
   88:711-750, 1976.

Orenstein DM, Henke KG, and Cerney FJ: Exercise and cystic
   fibrosis, *Phys Sports Med* 11:57-62, 1983.

Phillips S, Bohannon WE, Gayton WF, et al: Parent interview
   findings regarding impact of cystic fibrosis on families, *Dev
   Behav Pediatr* 6:122-127, 1985.

Pidgeon V: Compliance with chronic illness regimens: School
   aged children and adolescents, *J Pediatr Nurs* 4:36-47, 1989.

Quinton PM: Defective epithelial ion transport in cystic fibrosis,
   Clin Chem 35:726-730, 1989.

Rich DP, et al: Expression of cystic fibrosis transmembrane
   conductance regulator corrects defective chloride channel
   regulation in cystic fibrosis airway epithelial cells, *Nature,*
   347:358-363, 1990.

Rommens JM, Iannuzzi MC, Kerem B, et al: Identification of the cystic fibrosis gene: Chromosome walking and jumping, *Science* 245:1059-1065, 1989.

Rosenstein BJ and Eigen H: Risks of alternate date prednisone in patients with cystic fibrosis, *Pediatrics*, 87 (2):245-246, 1991.

Rosenstein B: (1990). Cystic fibrosis. In Oski FA, ed: *Principles and practice of pediatrics,* Philadelphia, 1990, JP Lippincott, pp 1362-1372.

Rosenstein BJ and Langbaum TS: Diagnosis. In Taussig LM, ed: *Cystic fibrosis,* New York, 1984, Thieme-Stratton, pp 85-114.

Rubin BK: Exposure of children with cystic fibrosis to environmental tobacco smoke, *N Engl J Med* 323 (12):782-788, 1991.

Rubinstein S, Moss R, and Lewiston N: Constipation and meconium ileus equivalent in patients with cystic fibrosis, *Pediatrics* 78:473-479, 1986.

Schwartz, RH: Cystic fibrosis. In Hoekelman RH, ed: *Primary pediatric care,* St Louis, 1987, CV Mosby, pp 1203-1210.

Shepherd R, Cooksley WGE, and Cooke WDD: Improved growth and clinical nutritional and respiratory changes in response to nutritional therapy in cystic fibrosis, *J Pediatr* 97:351-357, 1980.

Shepherd RW, Holt TL, Thomas BJ, et al: Nutritional rehabilitation in cystic fibrosis: Controlled studies of effects on nutritional growth retardation, body protein turnover, and course of pulmonary disease, *J Pediatr* 109:788-794, 1986.

Soutter VL, Kristidis P, Gruce MA, et al: Chronic undernutrition/growth retardation in cystic fibrosis, *Clin Gastroenterol* 15:137-155, 1986.

Stern RC: Cystic fibrosis: Recent developments in diagnosis and treatment, *Pediatr Rev* 7:276-286, 1986.

Stern RC: The primary care physician and the patient with cystic fibrosis, *J Pediatr* 114:31-36, 1989.

Stern RC, Byard PJ, Tomashefski JF, et al: Recreational use of psychoactive drugs by patients with cystic fibrosis, *J Pediatr* 111:293-299, 1987.

Taussig LM, Landau LI, and Marks MI: Respiratory system. In Taussig LM, ed: *Cystic fibrosis,* New York, 1984, Thieme-Stratton, pp 115-174.

Tavormina JB, Kastner LS, Slater PM, et al: Chronically ill children: A psychologically and emotionally deviant population? *J Abnorm Psychol* 4:99-110, 1976.

Venters M: Familial coping with chronic and severe illness: The case of cystic fibrosis, *Soc Sci Med* 15A:289-297, 1981.

Wall M: Update on the effects of passive smoking in children, *J Respir Dis* 8:31-36, 1987.

Wang EEL, Prober CG, Manson B, et al: Association of respiratory viral infections with pulmonary deterioration in patients with cystic fibrosis, *N Engl J Med* 311:1653-1658, 1984.

Wilfond BS and Fost N: The cystic fibrosis gene: Medical and social implications for heterozygote detection, *JAMA* 263:2777-2783, 1990.

Wood RE: Prognosis. In Taussig LM, ed: *Cystic fibrosis,* New York, 1984, Thieme-Stratton, pp 434-460.

13 *Diabetes Mellitus (Type I)*

••

Margaret Grey

ETIOLOGY

Diabetes mellitus was first described in the Egyptian *Ebers Papyrus* in 1500 BC. Type I, or insulin-dependent diabetes mellitus (IDDM), occurs most commonly in young people, and it is characterized by β-cell failure. In type II, or non–insulin-dependent diabetes mellitus (NIDDM), patients are often overweight, are usually more than 30 years of age, overproduce insulin, and have a receptor site defect. Thus, those with NIDDM can often be treated orally with hypoglycemic agents, whereas those with IDDM must be treated with insulin.

The etiology of IDDM is unknown, but many factors have been hypothesized to contribute to the cause of the disease. Genetic susceptibility is a necessary precursor to the development of IDDM (Drash, 1987). Certain histocompatibility leukocyte antigen (HLA) genes are believed to play a role in the genetic inheritance of the tendency to develop IDDM. Individuals with IDDM have an increased frequency of HLA genes B8, B15, DR3, and DR4 (Eisenbarth, 1986). The HLA-DR genes are known to be associated with autoimmunity. Evidence of autoimmunity is necessary but not sufficient for the development of IDDM. It is hypothesized that without genetic susceptibility, other factors will not initiate the autoimmune process. In autoimmunity, "self" antigens are no longer recognized as such, and a self-destructive process occurs. Islet cell antibodies can be detected in a majority of newly diagnosed patients with IDDM (Lendrum, Walker, and Gamble, 1975), and evidence of an autoimmune response may be present up to 9 years before the onset of clinical symptoms (Srikanto et al., 1983).

Other factors, such as host and environmental factors, may influence the development of the illness, because the concordance rate is only 50% in identical twins. Such factors include age, race, stress, and infectious agents (Vialettes et al., 1989).

INCIDENCE

Insulin-dependent diabetes mellitus is the most common metabolic disorder of childhood and it affects 1 child in 600 (LaPorte and Cruickshanks, 1985).

CLINICAL MANIFESTATIONS AT TIME OF DIAGNOSIS

Despite the fact that the autoimmune process may be long standing before the diagnosis of diabetes is made, the signs and symptoms of IDDM are usually present for a short period of time. Once the autoimmune process has destroyed enough of the pancreatic β, or islet cells to produce clinical evidence of illness, the classic symptoms (polydipsia, polyuria, polyphagia) of diabetes occur. As can be seen in Fig. 13-1, the lack of insulin production leads to disturbances in carbohydrate, protein, and fat metabolism.

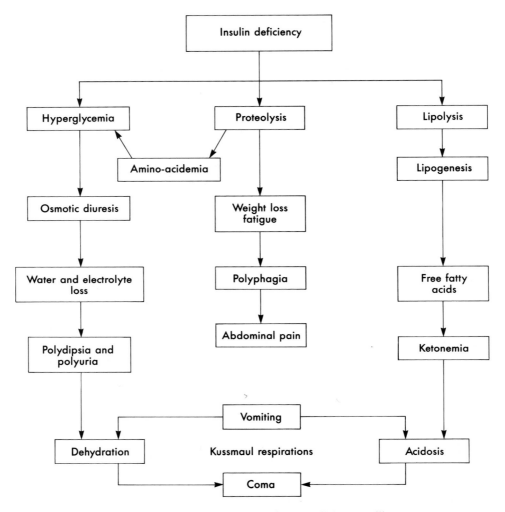

Fig. 13-1. Signs and symptoms of Type I diabetes mellitus.

The hormone insulin, produced by the pancreatic β cells, or islets of Langerhans, is responsible for the utilization of glucose in the cell. In its absence, there are three general alterations: (1) reduced entry of glucose into the cell; (2) unavailability of carbohydrate as a substrate for energy needs; and (3) utilization by the cell of alternate substrates, namely, fatty acids derived from adipose stores and amino acids from body protein. Thus, when there is lack of insulin, glucose cannot be used in the cell for energy, and hyperglycemia

results. The extraordinary concentration of glucose in the blood serves to promote an osmotic diuresis, so that large amounts of urine are produced. This osmotic diuresis is responsible for the symptom of polyuria, and as the body struggles to maintain homeostasis, polydipsia ensues.

If glucose is not available as a source of energy, alternative sources must be used. There is a reliance on lipolysis, as well as proteolysis. When this occurs, polyphagia becomes prominent as the body attempts to avoid starvation. Should these symp-

Table 13-1. Types and actions of insulin preparations

Class/name	Approximate action curves (hr)		
	Onset	Peak	Duration
Rapid acting			
Regular	0.5-1	2-4	4-6
Semilente	0.5-1.5	5-7	4-8
Biphasic	0.5-1	3-4/4-8	16-24
Intermediate acting			
NPH	1.5-2	6-12	18-24
Lente	1.5-2	6-12	16-24
Long acting			
Ultralente	4-8	10-20	24-36
PZI	4-8	14-24	>36

toms go uncorrected, the hyperglycemia and ketonemia secondary to increased lipolysis will progress to severe levels, and diabetic ketoacidosis will occur.

The diagnosis of diabetes is easily established. Any child with the classic symptoms should have levels of blood glucose and urinary glucose and ketones determined. If the blood glucose level is more than 180 mg/dl and glucose, ketones, or both are present in the urine, the diagnosis is established.

TREATMENT

Management of the illness has two major objectives: to return the blood glucose levels to near normal and to prevent complications (American Diabetes Association, 1989). Controversy exists about the relative roles of primary care providers and specialists in the care of children with diabetes. Current recommendations are that most children should be followed by the primary care giver for routine ongoing care but that the specialist team approach is best for education and ongoing oversight of the diabetes. This arrangement, of course, depends on many factors, including the proximity of the specialist and the expertise of the primary care provider.

Replacement of insulin results in dramatic reversal of the symptoms of the disease. At diagnosis, the majority of children are hospitalized, in part for correction of the metabolic derangement but also for education in the management of the illness.

Once any acidosis is corrected, subcutaneous treatment with insulin is the mainstay of therapy.

Table 13-1 shows the actions of the most common types of insulin. Insulin may be derived from beef or pork, or it may be genetically engineered as human insulin (Humulin). Most children are given two injections daily, one before breakfast and one before the evening meal. Although doses must be individually titrated, often two thirds of the daily dose is given in the morning as one-third short-acting insulin and two-thirds intermediate-acting insulin. The remaining one third is given in the evening, similarly divided between short- and intermediate-acting insulin. Based on the blood glucose response, the dose is altered as necessary for maintenance of blood glucose levels as close to normal as possible.

Shortly after the diagnosis is made, many children experience a sharp reduction in the insulin requirement. In some cases no insulin is necessary for a period of time, which may last up to 6 months, but some providers will continue a small dose to maintain the injection schedule. However, the insulin requirement will return, and children should be cautioned that this honeymoon period does not indicate that the diabetes has gone away. Once destruction of the β cells is complete, usually within 2 years of diagnosis, most children will require insulin replacement of approximately 1 U/kg of body weight (Travis, Brouhard, and Schreiner, 1987).

Because exogenous insulin cannot mimic the normal moment-to-moment response of the β cells to changes in blood glucose levels, regulation of both diet and exercise help to minimize the variation in blood glucose levels. The child with diabetes, unlike the individual with NIDDM, is often slender. Therefore, the goal of dietary therapy is to provide sufficient calories for normal growth and development distributed in three meals and two or three snacks. Such a meal plan, when concentrated sugars are limited or avoided, serves to help avoid hyperglycemia, prevent hypoglycemia, and maintain metabolic balance (Brink, 1988). Consistent with the current recommendations of the American Academy of Pediatrics, American and Canadian Diabetes Associations, and the American Dietetic Association (ADA), the composition of the diet should be 50% to 65% carbohydrate, 12% to 20% protein, and 25% to 30% fat. Caloric needs can be estimated to be 1000 calories for the first year of age with approximately 100 calories added per year of age until age 10 to 12 years. Thereafter, females may need a reduction in total calories to the common adult level of 1400 to 1600 calories daily unless they are exceptionally active on a regular basis, whereas males will continue to need approximately 2000 calories daily.

Maintenance of near-normal or normal blood glucose levels requires constant self-monitoring. Self-monitored blood glucose (SMBG) levels allow people with diabetes to have more precision in monitoring than is permitted with urine testing (Schiffrin and Belmonte, 1982). Glucose is not found in the urine until the blood glucose level rises above the renal threshold, usually about 180 mg/dl. Because the goal of therapy is to maintain blood glucose levels between 60 and 120 mg/dl, self-monitoring blood glucose levels allows the individual to know exactly what the blood glucose level is at any moment in time and allows the child to adjust the dose of insulin in response to their actual blood glucose level. Several methods can determine SMBG levels, all of which are similar. A droplet of capillary blood is obtained from a fingerstick and placed on a small glucose reagent strip. After the required period of time, the blood is either washed or wiped from the strip. The degree of color change on the strip is measured by inserting it in a meter or comparing it with a standardized color chart.

The pattern of testing varies with providers. Most children are advised to test a minimum of 2 times daily, at various times throughout the day, and when symptoms are present. However, some providers prefer that tests be done at times of peak insulin action (e.g., 3-5 PM, bedtime), whereas others prefer to see tests at varying times. In any case, the results of SMBG testing are used to identify asymptomatic hypoglycemia, to determine patterns in insulin action, and to make appropriate alterations in the insulin dose. For example, if a child consistently has high blood glucose levels before the evening meal, the morning intermediate-acting insulin (NPH or Lente) would be increased to prevent this effect.

Because these approaches do not provide a guarantee of normalization of blood glucose levels and prevention of complications, newer approaches to management are being tried. Such approaches are beyond the scope of this chapter, but primary care providers should be aware that researchers are working with artificial insulin delivery systems (Clark and Plotnick, 1990), transplantation of β cells, and immune suppression (Chase et al., 1990) as new methods of treatment.

PROGNOSIS

Diabetes is the fifth leading cause of death in the United States (National Center for Health Statistics, 1990). The life expectancy of a child with diabetes at the age of 10 is 44 years, whereas his or her peers can be expected to live 62 more years (Raskin and Rosenstock, 1987). For the most part, this early mortality is a result of the long-term complications of the illness.

Diabetic complications appear to be a function of the years of diabetes after puberty rather than the absolute number of years of diabetes (Rogers et al., 1986). Complications can range from asymptomatic mild proteinuria to blindness, renal failure, and painful neuropathies. The relationship between the degree of chronic hyperglycemia and complications is not clear, although a large multisite clinical trial is now underway to attempt to clarify this relationship. Raskin and Rosenstock (1987) suggest that hyperglycemia is a necessary but not sufficient factor for the development of complications. In addition to hyperglycemia, genetic factors appear to influence the development of complications. Epidemiologic evidence suggests that in the general diabetic population prevalence of microvascular complications is relatively high, with approximately 40% of patients experiencing renal failure and 50% of patients having diabetic retinopathy after 15 years.

ASSOCIATED PROBLEMS
Diabetic ketoacidosis and hypoglycemia

Fig. 13-1 shows the physiologic process that results in diabetic ketoacidosis (DKA) when there is a lack of insulin. Any potential stressor, such as illness, fever, injury, and psychosocial stress, can increase the risk of metabolic derangement caused by disturbances in counterregulatory hormones and lead to DKA. Thus, any stressor in a child with diabetes must be managed with care. Management of intercurrent illness is discussed later.

Children with well-controlled diabetes will occasionally experience mild to moderate hypoglycemia. Because the symptoms of DKA and hypoglycemia can sometimes be confused, they are compared in the box below. Hypoglycemia may be caused by too much insulin, too little food, too much exercise, or any combination of these factors. Although it is easily treated, prevention is the best approach. Again, SMBG determination is helpful. Using SMBG testing, children can identify patterns of lower blood glucose levels that may indicate

periods of increased risk. During these periods, the insulin dose can be altered to prevent the hypoglycemia. If the child anticipates unusual physical activity, both insulin and diet can be adjusted to prevent low glucose levels.

Hypoglycemia presents particular problems at different ages. Infants are unable to express the feelings associated with hypoglycemia, and they must be observed for listlessness, sleepiness, or irritability (Charron-Prochownik and Schwartz, 1984). Parents should be instructed that any unusual behavior at any time is an indication for blood glucose levels to be measured. If the result is less than 80 mg/dl, the conscious infant should be given 2 to 4 oz of sweet liquids or a small amount of cake frosting; the unconscious or convulsing infant should be given glucagon by injection (Lipman et al., 1989a). Older children can be taught the symptoms of hypoglycemia and how to prevent its occurrence. They should also be instructed to carry high-sugar foods with them at all times. All children with IDDM should wear medical identification so that they can be diagnosed and treated appropriately should they lose consciousness while away from home.

Some substances have the potential to increase the likelihood of hypoglycemia. Adolescents need to know that alcohol augments the glucose-lowering effects of insulin and that the symptoms of alcohol intoxication and hypoglycemia are similar. Low blood glucose levels can increase the body's sensitivity to alcohol. Many experimenting teens have found themselves in the emergency room with profound hypoglycemia. Stimulants such as amphetamines and cocaine may increase metabolism and decrease appetite, with a potential for hypoglycemia to occur (Lipman et al., 1989b).

Monilial infections

Once healthy girls are toilet trained, monilial infections of the perineum are rare until adolescence, when the estrogenation of the vagina provides a potential environment for monilial growth. Hyperglycemia also leads to increased glucose levels in vaginal secretions, which provides a healthy medium for monilia. Thus, girls with diabetes have an increased risk for monilial vaginitis, and any complaint of vaginal discharge and itching should be investigated with a potassium hydroxide preparation and treated appropriately.

SYMPTOMS OF HYPERGLYCEMIA AND HYPOGLYCEMIA

Hyperglycemia	Hypoglycemia
Slow onset	Rapid onset
Increased thirst and urination	Excessive sweating
High blood and urine glucose levels	Fainting
Urinary ketones	Headache
Weakness and abdominal pain	Trembling and shaking
Heavy, labored breathing	Hunger
Anorexia	Inability to waken
Nausea and vomiting	Irritability
	Personality change

PRIMARY CARE MANAGEMENT
Growth and development

Because IDDM is a metabolic disorder affecting carbohydrate metabolism, growth and sexual development may be slowed. Children and adolescents in poor control may fail to grow normally. Therefore, accurate measurement of height and weight and comparison with growth norms are imperative.

Even when children have normal linear growth, there may be delays in the onset and progression of puberty if glycemic control is not adequate. At each visit, Tanner stages of secondary sexual development should be assessed and recorded. Any deviation from the normal pattern should be investigated. In girls, menarche may be delayed. Loss of regular menses once cycling has been established may indicate a further degeneration in diabetic control and should be investigated.

Although it is not common unless the child receives too much insulin, obesity can occur in children and adolescents with IDDM. Rapid weight gain in the presence of high SMBG levels may suggest that a child is having undetected hypoglycemia with rebound of the blood glucose to high levels. This phenomenon is known as the "Somogyi phenomenon" and is frequently a cause of overtreatment with insulin. Management of the obesity should be done carefully, with attention to the need to maintain self-monitoring, because glucose levels may change dramatically when a weight loss diet is followed.

Another concern is the adolescent who manipulates overeating by reducing or omitting insulin. Some adolescents, especially girls, have learned that it is difficult to gain weight when the insulin dose is insufficient because of the huge losses of glucose and calories in the urine (Brink, 1988). Careful screening for eating disorders can sometimes lead to the identification of this problem.

Immunizations

Children and adolescents with diabetes should follow the immunization schedule recommended by the American Academy of Pediatrics. There is some controversy regarding the use of mumps vaccine in children with diabetes, because mumps and other viral infections have been repeatedly linked to the development of diabetes mellitus (Helmke, Otten, and Willems, 1980). It appears, however, that the vaccine or the active infection acts as a trigger for manifestation of the illness in susceptible individuals and therefore does not increase disease vulnerability (Helmke et al., 1986). Thus, the use of the measles, mumps, and rubella vaccine at the recommended ages is warranted.

Parents frequently ask about immunization for pneumococcus and influenza for children with diabetes, because the Public Health Service Advisory Committee on Immunization Practice (1978) recommends these immunizations for adult diabetic patients. The committee has not made recommendations regarding such immunizations for children with diabetes. Lederman and colleagues (1982) studied the response to polyvalent pneumococcal polysaccharide vaccine in diabetic children and concluded that DKA-prone children may derive some benefit from the vaccine, but the clinical efficacy was not established. They concluded that routine immunization with these vaccines should not be recommended.

Screening

Vision. Vision screening is of particular importance in children with diabetes as visual problems are not uncommon. A small number of children will develop cataracts early in the course of the illness, therefore observing the normalcy of the red reflex during the ophthalmic examination is very important. Fluctuations in blood glucose levels can also affect visual acuity. Children experiencing hypoglycemia may complain of visual disturbances, and those with hyperglycemia may also complain of blurred vision. Thus, it is important to relate the results of routine visual screening to the level of diabetic control, because improvement in metabolic control may improve the results of the visual testing.

Parents and children are often most concerned about the risk of diabetic retinopathy. Retinopathy of diabetes is the leading cause of blindness. Therefore, the ADA (1989) recommends that fundoscopic examination be performed at each visit in all individuals with diabetes. Further, in those children who are more than 12 years of age and who have had diabetes for at least 5 years, annual examination with dilation by a pediatric ophthalmologist is recommended.

Hearing. Routine screening is recommended.

Dental. Routine screening is recommended.

Blood pressure. Routine screening should be performed at each visit. Hypertension has been reported in up to 45% of all individuals with diabetes. Thus, the ADA (1989) recommends that orthostatic measurements be performed and recorded routinely.

Hematocrit. Routine screening is recommended.

Urinalysis. Routine screening is performed yearly, with examination for levels of ketones, glucose, and protein. After 5 years of diabetes or after puberty, total urinary protein excretion should be measured yearly by the microalbuminuria method to screen for renal complications. If proteinuria is detected, serum creatinine clearance or blood urea nitrogen concentration should be measured and glomerular filtration assessed.

Tuberculosis. Routine screening is recommended.

Condition-specific screening

GLYCOSYLATED HEMOGLOBIN. Children and adolescents with diabetes are routinely seen approximately every 3 months. Quarterly visits correspond to the rate at which the glycosylated hemoglobin levels can be expected to change. Glycosylated hemoglobin (Daneman et al., 1981), or hemoglobin A_{1c}, is a measure of the attachment of glucose to the circulating hemoglobin molecule. In nondiabetic individuals, glycosylated hemoglobin will comprise 3% to 6% of the total hemoglobin, whereas those with diabetes have levels in excess of 6%, varying in proportion to the blood glucose levels. The glycosylated hemoglobin level reflects the average blood glucose level over the most recent 3 months, because the life span of the hemoglobin molecule is approximately 120 days. It is not affected by short-term fluctuations and is considered to be an objective and accurate measure of long-term diabetes control (Gabbay et al., 1977).

THYROID FUNCTION. Because diabetes is an autoimmune disease, it is associated with other autoimmune diseases, especially Hashimoto's thyroiditis (Eisenbarth, 1986). Children and adolescents who demonstrate any change in growth pattern or who develop signs and symptoms of either hypothyroidism or hyperthyroidism should be tested with thyroid function studies (triiodothyronine, thyroxine, and thyroid-stimulating hormone levels).

Drug interactions

Many over-the-counter medications and antibiotics contain glucose, and some contain alcohol or traces of gluconeogenic substances such as sorbitol or glycerine (Kumar, Weatherly, and Beaman, 1991). In amounts usually ingested, these compounds may raise blood glucose levels slightly, but they should not markedly impair diabetic control. Pseudoephedrine has the potential to increase blood glucose levels because of its stimulant effect. This effect is minimal at usual doses, but all such products contain warnings that individuals with diabetes should consult their provider before taking the product, so primary care providers should be aware of the potential effect.

DIFFERENTIAL DIAGNOSIS AND MANAGEMENT OF COMMON PEDIATRIC CONDITIONS

When the classic symptoms of diabetes are present, there are few other diagnoses to consider. Polydipsia and polyuria may be caused by diabetes insipidus, but urinary and serum glucose levels will be normal. Urinary tract infections may also cause urinary frequency, but, again, glucose levels will be normal. Renal glycosuria is possible but unusual, and it will not be characterized by ketosis.

Illness management and prevention of diabetic ketoacidosis

Children and adolescents with diabetes are at no higher risk for most common infectious diseases of childhood than their peers, provided that the diabetes is under reasonable metabolic control. Because any stressor may lead to DKA in a child with diabetes, infections and other stressors must be managed with care.

Regardless of the insult, there are several important principles for management. Of utmost importance is the need to continue to take insulin even when the child is unable to eat the normal diet, because the excess of counterregulatory hormones released in response to the stressor will more than offset the decreased oral intake. Thus, even though dietary intake may be decreased, insulin requirement may be increased.

The principles of management include monitoring parameters of control, maintaining hydration, preventing hypoglycemia, and preventing DKA. For these principles to work effectively, it is imperative that the child and family know that any illness or insult involving fever, gastrointestinal symptoms, congestion in the head or chest, or urinary symptoms should be managed as a sick day (Ley and Goldman, 1990). Once a day is identified as a sick day, the usual rules for self-monitoring are altered to reflect the need for closer monitoring. Blood glucose levels should be tested every 4 hours, and those with blood glucose levels greater than 200 mg/dl should test urine for ketones. Blood glucose levels of more than 400 mg/dl on two determinations and moderate or high ketone levels in the urine that do not decrease with additional insulin should be viewed as an indication that the child should be seen and evaluated by either the primary care provider or the specialist.

Maintaining hydration is important in helping clear extra glucose and ketoacids. If children are unable to eat their usual diet, a large fluid intake should be maintained. In adolescents this amount should be more than 8 oz of fluid hourly. Such fluids should contain adequate amounts of carbohydrate (50-75 gm/6-8 hr) to maintain their usual caloric intake. Children will often drink nondiet sodas or flavored gelatin water when ill. If the child is vomiting or has diarrhea, broths may be helpful with replacing sodium losses.

INDICATIONS FOR EVALUATION BY A HEALTH CARE PROVIDER

Vomiting for more than 6 hours or more than 5 diarrheal stools in 1 day
Any change in mental status
Syncope
Temperature greater than 38.9°C for 12 hours
Blood glucose levels more than 400 mg/dl twice
Moderate or high ketone levels that do not decrease with extra insulin intake
Dysuria or other symptoms of urinary tract infection
Decrease in urinary output

To prevent DKA, the child may need additional insulin. In general, the family should administer the usual dose of insulin and add up to 20% of the total daily dose as regular insulin every 4 hours if the blood glucose level is greater than 300 mg/dl. Such management should be done in careful consultation with the child's diabetes team.

The box below lists those indications for which a child or adolescent should be seen and evaluated. Most important is the need for the child with any alteration in mental status to be evaluated. The provider should never assume that sleepiness in a child with diabetes is merely the result of the fatigue associated with an illness.

DEVELOPMENTAL ISSUES
Safety

The safety issues faced by families with a child or adolescent with diabetes are twofold. As discussed earlier, hypoglycemia is a significant risk for all affected children, and families and others in the child's social sphere should be prepared to respond appropriately. Older children need to know how to prevent severe hypoglycemia, especially when exercising. Children should be taught to eat a snack composed of complex carbohydrate and protein before exercise, not to inject insulin into exercising muscle, and to carry glucose with them at all times. When traveling, children or their parents should carry their supplies with them, not in checked baggage, and always have food available should a meal be delayed. Some airlines require a letter from a provider explaining the need for syringes to be carried on board an airplane.

The other important safety issue is the proper disposal of syringes. Children and parents need to be taught the importance of proper disposal of syringes to reduce the risk of injury to themselves and others. In addition, rendering of the syringe and needles useless immediately after injection helps to assure that the syringe will not be used for illicit drugs by someone else.

Child care

Toddlers and preschoolers with diabetes benefit from the socialization of preschool programs. They do not need specialized medical day care. Preschool teachers should be informed of parents' expectations. Snack and lunch intake is very important, so preschool teachers need to be aware of the child's need to eat and what should be served at each mealtime. They should be aware of appropriate food substitutions when food is refused. All care givers should be told how to manage symptoms of hypoglycemia. Emergency telephone numbers should always be available and should include telephone numbers of the parents, another emergency contact, the primary care provider, and the diabetes specialist.

Parents of children with diabetes often express concerns about the abilities of baby-sitters or day-care workers to manage a young child's diabetes (Hodges and Parker, 1987). Parents of young children can begin by leaving the child for only short periods of time, thus reassuring themselves that the sitter can successfully care for the child. Clear instructions regarding the child's diet and management of hypoglycemia should be provided in writing. Parents should be encouraged to train sitters in blood glucose monitoring and in recognition of hypoglycemic symptoms. Emergency telephone numbers should always be available.

Diet

Although insulin therapy is the cornerstone of treatment, a dietary plan is important in maintaining near-normoglycemia without wide swings in blood glucose levels. Long-term adherence to the dietary plan is probably the most difficult aspect of management for families (Hodges and Parker, 1987).

There are several different dietary philosophies, but no matter what the dietary philosophy, most meal plans are based on the exchange system. Current exchange lists can be obtained from the ADA (see the resources listed on p. 243), but the basic components are listed in Table 13-2. There are six food groups, including a "free" group. Within the groups, the nutritional composition of a serving of different foods is relatively constant. In the starch category, for example, one exchange is one slice of bread, ½ cup of white rice, or 1 medium, baked potato. The system helps families learn portion sizes and healthy childhood nutrition.

All dietary management plans have the goal of providing adequate calories and nutrients for normal growth. Daily consistency of intake with regular meals and snacks is important. There are three common approaches: the free diet, the rigid diet, and the constant carbohydrate diet (McMahan and Travis, 1987). The free diet allows most foods in unlimited amounts, but foods with concentrated carbohydrates (sweets) are restricted. The advantage of this dietary plan is that it allows for a more normal family life, and some advocates believe that such a plan leads to less difficulties with long-term adherence. Those who disagree with the plan note that children may get a mixed message about the importance of diet if a specific meal plan is not recommended.

Table 13-2. Dietary exchange system

| Food exchange | Calories | Approximate content gm/serving | | |
		Carbohydrate	Protein	Fat
Fruit	60	12	0	0
Starch	68	15	2	0
Milk				
Whole	170	12	8	10
Skim	90	12	8	Trace
Meat				
Lean	55	0	7	3
Medium fat	75	0	7	5
High fat	95	0	7	8
Fat	45	0	0	5
Free	0	Negligible	0	0

To the other extreme is the rigid diet. Proponents of this approach require eliminating all concentrated sweets from the diet and strict weighing and measuring all foods. Abraira, DeBartolo, and Myscofski (1980) found that individuals who follow the rigid diet plan have less fluctuation in blood glucose levels than do others. Some families find that such an approach is easier to follow, because the rules are clear. However, for most families, such rigid attention to food is not consistent with a healthy lifestyle, and battles at meal time may result.

Between these two approaches is the constant carbohydrate meal plan (McMahan and Travis, 1987). In this approach concentrated carbohydrates are discouraged, and exchanges of fruits, starches, and milk are kept relatively constant. Active participation of the family and the child in food decision making is encouraged. Protein or meat exchanges can be used to ensure that the child receives adequate food to satisfy hunger.

The selection of the appropriate meal plan should be made by the family in consultation with the diabetes team. The family is in the best position to judge the approach that will work for them. The imposition of a rigid approach on a nonwilling family will only lead to problems of nonadherence to the diet. In addition, for any child to adhere without question to a diet perceived as different from that of peers is clearly of concern. Thus providers need to be understanding in their approach and work with families to ensure as much dietary consistency as possible.

The wide availability of artificially sweetened foods and drinks has eased some of the difficulties children with diabetes faced in following the meal plan. Parents sometimes express concern, however, that extensive use of artificial sweeteners will be problematic for their children. Reviews of the literature by the Diabetes Task Force of the American Academy of Pediatrics (1985) have found no problems in long-term use of aspartame. In addition, adverse reactions to aspartame are no more frequent than with placebo (Nehrling et al., 1985).

It has been noted that an association between the eating disorders of anorexia nervosa and bulimia with IDDM exists. In some instances these children experienced extreme shifts in blood glucose levels. Wing and colleagues (1986) studied a large population of diabetic adolescents and found that diabetic subjects did not differ significantly from a comparison group in overall oral control or bulimic behaviors, but they did report more concern about diet than did the nondiabetic controls. Among the teens with diabetes, however, self-reported bulimic behaviors were associated with poorer diabetic control. Thus, adolescents with diabetes should also be screened using the usual techniques for eating disorders, particularly if diabetic control is poor (Littlefield et al., 1989).

Discipline

Although the issues related to discipline of a child with diabetes are not different from those of all children with a chronic condition, parents of children with diabetes report that their second most common concern in raising the child is discipline (Hodges and Parker, 1987). Parents most often worry that a hypoglycemic episode will be missed by attributing the unruly behavior to lack of discipline. It is appropriate for parents to test the blood glucose level at any time hypoglycemia is suspected. Then, if the result is within the normal range, the child can be disciplined appropriately. Some parents also worry that the stress of imposed discipline will raise the blood glucose level because of the presence of counterregulatory hormones. Although severe stressors may increase blood glucose levels (Chase and Jackson, 1981), no evidence suggests that usual disciplinary measures increase blood glucose levels or worsen diabetic control. Indeed, some studies (Grey, Tamborlane, and Genel, 1980) have suggested that parents who set reasonable limits for their children are more likely to have children in good diabetic control.

Toileting

Several issues related to toileting are important in the management of diabetes in children. Many children have secondary enuresis at the time of diagnosis. It is important to tell children who were previously dry that diabetes is the cause of their enuresis and that when the diabetes is adequately controlled, the enuresis should remit. It is also true that enuresis can occur with well-controlled diabetes. Other methods of diagnostic confirmation and treatment should be explored with these families.

Although testing urine for glucose is not as critical to management as it was before SMBG testing became available, urinary ketone levels are important indicators of status when a child is ill. Parents should know how to obtain such samples from infants and toddlers. Cotton balls tucked into a diaper can provide an adequate sample for use on a dipstick to determine ketone levels in pre-toilet-trained children. During toilet training when a child uses a potty chair, urine is readily obtainable. When the child moves onto the bathroom commode, the parent needs to teach the child to urinate into a paper cup so that the urine can be tested. Taught at a time when the child is feeling well, this task can be made into a game, so that, when necessary, the behavior has been learned.

Sleep patterns

Children with diabetes who are in good control should have no problems sleeping. However, those who are hyperglycemic overnight will have difficulty sleeping because of the recurrent need to urinate. This problem can be managed by improving diabetic control.

Hypoglycemia at night is a concern of parents. The child may not awaken with the usual early signs and symptoms, and the first sign may be a severe reaction with nightmares or seizures. Thus, prevention of nighttime hypoglycemia by adjusting the evening insulin dose appropriately and offering a bedtime snack is important. Parents should also be instructed in the use of the counterregulatory hormone glucagon in the event the child is not arousable.

Nightmares are common in young children and may be caused by hypoglycemia. Parents should determine the blood glucose level before assuming the cause of a nightmare. If the cause is hypoglycemia, treatment would include administration of glucose; if the nightmares are not related to hypoglycemia, appropriate comfort measures should be instituted. Prevention is the key, though, and significant nighttime hypoglycemia is to be avoided as much as possible by careful adjustment of diet and insulin.

School issues

Children and adolescents with diabetes should participate fully in school activities. Children whose diabetes is adequately controlled should attend school regularly and participate in any activity for which they are otherwise suited. Parents should be encouraged to inform the school nurse and the child's teachers when the diabetes is diagnosed. It is important that someone in the school be knowledgeable about the child's care so that hypoglycemia or illness can be managed appropriately. The need for other involvement, such as SMBG testing or injections, will depend on the child's usual regimen. Most professionals, however, suggest that monitoring and injections should not be necessary at school until the child is old enough to manage the regimen independently.

With older children, providers need to work with the child, family, and school personnel to arrange a school schedule that fits the child's diabetes regimen (Balik, Haig, and Moynihan, 1986). For example, a child who has had regular and NPH insulin at 7:00 AM should probably not have gym class immediately before a late lunch period. Arrangements need to be made so that the child can always have access to glucose-containing foods in the event of a hypoglycemic episode. For field trips the child should always have food available. A sack lunch with all food groups serves nicely as a substitute should a meal be unexpectedly delayed. Sports are also encouraged. Coaches should be aware of the diabetes and keep glucose-containing foods on hand. Depending on the degree of exercise, insulin dose may be lowered on extraactivity days, diet may be increased, or both in an attempt to prevent hypoglycemia. Hypoglycemia following exercise may occur up to 12 hours after the event, so children should be carefully monitored when any new activity is undertaken. Children should be advised that insulin is absorbed more rapidly from exercising muscle; thus, if a muscle is to be exercised, insulin should be injected in another site. For example, if a child will run track, the insulin could be administered in the arm or the abdomen rather than the leg.

Children whose diabetes is in poor control may experience difficulties in school performance. Because hypoglycemia can cause a child to lose the ability to concentrate when the blood glucose level is low, learning can be a problem. When the blood glucose level is consistently too high, many children experience difficulties in concentration and grades may suffer. Thus, any child with diabetes whose school performance changes should be carefully assessed for alterations in diabetic control.

As with all children who have a chronic condition, emphasis should be on the normality of the child, not the diabetes. Such an approach helps to minimize the sense of being different that is experienced by all affected children.

Sexuality

The achievement of normal growth and development is a goal of therapy. If the diabetes is adequately controlled, sexual development should be normal. If, on the other hand, sexual development is delayed, normal concerns about self and physical adequacy may be amplified. Providers need to monitor secondary sexual development carefully in children with diabetes, and any deviation from normal should be investigated. Often, tightening the diabetic control will improve growth. If not, the cause should be investigated.

All sexually active teens need information about birth control. Such information is especially important for those with diabetes because the risks of complications of pregnancy are at least 5 times greater than the already high risk for adolescents. Because of the risk of acquired immunodeficiency syndrome, many providers are encouraging condoms for birth control over all other methods. Unfortunately, as with healthy teens, proper and consistent use of condoms is variable. Other barrier methods, such as diaphragms, foams, and creams, may also be used by those with diabetes, but they share the same disadvantages as condoms and do not prevent sexually transmitted diseases.

Teenagers who are willing to use contraceptives often find the use of the birth control pill acceptable (Bartosch, 1983). The combination pill, containing both estrogen and progesterone, may have considerable risks for adolescents with diabetes. Side effects include cerebral ischemia, myocardial infarction, and rapid progression of retinopathy, so the combination pill is not recommended. The minipill, which is progesterone alone, appears to be reasonably well tolerated and is the oral contraceptive of choice.

Although the avoidance of adolescent pregnancy is clearly preferred, some teenagers will express the desire to become pregnant. It has been clearly demonstrated (Jovanovic, Druzin, and Peterson, 1981) that pregnancy outcomes can be dramatically improved if euglycemia is maintained both in the months preceding conception and throughout the pregnancy. Therefore, female adolescents who are at risk for pregnancy or who are contemplating pregnancy should be counseled regarding pregnancy outcomes and helped to achieve better diabetic control.

Male adolescents will often express concern about the well-known complication of impotence in diabetic men. This problem is thought to be a result of both vascular and neurologic compromise in those with long-standing diabetes. Fortunately, impotence caused by diabetes is very rare in adolescence, and most can be reassured.

SPECIAL FAMILY CONCERNS

Diabetes is a disease that requires ongoing active involvement of the child and the family in its management. Some children will neglect all aspects of care, even insulin injections, and be repeatedly hospitalized with DKA, whereas others will take their insulin but never perform SMBG testing or follow their dietary plan. Compliance is a behavioral coping strategy (Grey and Thurber, 1991) that is an issue in many chronic conditions and therefore is not discussed in depth here. However, any child or adolescent with repeated problems in management (poor control with or without repeated hospitalization) should be carefully questioned about adherence to the diabetic regimen.

Families worry about the appropriate assumption of self-care because of its importance in preventing long-term complications. Recommendations for understanding the levels at which children should assume various self-care activities are available (ADA, 1983). There is, however, broad disagreement among professionals as to the appropriate age for management of skills (Wysocki et al., 1990), and some authors (Ingersoll et al., 1986) have suggested that the too-early assumption of self-management is associated with poorer psychologic and metabolic outcomes. Therefore, decisions about assumption of self-care activities should be made by the family, by the child, and with the providers working together. Until more data on the impact of assuming self-care at different ages are available, the strict regulation by providers of such activities may be unwarranted.

In addition to the family issues that are common

to many chronic conditions, families with a child with diabetes face some unique problems. In studies of parents' concerns (Hauenstein et al., 1989; Hodges and Parker, 1987), several issues appear to be prominent. First is the adherence to the diabetes regimen, especially diet and the assumption of self-care. Second is the question of genetics and inheritance. In addition, psychosomatic issues may be of particular importance to families dealing with diabetes, because poorly functioning families have been shown to be associated with poorer diabetic control (Baker, 1970; Kovacs et al., 1989).

Guilt is often of concern to parents of children with diabetes, particularly because the disease is inherited. Families need to be provided with appropriate genetic counseling so that they are aware of the risks to other family members and the risks to offspring of the individual with diabetes. Such information will often help to assuage the guilt present at diagnosis, because the risk for first-degree relatives is low. The sibling of a child with IDDM has about a 5% to 10% risk, and the risk in an offspring of a single parent with diabetes is about 1% to 2%.

Considerable attention has been paid to family problems and their impact on metabolic control in children with diabetes. It is hypothesized that the well-functioning family facilitates a child's well-being by providing emotional support, advice, and practical help (Anderson and Auslander, 1980) and that poor family functioning interferes with self-care or causes stress-related metabolic deterioration (Baker, 1970). Results of studies of the influence of family life on diabetes control have been inconclusive (Kovacs et al., 1989). However, some families exhibit psychosomatic characteristics that have a clear adverse effect on the child with diabetes. Such families should be referred for family therapy.

SUMMARY OF PRIMARY CARE NEEDS FOR THE CHILD WITH
DIABETES MELLITUS (TYPE I)

Growth and development

Height and weight are normal unless control is
less than adequate.
Secondary sexual development may be delayed.
Rapid weight gain may signal overtreatment with
insulin.
Weight loss usually indicates poor control.

Immunizations

No special recommendations are necessary.

Screening

Vision

Check red reflex and perform fundoscopic examination at each visit.
Thorough pediatric ophthalmologic examination is
advised every 5 years.

Hearing

Routine screening is recommended.

Dental

Routine screening is recommended.

Blood pressure

Check blood pressure each visit and orthostatic
variation.

Hematocrit

Routine screening is recommended.

Urinalysis

Perform urinalysis yearly for ketones, glucose,
and protein determinations; measure total protein values after 5 years.

Tuberculosis

Routine screening is recommended.

Condition-specific screening

Check hemoglobin A_{1c} every 3 months.
Perform thyroid function studies if a change in
growth patterns occurs.
Perform other studies as indicated.

Differential diagnosis

During any illness prevent DKA with insulin,
monitor carefully, and maintain hydration.
Examine any child with altered hydration or mental status.

Developmental issues

Safety

Prevent hypoglycemia with careful monitoring; be
sure a glucose source is always available.
Dispose of syringes properly.

Child care

Teachers need training in management of dietary
needs and hypoglycemia.

Diet

Maintenance of normoglycemia is critical.
Stress the importance of regular distribution of
meals and snacks.
Of the various approaches to diet, all emphasize
consistency and low concentrated sweets.

Discipline

Unruly behavior may be caused by hypoglycemia.
The potential for conflict over diet, blood testing,
and insulin administration should be recognized.

Toileting

Enuresis may be present when control is poor.
Measurement of urinary ketones is important
when blood glucose levels are high or when
the child is ill.

Sleep patterns

Prevention of nighttime hypoglycemia is important.
Nightmares may be the result of hypoglycemia.

School issues

Full attendance and participation are expected.
School personnel must be aware of the child's
special needs.
If control is poor, performance may be affected.

Special family concerns

Assumption of self-care activities and adherence
to the regimen are of prime concern.
Parents often experience guilt concerning the inheritance of IDDM.
Psychosomatic families may have more problems
with diabetic management.

RESOURCES

Two national organizations provide help for families coping with diabetes in a child: the ADA and the Juvenile Diabetes Association (see the list of organizations that follows). The ADA is the largest such organization, composed of both lay individuals and professionals. They support research, education, fund raising, and camps, as well as provide lobbying efforts related to diabetes. They publish several pamphlets and books for families to use in understanding diabetes. At the local level, many affiliates provide support and educational programs for families and children. The ADA deals with all types of diabetes, not only IDDM.

The primary focus of the Juvenile Diabetes Foundation, on the other hand, is research toward a cure for IDDM. The organization does provide some support for families, but its major effort is devoted toward fund raising for research to find a cure for IDDM. Some families find that working toward the cure is helpful.

Organizations

American Diabetes Association
1660 Duke St
Alexandria, VA 22314
(800) ADA-DISC

Juvenile Diabetes Foundation
23 E 26th St
New York, NY 10010
(212) 689-7868

REFERENCES

Abraira C, DeBartolo M, and Myscofski JW: Comparison of unmeasured versus exchange diets in lean adults, *Am J Clin Nutr* 33:1064-1070, 1980.

American Diabetes Association: *Curriculum for youth education*, Alexandria, Va, 1983, The Association.

American Diabetes Association: Standards of medical care for patients with diabetes mellitus, *Diabetes Care* 12:365-368, 1989.

Anderson BJ and Auslander WF: Research on diabetes management and the family: A critique, *Diabetes Care* 3:696-702, 1980.

Baker L: Psychosomatic aspects of diabetes mellitus. In Hill OW, ed: *Modern trends in psychosomatic medicine*, ed 2, Stone Ram, Mass, 1970, Butterworth, pp 105-124.

Balik B, Haig B, and Moynihan PM: Diabetes and the school-aged child, *MCN* 11:324-330, 1986.

Bartosch J: Oral contraceptives: Selection and management, *Nurse Pract* 8:56-59, 1983.

Brink SJ: Pediatric, adolescent, and young-adult nutrition issues in IDDM, *Diabetes Care* 11:192-200, 1988.

Charron-Prochownik D and Schwartz S: Care of the infant with type I diabetes mellitus, *Diabetes Educ* 10:46-50, 1984.

Chase HP, Butler-Simon N, Garg SK, et al: Cyclosporine A for the treatment of new-onset insulin-dependent diabetes mellitus, *Pediatrics* 85:241-245, 1990.

Chase HP and Jackson GG: Stress and sugar control in children with insulin dependent diabetes mellitus, *J Pediatr* 98:1011-1013, 1981.

Clark LM and Plotnick LP: Insulin pumps in children with diabetes, *J Pediatr Health Care* 4:3-10, 1990.

Daneman D, Wolfson DH, Becker DJ, et al: Factors affecting glycosylated hemoglobin values in children with insulin-dependent diabetes, *J Pediatr* 99:847-853, 1981.

Diabetes Task Force: *Nutritional management of children and adolescents with insulin dependent diabetes mellitus*, Elk Grove Village, Ill, 1985, American Academy of Pediatrics.

Drash AL: The epidemiology of insulin-dependent diabetes mellitus, *Clin Invest Med* 10:432-436, 1987.

Eisenbarth GS: Type I diabetes mellitus: A chronic autoimmune disease, *N Engl J Med* 314:1360-1368, 1986.

Gabbay KH, Hasty K, Breslow JL, et al: Glycosylated hemoglobins and long-term blood glucose control in diabetes mellitus, *J Clin Endocrinol Metab* 44:859-864, 1977.

Grey M, Tamborlane WV, and Genel M: Psychosocial adjustment of latency-aged diabetics: Determinants and relationship to control, *Pediatrics* 65:69-72, 1980.

Grey M and Thurber FW: Adaptation to chronic illness in childhood: Diabetes mellitus, *J Pediatr Nurs* (1991).

Hauenstein EJ, Marvin RS, Snyder AL, et al: Stress in parents of children with diabetes mellitus, *Diabetes Care* 12:18-23, 1989.

Helmke K, Otten A, and Willems W: Islet cell antibodies in children with mumps infection, *Lancet* 2:211-212, 1980.

Helmke K, Otten A, Willems WR, et al: Islet cell antibodies and the development of diabetes mellitus in relation to mumps infection and mumps vaccination, *Diabetologia* 29:30-33, 1986.

Hodges LC and Parker J: Concerns of parents with diabetic children, *Pediatr Nurs* 13:22-24, 1987.

Ingersoll GM, Orr DP, Herrold AJ, et al: Cognitive maturity and self-management among adolescents with insulin-dependent diabetes mellitus, *J Pediatr* 108:620-623, 1986.

Jovanovic L, Druzin M, and Peterson CM: Effect of euglycemia on the outcome of pregnancy in insulin-dependent diabetic women as compared with normal control subjects, *Am J Med* 71:921-924, 1981.

Kovacs M, Kass RE, Schnell TM, et al: Family functioning and metabolic control of school-aged children with IDDM, *Diabetes Care* 12:409-414, 1989.

Kumar A, Weatherly M, and Beaman DC: Sweeteners, flavorings, and dyes in antibiotic preparations, *Pediatrics* 87:352-360, 1991.

LaPorte RE and Cruickshanks KJ: Incidence and risk factors for insulin-dependent diabetes. In National Diabetes Data Group, eds: *Diabetes in America,* Bethesda, Md, 1985, National Institutes of Health, No 85-1468, pp 1-12.

Lederman MM, Rodman HM, Schacter BZ, et al: Antibody response to pneumococcal polysaccharides in insulin-dependent diabetes mellitus, *Diabetes Care* 5:36-39, 1982.

Lendrum R, Walker SG, and Gamble DR: Islet cell antibodies in juvenile diabetes mellitus of recent onset, *Lancet* 1:880-882, 1975.

Ley B and Goldman D: Sick-day management: A partnership in preparation for the expected, *Clin Diabetes* 8:25-30, 1990.

Lipman TH, DiFazio DA, Meers RA, et al: A developmental approach to diabetes in children: Birth through preschool, *MCN* 14:225-259, 1989a.

Lipman TH, DiFazio DA, Meers RA, et al: A developmental approach to diabetes in children: School age–adolescence, *MCN* 14:330-332, 1989b.

Littlefield C, Rodin G, Craven J, et al: Eating disorders: A source of poor compliance and control in female adolescents, *Diabetes* 38(suppl 1):8A, 1989.

McMahan P and Travis LB: Dietary management. In Travis LB, Brouhard BH, and Schreiner BJ eds: *Diabetes mellitus in children and adolescents,* Philadelphia, 1987, WB Saunders, pp 73-92.

National Center for Health Statistics: Births, marriages, divorces, and deaths for 1989, *Monthly Vital Stat Rep* 38(12):1-20, 1990.

Nehrling JK, Kobe P, McLane MP, et al: Aspartame use by persons with diabetes, *Diabetes Care* 8:415-417, 1985.

Public Health Service Advisory Committee on Immunization Practices: Pneumococcal polysaccharide vaccine, *MMWR* 27:25-31, 1978.

Raskin P and Rosenstock J: Hyperglycemia, genetic susceptibility, and diabetic complications, *Clin Diabetes* 5:135-141, 1987.

Rogers DG, White NH, Santiago JV, et al: Glycemic control and bone age are independently associated with muscle capillary basement membrane width in diabetic children after puberty, *Diabetes Care* 9:453-459, 1986.

Schiffrin A and Belmonte M: Multiple daily self-glucose monitoring: Its essential role in long-term glucose control in insulin-dependent diabetic patients treated with pump and multiple subcutaneous injections, *Diabetes Care* 5:479-484, 1982.

Srikanto S, Ganda OP, Eisenbarth GS, et al: Islet cell antibodies and beta cell function in monozygotic triplets and twins initially discordant for type I diabetes mellitus, *N Engl J Med* 308:322-325, 1983.

Travis LB, Brouhard BH, and Schreiner BJ: *Diabetes mellitus in children and adolescents,* Philadelphia, 1987, WB Saunders.

Vialettes B, Ozanon JP, Kaplansky S, et al: Stress antecedents and immune status in recently diagnosed type I (insulin-dependent) diabetes mellitus, *Diabete Metab* 15:45-50, 1989.

Wing RR, Nowalk MP, Marcus MD, et al: Subclinical eating disorders and glycemic control in adolescents with type I diabetes, *Diabetes Care* 9:162-167, 1986.

Wysocki T, Meinhold P, Cox DJ, et al: Survey of diabetes professionals regarding developmental changes in diabetes self-care, *Diabetes Care* 13:65-68, 1990.

14   *Down Syndrome*

··

Judith A. Vessey

ETIOLOGY

Down syndrome, first described by Dr. John Langdon Down in 1866, is a condition associated with a recognizable phenotype and limited intellectual endowment because of extra chromosome 21 material. It is the most frequent autosomal chromosomal anomaly. The exact band of chromosomal material implicated in Down syndrome has been isolated, indicating that an entire replication of the 21st chromosome is not needed for expression. Down syndrome is found in all races and ethnic groups, occurring slightly more frequently in males than females (Verma and Huq, 1987).

Nondisjunction

Nondisjunction of the 21st chromosome is responsible for 95% of Down syndrome and is not inherited. Nondisjunction, or the uneven division of chromosomes, can occur during anaphase 1 or 2 in meiosis (reduction division of germ cells) or in anaphase of mitosis (somatic cell division). Although the exact mechanism remains unconfirmed, the pair of chromosomes fail to separate and migrate properly during cell division. When this occurs in meiosis, the haploid number for the respective daughter cells is unequal. If the cell receiving 24 rather than 23 chromosomes is fertilized, a trisomic zygote will result (Fig. 14-1).

Nondisjunction may also occur early in mitosis. The resulting zygote will possess two or more cell lines with varying chromosomal constitutions. The earlier nondisjunction occurs, the greater the percentage of affected cells. This inheritance pattern, referred to as mosaicism, is associated with fewer phenotypic features (Fig. 14-2).

Translocation

In Down syndrome caused by translocation, there are also three copies of the 21st chromosome. The third copy does not occur independently, however, but is attached to another chromosome, usually to one of the D group. The total chromosome count is 46 despite the fact that the material for 47 chromosomes is present. Although the phenotype for Down syndrome caused by translocation is the same as in nondisjunction, the inheritance pattern is quite different. In this form the disorder may reoccur in future pregnancies. If one parent has 45 chromosomes that include a translocation of the 21st chromosome, the gametes produced could result in a trisomic zygote. Although theoretically six combinations are possible, three of these are nonviable. Of the three that are viable, one is normal (N = 46), one results in a balanced translocation (N = 45), and one is an unbalanced translocation resulting in Down syndrome (N = 46) (Fig. 14-3). Although this would translate to a 33% chance of having a child with Down syndrome with each pregnancy, in clinical practice the actual distribution is different than the theoretical distribution. Risk of recurrence is 10% to 15% if the mother is the carrier and 5% to 8% if the father is the carrier.

INCIDENCE

Down syndrome occurs approximately once in every 650 to 1000 live births (Cohen, 1984), with

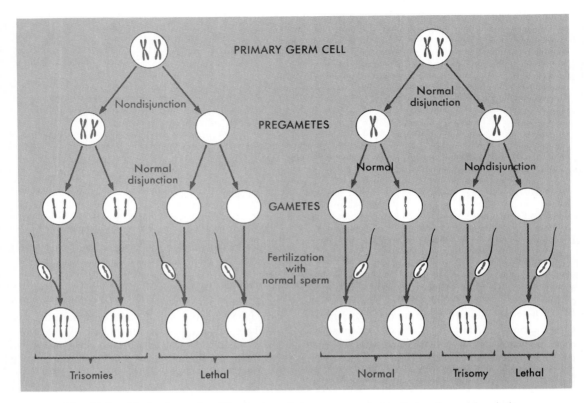

Fig. 14-1. Mechanisms of maldistribution of chromosomes during first and second meiotic divisions caused by nondisjunction.

the incidence varying by inheritance pattern. Down syndrome caused by translocation is independent of parental age, and the incidence remains stable across age cohorts. Advanced parental age, however, is implicated in nondisjunction. For women in their early twenties, the incidence is approximately 1 in every 1,500 births. The incidence rises gradually until maternal age surpasses 35, with the incidence then climbing to approximately 1 in 32 for 45-year-old women. Advanced paternal age has also been shown to correlate slightly with the incidence of Down syndrome in approximately 20% to 30% of the cases. Although the extra chromosome is paternal in origin, nondisjunction still occurs after fertilization. Because the overwhelming percentage of cases of Down syndrome are caused by nondisjunction, parental age directly affects the overall incidence.

CLINICAL MANIFESTATIONS AT TIME OF DIAGNOSIS

Down syndrome is most frequently diagnosed immediately following birth as a result of its distinctive phenotype. In infants of color or those born very prematurely, diagnosis may be delayed because the clinical features may not be as clearly recognized. Although more than 50 physical characteristics can be identified at birth (see the box on p. 248), no one feature is considered diagnostic. Features vary in their expression and are not always present. Some of the most commonly associated features, however, include generalized hypotonia, epicanthal folds, single transverse palmar creases, and diminished vigor.

A variety of congenital anomalies commonly occur in association with Down syndrome. Congenital cardiac disease is seen in approximately

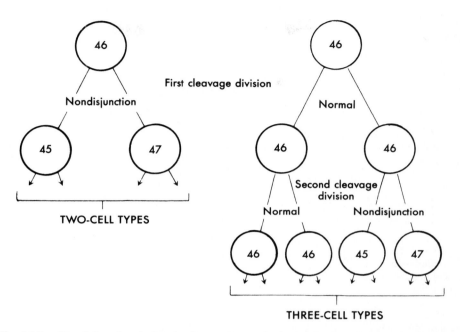

Fig. 14-2. Nondisjunction during the first and second mitotic division of the zygote, resulting in a mosaic phenotype. From Whaley, L. and Wong, D.: *Nursing care of infants and children,* ed. 4, St. Louis, 1991, Mosby–Year Book.

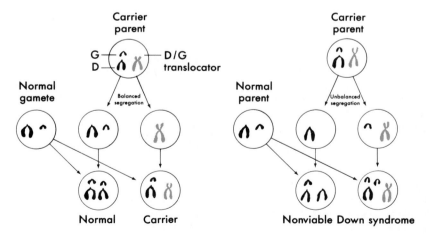

Fig. 14-3. Possible zygotes from the union of a somatically normal carrier of D/G translocation and with a genetically and somatically normal individual. From Whaley, L. and Wong, D.: *Nursing care of infants and children,* ed. 4, St. Louis, 1991, Mosby–Year Book.

COMMON FINDINGS IN DOWN SYNDROME

Skull

Flat occipital area
Brachycephaly
Hypoplasia of midfacial bones
Reduced interorbital distance
Underdeveloped maxilla
Obtuse mandibular angle

Eyes

Oblique narrow palpebral fissures
Epicanthic folds
Brushfield spots
Strabismus
Nystagmus
Myopia
Hypoplasia of the iris

Ears

Small, shortened ears
Low and oblique implantation
Overlapping helices
Prominent antihelix
Absent or attached earlobes
Narrow ear canals
External auditory meatus
Structural aberrations of the ossicles
Stenotic external auditory meatus

Nose

Hypoplastic
Flat nasal bridge
Anteverted, narrow nares
Deviated nasal septum

Mouth

Prominent, thickened and fissured lips
Corners of the mouth turned downward
High arched, narrow palate
Shortened palatal length
Protruding enlarged tongue
Papillary hypertrophy (early preschool)
Fissured tongue (later school years)
Periodontal disease
Partial anodontia
Microdontia
Abnormally aligned teeth
Anterior open bite

Neck

Short broad neck
Loose skin at nape

Chest

Shortened rib cage
Twelfth rib anomalies
Pectus excavation or carinatum
Congenital heart disease

Abdomen

Distended and enlarged abdomen
Diastasis recti
Umbilical hernia

Muscle tone and musculature

Hyperflexibility
Muscular hypotonia

Integument

Skin appears large for the skeleton
Dry and rough
Fine, poorly pigmented hair

Extremities

Short extremities
Partial or complete syndactyly
Clinodactyly
Brachyclinodactyly

Upper extremities

Short, broad hands
Single palmar transverse crease
Incurved short fifth finger
Abnormal dermatoglyphics

Lower extremities

Short and stubby feet
Gap between first and second toes
Plantar crease between first and second toe
Second and third toes grouped in a forklike position
Radial deviation of the third to the fifth toe

Physical growth and development

Short stature
Increased weight in later life

Other findings seen in the newborn

Enlarged anterior fontanel
Delayed closing of sutures and fontanels
Open sagittal suture
Nasal bone not ossified, underdeveloped
Reduced birth weight

40% of children, with endocardial cushion defects accounting for about 60% and septal defects comprising another 28% of cardiac malformations (Ferencz et al., 1989). Gastrointestinal (GI) malformations are seen, with duodenal atresia, congenital megacolon (Hirschsprung's disease), imperforate anus, annular pancreas, and pyloric stenosis among the most common problems. In males an increase in urogenital conditions, including micropenis, hypospadias, and cryptorchidism, has also been documented, although no rise in the incidence of anatomic abnormalities of the kidneys or ureters was noted (Lang et al., 1987). Surgical correction of anomalies can usually be undertaken in the neonatal period. Although many children experience total correction of the anomaly, others will suffer from untoward sequelae throughout their lives.

TREATMENT

No treatment can eliminate the chromosomal defect that causes Down syndrome. Extensive interdisciplinary services and research over the last 20 years has, however, transformed society's view of children with Down syndrome and accepted treatment protocols. Current accepted approaches include (1) genetic counseling, (2) prompt referral for surgical correction of congenital anomalies, and (3) enrollment in an early intervention program.

Genetic counseling

Validation of Down syndrome and its genotype by chromosomal analysis should be considered for all affected children. Although this will not affect the child's treatment or prognosis, it has significant implications for genetic counseling of family members. Because translocation is the cause in 4% to 6% of cases, parents and siblings will need to be tested to determine their carrier status and the risk of recurrence in future pregnancies carefully explained.

Surgery

Today surgical corrections of most major cardiac, GI, and genitourinary anomalies are performed routinely. Historically this was not the standard practice in some settings. Amidst moral and ethical controversy, however, the federal judiciary decreed in 1984 that treatment of life-threatening congenital

anomalies could not be refused only because a child was developmentally disabled (Mahon, 1990) (see Chapter 3).

In addition to life-saving surgeries, some children with Down syndrome are also undergoing plastic procedures to alter their phenotypic appearance. As these children continue to become more integrally mainstreamed into society, they are frequently stigmatized because of their physiognomy. Some parents, concerned about their child's social acceptance, will seek plastic surgery. Procedures include partial glossectomies, neck resections, Silastic implants for the chin and nose, and reconstruction of dysplastic helices. Some improvements have been reported; better articulation of speech, less mouth breathing, fewer and less severe upper respiratory tract infections, and improved mastication and swallowing may be realized (Olbrisch, 1982). Yet conflicting results on the success of corrective surgery have been reported by others (Katz and Kravetz, 1989; Klaiman and Arndt, 1989; Strauss et al., 1988). Plastic surgery is not indicated for all children. If after counseling it is still deemed appropriate, initial revisions begin when the child is approximately 3 years old.

Early intervention

Infant stimulation programs and continued early childhood education are designed to optimize a child's rate of development and minimize the amount of developmental lag that will occur between the child with Down syndrome and developmentally normal peers. Specific therapeutic exercises are devised to stimulate the infant's cognitive, social, motor, and language domains. Parents are usually taught these skills by special education teachers, physical therapists, occupational therapists, and speech pathologists so that they may be conducted at home. The child will later be referred to a specialized program designed to continue these intervention strategies and then mainstreamed into generic child care or school.

The research as to the results of early intervention programs has been extensive but as yet not conclusive. Short-term gains on children's developmental outcomes are often substantial. Although the long-term cognitive effects remain questionable (Gibson and Harris, 1988), improved family functioning and better social integration of the child are seen. It does appear that timing is a critical factor, with earlier interventions being correlated with greater developmental gains.

Numerous other approaches designed to improve these children's developmental outcomes such as patterning, megavitamin therapy, and the administration of butoctamide hydrogen succinate have also been tried. Unfortunately, the results of all of these interventions have been disappointing.

PROGNOSIS

Because of the association of Down syndrome with numerous anatomic and physiologic aberrations, life expectancy is reduced, with approximately a 12% mortality in the first year of life, rising to more than 20% by 12 years of age (Baird and Sadovnick, 1989). The number and severity of congenital anomalies significantly decrease life expectancy for some of these children. Premature aging and a high incidence of Alzheimer's disease are also seen in Down syndrome and reduce life expectancy for adults. With correct medical, educational, and social interventions, the majority of individuals live well into adulthood and have satisfying, productive lives (Miola, 1987). Successful outcomes appear to depend heavily on the early interventions children and their families receive. Aggressive, interdisciplinary management is paramount if a child with Down syndrome is to reach his or her full potential.

ASSOCIATED PROBLEMS
Mental retardation

Intellectual capabilities of children with Down syndrome vary dramatically. Most are moderately retarded (IQ 40-55, SD = 15), but a small percentage are either mildly affected (IQ 56-69, SD = 15) or severely impaired (IQ ≤39). For a few children, their intelligence quotients are not consistent with a diagnosis of mental retardation (Libb et al., 1983). Known correlates to children's intelligence and adaptive behavior skills are their physical condition, home environment, and individualized early intervention (Gibson and Harris, 1988; Libb et al., 1983). Unfortunately, cognitive function often deteriorates with aging, and significant losses in intelligence and social skills are seen earlier (frequently by age 40) than in persons who do not have Down syndrome (Brown et al., 1990).

Mental retardation may or may not be accompanied with behavior disorders. Depression, autistic-like behavior, and psychotic episodes have been reported. Neurologic deterioration, institutionalization, disturbed family life, stress associated with mainstreaming, and normal childhood stressors may have an effect on the mental health of children with Down syndrome.

Musculoskeletal and motor abilities

Orthopedic problems are second only to cardiac defects as a cause of morbidity in Down syndrome (Bennet et al., 1982). Flaccid muscle tone and ligamentous laxity occur to some extent in all affected children, possibly because of an intrinsic defect in their connective tissue. Among these conditions are pes planus, patellar subluxation, scoliosis, dislocated hips, atlantoaxial subluxation, joint and muscle pain, and rapid muscle fatigue. These problems may occur throughout the child's lifetime and should be carefully screened for by the examiner at each visit.

Surgical correction may be indicated for patellar hypermobility with subluxation, scoliosis, or dislocated hips. It should be noted that although the incidence of congenital dislocated hip in children with Down syndrome is similar to that of unaffected peers, approximately 1 in 20 will acquire dislocated hips between learning to walk and the end of the school-aged period (Bennet et al., 1982).

Another significant disorder is atlantoaxial instability. Atlantoaxial instability results from a "loose joint" between C1 and C2 and increased space between the atlas and odontoid process. It affects 15% to 20% of children with Down syndrome and is more common in boys than girls (Pueschel, 1983; Pueschel and Scola, 1987). The overwhelming majority of affected children are asymptomatic even though subluxation or dislocation may result. Early manifestations may include head tilt, torticollis, deteriorating gait, or changes in bowel or bladder function. If left untreated, they may progress to frank neurologic findings associated with spinal cord compression.

Vision

Increased prevalence of numerous ocular deviations is associated with Down syndrome. In order of decreasing frequency the most commonly occurring abnormalities are slanted palpebral fissures, spotted irises, blepharitis, strabismus, myopia, cataracts, keratoconus, and nystagmus (Caputo et al., 1989; Traboulsi et al., 1988). A significant loss in visual acuity will result if many of these conditions are not diagnosed and treated in early childhood.

Hearing

Structural deviations of the skull, foreface, external auditory canal, and middle and inner ears accompanied by eustacian tube dysfunction are associated with congenital and acquired hearing loss (Brown et al., 1989). The incidence of hearing loss in children with Down syndrome is estimated to range from 50% to 76% (Davies, 1988). Children with stenotic auditory canals are at particular risk for problems.

Immune system

It is well documented that children with Down syndrome have altered immune function, although the evidence is conflicting as to the exact nature of the changes (Levin, 1987). All areas of immune function appear to be altered in part because of changes in the thymus. Responsible for controlling many immunologic mechanisms, the thymus is histologically and functionally abnormal. Documented alterations include depressed neutrophil chemotaxis, numerous variations in phagocytosis, and a somewhat diminished complement system. The ability of B cells to produce immunoglobins to selected antigens is also impaired despite the relative normality in the number of cells. This is possibly the result of the influence of T-cell regulation, because qualitative and quantitative differences have been shown to exist in their number and function (Levin, 1987; Wysocki, Wysocki and Wierusz-Wysocka, 1987). Immune system deficits contribute directly to an increased incidence and severity of numerous other conditions. These include but are not limited to periodontal disease, respiratory problems, lymphocytic thyroiditis, leukemia, diabetes mellitus, alopecia areata, adrenal dysfunction, gluten enteropathy, and vitiligo (Sassaman, 1982).

Dental changes

Children with Down syndrome seem to develop fewer caries than unaffected children. Numerous other dental problems, however, including brux-

ism, malocclusion, defective dentition, and periodontal disease, are more prevalent in this population (Gullikson, 1973) because of a combination of anatomic anomalies of the oral cavity and immunologic dysfunction. Of particular significance is juvenile periodontitis, which is present in approximately 100% of children with Down syndrome. The disease progresses rapidly and may be noted even in deciduous dentition (Reuland-Bosma and van Dijk, 1986). Not accounted for merely by poor dental care, it is suspected that the altered immune function in conjunction with the extensive gingival inflammation seen in children with Down syndrome are responsible (Reuland-Bosma, van Dijk, and van der Weele, 1986). Mouth breathing and consumption of a diet high in soft foods, two common occurrences in children with Down syndrome, also contribute to their dental problems.

Respiratory functioning

Pulmonary hypertension and pulmonary hyperplasia, fewer alveoli, a decreased alveolar blood capillary surface area, and associated upper airway obstruction (lymphatic hypertrophy in the Waldeyer ring), combined with a compromised immune system, predispose children with Down syndrome to respiratory tract infections. If recurrent severe respiratory tract infections occur, they will have a significant impact on the child's development.

Thyroid function

Thyroid dysfunction in Down syndrome is commonly associated with autoimmune dysfunction (Pueschel, 1990). Usually it is an acquired rather than a congenital condition, and the prevalence may reach 40% in adults. Graves' disease, goiter, chronic lymphocytic thyroiditis, and hypothyroidism occur most frequently. Although thyroid dysfunction may remain subclinical for an extended period, alterations in thyroid-stimulating hormone, thyroid-binding globulin, iodine-131 uptake, and the presence of antithyroglobulin and antimicrosomal antibodies may be seen (Coleman and Abbassi, 1984; Mani, 1988).

Leukemia

Children with Down syndrome have approximately a fifteenfold risk of developing leukemia compared with other children. Neither acute lymphoblastic leukemia (ALL) nor acute nonlymphoblastic leukemia (ANL) predominate (Robison et al., 1984). Children with Down syndrome have the same prognosis as children without Down syndrome if they are able to achieve an initial remission. Unfortunately, remission is more difficult to achieve from both ALL and ANL, because children with Down syndrome may have a poor tolerance to antineoplastic drugs (Garré et al., 1987).

PRIMARY CARE MANAGEMENT
Growth and development

Infants with Down syndrome weigh less and are typically shorter than unaffected children at birth (Cronk, 1978). The velocity of linear growth is also reduced, with the most marked reductions seen between 6 and 24 months of age. This reoccurs during adolescence, when the growth spurt is less vigorous than what would normally be expected (Cronk et al., 1988).

Children with Down syndrome have a tendency toward being overweight. Beginning around 2 years of age (Chumlea and Cronk, 1981), untoward weight gain persists throughout the child's lifetime. For virtually every age, more than 30% of children with Down syndrome are above the 85th percentile for weight/height ratios (Cronk et al., 1988). Those of school age show the greatest propensity for weight/height percentile gain.

Differences by sex are noted, with boys being heavier and taller than girls from 3 to 24 months and again during the teen years (Cronk et al., 1988). No meaningful differences in weight, stature, or head circumference, however, have been seen between white and black children with Down syndrome (Ershow, 1986). Environment also plays a role, with a greater number of children raised by their families showing increased weight/height ratios than for those children raised in institutions (Cronk, Chumlea, and Roche, 1985). Significant differences have been seen between growth parameters of Down syndrome children with and without congenital heart defects, with the severity of growth delay being correlated to the severity of disease (Cronk et al., 1988).

When linear growth is assessed, the variations in velocity must be taken into account by the practitioner. Whereas growth adequacy is often determined by maintaining a particular percentile rank, variations in growth velocity affect these children's growth curves during early childhood. Growth velocities for children with and without Down syndrome are similar during the school-aged period, however, and stability will then be seen in percentile curves.

Measurements should be plotted on both the National Center for Health Statistics (NCHS) growth charts and growth charts specifically normed for children with Down syndrome (Figs. 14-4 to 14-7). The NCHS growth charts allow comparisons of children with Down syndrome to their chronologic-age peers and provide a frame of reference for parents. Weight/height percentiles found on the NCHS growth charts are independent of the child's age and are also useful in determining appropriate weight in children before adolescence. The specialty charts, where all percentiles for stature are less than their analogous percentiles on the NCHS charts, provide an excellent reference point for comparing growth among children with Down syndrome and in determining those at risk for failure to thrive or obesity (Cronk, 1978). Because inappropriate growth and excessive weight gain have ramifications for motor performance and social acceptance for children with Down syndrome, yearly assessments are required. Interventions for weight management may be introduced as necessary. Caloric reduction and increased exercise incorporated into a behavior management program is the approach most likely to be effective.

Development. Because Down syndrome is associated with global development delay, virtually all children with Down syndrome will have intelligence quotients below the second standard deviation on standardized tests such as the Weschler Intelligence Scale for Children—Revised or the Stanford-Binet Intelligence Test. Performance on other language, motor, and social aptitude tests will also be less than age norms for almost all children.

Children with Down syndrome will pass through the normal developmental milestones but at a much slower rate than expected. The practitioner can assist in the child's development by referring the family to an early intervention program as soon as possible after the child's birth. In the presence of significant congenital anomalies, pro-

Text continued on p. 258.

Boys with Down Syndrome:
Physical Growth: 1 to 36 Months

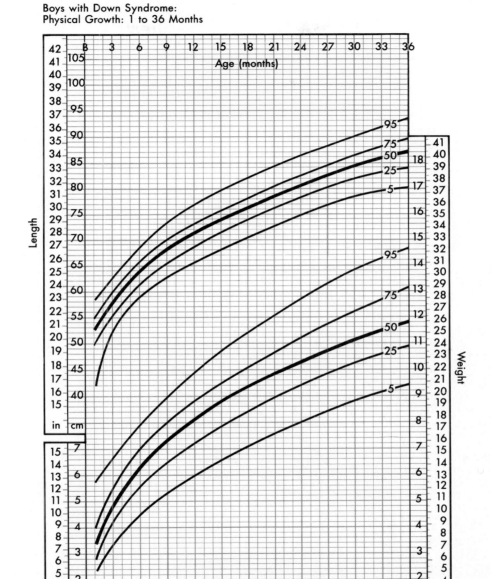

Fig. 14-4. Based on data from the Developmental Evaluation Clinic of the Children's Hospital, Boston, The Child Development Center of Rhode Island Hospital, and the Clinical Genetics Service of the Children's Hospital of Philadelphia. Supported by March of Dimes grant 6-449.

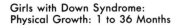

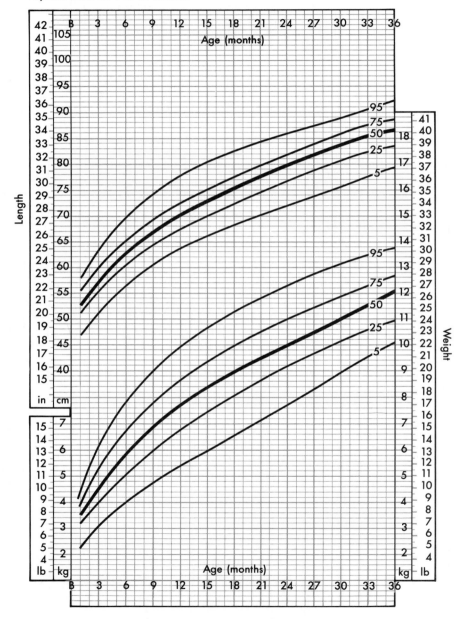

Fig. 14-5. Based on data from the Developmental Evaluation Clinic of the Children's Hospital, Boston, The Child Development Center of Rhode Island Hospital, and the Clinical Genetics Service of the Children's Hospital of Philadelphia. Supported by March of Dimes grant 6-449.

Boys with Down Syndrome:
Physical Growth: 2 to 18 Years

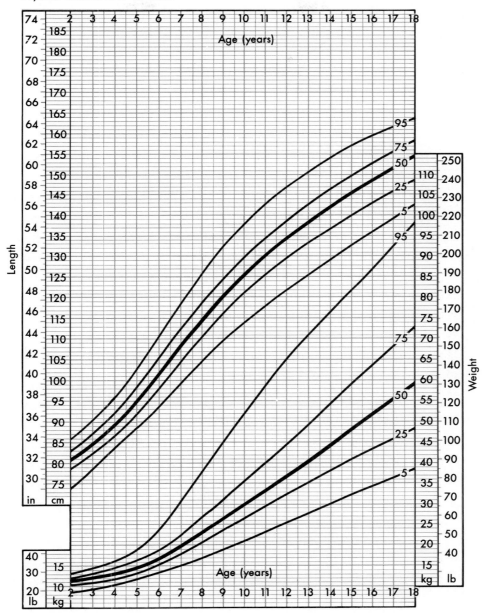

Fig. 14-6. Based on data from the Developmental Evaluation Clinic of the Children's Hospital, Boston, The Child Development Center of Rhode Island Hospital, and the Clinical Genetics Service of the Children's Hospital of Philadelphia. Supported by March of Dimes grant 6-449.

Girls with Down Syndrome:
Physical Growth: 2 to 18 Years

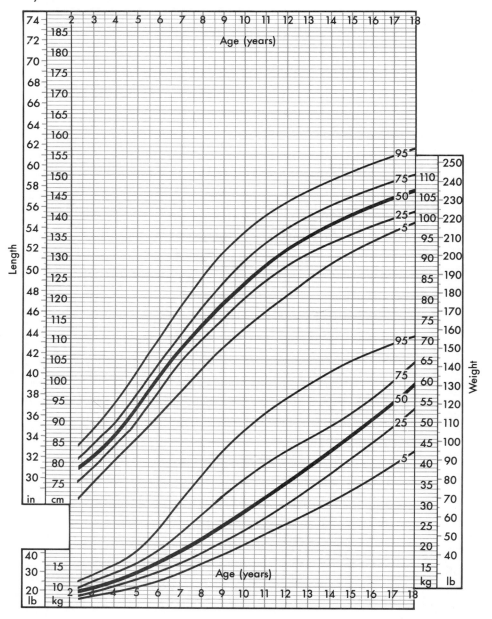

Fig. 14-7. Based on data from the Developmental Evaluation Clinic of the Children's Hospital, Boston, The Child Development Center of Rhode Island Hospital, and the Clinical Genetics Service of the Children's Hospital of Philadelphia. Supported by March of Dimes grant 6-449.

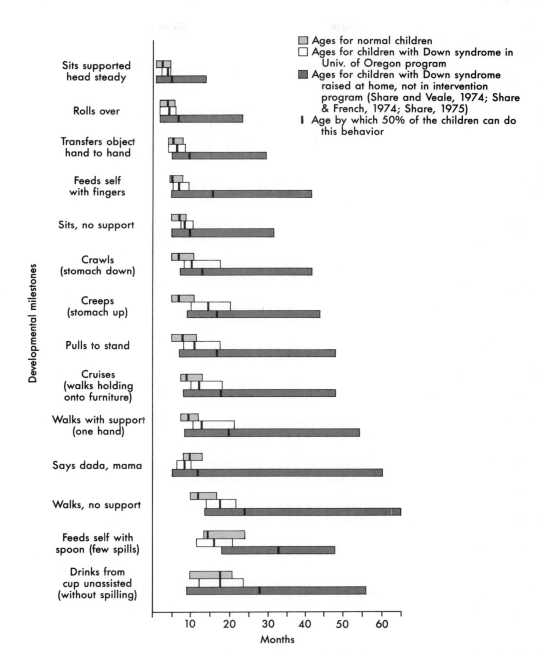

Fig. 14-8. Developmental milestones for children with Down syndrome. A new parents' guide. Kensington, MS, 1986, Woodbine House.

gram personnel will need guidance as to the intensity of activity the child is allowed. The child's progress should be carefully documented on standardized developmental schedules (Fig. 14-8) at each visit. Sharing the results of the child's developmental gains with the parents will objectively demonstrate the child's improvement, reinforcing their efforts.

Immunizations

Vaccination does not necessarily confer immunity in individuals with compromised secondary immune responses such as those seen in children with Down syndrome. Research that has investigated antibody response to immunization in children with Down syndrome is conflicting (Stiehm, 1989), and immunity should not be assumed by the practitioner. Additional immunizations may be necessary because this group of children is considered high risk for infection. In areas endemic for specific diseases, antibody titer levels may be assessed to determine a child's immune status. There are, however, no contraindications for immunizations for children with Down syndrome, and the national immunization schedule should be followed (Committee on Infectious Diseases, 1991).

Other immunizations. Pneumococcal polysaccharide vaccine (Pneumovax) is indicated for this population and is given at 2 years of age (Immunization Practices Advisory Committee, 1984). Yearly immunoprophylaxis for influenza should also be considered for all children more than 6 months of age. Current recommended dosages are two doses of 0.25 ml of split-virus vaccine for children 6 to 35 months of age and 0.50 ml of split-virus vaccine for children aged 3 to 12 years. Only split-virus vaccines should be given to children because they lessen the risk of postimmunization febrile episodes. Adolescents need only one 0.50-ml dose of either whole or split-virus vaccine (Immunization Practices Advisory Committee, 1989).

The hepatitis B exposure status of children who are or have been cared for in an institutional setting should be assessed because there is an increase in the prevalence of hepatitis B carriers among individuals with a history of institutionalization. For those who are surface antibody negative, immunization with hepatitis B vaccine (Recombivax) is highly recommended if they reside in an institu-

tional setting or are at other risk (Immunization Practices Advisory Committee, 1987). Children less than 11 years of age should receive three 5-μg doses at 1- and 5-month intervals, respectively. Family members, respite care providers, teachers, or other individuals working closely with children with Down syndrome may also be at increased risk of hepatitis B infection, depending on the child's status and their individual situation. Even though hepatitis B is not spread through casual contact, immunization for others is also recommended if circumstances warrant it.

Screening

Vision. Because of the large number of ocular defects associated with Down syndrome, all children should be evaluated by an ophthalmologist during infancy. Early referral is critical considering the synergistic effects that diminished vision and hearing have on development. Significant visual impairment is usually preventable because those conditions common in Down syndrome, such as strabismus and myopia are treatable (Caputo et al., 1989). Future screening recommendations should be determined in conjunction with the ophthalmologist according to the status of the child's eyes. At the minimum, the practitioner should screen for visual problems at each visit. Screening should include testing acuity, examining the red reflex and optic fundi, and checking alignment and oculomotor functions. Because children with Down syndrome may have difficulty using a Snellen or lazy E chart, acuity screening performed with the Titmus picture test or Allen picture cards will yield more valid results. The practitioner should note that some visual disorders, including cataracts and keratoconus, frequently do not develop until adolescence.

Many children with Down syndrome have difficulty keeping their glasses in place; therefore, parents should be counseled that purchasing glasses with lightweight plastic lenses and using an elastic strap around the child's occiput to secure them will help correct this problem. Contact lenses are not routinely recommended but may be appropriate for children with keratoconus.

Hearing. Because good hearing is a requisite for cognitive, social, and language development and because these children are at high risk for conductive hearing losses, careful assessment is needed. If the external ear orifice is so stenotic or other difficulties occur as to preclude adequate pneumootoscopic examination, alternate methods of evaluation must be used. Tympanometry provides one useful adjunct to assessment but is not reliable in children less than 1 year of age (Paradise, 1980). Because of the importance of early intervention, infants should be referred for microotoscopy between 9 and 12 months of age (Schwartz and Schwartz, 1978) if examination is difficult. Accumulation of cerumen leading to impacted canals is common; removal of cerumen every 6 months is recommended for children who have this problem. When middle ear disease occurs, it deserves aggressive intervention and close follow-up if further developmental insult is to be prevented.

If hearing aids are required, those that fasten onto the earpiece of eyeglasses may be useful alternatives. Hearing aids dependent on ear molds are difficult to fit for children who are just beginning to wear them. Frequently these children do not like the increased sound. Parents may need to be helped to find methods, such as behavior management, that will help improve their child's compliance for leaving the hearing aid in place. Parents must also be cautioned to devise mnemonic cues for remembering to change the batteries on a routine basis because it is unlikely that their child will be able to identify that their hearing aid is malfunctioning.

Dental. Because of the extremely high prevalence of dental problems in young children, aggressive dental care is necessary. The primary health care provider needs to document and carefully follow these children's dental problems. All children with Down syndrome should be evaluated before the age of 2 years by a dentist or pediadontist skilled in the care of children with developmental disabilities. Locating such dentists is often difficult for parents, and specific referrals to such professionals may be warranted.

Good dental hygiene, including frequent brushing and flossing, is indicated to reduce the amount of periodontal disease. If this is difficult, using a Water Pik should be considered. Effective toothbrushing techniques may be difficult to achieve because of the child's limited manual dexterity. Close supervision is required, and independent toothbrushing and mouth care may not be feasible

until the child is of school age or older (Hunter, 1987). Diets that contain low-sugar crunchy foods, such as fresh vegetables, will also help deter dental deterioration and should be encouraged. If periodontal disease is severe, chemical plaque control may be necessary. For children with congenital heart disease, prophylactic antibiotics should accompany all dental interventions (Dajani, 1990) (see Chapter 11).

Blood pressure. Routine screening is recommended. If there is a history of cardiac disease or a positive family history of hypertension more careful assessment is required.

Hematocrit. Routine screening is recommended.

Urinalysis. Routine screening is recommended.

Tuberculosis. Routine screening is recommended. No special precautions need to be taken unless the child is or has been institutionalized.

Condition-specific screening

THYROID DYSFUNCTION. Thyroid-stimulating hormone levels should be assessed yearly from birth. In the presence of any signs or symptoms suggestive of thyroid dysfunction, a complete thyroid panel should be drawn.

ATLANTOAXIAL INSTABILITY. In general, cervical spine x-ray studies should be considered for all children with Down syndrome after their second birthday (Pueschel, 1983). The risk of atlantoaxial subluxation must be appraised by the practitioner for all children who are planning on engaging in physically active exercise or sports (Committee on Sports Medicine, 1984) or are to undergo surgical or rehabilitative procedures (Msall et al., 1990).

HIP DISLOCATIONS. Assessing hip stability through age 10 years is indicated because early detection before the dislocation is fixed and acetabular dysplasia occurs will allow for optimal surgical correction. Early presenting signs of habitual dislocation are an increasing limp, decreasing activity, and an audible click. Pain does not usually occur unless the dislocation is acute. In older children, x-ray studies may be necessary for assessment.

Drug interactions

Down syndrome is associated with functional abnormalities in the neurotransmitter enzyme systems, with the cholinergic and noradrenergic systems particularly vulnerable (Coyle, Oster-Granite, and Gearhart, 1986). This may predispose children with Down syndrome to a hypersensitivity to cholinergic drugs, although the evidence is conflicting. Caution is advised if atropine, pilocarpine, or other related medications are to be given.

DIFFERENTIAL DIAGNOSIS AND MANAGEMENT OF COMMON PEDIATRIC CONDITIONS
Immune dysfunction

The significant changes in the immune systems of children with Down syndrome has significant implications for the practitioner. Specifically, all infections need to be treated aggressively because negative sequelae are more likely to develop. The incidence of many autoimmune diseases, including diabetes mellitus and juvenile rheumatoid arthritis, are also much greater in this population. Should a child exhibit signs and symptoms compatible with a diagnosis of any of these, thorough evaluation is indicated. Parents need to be educated about the signs and symptoms of conditions and the need to seek medical advice promptly (see Chapters 13 and 19).

Upper respiratory tract infections

Children with Down syndrome are prone to upper respiratory tract infections. These should be managed aggressively because untoward sequelae, including otitis media and pneumonia, are more apt to develop. Children with congenital heart disease should be examined at the first signs of illness; they are more likely to develop secondary problems, and parents may confuse an upper respiratory tract infection with early congestive heart failure. These children may also need to be given subacute bacterial endocarditis prophylaxis (see Chapter 11).

Behavioral changes

Behavioral changes may be caused by a variety of physiologic and psychologic problems, including (1) thyroid dysfunction, (2) obstructive sleep apnea, (3) neurodegeneration (primarily in older individuals), (4) declining physical competence (e.g., congestive heart failure), (5) disturbed home environment, and (6) overstimulation. Interventions must be cause specific. Trials with antide-pressants or antipsychotic drugs may be indicated in some cases after thorough evaluation.

Gastrointestinal symptoms

Because pyloric stenosis and Hirschsprung's disease are more common, the practitioner should carefully pursue complaints of persistent vomiting, constipation, or chronic diarrhea in infants. Constipation, a common problem, may also be related to inadequate peristalsis, poor diet, lack of exercise, or thyroid dysfunction. The cause of constipation must clearly be assessed so that the correct interventions are initiated.

Leukemia

Children with Down syndrome are at 15 to 20 times the risk for developing leukemia than other children. Easy bruising, unusual pallor, or listlessness, need to be fully evaluated. Parents must be alerted to not delay seeking health care for their child if any of these signs or symptoms develop.

DEVELOPMENTAL ISSUES
Safety

Safety issues for children with Down syndrome are the same as for their developmental, not chronologic, peers. Practitioners must adjust their normal schedule for providing anticipatory guidance to the development of the child with Down syndrome. If information is given too far in advance of the child's developmental progression, parents may forget or find it a painful reminder that their child is progressing more slowly than unaffected children.

Children with Down syndrome are more likely to sustain joint injuries as a result of their musculoskeletal problems. For children with atlantoaxial instability or those who have not yet been adequately evaluated, contact sports, somersaults, or other activities that may result in cervical injury should be restricted (Committee on Sports Medicine, 1984). Documentation that the child is not in danger of subluxation may be required for children participating in the Special Olympics.

Child care

Day care should provide appropriate social, cognitive, and physical stimulation for the child with Down syndrome. When selecting the type of day-care setting, parents should be encouraged to consider the child's personality and medical needs as well as their own philosophy about mainstreaming. Many generic day-care centers willingly mainstream children with Down syndrome into their programs and are sufficiently staffed to provide an excellent experience for the child. If the child has significant medical problems, specialized day care, often available through the school system, may be a better option. Practitioners should be aware of resources in their community to which parents may be referred to assist with day-care placement. The local affiliates of the Association of Retarded Citizens, the Association for the Care of Children's Health, or other specialty agencies may be helpful with this task.

All young children who attend group day care are more likely to experience a greater number of illnesses (Anderson et al., 1988; Wald et al., 1988), have more frequent hospitalizations (Bell et al., 1989; Johansen, Leibowitz, and Waite, 1988), and have a greater need for myringotomies (Wald et al., 1988) than children in home care.

If the individual child has proven to be highly susceptible to infections, a home care setting (less than six children) is recommended. As with all immunocompromised individuals, immunizations are an important component in prevention. If exposure to *Hemophilus influenzae* type b has occurred and the child is not immunized, rifampin prophylaxis may be considered (Committee on Infectious Diseases, 1984; Immunization Practices Advisory Committee, 1986).

Diet

Among the most significant concerns are feeding difficulties in young children and obesity in older children. Feeding problems may be encountered because of children's disproportionately large tongue, muscle flaccidity, poor coordination, significantly delayed social maturation, and congenital heart disease (Cullen et al., 1981).

For infants, breast-feeding should be encouraged. The immunogenic qualities offer additional protection against upper respiratory tract infections and other illnesses. The extra effort required of the child who is breast-feeding also helps develop the baby's orofacial muscles and tongue control and promotes greater jaw stability. Breast-feeding will take longer at first, and mothers will need to be encouraged in their efforts. In addition to standard guidance concerning breast-feeding, the practitioner may also suggest other helpful tips such as (1) awaking the infant for feeding, as necessary; (2) initially expressing some milk to encourage the infant to latch onto the breast; (3) assuring that the infant's nose and mouth are free of mucus; (4) checking that the infant's lip is turned out during feeding; and (5) holding the infant in an upright position during feeding (Danner and Cerutti, 1984, Riordan, 1983). For infants who are not breast-feeding, using soft, large-hole nipples may be helpful.

Blended and chopped foods and shallow-bowl, latex-covered spoons may be of some help in children who are learning to eat solids. If significant problems occur, consultation with an occupational therapist or other developmental therapist in designing an individualized feeding program is suggested.

For older children there are no routine dietary restrictions. Care should be taken to avoid excessive caloric intake if inappropriate weight gain is a problem.

Discipline

Children with Down syndrome are not usually more difficult to discipline than other children. Parents must be encouraged to remember that discipline needs to be appropriate for the child's developmental age, however, and not their chronologic age. Consistency in parental expectations and limit setting help prevent aberrant behavioral patterns from developing. Behavior management programs can be developed for specific discipline problems when the child has not been responsive to the parents' usual methods.

Toileting

The median age for toilet training children with Down syndrome is approximately 36 months. Parents need to be advised of this to reduce frustrations associated with unrealistic expectations. Routine toilet training techniques are effective. It will take longer, however, to train a child with Down syndrome, and additional positive reinforcement will be necessary.

Children with Down syndrome may suffer from constipation secondary to their generalized muscle flaccidity and low activity levels. Dietary corrections, occasional use of bulk laxatives, and increases in exercise can alleviate this problem.

Sleep patterns

Sleep disorders are uncommon in children with Down syndrome, with the exception of obstructive sleep apnea. Anatomic and immunologic differences predispose school-aged children in particular to this condition. A history of snoring, restless sleep, night terrors, and daytime somnolence should lead the practitioner to suspect that obstructive sleep apnea may be occurring, and referral to a sleep laboratory would be beneficial. Surgical interventions, including tonsillectomy, adenoidectomy, uvulopalatopharyngoplasty, and anterior reduction of the tongue, have been helpful in treating obstructive sleep apnea in this population (Donaldson and Redmond, 1988).

School issues

A variety of options for academic placement ranging from mainstreaming to residential placement exist. If circumstances permit, children with Down syndrome do best in a fully integrated environment with nondisabled peers. Families may need assistance in choosing the school setting that they think is most appropriate for their child. The primary care practitioner can be instrumental in helping the family locate the appropriate community services (e.g., mental health–mental retardation base service units) that will assist in educational placement.

All children with Down syndrome are eligible for educational provisions under Public Laws 99-457 and 94-142 (see Chapter 4). Parents should be encouraged to contact their social worker or local office of mental retardation shortly after the child's birth so that they can receive those educational, vocational, and supportive services for which the child is eligible.

Sexuality

Pubertal changes may occur earlier than normally expected in adolescents with Down syndrome (Evans and McKinlay, 1988). Accompanying these physical changes, adolescents will have similar social interests and biologic drives to their chronologic-age peers (Pueschel and Scola, 1988) and will need to be provided with the opportunity to participate in social activities with their peers. For parents who are highly protective, the social and sexual education that must accompany their children's increasing independence are often difficult and sensitive issues. The primary care provider needs to help parents recognize their responsibility in ensuring that their child can handle himself or herself in a socially and sexually appropriate manner.

Individualized instruction about self-care skills, biologic changes, social implications, and contraception is paramount so that both appearance of sexual impropriety and the risk of being sexually exploited may be minimized. Genetic counseling for both parents and child is necessary, because although men virtually always will be sterile, women are capable of reproducing. Planned Parenthood, the Association of Retarded Citizens, and parent support groups offer printed and audiovisual materials specifically designed for use with these families.

For some female adolescents, handling pubertal changes will be difficult. Family members need to be helped to recognize the behavior changes that may be related to normal hormonal cycles. For those who are menstruating and are unable to manage their own hygienic care, parents and other care givers must also take precautions in assisting if the adolescents are positive for hepatitis B.

Some parents may request sterilization of a daughter with Down syndrome. The right to procreative choice is protected by law, and statutes regarding sterilization vary dramatically from state to state (Williams, 1983). The practitioner is strongly suggested to consult with their state office of mental retardation for current guidelines, because in some jurisdictions sterilization is illegal. Professional practice standards from the American College of Obstetricians and Gynecologists and the American Academy of Pediatrics provide ethical guidelines for this difficult issue (Committee on Bioethics, 1990). If sterilization is to be pursued, the adolescent must participate in the decision to the extent possible and state and local laws strictly followed.

Special family concerns

Parenting a child with Down syndrome may be difficult. Because Down syndrome is associated with numerous health and developmental needs, raising these children can become overwhelming for some parents. Locating and coordinating acceptable medical, educational, and ancillary personnel may be highly stress producing. The primary care practitioner may be of tremendous assistance to the family in identifying appropriate resources and helping the parents become their child's lifelong case manager. Mothers in particular may find it difficult to balance their time and responsibilities among their children and spouse. Although many concerns are similar for all families with a special needs child, one notable issue for families of children with Down syndrome is the need for long-range planning. Some children with Down syndrome may never become totally self-sufficient, and families will need to plan for the child's lifetime. Others may marry and live semiindependent lives. The severity of the child's difficulty, internal family strengths, and the support offered from extended family and community networks all affect a family's adjustment.

Parents of children with Down syndrome will experience joy and pride in the child. They may also experience chronic sorrow. A natural response to an abnormal event, chronic sorrow is the prolonged sadness that parents may periodically experience at points throughout their child's lifetime (Olshansky, 1962). This occurs most commonly when developmental milestones, such as graduating high school, are missed (Wikler, Wascow, and Hatfield, 1981). For some parents this continued grief work is discomfiting, particularly if it is misinterpreted by professionals as pathologic grieving. Practitioners have the unique opportunity to assist families in recognizing that chronic sorrow is a normal extension of the grieving process and that their reactions are normal and healthy.

SUMMARY OF PRIMARY CARE NEEDS FOR THE CHILD WITH DOWN SYNDROME

Growth and development

Children usually have shorter stature and increased weight (after infancy).

Occipitofrontal circumference may be decreased.

Children should have height and weight measured at each visit and plotted on NCHS growth charts and normal growth charts for children with Down Syndrome.

Virtually all children will be mentally retarded and have global developmental delay.

Virtually all children will have hypotonia and joint laxity. Obesity compounds complications. Cognitive function often deteriorates with age. High incidence of early Alzheimer's disease.

Immunizations

Immunity may not be conferred from immunizations because of a compromised immune system. Titer analysis during outbreaks of communicable diseases is recommended.

Pneumococcal polysaccharide and influenza immunoprophylaxis should be considered.

Hepatitis B vaccine should be considered for all children who reside in an institutional setting.

Screening
Vision

High incidence of ocular defects. All infants should be evaluated by ophthalmologist.

Acuity and alignment testing and examination of the red reflex and optic fundi should be done at each visit.

Hearing

Anatomical abnormalities of ears common. Evaluation by specialist recommended during infancy.

Otoscopy and tympanometry should be performed at each visit.

50% to 76% have hearing loss. Many will require hearing aids.

Dental

Dental screening should be done a minimum of every 6 months from age 18 months because of the high incidence of periodontal disease.

Children with CHD may require antibiotic prophylaxis to prevent endocarditis.

Blood pressure

Routine screening is recommended.

Hematocrit

Routine screening is recommended.

Urinalysis

Routine screening is recommended.

Tuberculosis

Routine screening is recommended.

Condition-specific screening

Thyroid-stimulating hormone levels should be checked yearly if dysfunction is suggested.

Cervical spine x-ray studies to determine atlantoaxial stability should be done after age 2 years or before first surgery or athletic involvement.

Screening for hip dislocation is is necessary through age 10 years.

Drug interactions

Hypersensitivity to cholinergic drugs (e.g., atropine) is possible.

Differential diagnosis
Immune dysfunction

Children with Down syndrome are more susceptible to infections and autoimmune disorders.

Upper respiratory tract infections

Upper respiratory tract infections are often associated with otitis media and pneumonia and should be managed aggressively, especially when child has CHD.

Behavioral changes

Thyroid dysfunction, obstructive sleep apnea, neurodegeneration, declining physical competence, disturbed home environment, and overstimulation should be ruled out.

Gastrointestinal symptoms

Pyloric stenosis, megacolon, inadequate peristalsis, and thyroid dysfunction should be ruled out.

SUMMARY OF PRIMARY CARE NEEDS FOR THE CHILD WITH DOWN SYNDROME — cont'd

Leukemia

Unusual pallor, easy bruising, and listlessness should be fully evaluated.

Developmental issues
Safety

Anticipatory guidance needs to be based on the child's developmental level, not chronologic age.

Increased incidence of musculoskeletal injuries due to laxity.

Atlantoaxial instability a hazard. Must be ruled out before active sports program or surgery. Spine x-rays usually done at 2 yrs.

Child care

Small group day-care lessens the risk of repeated infections.

Eligible for special programs through 99-457 and 94-142.

Diet

Diets may need to be tailored to help correct constipation or obesity.

Discipline

Discipline must be developmentally appropriate; behavior management programs are often successful.

Toileting

Delayed bowel and bladder training may occur as a result of developmental lag; constipation is common because of low activity level, decreased peristalsis, poor diet.

Sleep patterns

Obstructive sleep apnea may occur; it is a problem of primarily school-aged children. Surgical intervention may be necessary.

School issues

Associated problems are covered by Public Laws 99-457 and 94-142; they assist families with school planning and mainstreaming.

Sexuality

Sex education must be taught so that children with Down syndrome are not abused and do not display inappropriate sexual behaviors.

Females may need assistance with menstrual hygiene.

Hepatitis B precaution advised.

Males are usually infertile but females may be fertile.

Special family concerns

Special family concerns include long-term care and chronic sorrow.

RESOURCES

Caring for a child with Down syndrome is a complex task because of the numerous physical, cognitive, and social concerns that must be addressed. Lists of additional resources for professionals and parents of children with Down syndrome follow.

Informational materials

Cunningham C: *Down's syndrome: An introduction for parents,* ed 2, Cambridge, Mass, 1988, Brookline Books. It is available from Brookline Books, Box 1046, Cambridge, MA 02238.

Hanson M: *Teaching the infant with Down syndrome: A guide for parents and professionals,* ed 2, Austin, Tex, 1988, Pro-Ed. It is available from Pro-Ed, 8700 Shoal Creek Blvd., Austin, TX 78758-6897.

Pueschel S, ed: *The young person with Down syndrome: Transition from adolescence to adulthood,* Baltimore, 1988, Brookes Publishing. It is available from Paul H. Brookes Publishing Co., Box 10624, Baltimore, MD 21285-0624.

Stray-Gundersen K, ed: *Babies with Down syndrome: A new parents guide,* Kensington, Md, 1986, Woodbine House. It is available from Woodbine House, Inc., 10400 Connecticut Ave., Kensington, MD 20895.

Tingey C: *Down syndrome: A resource handbook,* Waltham, Mass, 1988, College-Hill Press. It is available from College-Hill Press/Little, Brown, & Co., Order Dept., 200 West St., Waltham, MA 02254-9931.

Organizations

Association for Retarded Citizens
2501 Ave J
PO Box 6109
Arlington, TX 76011
(800) 433-5255

Commission on the Mentally Disabled
American Bar Association
1800 M St, NW
Washington, DC 20036
(202) 331-2240

National Down Syndrome Congress
1800 Dempster Rd
Park Ridge, IL 60068-1146
(800) 232-6372

National Down Syndrome Society
141 Fifth Ave
New York, NY 10010
(800) 221-4602

REFERENCES

Anderson LJ, Parker RA, Strikas RA, et al: Day-care center attendance and hospitalization for lower respiratory tract illness, *Pediatrics* 82:300-308, 1988.

Baird PA and Sadovnick AD: Life tables for Down syndrome, *Hum Genet* 82:291-292, 1989.

Bell DM, Gleiber DW, Mercer AA, et al: Illness associated with child day care: A study of incidence and cost, *Am J Public Health* 79:479-484, 1989.

Bennet GC, Rang M, Roye DP, et al: Dislocation of the hip in trisomy 21, *J Bone Joint Surg (Br)* 64:289-294, 1982.

Brown FR, Gree MK, Aylward EH, et al: Intellectual and adaptive functioning in individuals with Down syndrome in relation to age and environmental placement, *Pediatrics* 85(suppl 3):450-452, 1990.

Brown PM, Lewis GTR, Parker AJ, et al: The skull base and nasopharynx in Down's syndrome in relation to hearing impairment, *Clin Otolaryngol* 14:241-246, 1989.

Caputo AR, Wagner RS, Reynolds DR, et al: Down syndrome: Clinical review of ocular features, *Clin Pediatr* 28:355-358, 1989.

Chumlea WC and Cronk CE: Overweight among children with trisomy 21, *J Ment Defic Res* 25:275-280, 1981.

Cohen FL: *Clinical genetics in nursing practice,* Philadelphia, 1984, JB Lippincott.

Coleman M and Abbassi V: Down's syndrome and hypothyroidism: Coincidence or consequence, *Lancet* 1:(8376)69, 1984.

Committee on Bioethics: Sterilization of women who are mentally handicapped, *Pediatrics* 85:868-871, 1990.

Committee on Infectious Diseases, American Academy of Pediatrics: Revision of recommendation for use of rifampin prophylaxis of contacts of patients with *Haemophilus influenzae* infection, *Pediatrics* 74:301-302, 1984.

Committee on Sports Medicine, American Academy of Pediatrics: Atlantoaxial instability in Down syndrome, *Pediatrics* 74:152-153, 1984.

Coyle JT, Oster-Granite ML, and Gearhart JD: The neurobiologic consequences of Down syndrome, *Brain Res Bull* 16:773-787, 1986.

Cronk CE: Growth of children with Down's syndrome: Birth to age 3 years, *Pediatrics* 61:564-568, 1978.

Cronk CE, Chumlea WC, and Roche AF: Assessment of overweight children with trisomy 21, *Am J Ment Defic* 89:433-436, 1985.

Cronk C, Crocker AC, Pueschel SM, et al: Growth charts for children with Down syndrome: 1 month to 18 years of age, *Pediatrics* 81:102-110, 1988.

Cullen SM, Cronk CE, Pueschel SM, et al: Social development and feeding milestones of young Down syndrome children, *J Ment Defic* 85:410-415, 1981.

Dajani RS, Bisno AL, Chung KJ, et al: Prevention of bacterial endocarditis: recommendations by the American Heart Association, *JAMA* 264:2919-2922, 1990.

Danner SC and Cerutti ER: *Nursing your baby with Down's syndrome,* Rochester, NY, 1984, Childbirth Graphics.

Davies B: Auditory disorders in Down's syndrome, *Scand Audiol (Suppl)* 30:65-68, 1988.

Donaldson JD and Redmond WM: Surgical management of obstructive sleep apnea in children with Down syndrome, *J Otolaryngol* 17:398-403, 1988.

Ershow AG: Growth in black and white children with Down syndrome, *Am J Ment Defic* 90:507-512, 1986.

Evans AL and McKinlay IA: Sexual maturation in girls with severe mental handicap, *Child Care Health Dev* 14:59-69, 1988.

Ferencz C, Neill CA, Boughman JA, et al: Congenital cardiovascular malformations associated with chromosome abnormalities: An epidemiologic study, *J Pediatr* 114:79-86, 1989.

Garré ML, Relling MV, Kalwinsky D, et al: Pharmacokinetics and toxicity of methotrexate in children with Down syndrome and acute lymphocytic leukemia, *J Pediatr* 111:606-612, 1987.

Gibson D and Harris A: Aggregated early intervention effects for Down's syndrome persons: Patterning and longevity of benefits, *J Ment Defic Res* 32:1-17, 1988.

Hunter B: *Dental care for handicapped patients: A dental practitioner handbook,* Bristol, England, 1987, Wright.

Immunization Practices Advisory Committee: Update: Pneumococcal polysaccharide vaccine usage — United States, *MMWR* 33:273-281, 1984.

Immunization Practices Advisory Committee: Update: Prevention of *Haemophilus influenzae* type b disease, *MMWR* 35:170-180, 1986.

Immunization Practices Advisory Committee: Update on hepatitis B prevention, *MMWR* 36:355-366, 1987.

Immunization Practices Advisory Committee: Prevention and control of influenza: Part I. Vaccines, *MMWR* 38:297-311, 1989.

Johansen AS, Leibowitz A, and Waite LJ: Child care and children's illness, *Am J Public Health* 78:1175-1177, 1988.

Katz S and Kravetz S: Facial plastic surgery for persons with Down syndrome: Research findings and their professional and social implications, *Am J Ment Retard* 94:101-110, 1989.

Klaiman P and Arndt E: Facial reconstruction in Down syndrome: Perceptions of the results by parents and normal adolescents, *Cleft Palate J* 26:186-192, 1989.

Lang DJ, Van Dyke DC, Heide F, et al: Hypospadias and urethral abnormalities in Down syndrome, *Clin Pediatr* 26:40-42, 1987.

Levin S: The immune system and susceptibility to infections in Down's syndrome. In McCoy EE and Epstein CJ, eds: *Oncology and immunology of Down syndrome,* New York, 1987, Alan R Liss, pp 143-162.

Libb JW, Myers GJ, Graham E, et al: Correlates of intelligence and adaptive behaviour in Down's syndrome, *J Ment Defic Res* 27:205-210, 1983.

Mahon M: The nurse's role in treatment decision making for the child with disabilities, *Issues in Law and Medicine* 6, 247-268, 1990.

Mani C: Hypothyroidism in Down's syndrome, *Br J Psychiatry* 153:102-104, 1988.

Miola ES: Down syndrome: Update for practitioners, *Pediatr Nurs* 13:233-237, 1987.

Msall ME, Reese ME, DiGaudio K, et al: Symptomatic atlantoaxial instability associated with medical and rehabilitative procedures in children with Down syndrome, *Pediatrics* 85(suppl 3):447-449, 1990.

Olbrisch RR: Plastic surgical management of children with Down's syndrome: Indications and results, *Br J Plast Surg* 35:195-200, 1982.

Olshansky S: Chronic sorrow: A response to having a mentally defective child, *Soc Casework* 43:190-193, 1962.

Paradise JL: Otitis media in infants and children, *Pediatrics* 65:917-943, 1980.

Pueschel SM: Atlanto-axial subluxation in Down syndrome, *Lancet* 1:980, 1983.

Pueschel SM: Growth, thyroid function, and sexual maturation in Down syndrome, *Growth Genet Horm* 6:1-5, 1990.

Pueschel SM and Scola FH: Atlantoaxial instability in individuals with Down Syndrome: Epidemiologic, radiographic, and clinical studies, *Pediatrics* 80:555-560, 1987.

Pueschel SM and Scola PS: Parents' perception of social and sexual functions in adolescents with Down's syndrome, *J Ment Defic Res* 32:215-220, 1988.

Reuland-Bosma W and van Dijk LJ: Periodontal disease in Down's syndrome: A review, *J Clin Periodontol* 13:64-73, 1986.

Reuland-Bosma W, van Dijk LJ, and van der Weele L: Experimental gingivitis around deciduous teeth in children with Down's syndrome, *J Clin Periodontol* 13:294-300, 1986.

Riordan J: *A prenatal guide to breast feeding,* St Louis, 1983, CV Mosby.

Robison LL, Nesbit ME, Sather HN, et al: Down syndrome and acute leukemia in children: A 10-year retrospective survey from Childrens Cancer Study Group, *J Pediatr* 105:235-242, 1984.

Sassaman EA: Immunology. In Pueschel SM and Rynders JE, eds: *Down syndrome: Advances in biomedicine and the behavioral sciences,* Ware Press, Cambridge, MS, 1982, pp 229-232.

Schwartz DM and Schwartz RH: Acoustic impedance and otoscopic findings in young children with Down's syndrome, *Arch Otolaryngol* 104:652-656, 1978.

Stiehm ER: *Immunologic disorders in infants and children,* Philadelphia, 1989, WB Saunders.

Strauss RP, Mintzker Y, Feuerstein R, et al: Social perceptions of the effects of Down syndrome facial surgery: A school-based study of ratings by normal adolescents, *Plast Reconstruct Surg* 81:841-846, 1988.

Traboulsi EI, Levine E, Mets MB, et al: Infantile glaucoma in Down's syndrome (trisomy 21), *Am J Ophthalmol* 105:389-394, 1988.

Verma RS and Huq A: Sex ratio of children with trisomy 21 or Down syndrome, *Cytobios* 51:145-148, 1987.

Wald ER, Dashefsky B, Byers C, et al: Frequency and severity of infections in day care, *J Pediatr* 112:540-546, 1988.

Wikler L, Wascow M, and Hatfield E: Chronic sorrow revisited: Parent and professional depiction of adjustment of parents of mentally retarded children, *Am J Orthopsychiatry* 51:63-67, 1981.

Williams JK: Reproductive decisions: Adolescents with Down syndrome, *Pediatr Nurs* 9:43-44, 58, 1983.

Wysocki H, Wysocki J, and Wierusz-Wysocka B: The influence of thymus extract on the phagocytosis and the bactericidal capacity of polymorphonuclear neutrophils from children with Down's syndrome, *Ann NY Acad Sci* 496:740-742, 1987.

15 *Epilepsy*

Judith A. Farley

ETIOLOGY

Epilepsy is a chronic condition where there is repeated occurrence of seizure activity. Seizures are the abnormal discharge of electrical activity within the brain. When a sufficient number of neurons become overexcited, they discharge abnormally. This activity may or may not display clinical manifestations. If clinical manifestations do occur, the specific physical activity displayed will depend on the origin of the electrical activity and its expanse within the brain.

Epilepsy may be the result of an underlying disorder of the central nervous system (CNS) or a disorder that directly or indirectly effects the normal function of the CNS. Often, the true cause of epilepsy remains unknown (Hauser and Kurland, 1975).

Certain types of epilepsy have a familial predisposition, a genetic component, or both. Congenital structural anomalies of the CNS may cause epilepsy. Moreover, in the prenatal period, fetal infections, trauma, and maternal diseases have been identified as precipitating factors of epilepsy (American Association of Neuroscience Nurses [AANN], 1984; Newmark, 1984).

During the first month of life, asphyxia, intracranial hemorrhage, trauma, electrolyte imbalances, and inborn metabolic errors are thought to be potential causes of epilepsy. Primary infections of the CNS, including encephalitis and meningitis, or systemic infections resulting in persistent high fever have also been implicated as causative factors. Infants born to drug-addicted mothers with-draw during the neonatal period, which may also result in frequent reoccurring seizure activity (AANN, 1984; Newmark, 1984; Holmes, 1986).

The etiology of epilepsy in older children is generally the same as during the first month of life. In addition to those causes already discussed, this population of older individuals may have acute neurologic disorders or chronic conditions that have continued from earlier in life, such as infections (i.e., brain abscess), trauma, intracranial neoplasms, and degenerative disorders, all of which are associated with epilepsy (AANN, 1984; Gomez and Klass, 1982; Santilli and Sierzant, 1987).

INCIDENCE

The incidence of epilepsy varies greatly with age. The incidence is greatest in the population of infants less than 1 year of age, averaging roughly 1 per 1000 in the United States. Infants are particularly susceptible to developing epilepsy during the first 12 months of life. The incidence decreases with age. Seventy-five percent to 80% of epilepsy cases initially occur before 20 years of age, with 30% of the cases initially occurring within the first 4 years of life (Epilepsy Foundation of America, 1975). Approximately 50 per 100,000 individuals in the United States are newly affected each year (Holmes, 1986; Penry, 1986).

CLINICAL MANIFESTATIONS AT TIME OF DIAGNOSIS

The clinical manifestations at the time of diagnosis will vary depending on the primary cause and the

Table 15-1. Classification system of epileptic seizures

I. PARTIAL (FOCAL, LOCAL) SEIZURES

Partial seizures are those in which, in general, the first clinical and electroencephalographic (EEG) changes indicate initial activation of a system of neurons limited to part of one cerebral hemisphere. A partial seizure is classified primarily on the basis of whether or not consciousness is impaired during the attack. When consciousness is not impaired, the seizure is classified as a simple partial seizure. When consciousness is impaired, the seizure is classified as a complex partial seizure. Impairment of consciousness may be the first clinical sign, or simple partial seizures may evolve into complex partial seizures. In patients with impaired consciousness, aberrations of behavior (automatisms) may occur. A partial seizure may not terminate but instead progress to a generalized motor seizure. Impaired consciousness is defined as the inability to respond normally to exogenous stimuli by virtue of altered awareness and/or responsiveness.

There is considerable evidence that simple partial seizures usually have unilateral hemispheric involvement and only rarely have bilateral hemispheric involvement; complex partial seizures, however, frequently have bilateral hemispheric involvement.

Partial seizures can be classified into one of the following three fundamental groups:
- Simple partial seizures
- Complex partial seizures:
  With impairment of consciousness at onset
  Simple partial onset followed by impairment of consciousness
- Partial seizures evolving to generalized tonic-clonic convulsions:
  Simple evolving to generalized tonic-clonic convulsions
  Complex evolving to generalized tonic-clonic convulsions (including those with simple partial onset)

Clinical seizure type	EEG seizure type
A. Simple partial seizures (consciousness not impaired)	Local contralateral discharge starting over the corresponding area of cortical representation (not always recorded on the scalp)
1. With motor signs	
(a) Focal motor without march	
(b) Focal motor with march (jacksonian)	
(c) Versive	
(d) Postural	
(e) Phonatory (vocalization or arrest of speech)	
2. With somatosensory or special-sensory symptoms (simple hallucinations, e.g., tingling, light flashes, buzzing)	
(a) Somatosensory	
(b) Visual	
(c) Auditory	
(d) Olfactory	
(e) Gustatory	
(f) Vertiginous	
3. With autonomic symptoms or signs (including epigastric sensation, pallor, sweating, flushing, piloerection and pupillary dilation)	
4. With psychic symptoms (disturbance of higher cerebral function); these symptoms rarely occur without impairment of consciousness and are much more commonly experienced as complex partial seizures	
(a) Dysphasic	

Continued.

Table 15-1. Classification system of epileptic seizures—cont'd

Clinical seizure type	EEG seizure type
(b) Dysmnesic (e.g., dé-jà vu) (c) Cognitive (e.g., dreamy states, distortions of time sense) (d) Affective (fear, anger, etc.) (e) Illusions (e.g., macropsia) (f) Structured hallucinations (e.g., music, scenes)	

B. Complex partial seizures (with impairment of consciousness; may sometimes begin with simple symptoms)
 1. Simple partial onset followed by impairment of consciousness
  (a) With simple partial features, followed by impaired consciousness
  (b) With automatisms
 2. With impairment of consciousness at onset
  (a) With impairment of consciousness only
  (b) With automatisms
	Unilateral or, frequently, bilateral discharge; diffuse or focal in temporal or frontotemporal regions

C. Partial seizures evolving to secondarily generalized seizures (may be generalized tonic-clonic, tonic, or clonic) 1. Simple partial seizures (A) evolving to generalized seizures 2. Complex partial seizures (B) evolving to generalized seizures 3. Simple partial seizures evolving to complex seizures evolving to generalized seizures	Discharges listed earlier become secondarily and rapidly generalized

II. GENERALIZED SEIZURES (CONVULSIVE OR NONCONVULSIVE)

Generalized seizures are those in which the first clinical changes indicate initial involvement of both hemispheres. Consciousness may be impaired, and this impairment may be the initial manifestation. Motor manifestations are bilateral. The ictal EEG patterns initially are bilateral and presumably reflect neuronal discharge that is widespread in both hemispheres.

Clinical seizure type	EEG seizure type

A. Absence seizures
 1. Typical absence seizures
  (a) Impairment of consciousness only
  (b) With mild clonic components
  (c) With atonic components
  (d) With tonic components
  (e) With automatisms
  (f) With autonomic components (b-f may be used alone or in combination)
	Usually regular and symmetric 3-Hz, but may be 2 to 4-Hz, spike-and-slow-wave complexes; may have multiple spike-and-slow-wave complexes; abnormalities bilateral

2. Atypical absence seizures, which may have:
  (a) Changes in tone that are more pronounced
  (b) Onset and/or cessation that is not abrupt
	EEG more heterogeneous; may include irregular spike-and-slow-wave complexes, fast activity or other paroxysmal activity; abnormalities bilateral but often irregular and asymmetric

Table 15-1. Classification system of epileptic seizures—cont'd

Clinical seizure type	EEG seizure type
B. Myoclonic seizures (single or multiple myoclonic jerks)	Polyspike and wave or sometimes spike and wave or sharp and slow waves
C. Clonic seizures	Fast activity ($\geq$10 c/sec) and slow waves; occasional spike-and-wave patterns
D. Tonic seizures	Low voltage fast activity, a fast rhythm of 9-10 c/sec, or more decreasing in frequency and increasing in amplitude
E. Tonic-clonic seizures	Rhythm at $\geq$10 c/sec, decreasing in frequency and increasing in amplitude during tonic phase, interrupted by slow waves during clonic phase
F. Atonic seizures (astatic) (combinations of the above may occur, e.g., B and F, B and D)	Polyspikes and waves or flattening or low-voltage fast activity

III. UNCLASSIFIED EPILEPTIC SEIZURES

These include all seizures that cannot be classified because of inadequate or incomplete data and some that defy classification in hitherto described categories. They include some neonatal seizures (e.g., rhythmic eye movements, chewing, and swimming movements).

IV. ADDENDUM

Repeated epileptic seizures occur under a variety of circumstances:
1. As fortuitous attacks, coming unexpectedly and without any apparent provocation.
2. As cyclic attacks, at more or less regular intervals (e.g., in relation to the menstrual cycle, or the sleep-waking cycle).
3. As attacks provoked by (a) nonsensory factors (fatigue, alcohol, emotion, etc.) or (b) sensory factors, sometimes referred to as "reflex seizures."

The term "status epilepticus" is used whenever a seizure persists for a sufficient length of time or is repeated frequently enough that recovery between attacks does not occur. Status epilepticus may be divided into partial (e.g., jacksonian), or generalized (e.g., absence status or tonic-clonic status). When very localized motor status occurs, it is referred to as "epilepsia partialis continua."

Adapted from *Epilepsia* 22:489-501, 1981.

extent and involvement of abnormal electrical discharges within neuronal tissue. Because of the diversities and complexities that seizure activity invariably displays, an international classification system was adopted in 1970 and revised in 1981 (Table 15-1). This classification system groups seizures with similar clinical manifestations. The general purpose of this classification system is to assist the clinician with the assessment of the clinical course, the identification of appropriate treatment, and the evaluation of the individual's response to therapy (Bancaud et al., 1981; Gastaut, 1970).

The international classification system of epilepsy contains three major groupings: (1) partial seizures, (2) generalized seizures; and (3) unclassified epileptic seizures. Each major grouping is divided into subsets based on clinical manifestations and EEG findings.

Partial seizures are characterized by seizure activity that begins and is usually limited to one part of either the left or right cerebral hemisphere. A simple partial seizure refers to seizure activity that occurs without loss of consciousness. A complex partial seizure refers to seizure activity that occurs with impairment or loss of consciousness. The clinical activity displayed by the individual is contingent on the particular part of the cortex from which it is generated. For example, partial seizures may result in abnormal motor activity, such as muscle twitching or loss of tone, or sensory changes, such as tingling or numbness (Dreifuss, 1984; Holmes, 1986; Penry, 1986).

INTERNATIONAL CLASSIFICATION OF EPILEPSIES AND EPILEPTIC SYNDROMES

1. Localization-related (focal, local, partial) epilepsies and syndromes
1.1 Idiopathic (with age-related onset)
   At present the following syndromes are established, but more may be identified in the future:
   Benign childhood epilepsy with centrotemporal spike
   Childhood epilepsy with occipital paroxysms
   Primary reading epilepsy
1.2 Symptomatic
   Chronic progressive epilepsia partialis continua of childhood (Kojewnikow's syndrome)
   Syndromes characterized by seizures with specific modes of precipitation
1.3 Cryptogenic
   Presumed to be symptomatic; etiology unknown
2. Generalized epilepsies and syndromes
2.1 Idiopathic (with age-related onset; listed in order of age)
   Benign neonatal familial convulsions
   Benign neonatal convulsions
   Benign myoclonic epilepsy in infancy
   Childhood absence epilepsy (pyknolepsy)
   Juvenile absence epilepsy
   Juvenile myoclonic epilepsy (impulsive petit mal)
   Epilepsy with grand mal seizures on wakening
   Other generalized idiopathic epilepsies not already defined
   Epilepsies with seizures precipitated by specific modes of activation
2.2 Cryptogenic or symptomatic (in order of age)
   West's syndrome (infantile spasms, Blitz-Nick-Salaam Krämpfe)
   Lennox-Gastaut syndrome
   Epilepsy with myoclonic-astatic seizures
   Epilepsy with myoclonic absences

2.3 Symptomatic
   2.3.1 Nonspecific etiology
      Early myoclonic encephalopathy
      Early infantile epileptic encephalopathy with suppression burst
      Other symptomatic generalized epilepsies not already defined
   2.3.2 Specific syndromes
      Epileptic seizures may complicate many disease states; under this heading are diseases in which seizures are the presenting or predominant feature
3. Epilepsies and syndromes undetermined whether focal or generalized
3.1 With both generalized and focal seizures
   Neonatal seizures
   Severe myoclonic epilepsy in infancy
   Epilepsy with continuous spike-waves during slow-wave sleep
   Acquired epileptic aphasia (Landau-Kleffner syndrome)
   Other undetermined epilepsies not already defined
3.2 Without unequivocal generalized or focal features; all cases with generalized tonic-clonic seizures in which clinical EEG findings do not permit classification as clearly generalized or localization related (e.g., in many cases of sleep-grand mal) are considered not to have unequivocal generalized or focal features.
4. Special syndromes
4.1 Situations-related seizures (Gelegenheitsanfälle)
   Febrile convulsions
   Isolated seizures or isolated status epilepticus
   Seizures occurring only when there is an acute metabolic or toxic event caused by such factors as alcohol, drugs, eclampsia, nonketotic, hyperglycemic

Adapted from Commission on Classification and Terminology of the International League Against Epilepsy: *Epilepsia* 30:389-399, 1989.

In general, a simple partial seizure is confined to one cerebral hemisphere, whereas a complex partial seizure involves both hemispheres. A partial seizure (simple or complex) may evolve into a generalized tonic-clonic, tonic, or clonic convulsion (see Table 15-1) (Dreifuss, 1984; Holmes, 1986; Penry, 1986).

Generalized seizures are those in which the first clinical manifestations indicate that the seizure activity starts or involves both cerebral hemispheres. In this grouping of seizures, consciousness may be impaired. The clinical manifestations may include convulsive activity, although others, such as absence seizures, have nonconvulsive activity. Because both hemispheres are involved, the clinical manifestations are almost always bilateral (see Table 15-1) (Dreifuss, 1984; Holmes, 1986; Penry, 1986).

Not all seizure disorders fit neatly into a classified grouping. These seizures are referred to as unclassified epileptic seizures and characteristically have a wide variety of abnormal clinical activity. Examples of this activity may include rhythmic eye movements, chewing, and swimming movements. These activities are commonly seen in neonatal seizures (Dreifuss, 1984: Holmes, 1986; Penry, 1986).

Status epilepticus is defined as the state of continuing or recurring seizure activity in which recovery between seizures is incomplete. The seizure activity is unrelenting and usually lasts for 30 minutes or more. Any one of the seizure activities classified can evolve into status epilepticus. The state of status epilepticus should be considered a medical emergency and requires immediate intervention (AANN, 1984; Lederman, 1984; Pellock, 1984).

In addition to the seizures classified by the international system, there are several types of epileptic syndromes. These are seizure disorders that display a group of signs and symptoms that collectively characterize or indicate a particular condition. An additional classification system of these syndromes has been proposed by the International League Against Epilepsy and revised in 1989 (see the box on p. 272) (Dreifuss et al., 1985; International League Against Epilepsy, 1989). Several syndromes associated with epilepsy occur in infants and children. The three syndromes that occur most

often are infantile spasms, Lennox-Gastaut syndrome, and juvenile myoclonic epilepsy.

Infantile spasms are a form of epilepsy characterized by a variety of clinical manifestations. The infant may have episodes of sudden flexion or extension movements involving the neck, trunk, and extremities. Clinical manifestations of the resulting spasms may range from subtle head nods to violent body contractions, commonly referred to as "jacknife seizures." Onset of infantile spasms is usually between 3 and 12 months of age. They may be idiopathic or occur in response to a CNS insult. An EEG will display the classic hypsarrhythmia pattern of epileptic spike and wave discharges on a slow disorganized background (Gomez and Klass, 1982; Lombroso, 1983). Infantile spasms manifest a typical clinical course. The "spasms" usually occur in clusters and from 5 to 150 times daily, and they are usually worse when waking or falling asleep. Once it begins, the seizure activity increases in intensity and severity over time. Invariably there is a loss of developmental milestones associated with this syndrome (Gomez and Klass, 1982; Lombroso, 1983).

Lennox-Gastaut syndrome is an epileptic syndrome characterized by an onset of seizures early in childhood, usually around 1 to 5 years of age. This syndrome includes a variety of generalized seizures — predominantly tonic-clonic, atonic (drop attacks), akinetic, absence, and myoclonic activity. Mental retardation and delayed psychomotor development are often associated with this syndrome (Gomez and Klass 1982; Holmes, 1986).

Juvenile myoclonic epilepsy is a primary generalized epilepsy that usually affects adolescents and young adults. This is a relatively benign form of epilepsy involving myoclonic jerks of the neck, shoulders, and arms. The seizures may occur singularly or repetitively. This form of epilepsy is commonly associated with a normal neurologic examination, normal intelligence, and a positive family history of seizures (Delgado-Escueta and Enrile-Bacsal, 1984; Dreifuss, 1989).

TREATMENT

Specific treatment for epilepsy is directed at the particular clinical manifestations or syndrome of seizure activity and its underlying causes. Several other factors need to be considered in addition to

Table 15-2. Commonly used antiepileptic drugs*

Drug	Dosage/internal	Therapeutic plasma level	Seizure type	Common side effects	Adverse side effects
ACTH	Begin 40 units IM qd (taper gradually) Treatment course 2-4 mo		Infantile spasm	Hypertension GI distress Weight gain Electrolyte disturbance	Infection GI bleeding Sodium retention
Clonazapam (Clonopin)	0.1-0.2 mg/kg tid	0.01-0.08	Absence Generalized tonic-clonic Myoclonic Simple partial Complex partial	Drowsiness Ataxia GI distress	Behavioral changes Hyperactivity Cognitive dysfunction
Valproic acid (Depakote)	30-60 mg/kg qid	40-150	Absence Generalized tonic-clonic Myoclonic Simple partial Complex partial	Nausea-vomiting Fatigue with initiation Hair loss	Thrombocytopenia Pancreatitis Hepatic dysfunction Liver toxicity
Primidone (Mysoline)	10-25 mg/kg/day 3-4 times/day	5-12†	Tonic-clonic Complex partial Simple partial	Drowsiness Hyperactivity Ataxia Behavior changes	Oversedation Behavioral disturbances GI dysfunction
Phenytoin (Dilantin)	4-8 mg/kg bid	10-20	Generalized tonic-clonic Simple partial Complex partial	Gingival hyperplasia	Lethargy; ataxia; dizziness Skin reaction (rash) Hepatic dysfunction
Phenobarbitol	2-4 mg/kg qd; bid	15-40	Generalized tonic-clonic Myoclonic Simple partial Complex partial	Fatigue with initiation of treatment Hyperactivity Mood changes Irritability	Rash Lethargy Learning difficulties Behavioral changes Hepatic dysfunction
Carbamazepine (Tegretol)	10-30 mg/kg tid; qid	6-12	Generalized tonic-clonic Simple partial Complex partial	Drowsiness Ataxia; dizziness GI distress Irritability	Leukopenia Movement disorders Rashes Hepatic dysfunction Bone marrow suppression

Modified from *Physicians' Desk Reference*, ed 44, Oradell, NJ, 1990, Edward R Barnhart.
*ACTH, adrenocorticotropic hormone; IM, intramuscular; qd, every day; GI, gastrointestinal; tid, 3 times daily; qid, 4 times daily; bid, twice daily.
†When testing mysoline levels, always check phenobarbital levels as well.

the clinical manifestations presented at the time of diagnosis. The history, physical examination, and developmental examination present invaluable information needed to band the multitude of pieces that contribute to the diagnosis. The child's birth history and record of milestone achievement must also be considered. Family history must be explored for seizures. Report of presenting signs and symptoms, associated factors such as fever, or undisclosed head trauma (child abuse) are important considerations for the primary care practitioner to explore. Evaluation and testing, including an EEG to isolate the focus or origin and involvement of seizure activity in the brain and a computerized tomography scan or a magnetic resonance imaging (or both) of the brain to investigate the presence of a lesion or abnormal tissue, are also indicated. Finally, a complete metabolic work-up must be reviewed to explore the possibility of a deficiency or malabsorption (Dreifuss, 1984; Gomez and Klass, 1982; Holmes, 1986; Penry, 1986).

Treatment usually begins with the use of anticonvulsant medications (Table 15-2). Often the epileptic pattern and clinical course require the use of more than one drug in an effort to control the abnormal discharges. The child's age, classification of seizures, medication side effects, and compliance must be considered when a particular medication regimen is chosen (Dreifuss, 1984; Gomez and Klass, 1982; Holmes, 1986; Penry, 1986; Santilli and Sierzant, 1987).

Surgery is also a treatment for some forms of epilepsy. As with medical interventions, this form of treatment for epilepsy is directed at the particular clinical manifestations of seizure activity, the EEG findings, and underlying causes. If a site of origin or a seizure focus is identified, it may be possible to remove this area of the brain, eliminating seizure activity with no or little neurologic impairment. Certain forms of partial seizure disorders can be treated successfully with focal resective surgery (Brewer and Sperling, 1988; Santilli and Sierzant, 1987; Spencer, 1986).

The surgical removal of a cerebral hemisphere is a treatment available for children with unilateral hemispheric disease and medically intractable epilepsy. Total or partial hemispherectomies may be performed in effort to control localized epileptic conditions that are extremely complex and have a profound impact on the child's activities of daily living and life span (Bare, 1989; Spencer, 1986).

Corpus callosotomy is another neurosurgical treatment used to control generalized seizures (involving both hemispheres) that are medically intractable. Basically the corpus callosum is the bridge between the right and left cerebral hemispheres. In this classification of epilepsy, the abnormal electrical discharge begins in one hemisphere and crosses over the corpus callosum to the opposite hemisphere, creating a generalized response. This surgical procedure partially or completely severs this connecting bridge. The main objective of this treatment is to stop or decrease secondary generalization of seizure activity. A palliative procedure, it is done in an effort to minimize physical injury that may occur during seizure activity and decrease the need for anticonvulsant medications (Geoffroy et al., 1983; Luessenhop, dela Cruz, and Fenichel, 1970; Spencer and Spencer, 1989).

The ketogenic diet is a form of treatment for certain types of medically intractable epilepsies. This diet consists of foods with a high fat content and low carbohydrate and protein contents. The exact therapeutic mechanism is not completely known. It is thought, however, that the ketone bodies produced by this diet have an antiepileptic effect (DeVivo, 1983; Huttenlocher, 1976).

Both surgical and nutritional interventions almost always require concurrent medical treatment with antiepileptic drugs.

PROGNOSIS

The prognosis for epilepsy depends greatly on the type and severity of the disorder, the age of onset, coexisting disorders, and the type and success of medical, surgical, and nutritional therapy. Clearly, if a child's brain is active with abnormal electrical activity, the opportunity for normal growth, development and learning is limited. The convulsive disorders do not in themselves cause irreversible brain damage; rather, they take away the potential for normal brain and intellectual development.

As with the classification of epilepsy, clinical manifestations, treatment, and prognosis of epilepsy are dependent on many factors. Some seizure disorders cease or improve with age, others persist, and others become worse. The type of seizures and the age of onset help to determine treatment responsiveness and therefore the impact on the child's general prognosis. Epilepsies that start late in childhood and early adolescence usually have an excellent prognosis, with approximately 60% to 95% being controlled by drug treatment. However, the likelihood of continued freedom from seizures after withdrawal of medications varies greatly (Delgado-Esueta, Treiman, and Walsh, 1983; Thurston et al., 1982).

The forms of epilepsy that are more difficult to treat have a worse prognosis due to the impaired neurologic functioning and altered growth and development. The functional outcomes in seizure disorders that are more difficult to control are hard to predict but generally have a poorer prognosis (Dreifuss, 1984; Gomez and Klass, 1982; Holmes, 1986; Penry, 1986).

Several studies have estimated that approximately 40% to 50% of children diagnosed with epilepsy will eventually be seizure free. This remission state has been documented for as long as 5 to 20 years, and many of the children will stop taking all anticonvulsant medications during this time (Annegers, Hauser, and Elveback, 1979; Sofijanov, 1982; Thurston et al., 1982).

ASSOCIATED PROBLEMS

The etiology, age of onset, type of seizures, frequency of occurrence, and success of treatment all influence problems related to epilepsy.

Injury during seizures

There is the potential for injury during seizure activity. A child may sustain direct trauma, fall, or aspirate during a seizure. It is therefore vital for parents, care givers, and teachers to be knowledgeable about appropriate first-aid interventions to minimize injury in the event of a seizure.

Cognitive dysfunction

Children with epilepsy may also have various cognitive dysfunctions. In general, the intelligence quotients of these children are slightly lower than average (Holmes, 1986). Memory function is housed in the temporal lobe region of the left hemisphere. Children with complex partial seizures that emanate from the temporal lobe region have been reported to have difficulty with memory functions

(Lavadas, Umilta and Provinciali, 1979; Mayeux et al., 1980). Children with partial seizures manifested as staring spells may also have an impaired attention span. Specific antiepileptic drugs may further alter or impair selected facets of cognition, including memory and attention span (Dreifuss, 1984; Holmes, 1986).

Psychiatric problems

There is a greater incidence of psychiatric problems, emotional disturbances, and psychosocial and behavioral problems in children with epilepsy than in children with other chronic conditions or in the general population (Matthews, Barabas, and Ferrari, 1982; Rutter, Graham, and Yule, 1970).

PRIMARY CARE MANAGEMENT
Growth and development

The primary care practitioner must monitor body growth and total development for the child with epilepsy. It is particularly important to regularly obtain body heights and weights on these children, especially if there has been significant losses, gains, or dramatic growth spurts as in adolescence. It is critical that this information be kept current because antiepileptic drug dosages are calculated and prescribed for the child according to body weight to maintain therapeutic levels.

Primary care management and interventions related to the child's social, cognitive, and motor development depend greatly on the severity of the seizure disorder and underlying neurologic complications. Screening and assessment tools such as the Denver Developmental Screening Tool or Wechsler Intelligence Scale for Children, and regular neuropsychologic evaluations, help to identify the particular strengths and weaknesses or potential for weaknesses as the child matures.

If developmental delays are detected, these infants, children, and families may benefit from infant stimulation or early intervention programs. These programs are usually community based and provide therapy for the child and education for the parents focusing on developmental needs and appropriate child-centered interventions.

Immunizations

There is increased risk for infants and children with underlying seizure disorders of having a seizure after receiving either the diphtheria, tetanus, and pertussis (DTP) vaccine or the measles vaccine (Committee on Infectious Diseases, 1991). The present recommendations from the American Academy of Pediatrics regarding the DTP immunization in infants and children with neurologic disorders are as follows:

1. Administration of the pertussis vaccine may be, and in many cases should be, deferred in children with a progressive neurologic disorder (i.e., infantile spasm, uncontrolled epilepsy).

2. Infants and children with a history of seizures should have the pertussis vaccine deferred until the progress of the neurologic condition is determined. Children with well-controlled seizures or who are neurologically stable should receive the pertussis vaccine.

3. Children who are suspected or predisposed to developing a progressive neurologic condition with seizures should have the pertussis vaccine deferred until such time that the diagnosis can be determined.

4. A family history of seizures is not a contraindication for the child to receive the pertussis vaccine (Committee on Infectious Diseases, 1991).

If deferment of the pertussis vaccine is necessary, the American Academy of Pediatrics recommends that DTP vaccine be held completely until the child's first birthday. At this time a decision to administer either the complete DTP or just the DT vaccine can be made based on the previous criteria. Receipt of the DTP immunization frequently results in fever; therefore, the American Academy of Pediatrics also recommends that children who are predisposed to seizures and receive the DTP vaccine be given acetaminophen (15 mg/kg/dose) every 4-6 hours for 24 hours to control a fever and therefore possibly lower the child's seizure threshold. As with all difficult health care questions, the practitioner must view each infant and child in question individually and involve the family in the decision-making process.

Receipt of the measles vaccine frequently results in fever. The American Academy of Pediatrics recommends that the measles vaccine be administered to children who are predisposed to develop seizures or who have a positive history of seizures. Therefore, the same prophylactic therapy of acetaminophen (15 mg/kg/dose) every 4-6 hours for 24 hours after receipt of the vaccine is advised.

All other immunizations should be given according to routine schedule.

Screening

Vision. Routine screening is recommended.

Hearing. Routine screening is recommended.

Dental. Routine dental care is recommended. Gingival hyperplasia is a common occurrence in children receiving phenytoin (Dilantin) (PDR, 1990). Use of this antiepileptic drug may require more frequent brushing and flossing, with particular attention given to the child's gums. The dentist should be informed of the use of this antiepileptic drug.

Blood pressure. Infants treated with ACTH therapy require daily blood pressure monitoring for potential hypertension. Therefore, parents should be taught how to take and monitor the infant's blood pressure while receiving ACTH therapy.

Hematocrit. Routine screening is recommended.

Urinalysis. Routine screening is recommended.

Tuberculosis. Routine screening is recommended.

Condition-specific screening

DRUG TOXICITY SCREENING. Decreased hematocrit levels with increased bruising or bleeding in a child taking valproic acid (Depakene), carbamazepine (Tegretol), and phenytoin (Dilantin) may indicate thrombocytopenia, blood dyscrasia, and liver dysfunction. Complete blood cell counts with platelet, aspartate aminotransferase levels (SGOT), and alanine aminotransferase levels (SGPT) should be obtained every 2 weeks when the drug is initiated and then monthly for at least the first 6 months of treatment (PDR, 1990).

Drug interactions

Control of seizure activity is often enhanced with the use of more than one antiepileptic drug. It is important for the practitioner to know the particular regimen the child is on, the anticipated therapeutic serum levels, and common side effects (see Table 15-2). Several of these antiepileptic drugs have altered therapeutic effects when combined with common drugs used in pediatric care. Caution should be used in recommending or prescribing antihistamines, antidepressants, aspirin, oral contraceptives, and erythromycin.

Drugs such as antidepressants and antihistamines may alter the threshold of seizure activity and may interact with the therapeutic effects of antiepileptic medications. Because of the wide variety of antihistamines and antidepressants available, it is beyond the scope of this chapter to address each of the interactions specifically. The practitioner should review the individual therapeutic regimen prior to prescribing antihistamines or antidepressants to avoid potential complications.

The use of aspirin may decrease therapeutic plasma levels of phenytoin (Dilantin) by displacing the phenytoin from binding sites. This displacement causes an increased level of free phenytoin, which may result in toxic effects despite a decreased plasma level (Holmes, 1986; PDR, 1990). The use of aspirin may increase therapeutic plasma levels of valproic acid (Depakene) by displacing the valproate from the protein-binding sites. This would potentiate the drug's toxic side effect (Holmes, 1986; PDR, 1990). Acetaminophen is recommended instead of aspirin for mild analgesics and fever control.

The therapeutic effect of oral contraceptives may be altered when they are used in combination with antiepileptics. Failure rates have been reported to be higher in women taking certain antiepileptic drugs. As a result, a higher dose of oral contraceptive may be necessary in some women to achieve a full contraceptive effect (Mattson et al., 1986).

The use of erythromycin results in an increased plasma level of carbamazepine (Tegretol). Erythromycin decreases the metabolism or breakdown of carbamazepine, potentiating toxic effects (PDR, 1990).

DIFFERENTIAL DIAGNOSIS AND MANAGEMENT OF COMMON PEDIATRIC CONDITIONS
Seizurelike episodes

The practitioner will evaluate children with epilepsy who have common childhood illnesses that may or may not be related to this underlying disorder. These presenting signs and symptoms must be evaluated to provide appropriate treatment for the illness or to change the treatment regimen for the diagnosed seizure disorder.

Infants and young children frequently have a history of vomiting. Gastroesophageal reflux is a condition that produces vomiting. In this condition the reflux of stomach contents may enter only the lower esophagus, producing symptoms of choking, laryngospasm, apnea, arching, and occasionally loss of body tone (Herbst, 1981). This is a frightening, dramatic event for the parents to witness. Parents commonly report that the child has had a "seizure" or "convulsion." The diagnosis of gastroesophageal reflux can be confirmed through barium swallow and esophagram (Herbst, 1981).

Breath-holding spells are common occurrences in infants and young children that appear much like seizure activity. Such events usually begin with the child crying; the crying worsens, and the child may hold his or her breath and actually stop breathing. This causes cyanosis, and the child becomes unconscious and limp. Once the child loses consciousness, normal breathing returns. If persistent apnea occurs, the child may actually have seizure activity (Holmes, 1986; Pedley, 1983). The key to accurate diagnosis of breath-holding spells versus seizure activity is meticulous history taking on the part of the practitioner. This is dependent on reliable reporting by the parents of a witnessed event. These attacks are always associated with crying, and the apnea and cyanosis occur before there is loss of consciousness (Holmes, 1986; Pedley, 1983).

Severe headaches or migraine headaches often are difficult to differentiate from seizure activity. Migraine headaches are frequently associated with clinical manifestations similar to those seen with simple partial seizures (i.e., visual changes, weaknesses, nausea, flushing). A complete history of presenting signs and symptoms, family history, and EEG findings may help to confirm the differential diagnosis of migraine headaches (Holmes, 1986; Pedley, 1983).

Cardiac dysfunction, such as arrhythmias and syncopal episodes, may be mistaken for seizure activity. The child may have a loss of consciousness, manifesting much like "drop attacks," or an atonic seizure. These events are different from seizure activity in that there is usually a gradual change in consciousness accompanied by dizziness, decreased or irregular pulse, pale clammy appearance, and mild neurologic impairment after the event (confusion, lethargy). An EEG performed during an event is usually normal. In addition, there may be a positive family history of cardiac anomalies or syncopal attacks (Holmes, 1986; Pedley, 1983).

Pseudoseizures are behavioral manifestations that closely resemble seizures but do not correlate with epileptic activity on the EEG. Frequently, pseudoseizures occur in children and adolescents with a diagnosed seizure disorder. These "spells" are sometimes quite convincing and are not necessarily intentional. A psychiatric referral in combination with medical therapy is appropriate to evaluate, differentiate, and treat this diagnosis separate from electrically discharged seizures (Cohen and Sutter, 1982; Pedley, 1983).

Unusual body movements in infants and children, such as a hyperstartle response to stimuli, muscle tics, muscle spasticity, and altered gait pattern, are conditions that may be confused with epileptic patterns. Again, the diagnosis can usually be differentiated by careful testing, assessment, precise history taking, and accurate reporting of signs and symptoms experienced by the child and witnessed by the parent.

Differential diagnosis of common pediatric problems is sometimes very difficult and may require additional testing to rule out seizure activity. Referral to other specialists such as pediatric neurologist, cardiologist, gastroenterologist, or psychologist may also be necessary for supportive consultation and diagnostic confirmation.

Fever

The presence of infection and fever in a child with epilepsy may alter the serum levels and therapeutic effects of antiepileptic drugs. Moreover, fever may lower a child's seizure threshold. Parents should be advised by the practitioner of methods of fever management, including increasing fluid intake, controlling environmental factors, and using antipyretics appropriately. Parents should be advised not to increase antiepileptic drug therapy without consulting the health care provider.

DEVELOPMENTAL ISSUES
Safety

There are many issues regarding safety that are particular to the infant and child with epilepsy. Parents must be educated to the changes that may occur and threaten their child's safety. This includes instruction of how to intervene safely and appropriately during frequent or prolonged seizure activity. Parents, teachers, and caretakers must know these steps to follow in the event of such an occurrence. It is crucial to (1) maintain an adequate airway, (2) lower the child to the ground, (3) turn and keep the child on his or her side to prevent aspiration, (4) protect the child from injury to the head and limbs, and (5) stay with the child and call for help. The practitioner should emphasize to the parent that never at any time should one attempt to put anything in the child's mouth. Also, a child's tonic-clonic movements should not be restrained during the seizure activity unless the child is in danger of greater injury. Parents should also be certified to perform cardiopulmonary resuscitation in the event of an arrest.

Certain seizure types (i.e., complex partial seizures, atonic seizures, Lennox-Gastaut syndrome) often result in a sudden loss of consciousness and change in body muscle tone. With these seizures there is loss of muscle tone (atonic) or extreme tension of muscle groups (tonic). These changes may occur independently or just before a generalized body convulsion. Because the onset of this seizure activity is unpredictable, the actual clinical manifestation is the child suddenly dropping to the floor. There is great potential for injury, especially to the head. For this reason the practitioner should advise the parents to have their child wear a helmet in an effort to protect the child's head in the event of such seizure activity. A hockey or bicycle helmet provides adequate protection to the areas (forehead, back of head) most commonly hit during these drop attacks. These helmets are lightweight, come in various colors and sizes, and are available wherever sports equipment is sold. The child's individuality and cooperation may be fostered by placing creative designs, stickers, and labels on the helmet.

For similar reasons consideration must be given to the child's participation in certain activities that may increase the risk of injury should a seizure occur. Participation in activities such as swimming and gymnastics are commonly questioned by parents and school teachers. It is not necessary to restrict the child from taking part in these exercises, provided there is adequate supervision by a responsible adult who is able to intervene appropriately should an emergency arise.

There are tremendous safety issues for the adolescent with epilepsy related to the use of various machinery (e.g., lawn mowers; machines in shop classes). The same principles should pertain to decisions regarding participation in such activities. Each state has its own laws pertaining to an individual with epilepsy securing a license to operate a motor vehicle. Compliance with antiepileptic drugs presents another safety issue for the adolescent. This is a time of tremendous peer pressure and challenges. Alcohol use and experimentation with other drugs are common occurrences in today's society. Intake of these substances often lowers the anticonvulsant's therapeutic effects and therefore lowers the seizure threshold. Education on the individual's personal responsibility for health maintenance may minimize these complications.

As discussed in the previous section, there is potential for limited cognitive ability and altered judgment in these children. This is an important concept to discuss with parents when they are considering independence issues.

Child care

Finding appropriate day care often presents a challenge for parents. This challenge is even greater for parents of children with a chronic condition such as epilepsy. The primary care practitioner can assist the family in this endeavor by helping to identify local agencies familiar with the care involved with a child with epilepsy or by providing the education needed about epilepsy to the child care agencies who are able to support these children's special needs.

Specific needs of the child in child care are dependent on the individual seizure disorder. The child care providers must be educated in the same manner as the parents regarding emergency aid and interventions during seizures. They must have an understanding of the clinical manifestations and what type of seizure activity to expect and monitor. Frequently medications must be administered

during the hours a child is at day care. It is therefore necessary for the day-care providers to have information regarding the rationale for the anticonvulsant, potential side effects, and proper administration of the prescribed drugs. All medications should be stored in a safe, locked location to prevent accidental ingestion.

Diet

Infants with epilepsy may have difficulty with feeding because of the frequency of their seizure activity or because of increased lethargy from anticonvulsant therapy or the postictal state. In addition, seizure activity may produce a temporary state of increased metabolism. This in combination with poor intake may result in an inadequate nutritional balance for growth and development. Assessment of growth curves over time in combination with the parents' reports of intake help to determine if interventions such as increased calories per feeding and supplemental feedings are necessary. Temporary assistance and supplementation can be supported with use of a nasogastric tube. Children with persistent weight loss, poor oral feeding abilities, and failure to thrive may require a gastric tube for calorie, fluid, and medication intake.

Conversely, excessive weight gain may occur in infants and children with epilepsy. The neurologic impairments that may accompany epilepsy may result in poor motor function leading to decreased physical activity, which requires less caloric intake for normal body growth. Again, assessment of growth curves over time in addition to the parents' reports of intake help to determine if interventions such as decreased calories per feeding are necessary.

Weight gain is a significant issue in infants with infantile spasms. First, infants with this epileptic syndrome commonly are extremely irritable. This irritability is frequently quieted with feeding, and in an effort to soothe their distressed infant, parents may overfeed the infant. In addition, the treatment of choice for this seizure disorder is administration of ACTH. A major side effect of this drug is weight gain. The child's weight and growth must be monitored closely while the child is taking this medication.

An accepted form of therapy to control intractable seizures in children is the ketogenic diet with the objective of producing ketosis. This is an extremely difficult diet for a child to maintain and is often associated with weight loss and hypoglycemia. Careful monitoring of these children's nutritional status is necessary.

Discipline

Children with epilepsy have an increased risk of psychosocial adjustment problems. In fact, there is a reported greater incidence of psychiatric problems, emotional disturbances, psychosocial problems, and behavioral problems in children with epilepsy than in children with other chronic conditions or in the general population (Matthews, Barabas, and Ferrari, 1982; Rutter, Graham, and Yule, 1970). This invariably influences the parents' and family members' response to discipline (Kessler, 1977). Guidance on discipline should be provided to parents early in the child's life and should always reflect the child's cognitive ability. The need for parents to provide discipline and direction, and to encourage the child's independence should be emphasized frequently. Referral for parent counseling may be necessary to assist with the particular needs and challenges that may arise (Austin, McBride, and Davis, 1984; Austin and McDermott, 1988).

Toileting

There are usually no particular concerns related to toileting the child with epilepsy. Standard developmental counseling is recommended.

Sleep patterns

Sleep patterns may be altered if seizure activity occurs at night. These infants and children are at increased risk for apnea or respiratory difficulties since the seizure activity may be unwitnessed and therefore prolonged during the night. These children should wear a cardiac or apnea monitor during sleep. Pillows should also be used with caution. If the child does not have a history of respiratory difficulties during sleep, a room intercom monitor may be used to alert the parents of seizure activity. Early recognition of seizure activity helps to limit complications.

Seizure activity during the day may result in prolonged postictal states interfering with the child's sleep pattern at night. Parents should be instructed not to allow their child to sleep for extended periods during the daytime hours. The postictal state often cannot be interrupted, however, and even the greatest effort to keep a child awake may not be successful.

School issues

Children with epilepsy may have social, intellectual, and cognitive difficulties. These must be assesssed and identified so that interventions for the child's particular learning needs can be individualized and addressed. Early intervention programs or infant stimulation programs should be consulted if the seizure disorder begins during infancy or early childhood. These children are at risk for developmental delay, and early assessment allows for appropriate interventions to begin, which maximizes learning potentials.

If needed, this preschool plan can be carried into the formal educational program as a child ages. Core evaluations by the individual school systems are necessary and appropriate for children at risk.

It is important to establish a supportive, well-informed environment for the child (Dreifuss, 1984). School staff should be informed of the child's medical diagnosis even if the child progresses well and does not require special educational classes. This information allows the teachers to be helpful in assessing behavioral side effects of anticonvulsant therapy. Also, a teacher who is informed of the potential for seizure occurrence and who has been instructed by the parents and the primary care practitioner on proper interventions is more apt to be calm and intervene appropriately if needed.

A tremendous social stigma accompanies the diagnosis of epilepsy. It is very important that the practitioner recognize the stress this diagnosis places on the child and its impact on the child's self-concept, relationships with peers, and the educational system. The unpredictability and lack of control of seizure activity is part of this stress. Misconceptions, fears, apprehensions, and judgments of the peer group commonly have a negative effect on the child's self-esteem (Matthews, Barabas, and Ferrari, 1982; Rutter, Graham, and Yule, 1970). The primary care practitioner should explore opportunities to educate the community and increase knowledge and understanding concerning this condition. Greater understanding of epilepsy may yield compassion and acceptance rather than ridicule and fear of these children.

The practitioner should inquire about school performance and peer interactions at each well child visit. It may be appropriate to refer the child for additional counseling and professional support to help manage with these ongoing stresses (Hoare, 1984).

Sexuality

In the female adolescent with epilepsy, the seizure threshold may fall with the cyclic changes induced by the menstrual cycle. This is presumably related to the water retention, electrolyte imbalances, and decreased levels of progesterone. If this occurs, cyclic adjustments of the antiepileptic medications should be made (DaSilva, Binne, and Meinardi, 1984; Dana-Haeri and Richens, 1983; Lechtenberg, 1985). The type of oral contraceptives should be considered on an individual basis (Mattson et al., 1986).

Caution should be taken if the woman with epilepsy becomes pregnant, because certain anti-epileptic drugs are potentially teratogenic. Anti-epileptic drugs such as phenytoin, carbamazepine, primidone, and phenobarbital have been associated with birth defects and fetal loss. The use of particular antiepileptic drugs may need to be altered during pregnancy (Bossi, 1983; Yerby, Koepsell, and Daling, 1985).

SPECIAL FAMILY CONCERNS

All of these families experience some sense of grief as parents mourn the loss of the "normal" child (Lessman, 1982). Societal stigma and misconceptions concerning epilepsy are particularly stressful to the family. The diagnosis has implications for all aspects of growth and development; child care, health care, recreation, education, transportation, employment, and insurance coverage (life and health).

This condition presents a chronic and intense stress on the family system. This, in addition to the unpredictability of seizure occurrence, often results in overprotective parents and dependent children (Austin, McBride, and Davis, 1984; Austin and McDermott, 1988; Lerman, 1977).

SUMMARY OF PRIMARY CARE NEEDS FOR THE CHILD WITH EPILEPSY

Growth and development

Obtain height and weight at each visit. Medications must be based on current accurate measurements.

Regularly screen and assess cognitive and motor skills.

Perform regular neuropsychologic screening.

If developmental delay is present, recommend early intervention with an infant stimulation program.

Immunizations

Children with underlying seizure disorders are at increased risk of having a seizure after DPT or measles vaccine. Pertussis may be deferred and DT used. Measles vaccine continues to be recommended.

Screening
Vision

Routine screening is recommended.

Hearing

Routine screening is recommeded.

Dental

Routine screening is recommended. Phenytoin may cause gingival hyperplasia. Children taking phenytoin require more frequent cleaning by the dental hygienist.

Blood pressure

Routine screening is recommended.

Infants receiving ACTH therapy may require daily monitoring of blood pressure.

Hematocrit

Routine screening is recommended.

Urinalysis

Routine screening is recommended.

Tuberculosis

Routine screening is recommended.

Condition-specific screening
  Drug toxicity screening

Drug toxicity screening is necessary the first 6 months of therapy for valproate, carbamazepine, and phenytoin.

Drug interactions

Several antiepileptic drugs have altered therapeutic effects when combined with antihistamines, aspirin, antidepressants, oral contraceptives, and certain antibiotics. Careful monitoring is required.

Differential diagnosis

Rule out seizurelike symptoms:
  Gastrointestinal symptoms—rule out gastroesophageal reflux.
  Respiratory symptoms—rule out breath-holding spells and apnea.
  Visual changes, nausea—rule out severe headaches and migraines
  Cardiac symptoms (arrhythmias, syncopal episodes)—rule out cardiac arrhythmias
  Pseudoseizures
  Movement disorders, hyperstartle, muscle tics, muscle spasticity, altered gait patterns—rule out restor movement

Management of illness with fever—Risk of seizures is increased. Observe closely and provide antipyretic therapy.

Developmental issues
Safety

Provide instructions regarding emergency interventions for seizure activity.

Use helmet for certain seizure types.

Use caution with certain sports and activities.

Use caution with use of machinery, including motor vehicles.

Alcohol may lower seizure threshold.

Child care

Provide instructions to agency regarding emergency interventions for seizure activity.

Provide instructions for medication given at day care.

Diet

Diets may be tailored to meet the child's caloric needs.

The ketogenic diet is difficult to maintain.

Discipline

Standard developmental counseling is recommended.

Toileting

Toileting is reflective of child's cognitive and developmental ability.

Continued.

SUMMARY OF PRIMARY CARE NEEDS FOR THE CHILD WITH EPILEPSY — cont'd

Sleep patterns

The child may require use of cardiac or apnea monitor.

Sleep patterns may be altered with prolonged or frequent seizure activity.

School issues

Learning needs must be individualized and addressed. Teachers should be informed of seizure history, and instructions regarding emergency interventions for seizure activity should be given.

Social stigma of epilepsy may adversely affect the child's self-concept.

Sexuality

Cyclic changes induced by the menstrual cycle may alter antiepileptic effects.

Some antiepileptic drugs are teratogenic. Counseling may be necessary.

Special family concerns

Chronic sorrow and stress
Social stigma
Unpredictability of seizure activity

RESOURCES

The health care system must be empathetic to the multiple needs of children with epilepsy and their families. Health care workers provide the physical, emotional, and social care that these individuals very much need. Nevertheless, no one understands or feels the problems these children and families face during their day-to-day lives as well as another child or family with the same disorder. For this reason, parent and peer support groups are available to provide a network of help and comfort within the community. Such resources not only are necessary but have proved to be a major factor in coping and adaptation for affected families (Wallander and Varni, 1989).

Epilepsy Foundation of America
    National Epilepsy Library and Resource Center
    4351 Garden City Dr
    Landover, MD 20785-2267
    (301) 459-3700
    (800) EFA-4050

National Easter Seal Society
    2023 W Ogden Ave
    Chicago, IL 60612

REFERENCES

American Association of Neuroscience Nurses: *Core curriculum for neuroscience nursing,* ed 2, Park Ridge, Ill, 1984, The Association.

Annegers JF, Hauser WA, and Elveback LR: Remission of seizures and relapse in patients with epilepsy, *Epilepsia* 20:729-737, 1979.

Austin JK, McBride AB, and Davis H: Parental attitude and adjustment to childhood epilepsy, *Nurs Res* 33:92-96, 1984.

Austin JK, and McDermott N: Parental attitude and coping behaviors in families of children with epilepsy, *J Neurosci Nurs* 20:174-179, 1988.

Bancaud J, Henriksen O, Rubio-Donnadieu Seino M., et al: Proposal for revising clinical electroencephalographic classification of epileptic seizures, *Epilepsia* 22:489-501, 1981.

Bare MA: Hemispherectomy for seizures, *J Neurosci Nurs* 21:18-23, 1989.

Bossi L: Fetal effects of anticonvulsants. In Morselli PL, Pippenger CE, and Penry JK, eds: *Antiepileptic drug therapy in pediatrics,* New York, 1983, Raven Press, pp 37-64.

Brewer K and Sperling MR: Neurosurgical treatment of intractable epilepsy, *J Neurosci Nurs* 20:366-372, 1988.

Cohen RJ and Sutter C: Hysterical seizures: Suggestion as a provocative EEG test, *Ann Neurol* 11:391-395, 1982.

Committee on Infectious Diseases: *Report on the committee of infectious diseases,* ed 22, Elk Grove Village, 1991, The Academy of Pediatrics.

Dana-Haeri J and Richens A: Effect of norethisterone on seizures associated with menstruation, *Epilepsia* 24:377-381, 1983.

DaSilva AM, Binne CD, and Meinardi H: *Biorhythm and epilepsy,* New York, 1984, Raven Press.

Delgado-Escueta AV and Enrile-Bacsal F: Juvenile myoclonic epilepsy of Janz, *Neurology* 34:285-294, 1984.

Delgado-Escueta AV, Treiman DM, and Walsh GO: Treatable epilepsies, *N Engl J Med* 308:1508-1514, 1983.

DeVivo DC: How to use other drugs (steroids) in the ketogenic diet. In Morselli PL, Pippenger CE and Penry JK eds: *Antiepileptic drug therapy in pediatrics,* New York, Raven Press.

Dreifuss FE: *Pediatric epileptology,* Boston, 1984, Wright.

Dreifuss FE: Juvenile myoclonic epilepsy: Characteristics of a primary generalized epilepsy, *Epilepsia* 30:S1-S7, 1989.

Dreifuss FE, Martinez-Lage M, Roger J, et al: Proposal for classification of epilepsies and epileptic syndromes, *Epilepsia* 26:268-278, 1985.

Epilepsy Foundation of America: *Basic statistics on the epilepsies,* Philadelphia, 1975, FA Davis.

Gastaut H: Clinical and electroencephalographic classification of epileptic seizures, *Epilepsia* 11:102, 1970.

Geoffroy G, Lassonde M, Delisle F, et al: Corpus callosotomy for control of intractable epilepsy in children, *Neurology* 33:891-897, 1983.

Gomez MR and Klass DW: Epilepsies of infancy and childhood, *Ann Neurol* 13:113-124, 1983.

Hauser WA and Kurland LT: *The epidemiology of epilepsy in Rochester, Minnesota, 1935 through 1967, Epilepsia,* 16, 1975.

Herbst JJ: Gastroesophageal reflux, *J Pediatr* 98:24-30, 1981.

Hoare P: The development of psychiatric disorders among school children with epilepsy, *Dev Med Child Neurol* 26:3-13, 1984.

Holmes GL: *Diagnosis and management of seizures in children,* Philadelphia; 1986, WB Saunders.

Huttenlocher PR: Ketonemia and seizures: Metabolic and anticonvulsant effects of two ketogenic diets in childhood epilepsy, *Pediatr Res* 10:536-540, 1976.

International League Against Epilepsy: Proposal for revised classification of epilepsies and epileptic syndromes, *Epilepsia* 30:389-399, 1989.

Kessler JW: Parenting the handicapped child, *Pediatr Ann* 10:654-661, 1977.

Lavadas E, Umilta C, and Provinciali L: Hemisphere-dependent cognitive performances in epileptic patients, *Epilepsia* 20:493-502, 1979.

Lechtenberg R: *The diagnosis and treatment of epilepsy,* New York, 1985, Macmillan Publishing.

Lederman RJ: Status epilepticus, *Cleve Clin Q* 51:261-266, 1984.

Lerman P: The concept of preventive rehabilitation in childhood epilepsy: A plea against overprotection and overindulgence. In Penry JK, ed: *Epilepsy, the eighth international symposium.* New York, 1977, Raven Press.

Lessman SE: Accepting epilepsy: Social and emotional issues for patients and their families. In Black RB, Herman PP, and Shope JT eds: *Nursing management of epilepsy,* Rockville, MD, 1982, Aspen Systems.

Lombroso CT: A prospective study of infantile spasms: Clinical and therapeutic correlations, *Epilepsia* 24:135, 1983.

Luessenhop AJ, dela Cruz TC, and Fenichel GM: Surgical disconnection of the cerebral hemispheres for intractable seizures: Results in infancy and childhood, *JAMA* 213:1630-1636, 1970.

Matthews WS, Barabas G, and Ferrari M: Emotional concomitants of childhood epilepsy, *Epilepsia* 23:671-681, 1982.

Mattson RH, Cramer JA, Darne PD, et al: Use of oral contraceptives by women with epilepsy, *JAMA* 256:238-240, 1986.

Mayeux R, Brandt J, Rosen J, et al: Interictal memory and language impairment in temporal lobe epilepsy, *Neurology* 30:120-125, 1980.

Newmark M: Genetics of the epilepsies. In Dreifuss FE: *Pediatric epileptology:* Classification and management of seizures in the child, Boston, 1984, Wright.

Pedley TA: Differential diagnosis of episodic episodes, *Epilepsia* 24:S31-S44, 1983.

Pellock JM: Status epilepticus. In Pellock JM and Meyer EC, eds: *Neurologic emergencies in infancies and childhood,* Philadelphia, 1984, Harper & Row Publishers.

Penry JK: *Epilepsy: Diagnosis, management. quality of life,* ed 2, New York, 1986, Raven Press.

Physicians' desk reference, ed 44, Oradell, NJ, 1990, Edward R Barnhart.

Rutter M, Graham P, and Yule W: A neuropsychiatric study in childhood, *Clin Dev Med,* 35-36, 1970.

Santilli N and Sierzant TL: Advances in the treatment of epilepsy, *J Neurosci Nurs* 19:141-157, 1987.

Sofijanov N: Clinical evolution and prognosis of childhood epilepsies, *Epilepsia* 23:61-69, 1982.

Spencer DD and Spencer SS: Corpus callosotomy in the treatment of medically intractable secondarily generalized seizures of children, *Cleve Clin J Med* 56:69-78, 1989.

Spencer SS: Surgical options for uncontrolled epilepsy, *Neurol Clin* 4:669-695, 1986.

Thurston JH, Thurston DL, Hixon BB, et al: Prognosis in childhood epilepsy: Additional follow-up of 148 children 15-23 years after withdrawal of anticonvulsant therapy, *N Engl J Med* 306:831-836, 1982.

Wallander JL and Varni JW: Social support and adjustment in chronically ill and handicapped children, *Am J Community Psychol* 17:185-201, 1989.

Yerby M, Koepsell T, and Daling J: Pregnancy complications and outcomes in a cohort of women with epilepsy, *Epilepsia* 26:631-635, 1985.

16 *Fragile X Syndrome*

••

Amy Cronister Silverman and *Randi J. Hagerman*

ETIOLOGY

Fragile X syndrome is a relatively newly recognized condition that causes cognitive impairment ranging from mild learning disabilities to severe mental retardation. This condition derives its name from the presence of a fragile site or break in the X chromosome at Xq27.3 (Fig. 16-1) which is identifiable by chromosome analysis. Because of the phenotypic variability among children with fragile X syndrome and because this condition was only recently discovered, the majority of individuals with fragile X syndrome remain undiagnosed.

Fragile X syndrome is caused by an abnormal gene or genes on the long arm of the X chromosome. Inherited in an X-linked fashion, this condition commonly affects multiple family members throughout several generations. Unlike other X-linked conditions, females can be affected by fragile X syndrome but usually to a lesser extent than males. More commonly, females are cognitively normal without physical features typical of fragile X syndrome. In addition, 20% of all males who carry the fragile X gene escape any manifestations of this condition. Women who carry the fragile X gene have a 50% chance with each pregnancy of passing this gene to their children.

INCIDENCE

Fragile X syndrome is the most common cause of inherited mental retardation known. Down syndrome, which rarely is inherited, has an incidence of approximately 1 per 700. In comparison, fragile X syndrome affects 1 per 1,000 males (Herbst and

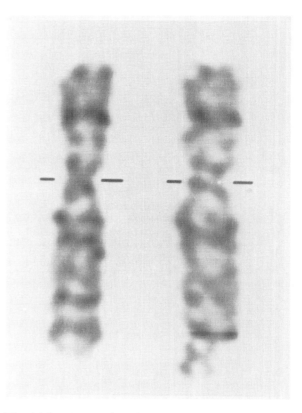

Fig. 16-1. A normal X chromosome and a fragile X chromosome demonstrating the fragile X site at Xq27.3.

Miller, 1980; Webb, Thake, and Todd, 1986), and perhaps as many as 1 per 750 females carry the fragile X gene (Opitz, 1986). Screening of individuals with mental retardation in institutional and other residential settings has shown that 2% to 15% (Hagerman et al., 1988) of this high-risk population have fragile X syndrome as the cause of their mental impairment.

Population studies of such diverse groups as the Aborigines in Australia, the Zulus of Africa, and individuals screened in Sweden, Finland, New South Wales, England, and France suggest that fragile X is equally common among all racial and ethnic groups (Sherman, 1991). As mentioned earlier, however, the majority of families affected by this syndrome are still undiagnosed and therefore remain unaware of available treatment and intervention.

CLINICAL MANIFESTATIONS AT TIME OF DIAGNOSIS

When most health care practitioners hear the word syndrome, they think of an individual who appears phenotypically abnormal. Similarly, most syndromes have consistent cognitive and physical features that succinctly describe the clinical manifestations. Although the majority of individuals with fragile X syndrome share certain clinical findings, there is much variability. The health care practitioner should note that children with this syndrome may not be immediately recognizable by their phenotype.

Males

The majority of males with fragile X syndrome have IQs in the mild to moderate range of mental retardation. A significantly smaller percentage are severely to profoundly retarded. Hagerman, Kemper, and Hudson (1985) have described learning disabled boys with fragile X who have IQs in the normal range. This may not be a rare occurrence but instead a continuum of the cognitive spectrum of involvement (Chudley de von Flint, and Hagerman, 1987). The cognitive profile of males with fragile X includes difficulty with abstract reasoning, math, and attention.

Delayed onset of language is present in nearly all males with fragile X. In some children difficulties are evidenced by only language problems

related to weaknesses in abstract reasoning. Other children as young as 18 months of age have delayed speech and significant deficits in receptive and expressive language. Perseveration and echolalia, or repetitive speech, are common speech characteristics of the individual with fragile X. A fast rate of speech, cluttering, mumbling, rambling, and poor topic maintenance are also frequent findings (Madison, George, and Moeschler, 1986; Newell, Sanborn, and Hagerman, 1983; Scharfenaker and Schreiner, 1989).

The three classic physical features associated with the fragile X syndrome phenotype are a long narrow face, prominent or large ears, and, in males, enlarged testicles. Approximately 80% of all males with fragile X will exhibit one or more of these features (Hagerman, 1987; Sutherland and Hecht, 1985). A long narrow face is a more subjective measurement, although Butler and colleagues (1991) and others (Hockey and Crowhurst, 1988; Simko et al., 1989) have described an anthropometric method which may lead to better characterization of facial features.

Large ears (>2 SD above the norm) are seen in 50% of boys with fragile X (Fig. 16-2). Prominent or cupped ears are often a more useful discriminating feature among this younger group. This finding is observed in 60% to 70% of boys and is frequently the only obvious physical feature associated with fragile X syndrome (Simko et al., 1989; Hagerman, 1991a).

Enlarged testicles are frequently observed in the mentally retarded population; 70% to 90% of men with fragile X have a testicular volume greater than 30 ml (Sutherland and Hecht, 1985). An orchidometer (Fig. 16-3) consisting of ellipsoid shapes of varying size is a useful instrument to measure testicular volume, especially in prepubescent boys in whom testicular volume may be less obvious (4 ml or greater in approximately 30% of fragile X boys compared with a normal testicular volume of 2 ml in those up to age 8 years).

Other more subtle physical features noted among the fragile X population include a prominent jaw, prominent forehead, and long palpebral fissures (Brondum-Nielsen et al., 1983; Butler et al., 1991; Hagerman, 1991a). A high arched palate, mitral valve prolapse, hypotonia, hyperextensible finger joints and flat feet suggest these individuals

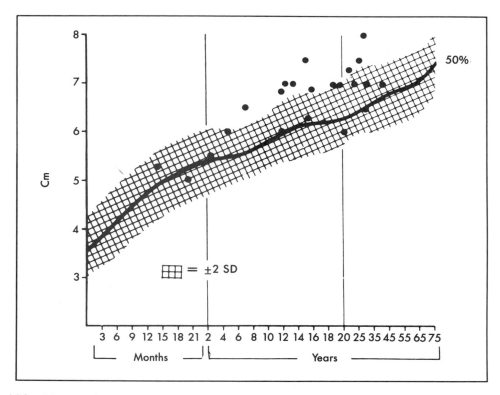

Fig. 16-2. Mean ear length. From Hagerman, R., Smith, A.C.M., and Manner, R.: Clinical features of the fragile X syndrome. In Hagerman, R., McBogg, P. (Eds.): The Fragile X Syndrome: Diagnosis, Biochemistry and Intervention, Dillon, CO, 1983, Spectra Publishing Co.

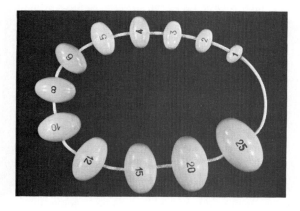

Fig. 16-3. Prader orchidometer used to measure testicular volume.

may have an underlying connective tissue disorder (Opitz, Westphal, and Daniel, 1984; Hagerman et al., 1984).

It is very important to recognize that the majority of males with fragile X, especially the younger boys, appear quite normal (Fig. 16-4). Often what is more concerning to the parents are the behavioral characteristics. Hyperactivity is observed in more than 70% of boys with fragile X syndrome yet frequently disappears after puberty. Poor attention span, often combined with impulsivity, is also problematic for all boys with fragile X regardless of their level of cognitive functioning (Hagerman, Kemper, and Hudson, 1985; Fryns et al., 1984). Approximately 90% have poor eye contact (Hagerman, 1991a; Pueschel and Finelli,

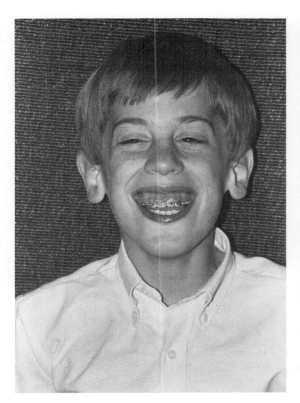

Fig. 16-4. Prepubertal fragile X male.

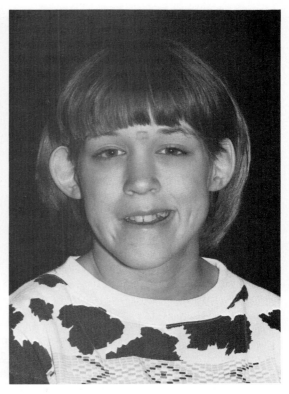

Fig. 16-5. Young heterozygous fragile X female who is affected physically and cognitively by fragile X syndrome.

1984), and 60% to 70% display unusual hand mannerisms, including hand flapping and hand biting (Hagerman, 1987).

Females

Overall, females who are affected by fragile X syndrome display milder phenotypic features than males, although some have been described with moderate and severe retardation (Fig. 16-5).

Approximately 35% of all females who carry the gene (also referred to as heterozygotes) have an IQ less than 85 (Sherman et al., 1984, 1985). Of the remaining two thirds, as many as one half demonstrate significant learning disabilities. A specific cognitive profile has been described in fragile X females. Areas of weakness demonstrated in females of all functioning abilities include math and abstract reasoning. Attentional problems are also

common (Kemper et al., 1986; Madison, George, and Moeschler, 1986; Miezejeski et al., 1986).

Speech and language difficulties are noted in some heterozygotes. Although more work is needed in this area, receptive and expressive language deficits, including difficulties with auditory processing, inappropriate and tangential speech, poor topic maintenance, and written language difficulties, have been reported (Hagerman, 1987; Madison, George, and Moeschler, 1986; Scharfenaker and Schreiner, 1989).

The physical characteristics are less obvious than those described in males with fragile X. Prominent ears, a long narrow face, a prominent forehead and jaw, and hyperextensible finger joints have been described by several authors (Cronister et al.,

1991, Fryns, 1986). Phenotypic expression is more frequently observed in the mentally impaired population; however, penetrance of the fragile X gene or genes is seen in normal functioning heterozygous females also (Cronister et al., 1991; Loesch and Hay, 1988).

To improve diagnosis in fragile X syndrome, the health care provider needs to be familiar with the characteristic gestalt that defines this very common condition. It is important to recognize that none of the physical, behavioral, or psychologic characteristics looked at individually is diagnostic of fragile X syndrome. However, the finding of one or more of these features in combination with developmental delay or mental retardation of unknown cause should alert the clinician to order chromosome studies. The fragile X checklist (see the box below) was designed to assist the health care professional with screening developmentally delayed or mentally retarded children and adults.

A child receives a zero for each feature not present, 1 point for those present in the past or questionably present, and 2 points for those definitely present. The higher the score, the greater the risk for fragile X syndrome (Hagerman, Amiri, and Cronister, 1991).

TREATMENT

To date few health care professionals are knowledgeable about the diagnosis and treatment of individuals with fragile X syndrome. It is not uncommon, however, for an undiagnosed child with fragile X to be seen by the health care practitioner with one of several associated medical problems, including repeated ear infections, strabismus, hyperactivity, delayed language, tantrums, violent outbursts, seizures, or hypotonia. Although much of the medical intervention is approached as it would be with any child, certain treatment options specific to the fragile X diagnosis can significantly

---

FRAGILE X CHECKLIST

	Score		
	0 (Not present)	1 (Borderline or present in the past)	2 (Definitely present)
Mental retardation	_____	_____	_____
Perseverative speech	_____	_____	_____
Hyperactivity	_____	_____	_____
Short attention span	_____	_____	_____
Tactile defensiveness	_____	_____	_____
Hand flapping	_____	_____	_____
Hand biting	_____	_____	_____
Poor eye contact	_____	_____	_____
Hyperextensible finger joints	_____	_____	_____
Large or prominent ears	_____	_____	_____
Large testicles	_____	_____	_____
Simian crease or Sydney line	_____	_____	_____
Family history of mental retardation	_____	_____	_____
TOTAL SCORE: _____			

Adapted from Hagerman RJ: Fragile X syndrome, *Curr Probl Pediatr* 17:621-674, 1987.

improve the developmental outcome of these children.

Any signs that indicate developmental delay, sensory integration dysfunction, or language delays deserve immediate and aggressive treatment in a child with fragile X. All areas of a child's presenting signs and symptoms should be addressed, and thus a multidisciplinary approach to evaluation and therapy is essential.

Medication

Medical management of hyperactivity and attentional problems can augment learning and behavioral management at home and in the school. Central nervous system stimulant medication has proved the most reliable, with improvements in as many as two-thirds of affected children (Hagerman, Murphy, Wittenberger, 1988). No one drug is effective for all children. Most commonly children will be prescribed methylphenidate (Ritalin), but pemoline (Cylert) and dextroamphetamine (Dexedrine) have also proved beneficial (Hagerman, 1991b) (see Chapter 20).

Folic acid therapy has been reliably helpful in managing behavioral problems in the adult, although it may be helpful for only approximately 50% of prepubertal boys with fragile X (Hagerman, 1991b). Its use is controversial, and several studies have shown a lack of efficacy. Other studies have shown noticeable improvements in activity level, attention span, unusual mannerisms and coping skills. The mechanism of action of folate is unclear, but it does not appear to be specific to fragile X syndrome. Because harmful side effects are rare, many families request that their child be given folic acid as a trial. Routinely a prepubescent child is placed on a regimen of 10 mg/day (divided twice daily) for 3 to 6 months. Regardless of the dosage, careful follow-up is warranted to monitor vitamin B_6 and zinc serum levels, which may become deficient. If, however, improvements are not noticeable within the trial period, the clinician should consider an alternative treatment. Clonidine (Catapres) has shown beneficial results, but the number of children placed on this treatment protocol is extremely limited (Bregman, Ort and Leckman, 1989). Research is ongoing to determine what other medication may be optimal for treating the individual with fragile X.

Educational intervention

Several studies have indicated that IQ declines with age (Borghgraef et al., 1987; Dykens et al., 1989; Lachiewicz et al., 1987). Some males, however, whose IQs have remained stable over time have been followed (Hagerman et al., 1989). There is a tendency for the individual with fragile X to perform better on some academic tests than the IQ score would predict. Children with fragile X syndrome typically are better visual learners than auditory learners. Significant memory abilities and well-developed skills in recognizing visual gestalts make reading, spelling, and vocabulary obvious areas of strength for many (Kemper et al., 1987; Scharfenaker and Schreiner, 1989).

When developing an educational program, one must consider the child's overall intellectual abilities. Mainstreaming is a realistic goal for some children, whereas others may need a more structured and specialized program. The child with fragile X will improve most significantly if he or she is shown appropriate role models. Educational intervention strategies should emphasize a child's strengths, such as imitating abilities, memory, visual skills, and vocabulary. The curriculum should also be focused on areas of interest (Scharfenaker and Schreiner, 1989; Scharfenaker, Hickman, and Braden, 1991). Logo reading is an example of a learning tool developed to capitalize on the child's interesting sense of incidentally acquired knowledge (Braden, 1988). The idea is to use logos from popular television commercials and advertisements as the basis for a sight word vocabulary. The logos are gradually faded away such that only the word, phrase, or number remain.

Another learning tool that has proved successful is the use of computers for learning enhancement. This medium may be used to enhance language ability and academic progress in reading, spelling, and math. It can utilize visual matching skills and can help focus attention with colorful programs.

Speech and language and occupational therapy intervention are critical components of the education program and are recommended for all children with fragile X syndrome. Therapy is most effective when it incorporates a child's primary areas of interest. When possible, speech and language therapy sessions should include one or two other children who function at a higher level. Again, early intervention and vigorous treatment can optimize a child's speech and language abilities (Scharfenaker and Schreiner, 1989; Scharfenaker, Hickman, and Braden, 1991). Occupational therapy can be combined with speech and language therapy so that attention is maintained and the child is provided with an experiential approach to language (Windeck and Laurel, 1989).

Because the child with fragile X is easily overstimulated, occupational therapy should be geared toward helping a child reorganize, interpret, and adjust to sensory stimulation. For this reason, sensory integration therapy is the method of choice when one is working with these children. With this form of treatment, improvements should be noticeable in motor skills, balance, coordination, movement, sequencing, and attention (Scharfenaker, Hickman, and Braden, 1991).

Genetic counseling

Fragile X syndrome is known to affect generation after generation, and many families have two or more children affected by this condition. Early diagnosis can provide relatives with important information regarding fragile X inheritance, recurrence risks, carrier testing, and family planning options.

Fragile X syndrome is inherited in an X-linked fashion. Males are typically affected by any deleterious gene they carry on the X chromosome. Females, on the other hand, are usually normal because the abnormal gene on one X chromosome is compensated for by the normal gene on the other X chromosome. Heterozygous females have a 50% chance to pass the abnormal gene to their children. Males who carry the fragile X gene, on the other hand, will pass the abnormal gene to all of their daughters but none of their sons.

For reasons not clearly understood, fragile X syndrome does not conform to the classic pattern of X-linked inheritance. Obvious fragile X expression in heterozygotes is common, with approximately one third of the females being mentally impaired. Moreover, mental impairment appears to influence a woman's risk of having mentally impaired children. For example, a woman with an IQ less than 85 has a 25% chance of having an affected son compared with a 19% chance for a woman with a normal IQ (Sherman et al., 1985; Weaver and Sherman, 1987).

Another important exception to the rule is that not all males who carry the fragile X gene are affected. In fact, approximately 20% of male gene carriers are perfectly normal mentally and physically (Sherman et al., 1985). These males are referred to as nonpenetrant, or transmitting, males. Curiously, nonpenetrant males tend to have perfectly normal daughters, but all are heterozygotes. These daughters can go on to have sons affected by fragile X syndrome. Large family studies have shown that brothers of nonpenetrant males are less likely to be affected by fragile X syndrome.

Recurrence risks for individuals who carry the fragile X gene are listed in Table 16-1. A heterozygous female can have a son or daughter who is not a carrier or a son or daughter who carries the gene and is affected, or a son or daughter who carries the gene and is perfectly normal. Again, mental impairment of the parent will influence recurrence risk figures.

Because fragile X syndrome is inherited, it is essential that a thorough family history or pedigree be taken. A list of signs and symptoms to consider when the pedigree is taken are provided in the box on p. 290. Any relative with one or more of these findings should be suspected as either a carrier or an affected individual.

Once the pedigree is complete and at-risk relatives identified, carrier testing and other testing options can be presented to these individuals. The most common testing to diagnose fragile X syndrome, chromosome analysis or cytogenetic testing, is also used to determine carrier status. It is important to understand that an individual can be a carrier of the fragile X gene but not demonstrate the fragile X site on chromosome analysis. Any relative who tests negative for fragile X syndrome on chromosome analysis should be offered DNA linkage analysis to more clearly define his or her true carrier status.

Prenatal diagnosis is available to all families with a confirmed diagnosis of fragile X syndrome. This testing includes amniocentesis (performed at 14-18 weeks' gestation), chorionic villi sampling (performed at 9½-12 weeks' gestation) and percutaneous umbilical blood sampling (18-22 weeks' gestation). Each procedure has specific benefits and drawbacks that should be carefully discussed with a genetic counselor before a pregnancy or testing

Table 16-1. Recurrence risks for offspring of known fragile X gene carriers

Heterozygous female	Mentally impaired son (%)	Nonpenetrant son (%)	Noncarrier son (%)	Mentally impaired daughter (%)	Normal IQ heterozygous daughter (%)	Noncarrier daughter (%)
IQ ≥ 85	19	6	25	8	17	25
IQ < 85	25	0	25	14	11	25
Nonpenetrant male	0	0	50	0	50	0

Data from Wearer and Sherman, 1987.

is pursued. Currently the accuracy of this testing ranges from 95% accurate when cytogenetic testing is performed alone to 99% if cytogenetic testing is combined with prenatal DNA linkage studies (Brown et al., 1988; Jenkins et al., 1986; Shapiro, Wilmont, and Murphy, 1991; Silverman, 1991.)

PROGNOSIS

Individuals with fragile X syndrome are expected to live a normal life span regardless of intellectual functioning.

ASSOCIATED PROBLEMS
Otitis media

Recurrent otitis media has been reported in 45% to 60% of all children with fragile X syndrome. Approximately 40% of these children will require myringotomy tube insertions (Hagerman, Altshul-Stark, and McBogg, 1987; Simko et al., 1989). There has been some speculation that this may be caused by an unusual angle or collapsibility of the eustachian tube (Hagerman, 1991a). Appropriate intervention is critical to avoid conductive hearing loss and a compounding of language deficits typical for fragile X (Rapin, 1979).

Connective tissue problems

Fifty percent of all individuals with fragile X will have pes planus (Davids, Hagerman, and Eilert, 1990). Clubfoot has also been reported and may be related to hypotonia in utero. In the study by Davids and associates (1990), joint laxity was documented in approximately 70% of children 10 years or younger. For reasons not clearly understood, hypotonia tends to disappear with age. Scoliosis

may be present, and hernias appear to be more common in children with fragile X than in the general population. These problems may also be related to an underlying connective tissue disorder. Routine intervention is recommended.

Cardiac problems have also been noted in persons with fragile X syndrome. These may be secondary to a connective tissue disorder. Mitral valve prolapse has been diagnosed in 22% to 55% of individuals affected (Loehr et al., 1986; Sreeran et al., 1989). Although usually benign, mitral valve prolapse can predispose a person to arrhythmias. Thus far this has not been noted in males with fragile X, but 30% of heterozygous females complain of heart palpitations (Cronister et al., 1991). Mild dilation of the base of the aorta has also been observed with ultrasound studies in as many as 50% of this population. It does not appear to be progressive (Loehr et al., 1986; Sreeran et al., 1989).

Vision problems

Strabismus (either esotropia or exotropia) appears to be present in approximately 30% to 56% of those with fragile X syndrome. Other eye problems such as myopia, nystagmus, and ptosis have been observed with and without strabismus (Schnizel and Largo, 1985; Storm et al., 1987).

Seizures

Seizures have been documented in approximately 20% of all individuals with fragile X. Generalized seizures and partial complex seizures have been reported (Musumeci et al., 1991; Wisniewski et al., 1991). A careful history should be taken and if clinical seizures are present, treatment with an anticonvulsant such as carbamazepine (Tegretol) is warranted.

Oral problems

A high arched palate is seen with greater frequency among the fragile X population and can explain the increased incidence of dental malocclusion (Partington, 1984). Several reports have also noted Pierre Robin syndrome (micrognathia and cleft palate) in combination with the fragile X syndrome.

Autistic-like tendencies

Much has been written in the literature to suggest an association between autism and fragile X syndrome. Studies have estimated that 5% to 53% of all individuals with fragile X meet *Diagnostic and Statistical Manual of Mental Disorders DSM-III-R* criteria for autism (Benezech and Noel, 1985; Brown et al., 1982, 1986; Partington, 1984). The majority of individuals, however, are more appropriately described as autistic-like. In addition to poor eye contact and unusual hand mannerisms, many children have fascinations with certain objects, such as vacuum cleaners and record players. What differentiates the majority of individuals with fragile X from those with autism is they characteristically lack a pervasive inability to relate. Although social anxiety is obvious at times, many children with fragile X can be intermittently quite sociable, demonstrating a spontaneous and natural sense of humor (Hagerman, 1987; Scharfenaker, Hickman, and Braden, 1991).

Psychiatric manifestations

Researchers have only recently investigated the psychiatric manifestations of the fragile X gene in females. As with males with fragile X, social anxiety is a common complaint. Many of the affected girls appear shy, are withdrawn, and have poor eye contact. Occasional cognitively normal women recall their childhood burdened by similar types of problems. Poor self-image and depression have also been described (Hagerman and Sobesky, 1989; Reiss et al., 1988). Reiss and colleagues (1988) have reported an increased incidence of schizotypal features, including emotional withdrawal and odd communication patterns. Further work is necessary to define the true relationship between the genetic defect and the neuropsychiatric phenotype.

Sensory integration difficulties

Other behavioral concerns include an inability to calm when the child is overstimulated or overwhelmed. New stimuli or novel situations can be frightening. Many parents describe their child as being hypersensitive to touch or tactilely defensive. Sensory integration difficulties are evidenced by an inability to screen out noises, lights, or confusion. Common responses to this overloading can include tantrums or outburst behavior, aggressive behavior, emotional instability, and, rarely, psychotic behavior (Scharfenaker and Schreiner, 1991; Scharfenaker, Hickman, and Braden, 1991; Hagerman, 1991b).

PRIMARY CARE MANAGEMENT
Growth and development

Increased head circumference (greater than the 75th percentile) at birth and throughout childhood has been reported by several authors (Borghagraef, Fryns, and Van den Berghe, 1990; Turner, Daniel, and Frost, 1980; Turner et al., 1986). This may lead to a possible misdiagnosis of Sotos' syndrome (cerebral gigantism). Others, however, have concluded that this deviance of head circumference into the upper range of normal occurs only occasionally and therefore is not a consistent finding (Partington, 1984). No special intervention is necessary for a large head circumference.

Controversy also exists regarding birth weights and growth. Prouty and others (1988) found growth to be normal and noted only a mild increase in growth percentiles from childhood into adult life. Partington (1984) reported similar findings. Sutherland and Hecht (1985), on the other hand, reported that 9 of 29 (31%) boys studied were above the 95th percentile.

In addition to deficits in cognitive functioning and speech, children with fragile X may be delayed in meeting other age-appropriate developmental milestones. Developmental delay will be evident with early developmental testing, such as the Bayley Scales of Infant Development (see Chapter 3). Other early warning signs are clumsiness and poor balance. Toe walking, an unusual gait, lack of flow of movement, and trouble with motor planning may also occur secondary to hypotonia, joint laxity, and sensory integration difficulties (Scharfenaker, Hickman, and Braden, 1991).

Immunizations

Vaccination regimen is the same as it would be for any infant or child. Should a child have a seizure disorder, the American Academy of Pediatrics guidelines for administering pertussis and measles vaccinations to those with seizures should be followed (see Chapter 15). (Committee on Infectious Diseases, 1991).

Screening

Vision. An eye examination is recommended as early as possible after the fragile X diagnosis is made to rule out strabismus and the less frequent findings of myopia, hyperopia, astigmatism, nystagmus, and ptosis. The evaluation should include a complete case history, visual acuity evaluation, refractive error determination, oculomotor assessment, and fundoscopy. Other testing may include an assessment of focusing function and visual developmental-perceptual skills. Yearly screening is sufficient unless visual difficulty is suspected. Early intervention is encouraged to avoid the development of blurred vision, amblyopia, or diplopia as a result of an uncorrected refractive error or strabismus. Treatment for many of the ophthalmologic problems includes corrective lenses, patching, or both—treatment that is relatively inexpensive and noninvasive. For some cases of strabismus, however, surgery may be the treatment of choice. Although early intervention may not dramatically influence cognitive functioning, corrected vision will maximize a child's learning potential.

Hearing. Because of the increased risk for recurrent ear infections, hearing evaluations are strongly recommended in the newly diagnosed child. Audiometry testing is usually sufficient to assess hearing. Any child who has a history of recurrent ear infections is best referred to an ear, nose, and throat (ENT) specialist to determine whether pressure equalizing (PE) tubes are warranted.

Dental. A routine dental screening by the practitioner may reveal a high arched palate, cleft palate, or dental malocclusion, all of which compound speech problems. Any child requiring dental work should be evaluated for mitral valve prolapse. If it is present, prophylactic antibiotic treatment to avoid subacute bacterial endocarditis is warranted

(see Chapter 11). Although it is not always possible, families should be referred to a pedodontist experienced in working with developmentally delayed and hyperactive children.

Blood pressure. Routine screening is recommended.

Hematocrit. Routine screening is recommended.

Urinalysis. Routine screening is recommended.

Tuberculosis. Routine screening is recommended.

Condition-specific screening

MITRAL VALVE PROLAPSE. Children with fragile X syndrome are at increased risk of mitral valve prolapse. Careful screening to detect a click or murmur is essential to detect this problem or any other cardiac involvement. Any child with an abnormal cardiac examination should be referred to a cardiologist for formal evaluation.

SPEECH AND LANGUAGE. Some children will have early speech delays that may be so subtle that they go undetected by the parents or teachers. An early and annual speech and language evaluation should be performed to detect any speech or language deficit that can be improved through early intervention. Because of the diversity of speech and language difficulties in children with fragile X, no one screening tool is recommended, and thus each child should be approached on an individual basis. Because routine screening tools such as the Denver Developmental Screening Test are usually not sensitive enough, children identified with fragile X syndrome should have a formal evaluation by a licensed speech and language pathologist preferably experienced with fragile X syndrome.

CONNECTIVE TISSUE PROBLEMS. Early detection of flat feet and scoliosis can prevent further sequelae. Screening should also include a careful examination for excessive joint laxity and other complications of loose connective tissue, such as hernias.

SEIZURES. When the clinical history suggests seizures, an electroencephalogram is indicated. Unusual findings can include a slow background rhythm and spike-wave discharges that are often similar to rolandic spikes (Musumeci et al., 1988a, 1988b). Any child who appears to be having seizures should be treated with anticonvulsant medication and be followed closely by a pediatric neurologist. If a child is taking medication to control seizures, anticonvulsant serum levels should be followed (see Chapter 15).

Drug interactions

Carbamazepine is a commonly prescribed anticonvulsant and is also used to control behavior problems such as violent outbursts, aggression, and self-injurious behavior. Concurrent treatment with macrolide antibiotics, cimetidine (Tagamet), propoxyphene (Darvon), and isoniazid (INH) can interfere with the breakdown of carbamazepine, causing nausea, vomiting, and lethargy. Folic acid therapy may worsen the seizure frequency in the child with epilepsy.

DIFFERENTIAL DIAGNOSIS AND MANAGEMENT OF COMMON PEDIATRIC CONDITIONS
Recurrent otitis media

As mentioned earlier, a frequent pediatric health problem in the child with fragile X is ear infections. It is imperative that these children be vigorously monitored and treated for recurrent otitis media to avoid sequelae that could further compromise language development and learning. In young children parents may not recognize otitis as the cause of their child's irritability. It may be helpful to inform parents of children with fragile X that recurrent otitis media is a common problem and review for them which signs or symptoms are indicators of infection.

To best determine a child's individualized medical management, newly diagnosed families should be referred to a health care team with expertise in fragile X syndrome for a thorough evaluation and consultation.

DEVELOPMENTAL ISSUES
Safety

Families and educators should not expect every child with fragile X to be able to learn age-appropriate safety. It will depend on each child's individual strengths and weaknesses. With strong visual and mimicking abilities and through the use of repetition, many children can be taught to follow safety tips.

Hyperactivity may lead to more accidents, so these children should be monitored closely. Because children with fragile X can be overstimulated by their environment, the home setting and particularly the child's playroom and bedroom should be a calm and uncluttered environment. The use of bean bag chairs, vibrating pillows, musical tapes, and appropriate environmental changes can be discussed with an occupational therapist.

Parents may also be concerned about their child's safety if they display self-injurious behavior. Head banging is rare but can be harmful to the child. Hand biting, despite its frequency, does not commonly cause scarring. Nevertheless, parents may wish to pursue behavior management therapies to decrease the frequency of these behaviors. Parents and professionals should also be advised of possible seizure activity and taught appropriate intervention.

Child care

Issues related to child care are common concerns for parents of a child with fragile X. Because of the short attention span and hyperactivity, child care providers should be knowledgeable about behavior modification techniques. The environment in which the child is placed is also important. Colors, noise level, and the amount of light can be altered to avoid overstimulation. Slowly but gradually new events can be programmed into the child's day. Setting a common time each week to introduce a new game, playing in a new space, or meeting a new day-care provider can help a child anticipate and deal more effectively with change. If these aspects of day care are well managed, there is no reason why a child with fragile X cannot be placed in full-day or half-day programs. Placement with nonaffected children is very helpful for modeling appropriate behavior.

Diet

Obsessive-compulsive behavior can be seen in children with fragile X syndrome, and this may involve food cravings. Obesity has been a problem for a small subgroup of children with fragile X (Fryns et al., 1987). This may, in fact, be secondary to perseverative eating or hypothalamic dysfunction (Fryns et al., 1987). Parents of obese children should be encouraged to place their children on appropriate diets. Exercise programs for older children may also be beneficial, and the use of exercise videos, which uses their visual and mimicking abilities are helpful. Failure to thrive is not uncommon in infants with fragile X syndrome. On the other hand this may be due to aversion to some food textures, frequent infections, or problematic mothering skills if the mother herself is affected by the syndrome.

Discipline

Children with fragile X syndrome are especially noncompliant in response to an unexpected event or change in routine and therefore need a highly structured environment. Sending the child to school the same way each day, having meals on a scheduled basis, and using the same nightly routines are encouraged. Behavior problems should be anticipated if the child is faced with an unexpected event. The prevention of unpredictable events in the home or at school is obviously an unrealistic expectation and should not be overemphasized. On the other hand, change and transitions should be gradually programmed into the child's learning and home environment. Setting limits, giving the child time-outs, and being consistent are appropriate responses when disciplinary action is required.

Toileting

Parents of children with fragile X often need help in setting realistic expectations regarding toilet training. Some children achieve this milestone on time, but delayed training is more common. Parents should not be discouraged if a child takes longer to learn. The establishment of a predictable routine and consistent positive reinforcement are general principles that are helpful for children with fragile X. As with parents of any child having toileting-training difficulties, parents are discouraged from being overly critical or reprimanding.

Sleep patterns

Frequent wakefulness in early childhood is a common problem in children with fragile X. Overstimulation can often interfere with sleeping, and calming techniques such as music are useful in quieting the child in preparation for bedtime.

School issues

Most children with fragile X syndrome identified thus far are receiving special education. Mainstreaming is a potential goal as described under the treatment section. Children can be mainstreamed in preschool programs as well, but child care providers should be experienced in specialized education. A program that provides for individualized attention and a high teacher/student ratio is best. The success of any approach will depend on a number of factors specific to each child, including the child's level of cognitive functioning, distractibility, impulsivity, the structure of the class, classroom environment, and appropriate role models.

Because few educators are knowledgeable about fragile X syndrome, the health care professional can play an active role in helping families educate the teachers and therapists about the specialized needs of their child and why an integrative approach that emphasizes a child's overall strengths and weaknesses is essential for effective learning.

Sexuality

Masturbation and other forms of self-stimulatory behavior are common among the mentally retarded population and are occasionally problematic for the adolescent with fragile X. Families can be supportive by providing appropriate sex education and by talking openly about sexuality issues. This need can also be met through family or individual counseling (Brown, Braden, and Sobesky, 1991). Counseling or therapy can also train new behaviors that can replace socially inappropriate behavior, such as masturbation in public. Most important, counseling can provide an environment in which the adolescent can discuss and deal with issues of sexuality in a supportive environment.

Fertility is usually normal in men with fragile X, although reproduction is rare because of cognitive deficits (Cantú, et al., 1976). Ovarian problems and premature menopause have been reported in heterozygous women (Cronister et al., 1991). Fryns (1986) has reported increased fertility and twinning in heterozygous fragile X women. Mildly retarded individuals will require support in parenting. Sex education and genetic counseling should therefore be available to them.

SPECIAL FAMILY CONCERNS

Perhaps the most frustrating aspect of having a child diagnosed with fragile X syndrome is realizing that so few professionals have a good understanding of this disorder and how it can affect a child and other family members. As a consequence many parents become the main advocate for their child in both the educational and medical settings. Health care professionals who are unfamiliar with fragile X syndrome should make every effort to listen carefully to families. It is also the parents' responsibility to (1) educate themselves about this unique disorder so that they too appreciate these children's specialized needs and (2) recognize their own needs if they require additional support because they themselves are affected by the syndrome.

AUTHOR'S NOTE

Exciting advances in the molecular biology of the fragile X gene were made in May of 1991. Oberle et al. (1991) and Yu et al. (1991) found the existence of the repetitive CGG sequences at the fragile X site. The length of the repetitive sequences has correlated with the degree of involvement from the fragile X syndrome. That is, normal transmitting males were found to possess a 150 to 400 base pair insertion and mentally retarded individuals with the full fragile X syndrome had a sequence length of over 1,000 base pairs. Subsequently, Verkerk et al. (1991) identified a candidate gene for the fragile X syndrome which was named the FMR 1 gene (fragile X mental retardation — 1 gene). This gene codes for a protein which is rich in arginine because of a lengthy CGG repeat. In affected individuals this CGG region will expand in length as previously reported to over 1,000 base pairs. There is also evidence for hypermethylation within this gene that also correlates with the degree of involvement from the fragile X syndrome. This significant advance will lead to a better DNA diagnostic tool for identifying carriers who are cytogenetically fragile X negative and also identifying individuals affected by the syndrome. Further work in this area will help to clarify the correlation between degree of clinical involvement and the structure of the gene, including the number of repetitive sequences and the focal areas of hypermethylation.

Oberle I, Rousseau F, Heitz D, Kretz C, Devys D, Hanauer A, Boue J, Bertheas MF, and Mandel JL: Instability of a 550-base pair DNA segment and abnormal methylation in fragile X syndrome, *Science* 252:1097-1102, 1991.

Verkerk AJMH, Plerettl M, Sutcliffe JS, Fu Y-H, Kuhl DPA, Pizzuti A, Reiner O, Richards S, Victoria MF, Zhang F, Eussen BE, van Ommen G-JB, Blonden LAJ, Riggins GJ, Chastain JL, Kunst CB, Galjaard H, Caskey CT, Nelson DL, Oostra BA, and Warren ST: Identification of a gene (FMR-1) containing a CGG repeat coincident with a breakpoint cluster region exhibiting length variation in fragile X syndrome, *Cell* 65(5):905-914, 1991.

Yu S, Pritchard M, Kremer E, Lynch M, Nancarrow J, Baker E, Holman K, Mulley JC, Warren ST, Schlessinger D, Sutherland GR, and Richards RI: Fragile X genotype characterized by an unstable region of DNA, *Science* 252:1179-1181, 1991.

SUMMARY OF PRIMARY CARE NEEDS
FOR THE CHILD WITH FRAGILE X SYNDROME

Growth and development

Physical growth is usually within normal limits.
Some children are reported to have large heads
for body size.
Deficits in cognitive function and speech are
common.
Developmental delays in gross motor skills are
common.

Immunizations

Routine immunizations are recommended.
AAP guidelines for immunizations in children
with seizures should be followed where indicated.

Screening
Vision

Eye examination for strabismus, refractive errors,
and visual perceptual skills is recommended at
the time of diagnosis. If no problems are
found, annual vision screening is recommended.

Hearing

An increased risk of otitis media warrants audiometric testing. The child may need referral to
an ENT specialist for PE tubes.

Dental

Screening for palate and dental abnormalities is
recommended. If mitral valve prolapse is present, prophylactic antibiotics will be needed for
dental work.

Blood pressure

Routine screening is recommended.

Hematocrit

Routine screening is recommended.

Urinalysis

Routine screening is recommended.

Tuberculosis

Routine screening is recommended.

Condition-specific screening
Mitral valve prolapse

In the presence of an abnormal cardiac examination, mitral valve prolapse must be ruled out
by a cardiologist.

Speech and language

Speech and language evaluation should be done
annually, with early intervention if a problem
is detected.

Connective tissue problems

The child should be screened for flat feet, scoliosis, and excessive joint laxity.

Seizure disorders

A clinical history suggestive of seizures must be
evaluated by electroencephalography. If the
child is taking anticonvulsants, blood levels
must be monitored.

Drug interactions

Carbamazepine is altered by macrolide antibiotics, cimetidine, propoxyphene, and isoniazid.
See Chapter 15 for drug interactions with seizure
medications.

Differential diagnosis

Recurrent otitis media is common.

Developmental issues
Safety

Cognitive dysfunction may limit the child's
awareness of safety issues.
Hyperactivity may make the child more accident
prone.
Self-injurious behavior may occur, and parents
can be taught behavior management therapies.
If seizures are present, seizure precautions are
necessary.

Child care

Short attention span and hyperactivity may be
modified by subdued environments. New activities must be introduced slowly.

Diet

Obsessive eating may result in obesity in older
children.
Infants may have failure to thrive.

Continued.

**SUMMARY OF PRIMARY CARE NEEDS
FOR THE CHILD WITH FRAGILE X SYNDROME — cont'd**

Discipline

Children behave better in highly structured environments.
Consistent limit setting is beneficial.
Positive reinforcement is essential.

Toileting

Delayed continence is not uncommon.

Sleep patterns

Frequent wakefulness in early childhood is not uncommon.
Overstimulation should be avoided.

School issues

Most children are placed in special education.
The provider can help educate the school system personnel on condition and treatment.

Sexuality

Self-stimulatory behaviors are common. Counseling may help decrease inappropriate behavior.
Fertility is normal in men; reports on women vary.
Sex education, birth control, and genetic counseling are necessary.

Special family concerns

The family may have difficulty adjusting to the diagnosis; parents may also be affected.
Genetic counseling is warranted.
Because the condition is not well known, care may be nonspecific.

RESOURCES

The National Fragile X Foundation was established to educate parents, professionals, and the lay public regarding the diagnosis and treatment of fragile X syndrome and other forms of X-linked mental retardation. In addition, the National Fragile X Foundation promotes research pertaining to fragile X syndrome in the areas of biochemistry, genetics, and clinical applications. All parents who have a child diagnosed with fragile X syndrome and interested professionals working with the developmentally delayed population are encouraged to write or call the foundation so they may receive the quarterly newsletter and other services available to them.

Organizations

National Fragile X Foundation
   1441 York St, Suite 215
   Denver, CO 80206
   (800) 688-8765
   (303) 333-6155

REFERENCES

Benezech M and Noel B: Fra(X) syndrome and autism, *Clin Genet* 28:93, 1985.

Borghgraef M, Fryns J, Dielkens A, et al: Fragile X syndrome: A study of the psychological profile in 23 patients, *Clin Genet* 32:179-186, 1987.

Borghgraef M, Fryns JP, and Van den Berghe H: The female and the fragile X syndrome: Data on clinical and psychological findings in fragile X carriers, *Clin Genet* 37:341-346, 1990.

Braden M: *Optimal educational strategies to maximize learning potential in the fragile X patient,* Unpublished manuscript, 1988.

Bregman J, Ort S, and Leckman J: Controlled study of Ritalin, Clonidine, and placebo, Personal communication, 1989.

Brondum-Nielsen K, Tommerup N, Frillis B, et al: Diagnosis of the fragile X syndrome (Martin-Bell syndrome): Clinical findings in 27 males with the fragile site at Xq28, *J Ment Defic Res* 27:211-226, 1983.

Brown J, Braden M, and Sobesky W: Treatment of behavioral and emotional problems. In Hagerman RJ and Silverman AC, eds: *The fragile X syndrome: Diagnosis, treatment, and research,* Baltimore, 1991, Johns Hopkins University Press.

Brown WT, Gross A, Chan C, et al: Clinical use of DNA markers in the fragile X syndrome for carrier detection and prenatal diagnosis. In Willey AM, ed: *Nucleic acid probes in diagnosis of human genetic diseases,* New York, 1988, Wiley & Sons.

Brown WT, Jenkins EC, Cohen IL, et al: Fragile X and autism, *Am J Med Genet* 23:341-352, 1986.

Brown WT, Jenkins EC, Friedman E, et al: Autism is associated with the fragile X syndrome, *J Autism Dev Disord* 12:303-307, 1982.

Butler MG, Allen GA, Slingh D, et al: Preliminary communication: Photoanthropometric analysis of individuals with the fragile X syndrome, *Am J Med Genet* 30:165-168, 1988.

Butler MG, Allen GA, Haynes JL, et al: Anthropomorphic comparisons in mentally retarded males with and without the fragile X syndrome, *Am J Med Genet* 38:260-268, 1991.

Cantu JM, Scaglia HE, Medina M, et al: Inherited congenital normofunctional testicular hyperplasia and mental deficiency, Hum Genet 33:23-33, 1976.

Chudley AE, de von Flindt R, and Hagerman RJ: Cognitive variability in the fragile X syndrome, *Am J Med Genet* 28:13-15, 1987 (invited editorial comment).

Committee on Infectious Diseases: *Report of the Committee on Infectious Diseases,* ed 22, Elk Grove Village, Il, The American Academy of Pediatrics, 1991.

Cronister A, Schreiner R, Wittenberger M, et al: The heterozygous fragile X female: Historical, physical, cognitive and cytogenetic features, *Am J Med Genet* (in press).

Davids JR, Hagerman RJ, and Eilert RE: The orthopaedic aspects of the fragile X syndrome, *J Bone Joint Surg BR* 72:889-896.

Dykens E, Hodapp R, Ort S, et al: The trajectory of cognitive development in males with the fragile X syndrome, *J Am Acad Child Adolesc Psychiatry* 28:422-426, 1989.

Fryns JP: The female and the fragile X: A study of 144 obligate female carriers, *Am J Med Genet* 23:157-169, 1986.

Fryns JP, Haspeslagh M, Deneymaeker AM, et al: A peculiar subphenotype in the fragile X syndrome: Extreme obesity, short stature, stubby hands and feet, diffuse hyperpigmentation. Further evidence of disturbed hypothalamic function in the fragile X syndrome? *Clin Genet* 32:388-392, 1987.

Fryns JP, Kleczkowska A, and Van den Berghe H, et al: The psychological profile of the fragile X syndrome, *Clin Genet* 25:131-134, 1984.

Hagerman RJ: Fragile X syndrome, *Curr Probl Pediatr* 17:621-674, 1987.

Hagerman RJ: Physical and behavioral phenotype. In Hagerman RJ and Silverman AC eds: *The fragile X syndrome: Diagnosis, treatment, and research,* Baltimore (1991a), Johns Hopkins University Press.

Hagerman RJ: Medical follow-up and pharmacotherapy. In Hagerman RJ and Silverman AC, eds: *The fragile X syndrome: Diagnosis, treatment, and research,* Baltimore (1991b), Johns Hopkins University Press.

Hagerman RJ, Amiri K, and Cronister A: The fragile X checklist, *Am J Med Genet* 38:283-287.

Hagerman RJ, Berry R, Jackson III AW, et al: Institutional screening for the fragile X syndrome, *Am J Dis Child* 142:1216-1221, 1988.

Hagerman RJ, Kemper M, and Hudson M: Learning disabilities and attentional problems in boys with the fragile X syndrome, *Am J Dis Child* 139:674-678, 1985.

Hagerman RJ, Murphy M, and Wittenberger M: A controlled trial of stimulant medication in children with fragile X syndrome, *Am J Med Genet* 30:377-392, 1988.

Hagerman RJ, Schreiner R, Kemper M, et al: Longitudinal IQ changes in fragile X males. *Am J Med Genet* 33:513-518, 1989.

Hagerman RJ, Altshul-Stark D, and McBogg P: Recurrent otitis media in boys with the fragile X syndrome, *Am J Dis Child* 142:1216-1221, 1987.

Hagerman RJ, Smith ACM, and Mariner R: Clinical features of the fragile X syndrome. In Hagerman RJ and McBogg PM, eds: *The fragile X syndrome: Diagnosis, biochemistry and intervention,* Dillon, Colo, 1983, Spectra Publishing, pp 83-94.

Hagerman RJ and Sobesky WE: Psychopathology in fragile X syndrome, *Am J Orthopsychiatry* 59:142-152, 1989.

Hagerman RJ, Van Housen K, Smith ACM, et al: Consideration of connective tissue dysfunction in the fragile X syndrome, *Am J Med Genet* 17:111-121, 1984.

Herbst D and Miller J: Non specific X-linked mental retardation: II. The frequency in British Columbia, *Am J Med Genet* 7:461-469, 1980.

Hockey A and Crowhurst J: Early manifestations of the Martin-Bell syndrome based on a series of both sexes from infancy, *Am J Med Genet* 30:61-71, 1988.

Jenkins EC, Brown WT, Krawczun CJ, et al: Recent experience in prenatal fra(X) detection, *Am J Med Genet* 30:329-336, 1988.

Kemper MB, Hagerman RJ, Ahmad RS, et al: Cognitive profiles and the spectrum of clinical manifestations in heterozygous fra(X) females, *Am J Med Genet* 23:139-156, 1986.

Kemper MB, Hagerman RJ, and Altshul-Stark D: Cognitive profiles of boys with the fragile X syndrome, *Am J Med Genet* 30:191-200, 1987.

Lachiewicz AM, Gullion CM, Spiridigliozzi GA, et al: Declining IQ scores of young males with fragile X syndrome, *Am J Med Genet* 30:272-278, 1987.

Loehr JP, Synhorst DP, Wolfe RR, et al: Aortic root dilatation and mitral valve prolapse in the fragile X syndrome, *Am J Med Genet* 23:189-194, 1986.

Loesch DZ and Hay DA: Clinical features and reproductive patterns in fragile X female heterozygotes, *J Med Genet* 25:407-414, 1988.

Madison LS, George C, and Moeschler JB: Cognitive functioning in the fragile X syndrome: A study of intellectual, memory and communication skills, *J Ment Defic Res* 30:129-148, 1986.

Miezejeski CM, Jenkins EC, Hill AL, et al: A profile of cognitive deficit in females from fragile X families, *Neuropsychologia* 24:405-409, 1986.

Musumeci SA, Colognola RM, Ferri R, et al: Fragile X syndrome: A particular epileptogenic EEG pattern, *Epilepsia* 29:41-47, 1988b.

Musumeci SA, Ferri R, Colognola RM, et al: Prevalence of a novel epileptogenic EEG pattern in the Martin-Bell syndrome, *Am J Med Genet* 30:207-212, 1988a.

Musumeci SA, Hagerman RJ, Amiri K, Cronister A: Epilepsy, EEG findings and associated complaints in fragile X syndrome. Submitted for publication.

Newell K, Sanborn B, and Hagerman RJ: Speech and language dysfunction in the fragile X syndrome. In Hagerman RJ and McBogg P, eds: *The fragile X syndrome: Diagnosis, biochemistry and intervention,* Dillon, Colo, 1983, Spectra Publishing, pp 175-200.

Opitz JM: On the gates of hell and a most unusual gene, *Am J Med Genet* 23:1-10, 1986.

Opitz JM, Westphal JM, and Daniel A: Discovery of a connective tissue dysplasia in the Martin-Bell Syndrome, *Am J Med Genet* 17:101-109, 1984.

Partington MW: The fragile X syndrome: Preliminary data on growth and development in males, *Am J Med Genet* 17:175-194, 1984.

Prouty LA, Rogers C, Stevenson RE, et al: Fragile X syndrome: Growth development and intellectual function, *Am J Med Genet* 30:123-142, 1988.

Pueschel SM and Finelli PV: Neurologic investigations in patients with fragile X syndrome. Proceedings of the American Academy of Cerebral Palsy and Developmental Medicine, Washington, DC, April 1984 (abstract).

Rapin I: Conductive hearing loss effects on children's language and scholastic skills: A review of the literature, *Ann Otol Rhinol Laryngol* 88:3-12, 1979.

Reiss AL, Hagerman RJ, Vinogradov S, et al: Psychiatric disability in female carriers of fragile X chromosome, *Arch Gen Psychiatry* 45:25-30, 1988.

Scharfenaker S, Hickman L, and Braden M: An integrated approach to intervention with fragile X individuals. In Hagerman RJ and Silverman AC eds: *Fragile X syndrome: Diagnosis, treatment, and research,* Baltimore, (1991), Johns Hopkins University Press.

Scharfenaker S and Schreiner R: Cognitive and speech language characteristics of the fragile X syndrome, *Rocky Mountain J Commun Disorders,* 1989.

Schnizel A and Largo RH: The fragile X syndrome (Martin-Bell syndrome) clinical and cytogenetic findings in 16 prepubertal boys and in 4 of their 5 families, *Helv Paediatr Acta* 40:133-152, 1985.

Shapiro LR, Wilmot PL, Murphy PD: Prenatal diagnosis of the fragile X syndrome: Possible end of the experimental phase for amniotic fluid, *Am J Med Genet* 38:453-455, 1991.

Sherman SL: Introduction and epidemiology of the fragile X syndrome. In Hagerman RJ and Silverman AC, eds: *Fragile X syndrome: Diagnosis, treatment and research,* Baltimore, (1991), Johns Hopkins University Press.

Sherman SL, Jacobs PA, Morton NE, et al: Further segregation analysis of the fragile X syndrome with special reference to transmitting males, *Hum Genet* 69:289-299, 1985.

Sherman SL, Morton NE, Jacobs PA, et al: The marker (X) syndrome: A cytogenetic and genetic analysis, *Ann Hum Genet* 48:21-37, 1984.

Silverman AC: Genetic Counseling. In Hagerman RJ and Silverman AC, eds: *Fragile X syndrome: Diagnosis, treatment, and research,* Baltimore (1991), Johns Hopkins University Press.

Simko A, Hornstein L, Sonkup S, et al: Fragile X syndrome: Recognition in young children, *Pediatrics* 83:547-552, 1989.

Sreeran N, Wren C, Bhate M, et al: Cardiac abnormalities in the fragile X syndrome, *Br Heart J* 61:289-291, 1989.

Storm RL, De Benito R, and Ferretti C: Ophthalmologic findings in the fragile syndrome, *Arch Ophthalmol* 105:1099-1102, 1987.

Sutherland GR and Hecht F: *Fragile sites on human chromosomes,* New York, 1985, Oxford University Press.

Turner G, Daniel A, and Frost M: X-linked mental retardation, macroorchidism, and the Xq27 fragile site, *J Pediatr* 96:837-841, 1980.

Turner G, Opitz JM, Brown TW, et al: Conference report: Second international workshop on the fragile X and on X-linked mental retardation, *Am J Med Genet* 23:11-67, 1986.

Wearer DD and Sherman SL: Letter to the Editor: A counseling guide to the Martin-Bell syndrome, *Am J Med Genet* 26:39-44, 1987.

Webb TD, Thake A, and Todd J: Twelve families with fragile Xq27, *J Med Genet* 23:400-406, 1986.

Windeck SL and Laurel M: A theoretical framework combining speech-language therapy with sensory integration treatment, *Am Occup Ther Assoc Sensory Integration Spec Interest Sect Newslett* 12:1-5, 1989.

Wisniewski KE, Segan SM, Miezejeski CM, et al: The fragile X syndrome: Neurological, electrophysiological and neuropathological abnormalities, *Am J Med Genet* 38:476-480, 1991.

17 *Hydrocephalus*

···

Patricia Ludder Jackson

ETIOLOGY

Hydrocephalus results from an imbalance between the production and absorption of cerebrospinal fluid (CSF), resulting in the enlargement of the ventricular system and increased CSF pressure. It is most frequently caused by an intraventricular or extraventricular blockage in the normal circulation and absorption of CSF (Fig. 17-1 and the box on p. 304).

In *congenital obstructive hydrocephalus* the flow of CSF to the arachnoid spaces is blocked, resulting in enlargement of the ventricular system proximal to the site of obstruction. The most common obstruction is congenital aqueductal stenosis usually at the aqueduct of Sylvius. This may occur as the result of a perinatal infection (toxoplasmosis, cytomegalovirus, mumps, syphilis, meningitis) or as a result of compression and obstruction of the aqueduct by a lesion (congenital aneurysm, arachnoid cyst, subdural hematoma caused by birth injury, intraventricular or subarachnoid hemorrhage or early neonatal brain tumors) (Bell and McCormick, 1978; Volpe, 1987). Congenital malformations of the brain, such as Dandy-Walker malformation, which causes atresia of the foramina of Luschka and Magendie, also result in hydrocephalus. In addition, there is a sex-linked recessive form of aqueductal stenosis. Hydrocephalus may also be a component of numerous syndromes (Bell and McCormick, 1978; Volpe, 1987).

Outside of the newborn period, obstructive hydrocephalus may occur as a result of CNS infections, tumors, trauma, arteriovenous malforma-

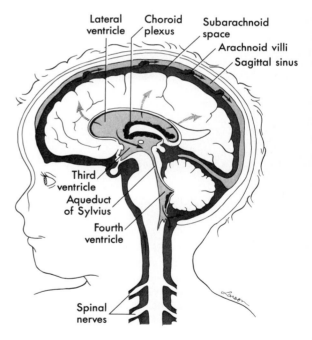

Fig. 17-1. Cerebrospinal fluid (CSF) circulatory pathway. Drawing shows a view of the center of the brain. *Solid arrows* show major pathway of CSF flow; *broken arrows* show additional pathways. *From About hydrocephalus: A book for parents (p. 9) Edwards MS and Derechin M, (eds) Drawings by Lynne Larson. 1986, San Francisco, University of California. Reprinted with permission.*

303

CLASSIFICATION OF HYDROCEPHALUS

I. Noncommunicating (intraventricular obstructive) hydrocephalus
   A. Maldevelopment of the aqueduct
   B. Obstruction caused by a mass (i.e., neoplasm, cyst, hematoma, aneurysm)
   C. Obstruction secondary to exudate, hemorrhage, or parasites
   D. Obstruction of the fourth ventricle outlet (i.e., Dandy-Walker malformation)
II. Communicating (extraventricular obstructive) hydrocephalus
   A. Secondary to central nervous system (CNS) infection or hemorrhage
   B. Arachnoid villi obstruction by erythrocytes
   C. Arnold-Chiari malformation
   D. Congenital malformation of arachnoid villi
III. Communication hydrocephalus caused by excessive CSF formation
   A. Choroid plexus papilloma

Adapted from Bell WE and McCormick WF: *Increased intracranial pressure in children: Diagnosis and treatment*, Philadelphia, 1978, WB Saunders.

---

tions, or systemic bleeding disorders (Bell and McCormick, 1978).

Communicating hydrocephalus occurs when blockage of normal CSF reabsorption in the subarachnoid area develops. It may be the result of CNS infection, bacterial or viral, subarachnoid hemorrhage, or as the result of congenital malformation of the subarachnoid spaces. In communicating hydrocelphalus both the lateral and fourth ventricles are enlarged.

INCIDENCE

The overall incidence of hydrocephalus may be as high as 2 per 1000. The incidence of hydrocephalus, excluding the hydrocephalus associated with myelomeningocele, is estimated to be 0.5 to 1 per 1000, with aqueductal stenosis responsible for approximately one third of the cases (Stein et al., 1981). The incidence of myelomeningocele varies dramatically from region to region. In the United States the incidence is approximately 1 per 1000

births. Eighty percent of these children will develop hydrocephalus during the first year of life as a result of either an Arnold-Chiari II malformation of the subarachnoid pathway or an associated aqueductal stenosis.

CLINICAL MANIFESTATIONS AT TIME OF DIAGNOSIS

Although the signs and symptoms of hydrocephalus may be somewhat varied as a result of the specific cause of the condition, there are common clinical manifestations associated with the increased intracranial pressure. If the accumulation of excessive CSF occurs slowly, the infant or young child may be asymptomatic until the hydrocephalus is quite advanced (Bell and McCormick, 1978). Significant dilation of the ventricle may occur before abnormal head growth is apparent. Full or distended fontanels, frontal bossing, prominent scalp veins, vomiting, irritability, and even opisthotonic posturing may be observed by the practitioner before dramatic changes are noted in head circumference.

In the child more than 18 to 24 months of age with fused cranial sutures, the development of hydrocephalus may result in the nonspecific symptoms of headache, nausea, vomiting, and personality changes, including irritability, lethargy, and loss of interest in normal daily activities. Spasticity or ataxia of the lower extremities, as well as urinary incontinence, may occur. These children frequently complain of vision problems because increased intracranial pressures on the second, third, or sixth cranial nerves result in extraocular muscular paresis and papilledema (Bell and McCormick, 1978). Alterations in growth, sexual development, and fluid and electrolyte imbalance may occur if there is increased pressure at the site of the hypothalamus.

TREATMENT

Treatment for hydrocephalus must be aimed at the individual cause and corrected if possible. Shunting of the CSF away from the closed cranial space is usually necessary (Olsen and Frykberg, 1983; Post, 1985). Ventriculoperitoneal shunts are most commonly used, but ventriculoatrial shunts are also used when the peritoneal cavity is inaccessible (Fig. 17-2). The ventricular portion of the shunt is inserted into the anterior horn of the lateral ventricle via a parietal or occipital burr hole. The peritoneal

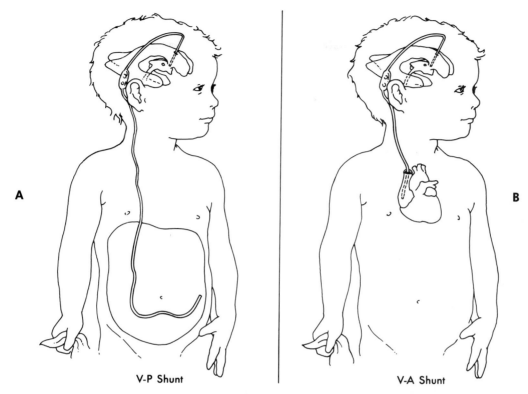

A

B

V-P Shunt   V-A Shunt

Fig. 17-2. Pathway used for **A,** ventriculoperitoneal shunt and **B,** ventriculoatrial shunt. *From About hydrocephalus: A book for parents (p. 21) Edwards MS and Derechin M, (eds) Drawings by Lynne Larson, 1986, San Francisco, University of California. Reprinted with permission.*

or atrial portion is tunneled under the child's skin to the designated location where a small incision is made and the distal portion of the shunt is either inserted through the peritoneum into the peritoneal cavity or through the neck into the superior vena cava and into the right atrium. The reservoir and tubing are palpable from the burr hole to its insertion at either the peritoneum or superior vena cava.

Although the advent of CSF shunting dramatically improved the prognosis for children with hydrocephalus, shunts continue to have inherent problems. Shunt malfunction may occur because of chronic or acute inflammation, accumulation of cellular debris or blood, or occlusion of either the distal or proximal end of the shunt as a result of growth (Sekhar, Moossy, and Guthkelch, 1982). Shunts in children with cranial neoplasms were found to have the highest rate of complications in

a recent study (Serlo, Fernell, Heikkinen, et al., 1990). The need for shunt revisions occurs at some point in almost all children treated for hydrocephalus from infancy and averages three to five revisions during childhood (Amacher and Wellington, 1984; Dennis et al., 1981; McCullough and Balzer-Martin, 1982). Although shunt revisions are traumatic for the child and family and pose physical risk because of surgery and increased intracranial pressure, the number of revisions has not been adversely associated with intellectual activity (Dennis et al., 1981).

The incidence of shunt infection has decreased significantly in the past decade but continues to be a major source of shunt malfunction and potential morbidity for the child. Shunts create a medium in the host where normal phagocytosis is impaired, allowing the child to be more susceptible to CNS infections (Borges, 1982). Reported rates of infection range from 2% to 17.8% (Andretta, 1987; Odio, McCraken, and Nelson, 1984; Serlo, Fernell, Heikkinen, et al., 1990; Yogev, 1985), with infants less than 1 year of age having a higher incidence than older children and children with hydrocephalus due to perinatal intracranial hemorrhage having the highest rate of infection. Staphylococcal organisms are responsible for 60% to 75% of infections, with gram-negative bacilli being the second most common organism associated with peritoneal shunts. More than 50% of staphylococcal infections occur within 2 weeks of the operation, and 70% of all infections occur within 2 months of surgery, probably from a slow-growing contaminate such as *Staphylococcus epidermidis* (Yogev, 1985). *Haemophilus influenzae* meningitis is also believed to be more common in children with shunts (Patriarca and Lauer, 1980; Rennels and Wald, 1980).

Due to the increased risk of even transient bacteremia causing shunt infections it is generally recommended that children with shunts receive antibiotic prophylaxis prior to dental work with anticipated bleeding, oral or upper respiratory tract procedures, and genitourinary and gastrointestinal procedures. The recommended prophylaxis is the same used for prevention of bacterial endocarditis in children with CHD (see the box on p. 196, Chapter 11) (Dajani, Bisno, Chung, et al., 1990). In children with ventriculoatrial shunts, the possibility of bacterial endocarditis as a complication must not be overlooked. Cardiac complications from atrial shunts is a major reason peritoneal shunts are more popular today.

Approximately 20% of the children with congenital hydrocephalus outgrow the need for a shunt (Epstein, 1985). This compensated or resolved hydrocephalus usually occurs during the first year of life with rapid growth of the brain structures, though it may not be identified until later when revision of the shunt because of growth would normally occur. Compensated hydrocephalus is accompanied by stable moderate or advanced ventriculomegaly. In this situation the shunt is left in place until needed to be removed, and the child is followed by periodic computerized tomography scans and neuropsychologic examinations. Annual neuropsychologic testing is recommended because intellectual deterioration has been associated with

arrested hydrocephalus (Whittle, Johnston, and Besser, 1985).

PROGNOSIS

The outlook for children with hydrocephalus continues to improve. Five-year survival usually is greater than 80%, with the majority of deaths occurring as a result of severe congenital malformations or progressive brain tumors during the first year of treatment (Amacher and Wellington, 1984; Fernell, Hagberg, and Hagberg 1988a, 1988b; McCullough and Balzer-Martin, 1982). Congenital hydrocephalus ranks eighth in congenital anomalies for years of potential life lost as measured by the National Center for Health Statistics (Centers for Disease Control 1988). It is important for the primary care provider to remember that children with hydrocephalus remain at risk for increased morbidity and early mortality even after years of excellent progress and shunt function (Amacher and Wellington, 1984).

ASSOCIATED PROBLEMS
Intellectual problems

Intellectual function is difficult to predict early after diagnosis. The etiology of the hydrocephalus appears to be the most important determining factor, with uncomplicated hydrocephalus having a better cognitive prognosis than hydrocephalus associated with brain injury. In recent studies, two thirds of the children with hydrocephalus had normal or borderline normal intelligence (Amacher and Wellington, 1984; Dennis et al., 1981; McCullough and Balzer, 1982). In children with IQs greater than 70, performance IQs were lower than full-scale and verbal IQs (Amacher and Wellington, 1984; Dennis et al., 1981; McCullough and Balzer, 1982). This discrepancy indicates a need for preschool and school counseling and testing to identify areas of learning disability.

Ocular problems

As reported earlier, ocular abnormalities are often found at the time of diagnosis or during episodes of shunt malfunction. Increased intracranial pressure results in optic nerve pressure, limited upward gaze, extraocular muscle paresis, and papilledema (Dennis et al., 1981; Rudolph, 1987).

Even with a functioning shunt and controlled

hydrocephalus, however, visual problems are common. Gaze and movement problems such as strabismus, astigmatism, nystagmus, and amblyopia are found in approximately 25% to 33% of the children (Mankinen-Heikkinen and Mustonen, 1987). Refractive and accommodation errors are found in about the same percentage of children but not necessarily the same children. The optic disk is frequently found to be abnormally light or pale but papilledema is not found under normal conditions (Mankinen-Heikkinen and Mustonen, 1987). Abnormalities in vision are associated with lower intelligence scores and may help identify the child at higher risk for mental retardation and need for more careful followup and referral to infant stimulation programs (Dennis et al., 1981; Donders, Canady, and Rourke, 1990). Correctable visual problems should be attended to as soon as possible so that poor vision does not interfere with learning potential.

Motor disabilities

Unfortunately as many as 75% of the children with hydrocephalus will have some form of motor disability (Dennis et al., 1981, Fernell, Hagberg, and Hagberg 1988a, 1988b). These disabilities vary from severe paraplegia to mild imbalance or weakness. The severity of the motor deficit is most often diagnosis related, with conditions such as porencephaly, Dandy-Walker malformation, and myelomeningocele having more serious motor defects than simple congenital hydrocephalus.

Hydrocephalus also affects fine motor control (Dennis et al., 1981). Kinesthetic-proprioceptive abilities of the hands are often negatively affected, and this, coupled with the impaired bimanual manipulation and frequent visual deficits, makes it difficult for the child with hydrocephalus to perform well on time-limited, nonverbal intelligence tests (Dennis et al., 1981).

Seizures

Because of the increased intracranial pressure, seizures in infancy are common at the time of initial diagnosis. Fortunately, only 20% to 33% of the infants with hydrocephalus continue to have seizures after the first year of life (Dennis et al., 1981; Fernell, Hagberg, and Hagberg, 1988a, 1988b). These seizures may be simple or complex, partial or generalized, and usually can be well managed with standard anticonvulsant therapy. Acquired hydrocephalus is more often associated with seizure activity because of the underlying reason for the development of hydrocephalus (e.g., brain tumor, CNS trauma, or infection). These seizures may be more focal in origin and more difficult to control. (For further discussion on seizure disorders, see Chapter 15.)

PRIMARY CARE MANAGEMENT
Growth and development

Both precocious puberty and short stature have been reported in children with hydrocephalus (Greenspan and Forsham, 1986). Sexual development before the age of 8 years in girls and 10 years in boys is considered precocious and warrants further diagnostic study. Heights below the fifth percentile, if not compatible with family stature, indicate growth retardation. Treatment is available for both of these conditions, and children should be referred to an endocrinologist if these signs occur.

Typically, measurements of a child being seen in a primary care practice are done by minimally trained office or clinic personnel. In the case of the child suspected of having hydrocephalus or known to have hydrocephalus, the head circumference should be measured by the practitioner. Until the cranial sutures are completely fused, which is often delayed in these children, growth of head size is a major diagnostic tool in evaluating the child's condition.

Once the diagnosis of hydrocephalus has been made and a shunt inserted, the head circumference may decrease 1 to 2 cm as the pressure is relieved. After this initial decrease the head should grow only in proportion to the child's body. Therefore, a newborn infant whose weight and height are in the fiftieth percentile for age and who has a head size of 40 cm when a shunt is placed shortly after birth may not resume head growth for 2 to 4 months (Fig. 17-3). Resumption of growth prior to that time might indicate shunt malfunction. The significance of head size measurements in the shunted child cannot be overestimated, and daily measurements may be necessary during evaluation of the shunt-dependent infant for possible shunt malfunction.

Standard early infant developmental assessment

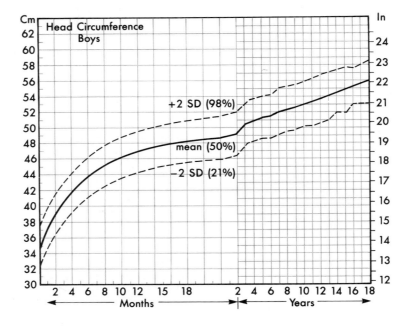

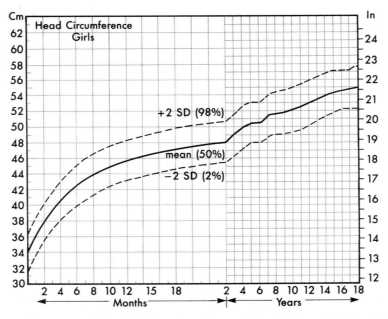

Fig. 17-3. Head circumference charts from birth to age 18 years. From Neilhaus, G.: Head circumference from birth to eighteen years, Pediatrics 41:106-114, 1968.

tools used in primary care practice, such as the Denver Developmental Screening Test, are of little help is assessing these infants. Tasks that require head control, such as elevating the head while in the prone position, rolling over, pulling to a sitting position without head lag, and even sitting unassisted, will be delayed in the infant with macrocephaly. It is important for the practitioner to interpret developmental findings in light of other clinical observations to assist the parents in setting reasonable expectations for their infant.

Other motor delays can be expected during infancy and childhood given that approximately 75% of children with hydrocephalus have some form of motor disability. The primary care provider must carefully document motor skill acquisition, because a loss of skill may indicate shunt malfunction or progression of the primary etiology. This applies to the older school-aged child and the infant. Ataxia, slurred speech, lack of progression in school, incontinence, and so forth may indicate a deterioration in neurologic status and the need for further evaluation.

Often these children will benefit from infant stimulation programs or physical therapy, and the health care provider must be familiar with the program offerings in the family's community to help them identify services that would be most beneficial for their child.

Immunizations

Diphtheria, tetanus, and pertussis. Pertussis poses a special problem for infants with hydrocephalus. Infants and children with a history of seizures are at increased risk of seizures following receipt of pertussis (Committee on Infectious Diseases, 1991). As stated earlier, seizures at the time of diagnosis during the newborn period are often present in infants with hydrocephalus. It is difficult to determine which of these infants will continue to have recurrent seizures and which will not. Hence, deferral of diphtheria-tetanus-pertussis immunization may be prudent until neurologic stability is ascertained. The risk of contracting pertussis is low, but because "neurologically impaired children may be at an increased risk of morbidity and morality from illness caused by *Bordetella pertussis*, immunization is not absolutely contraindicated, and in some patients (such as those with well-controlled seizures, corrected hydrocephalus, or cerebral palsy) will be indicated" (Committee on Infectious Diseases, 1991).

Outbreaks of pertussis continue to occur in the United States; the decision to defer vaccination should be reassessed with the parents at each visit. Children in day care, attending special developmental programs, or receiving care in residential centers are exposed to other children who also may not be immunized and therefore are at increased risk of developing pertussis. The primary care provider will need to weigh the risk of disease against the risk of the vaccine's side effects. In these difficult situations consultation with the child's neurosurgeon or neurologist may be advisable to help assess the child's seizure potential.

If the primary care provider, with parental consent, decides early in infancy that the pertussis immunization will be withheld, diphtheria and tetanus vaccines should be given on schedule. When an acellular pertussis vaccine becomes available, the incidence of neurologic side effects may be decreased. Hopefully infants with a history of seizures may then be immunized on schedule without increased risk.

Measles. Measles vaccine has also been implicated in postvaccination seizures, with a higher incidence occurring in infants and children with a personal history of convulsions (Committee on Infectious Diseases, 1991). It is not believed these postvaccine seizures produce permanent neurologic damage, and the high ongoing risk of natural measles with its high morbidity rate justifies measles immunization in children with a personal history of convulsions (Committee on Infectious Diseases, 1991).

Haemophilus influenzae type b. The use of Hib vaccine is variable but generally much lower than the other recommended vaccinations (Gururaj and Rogers, 1987). Because of the increased risk of *Haemophilus influenza* type b CNS infections in children with shunts (Borges, 1982; Patriarca and Lauer, 1980; Rennels and Wald, 1980), children with shunted hydrocephalus should definitely receive the new conjugated vaccine starting at 2 months of age (Centers for Disease Control, 1991). Children who have had a history of documented Hib disease before 2 years of age may not produce adequate antibodies to prevent a second infection and should therefore also be immunized. Chemoprophylaxis of household or day-care contacts of children with Hib disease is required even with adequate immunization (Centers for Disease Control, 1991).

Other immunizations. Vaccination for polio, mumps, and rubella should be given as routinely scheduled. At this time there is no research on the efficacy of giving pneumococcal or influenza vaccines to these children (AAP, 1988), but the primary care provider may elect to administer these additional vaccines to children with multiple shunt infections or severe motor disabilities. As soon as varicella vaccine is licensed, it is recommended that these children be given it to lessen the chance of varicella encephalitis.

Screening

Vision. Because of high incidence of visual defects in children with hydrocephalus, the practitioner must pay particular attention to visual screening. The Hirschberg light reflex, cover test, tracking, and fundoscopic examinations should be performed at each office visit and the results carefully documented in the record. At approximately 6 months of age the child should be referred to a pediatric ophthalmologist for a thorough examination. Yearly examinations should be scheduled thereafter.

Frequently these children will need eye muscle surgery to correct esotropia or exotropia. The practitioner can be instrumental in completing preoperative examinations and preparing the family for surgery.

Hearing. In addition to routine office screening for hearing acuity, an auditory evoked response test should be ordered if the infant has had a history of CNS infection or antibiotic treatment with aminoglycocides. Subsequent shunt malfunctions or CNS infections require reassessment of hearing. Periodic evaluation by an audiologist is recommended.

Dental. Routine dental care is recommended. If the child is taking phenytoin (Dilantin) for seizure control, dental care may need to be more frequent because of hyperplasia of the gums. Poor dental hygiene and peridontal infections may produce bacteremia even in the absence of dental procedures (Dajani et al., 1990). Prophylaxis with penicillin

is recommended for all dental work likely to cause gingival bleeding including routine cleaning of teeth. The spontaneous shedding of primary teeth or simple adjustment of orthodontic appliances do not require prophylaxis (Dajani, et al., 1990), to prevent bacterial endocarditis (see Chapter 11).

Blood pressure. Blood pressure readings should be recorded on each clinic or office visit. Elevations in blood pressure occur in conjunction with elevations in intracranial pressure. Having an established baseline reading can help the practitioner assess the child for possible shunt malfunctions or progression of disease process.

Hematocrit. Routine screening is recommended.

Urinalysis. Routine screening is recommended.

Tuberculosis screening. Routine screening is recommended.

Condition-specific screening

HEAD CIRCUMFERENCE. Head circumference measurements should be taken at every clinic or office visit until the child's sutures are completely fused (see the discussion of growth and development).

Drug interactions

No routine medications are prescribed for children with hydrocephalus. (See Chapter 15 for drug interactions with anticonvulsant therapy.)

DIFFERENTIAL DIAGNOSIS AND MANAGEMENT FOR COMMON PEDIATRIC CONDITIONS

Unfortunately for the primary care provider, many of the symptoms of shunt malfunction or infection are the same symptoms commonly found with routine childhood illness. It is important to remember that these children will develop otitis media, gastrointestinal (GI) illnesses, and viral infections with fever just like their unaffected peers. The practitioner must approach these children as children first. A calm manner, accompanied by a thorough history and examination, will be most reassuring to parents and most productive for the practitioner.

Fever

Fevers associated with shunt malfunction or infection can be chronic or acute, mild or severe. The greater the time that has elapsed since the child's last shunt surgery, the less likely the fever is associated with shunt malfunction. Other symptoms, especially a change in sensorium or continued irritability after the fever has been controlled, are the most critical observations when one is trying to rule out shunt malfunction.

During the infant's first year when shunt infections are most common, parents should be encouraged to consult with the primary care provider whenever a temperature greater than 38.5° C occurs. The practitioner, with the consulting physician, can then evaluate the child early in the course of illness and note progression of symptoms.

If a focus of infection other than the shunt is identified, it should be treated appropriately. No studies indicate frequent antibacterial therapy for illnesses of questionable origin reduces the incidence of shunt malfunction. Children being treated for such bacterial infections as otitis media, pneumonia, or streptococcal sore throat should be seen in the office or clinic 24 to 48 hours after treatment is initiated to be carefully reassessed. Continued or worsening symptoms may indicate progression of the infection into bacteremia or a CNS infection caused by the increased susceptibility as a result of the shunt (Schutzman, Petryki, and Fleisher, 1991). Close follow-up is required.

If the child has a mild or moderate fever of unknown origin with other symptoms compatible with a common childhood illness and no obvious signs of shunt malfunction, such as erythema or edema along the tubing track, changes in sensorium, or meningeal signs, the practitioner can assume a wait and see attitude. Arrangements for telephone follow-up or a return appointment in 24 hours should be made. The parents must be instructed on symptoms, such as developing lethargy or recurrent vomiting, that need to be reported immediately should they occur.

Children who have very high temperatures (>40° C) and symptoms of moderate to severe illness must be assumed to have a shunt infection until proved otherwise. Consultation with the neurosurgeon or neurologist is advised. Blood cultures for both aerobic and anaerobic organisms should be drawn, though they often are not initially positive. A complete blood cell count is also indicated, but minimal leukocytosis does not rule out shunt infection. Cerebrospinal fluid can be obtained for culture via a lumbar puncture or through the shunt reservoir. A chest x-ray film and urine culture are recommended to rule out pneumonia or urinary tract infection, but if the history and physical findings strongly suggest shunt involvement, those may be omitted. The neurosurgeon may prefer that all tests be done at the hospital because hospitalization is often required to complete the evaluation and treatment process.

Gastrointestinal symptoms

Nausea and vomiting are common clinical symptoms during childhood, often accompanying such diverse conditions as influenza, otitis media, and urinary tract infections. Diarrhea and abdominal pain are also frequent complaints in childhood. Children with hydrocephalus can be expected to have these common complaints as frequently as their unaffected counterparts.

When the child has mild GI symptoms, the practitioner must assess the presence or absence of other symptoms and history of exposure to GI illness. Mild to moderate fever is often present with both GI infections and shunt malfunction and therefore is not a good differentiating symptom. The presence or absence of swelling or inflammation along the catheter line or at the incision site is highly suggestive of shunt involvement. In addition, with a shunt malfunction the shunt reservoir will frequently not pump and drain as expected and may be a key observation. Probably most important to assess is a change in the child's sensorium and behavior, which indicates increased intracranial pressure. If the child appears normal to the parents or only a "little under the weather," the practitioner can again take a wait and see attitude as long as close follow-up can be maintained.

In children with shunts the primary care provider must recognize that abdominal symptoms may be the presenting symptom of peritoneal shunt malfunction. Abdominal pain, acute diarrhea, peritonitis, and tenderness associated with malfunctioning of the peritoneal tubing may mimic an acute condition of the abdomen (Hubschmann and Countee, 1980; Odio, McCracken, and Nelson, 1984; Reynolds, Sherman, and Mclone, 1983). It may be impossible for the practitioner to differentiate the symptoms of an acute condition of the abdomen from peritoneal shunt malfunction, and consultation with and referral to the attending neurosurgeon are advised.

One unfortunate possible side affect of ventriculoperitoneal shunts is metastasis of brain tumor cells from the ventricular cavities into the abdominal cavity (Epstein, 1985). This must be considered when one is making a differential diagnosis in a child with more chronic or recurring abdominal complaints if the child has a history of a brain tumor. Appropriate referral is required to rule out this possibility after more common reasons for the complaint have been proved negative.

Headaches

Older children frequently complain of headaches. This too can occur in the child with a shunt and may have the same origin as in children without hydrocephalus. But if routine treatment with mild analgesics does not relieve the symptom, or if the headaches become frequent or chronic, evaluation by the neurologist and neurosurgeon is required. Shunt malfunction can be partial or variable, depending on cerebral blood flow, CSF production, and the child's activity, and may result in periodic episodes of increased intracranial pressure (Epstein, 1984).

Children with hydrocephalus occasionally experience headaches and vomiting in the early morning after sleeping all night. Usually these symptoms subside after the children have been up for a few hours; they may be caused by temporary partial blockage of the shunt from cellular debris, inactivity, and the horizontal sleeping position, which negates the beneficial affect of gravity for ventricular drainage. If these episodes are infrequent and self-limited, they do not require treatment other than acetaminophen for pain and possibly promethazine hydrochloride (Phenergen) or trimethobenzamide hydrochloride (Tigan) for nausea and vomiting. If the parents are reliable, prescriptions for these medications can be given in advance so that the parents will have them available when an episode occurs. They should be instructed to call the primary provider if these symptoms continue for more than 6 hours or are associated with a decrease in the level of consciousness or loss of motor ability.

DEVELOPMENTAL ISSUES
Safety

The primary care provider plays a major role in educating parents and children about safety. Families may be so overwhelmed with the task of parenting a child with a chronic condition that routine safety measures are overlooked.

The prolonged lack of head control in the child with hydrocephalus predisposes them to accidental head injury. In addition, car seat safety studies indicate infants should be positioned facing the rear in a semireclined position until the infant is able to sit upright fully supporting his or her head. Infants with hydrocephalus may not be able to attain head control or sit upright until late in their first year of life. This must be reviewed and parents encouraged to use the infant car seats properly to decrease the risk of head, neck, and abdominal injury (Bull, Stroup, and Gerhart, 1988).

As the child grows, activities should be limited as little as possible to encourage normal development and peer relationships. Helmets should be strongly recommended for all activities which frequently result in falls, such as bike and skateboard riding.

Child care

The majority of mothers are currently working outside the home. Child care and preschool placement are major issues for all working parents but even more so when the child has a chronic condition. Fortunately the current shunt systems are self-maintained and do not require special care such as pumping periodically throughout the day. There are no special care needs for the child with hydrocephalus unless other disabilities, such as cerebral palsy, seizures, or mental retardation, are present.

Children with hydrocephalus, however, are at greater risk for CNS infections than their peers because of the presence of the shunt (Andretta, 1987; Borges, 1982; Yogev 1985). Parents must understand that children who attend day care or preschool will have more frequent exposure to childhood infections and will have more illnesses, usually respiratory or GI than those who stay at home (Hurwitz, Gunn, Pinsky, et al., 1991). Children less than 1 year of age have a higher shunt infection rate than older children (Odio,

McCracken, and Nelson, 1984; Yogev, 1985). For this reason it is advisable for the infant up to 1 year of age to receive child care at home or in a small home care program to minimize exposure to common pediatric pathogens.

Diet

There are no special dietary requirements for children with hydrocephalus. Many parents become overly concerned about episodes of regurgitation or vomiting common in all infants, and clarification as to what is normal and what is pathologic vomiting should be made early after the diagnosis of hydrocephalus. The parents may be hesitant to burp the infant because of poor head control or concern over dislodging the shunt. Alternate positions for burping can be demonstrated. If repeated regurgitation does occur, parents should be advised about using an infant seat for postfeeding positioning and introducing solids if age appropriate.

Discipline

Discipline for children with hydrocephalus should be managed as for normal children, recognizing the limitations of cognitive and motor development of the individual child. Some parents may have difficulty understanding the discrepancy between their child's verbal and performance skills and may have expectations that are too high for the child to attain. This may lead to inappropriate discipline. On the other hand, parents may be afraid to discipline their child and must be encouraged to set appropriate limits.

The practitioner must always be concerned with the increased possibility of child abuse in children with chronic conditions. Head injuries and abdominal injuries are common in child abuse and may result in further brain injury or shunt malfunction.

Toileting

Children with neurologic deficits associated with hydrocephalus may have delayed ability to develop bowel and bladder control (Bell and McCormick, 1978). Parents need to be counseled on the possibility of this difficulty and methods of toilet training reviewed. The neurologist and neurosurgeon following the child's development should be consulted concerning the neurologic capability of the child to attain satisfactory toilet training. If necessary, special bowel training and clean intermittent catheterization education should be provided and can usually be obtained through referral from the neurologist or neurosurgeon (see Chapter 21).

Sleep patterns

Parents may be concerned about their infant or child sleeping in a position that might adversely affect the shunt. They need to be reassured their child can sleep in any position that is comfortable without fear of affecting the shunt. Infants and young children should be encouraged to assume a normal sleeping pattern at night.

School issues

Most school-aged children with hydrocephalus will be eligible for special educational programs under Public Law 94-142. Some states in addition now offer preschool assessment and therapy for at-risk infants. The practitioner can be of great assistance in helping the family plan the child's individualized educational program (IEP) to assure appropriate interventions for the child. Although Public Law 94-142 requires the school district to assess the child's needs, financial constraints of the school district may limit neuropsychologic testing; therefore, any testing done before school may be very beneficial and should be forwarded to the school district on request. Parents may need assistance in obtaining medical records that would help in formulating the child's IEP.

Because of physical or intellectual limitations, some children with hydrocephalus will qualify for separate special education classes. Other children will be able to be mainstreamed into the regular classrooms and receive special services, such as adaptive physical education, to help with motor control and balance, occupational therapy to assist with kinesthetic-proprioceptive deficits, or psychologic counseling to address emotional issues.

As the child reaches junior high school and high school some limitations should be made on competitive, high-impact sports. Tackle football, soccer, and ice hockey have a much higher risk of head injury than track, swimming, or tennis. If the child has mild-moderate neuromotor deficits, an evaluation by a sports medicine professional may help identify sports activities the child will be able to perform with success. This is often beneficial to the child's self-esteem and encourages peer relationships, both of which may be problematic areas for the child with hydrocephalus.

The practitioner should routinely ask the parents and child about school progress. If academic difficulties develop, the child should be referred for repeat neuropsychologic testing to rule out medical reasons for these problems (Whittle, Johnston, and Besser, 1985). If the difficulty is assessed to be more emotional, which often happens during the adolescent years when the child struggles with his or her body image and identity, a referral for counseling should be made. It is advisable that the referral be made to a professional experienced in working with disabled children.

Sexuality

No special sexual problems are associated with hydrocephalus. Sexuality and reproductive issues should be managed as with other children. Female adolescents receiving anticonvulsive therapy should be informed of the possible teratonogenic effects of the medications they are taking (see Chapter 15). Adolescents with associated motor disabilities may have additional needs (see Chapters 9 and 21).

SPECIAL FAMILY CONCERNS

Parents of children with hydrocephalus constantly worry about continued shunt function. With every malfunction there is the need for surgery and the perceived threat of further brain damage. This constant worry and the daily responsibility and stress of caring for a child who may have multiple medical problems are very hard on families (Jackson, 1985). Financial strain from numerous medical visits or surgical procedures may deplete a family's financial reserve. Private insurance may not be obtainable unless offered through a large group employment policy. Concern about the child's ability to be self-supporting and independent in the future are also an issue for parents as the child grows into adolescence.

SUMMARY OF PRIMARY CARE NEEDS FOR THE CHILD WITH HYDROCEPHALUS

Growth and development

Both precocious puberty and short stature are reported.

Height and weight are usually within normal range unless the child is severely handicapped.

If enlarged head size is diagnosed in infancy and a shunt is placed, head size should follow normal growth curve.

The head should be measured at each visit until the sutures are fused.

Standard infant development tests may indicate delay because of poor head control.

Seventy-five percent of children will have some motor disability.

Immunization

Pertussis vaccine may be deferred in infants with seizures.

Measles vaccine may cause seizures in children with seizure disorders but is recommended because of the prevalence of measles.

Haemophilus influenzae type b conjugated vaccine is strongly recommended.

Pneumococcal vaccine and influenza vaccine should be considered for children with multiple shunt infections.

Screening
Vision

Hirschberg's examination, cover test, ability to track, and fundoscopic examination should be done at each visit. The child should be examined by an ophthalmologist at 6 months of age and then yearly thereafter.

Hearing

Routine office screening is recommended. Auditory evoked response test should be given to children with a history of CNS infection or who have been treated with aminoglycosides.

Dental

Routine dental care is recommended.

Children on phenytoin therapy require more frequent dental care.

Prophylactic antibiotics are recommended for dental procedures likely to cause bleeding.

Blood pressure

Blood pressure should be recorded at each visit.
Blood pressure increases with increased intracranial pressure.

Hematocrit

Routine screening is recommended.

Urinalysis

Routine screening is recommended.

Tuberculosis

Routine screening is recommended.

Condition-specific screening
   Head circumference

Head circumference should be measured at each visit until the sutures are completely fused.

Drug interactions

No routine medications are prescribed.

Differential diagnosis
Fever

Rule out shunt infection or CNS infection.

Gastrointestinal symptoms

Rule out increased intracranial pressure with nausea and vomiting.

Rule out peritonitis with abdominal pain or acute diarrhea.

Rule out metastatic abdominal tumor in children with primary brain tumors and ventriculoperitoneal shunts.

Headaches

Rule out shunt malfunction as the cause of acute or chronic headaches.

Developmental issues
Safety

The risk of head injury is increased because of poor head control.

A rear-facing car seat should be recommended until the child is able to sit unsupported.

A helmet should be used for bike and skateboard riding.

Continued.

SUMMARY OF PRIMARY CARE NEEDS FOR THE CHILD WITH HYDROCEPHALUS — cont'd

Low impact sports should be selected to prevent head trauma.

Child care

No special care needs are required except when the child has a severe motor disability or seizures.

Home care or small day-care programs are recommended during the child's first year of life to reduce infections.

Discipline

Expectations are normal, with recognition of the possible discrepancy between verbal and motor abilities. Physical punishment is a hazard because it may cause head or abdominal injury.

Toileting

Delayed bowel and bladder training may occur because of neurologic deficit.

Sleep patterns

Standard developmental counseling is advised.

School issues

Associated problems are often covered by Public Law 94-142.

Families should be assisted in IEP hearings.

Children may have possible adjustment problems during adolescence.

Children may need psychometric testing for poor school performance.

Sexuality

Standard developmental counseling is advised unless associated problems warrant additional care.

Special family concerns

Families are concerned about continued shunt function and the possibility of brain damage caused by shunt failure or infection.

RESOURCES

Parent-to-parent support groups can be very helpful offering parent support, publishing newsletters, and even hosting major medical conferences for both health professionals and parents. These organizations also enable a network for children with hydrocephalus, offering them the opportunity to make new friends, develop peer support, and exchange knowledge. The practitioner should become familiar with the organizations in the community so that appropriate referrals can be made. It is better to make such a referral early after the child's diagnosis than to wait to see how the parents cope. All parents need support above and beyond what is reasonable for the physician or nurse to provide.

Organizations
National organizations

Hydrocephalus Association
2040 Polk St, Box 342
San Francisco, CA 94109
(415) 776-4713

HOPE (Hydrocephalus Opens People Eyes)
104-47 120th St
Richmond Hill, NY 11419

National Organization for Rare Disorders (NORD)
PO Box 8923
New Fairfield, CT 06812
(203) 746-6518

Spina Bifida Association of America
1700 Rockville Pike
Rockville, MD 20852

United Cerebral Palsy Association, Inc
Seven Penn Plaza, Suite 804
New York, NY 10016
(800) 872-1827

REFERENCES

Amacher AL and Wellington J: Infantile hydrocephalus: Long-term results of surgical therapy, *Child Brain* 11:217-229, 1984.

American Academy of Pediatrics: Policy Statement: *Haemo-*

philus influenzae type b conjugated vaccines: Immunization of children at 15 months of age, *AAP News*, 1990, July p 10.

American Committee on Immunization Practices: New *Haemophilus influenzae* type b (HIB) vaccine recommendations, *MMWR* 37:13-16, 1988.

Andretta G: Shunt infections in hydrocephalic children, *Int Pediatr* 2:242-244, 1987.

Bell WE and McCormick WF: *Increased intracranial pressure in children: Diagnosis and treatment*, Philadelphia, 1978, WB Saunders.

Borges LF: Cerebral spinal fluid shunts interfere with host defenses, *Neurosurgery* 10:55-60, 1982.

Bull MJ, Stroup KB, and Gerhart S: Misuse of car safety seats, *Pediatrics* 81:98-101, 1988.

Centers for Disease Control: Haemophilus b conjugated vaccines for prevention of Haemophilus influenzae type b disease among infants and children two months of age and older: Recommendations of the Immunization Practice Advisory Committee (ACIP), *MMWR*, 40:1-7, 1991.

Centers for Disease Control: Premature mortality due to congenital anomalies—United States, *MMWR* 37:505-506, 1988.

Committee on Infectious Diseases: *Report of the Committee on Infectious Diseases,* ed 22, Elk Grove Village, Il, 1991, The American Academy of Pediatrics.

Dajani AS, Bisno AL, Chung KJ, et al: Prevention of bacterial endocarditis: Recommendations by the American Heart Association, *JAMA* 264(22) 2919-2922.

Dennis M, Fitz C, Netley C., et al: The intelligence of hydrocephalic children, *Arch Neurol* 38:607-615, 1981.

Donder J, Canady AI, and Rourke BP: Psychometric intelligence after infantile hydrocephalus, *Child's Nervous System* 6:148-154, 1990.

Epstein F: Increased intracranial pressure in hydrocephalic children with functioning shunts: A complication of shunt dependency. In Shapiro K and Marmarou M, Raven Press, *Hydrocephalus*, New York, 1984, p 315-321.

Epstein F: How to keep shunts functioning, or "The impossible dream," *Clin Neurosurg* 32:608-631, 1985.

Fernell E, Hagberg B, and Hagberg G: Epidemiology of infantile hydrocephalus in Sweden: I. A clinical follow-up study in children born at term, *Neuropediatrics* 19:135-142, 1988a.

Fernell E, Hagberg B, and Hagberg G: Epidemiology of infantile hydrocephalus in Sweden: II. Current aspects of the outcome in preterm infants, *Neuropediatrics* 19:143-145, 1988b.

Greenspan FS and Forsham PH: *Basic and clinical endocrinology*, Los Altos, Calif, 1986, Lange Medical Publications.

Gururaj VP and Rogers PF: *Haemophilus influenzae* type b vaccine: Use in the pediatric population, *Pediatrics* 80:731-735, 1987.

Hubschmann OR and Countee RW: Acute abdomen in children with infected ventriculoperintoneal shunts, *Arch Surg* 115:305-307, 1980.

Hurwitz ES, Gunn WJ, Pinsky PF, et al: Risk of respiratory illness associated with day-care attendance: a nationwide study, *Pediatrics* 87(1) 62-69, 1991.

Jackson PL: When the baby isn't perfect, *Am J Nurs* 85:396-399, 1985.

Mankinen-Heikkinen A and Mustonen E: Ophthalmic changes in hydrocephalus: A follow-up examination of 50 patients treated with shunts, *Acta Ophthalmol* 65:81-86, 1987.

McCullough D and Balzer-Martin LA: Current prognosis in overt neonatal hydrocephalus, *J Neurosurg* 57:378-383, 1982.

Odio C, McCracken G, and Nelson J: CSF shunt infections in pediatrics, *Am J Dis Child* 138:1103-1106, 1984.

Olsen L and Frykberg T: Complications in the treatment of hydrocephalus in children: A comparison of ventriculoatrial and ventriculoperitoneal shunts in a 20-year material, *Acta Paediatr Scand* 72:385-390, 1983.

Patriarca P and Lauer B: Ventriculoperitoneal shunt-associated infections due to Haemophilus influenza, *Pediatrics* 65:1007-1009, 1980.

Post E: Currently available shunt systems: A review, *Neurosurgery* 16:257-260, 1985.

Rennels MB and Wald ER: Treatment of *Haemophilus influenzae* type b meningitis in children with cerebrospinal fluid shunts, *J Pediatr* 97:424-426, 1980.

Reynolds M, Sherman J, and Mclone D: Ventriculoperitoneal shunt infection masquerading as an acute surgical abdomen, *J Pediatr Surg* 18:951-954, 1983.

Rudolph A: *Pediatrics*, New York, 1987, Appleton-Century-Crofts.

Schutzman SA, Petryck S, Fleisher GR: Bacteremia with otitis media, *Pediatrics* 87(1)48-53, 1991.

Sekhar L, Moossy J, and Guthkelch N: Malfunctioning ventriculoperitoneal shunts, *J Neurosurg* 56:411-416, 1982.

Serlo W, Fernell E, Heikkinen E, et al: Functions and complications of shunts in different etiologies of childhood hydrocephalus, *Child's Nervous System* 6:92-94, 1990.

Stein S, Feldman J, Apfel S, et al: The epidemiology of congenital hydrocephalus: A study in Brooklyn, N.Y., 1968-1976, *Child Brain* 8:253-262, 1981.

Volpe J: *Neurology of the Newborn*, Philadelphia, 1987, WB Saunders.

Whittle IK, Johnston IH, and Besser M: Intracranial pressure changes in arrested hydrocephalus, *J Neurosurg* 62:77-82, 1985.

Yogev R: Cerebrospinal fluid shunt infections: A personal view, *Pediatr Infect Dis* 4:113-118, 1985.

18 *Inflammatory Bowel Disease*

Veronica E. Perrone

ETIOLOGY

The term inflammatory bowel disease (IBD) encompasses the diagnoses Crohn's disease and ulcerative colitis. These two diseases are distinct entities but are commonly discussed together because they share many of their presenting signs and symptoms, as well as approaches to diagnosis and treatment.

Crohn's disease is a chronic inflammatory disease of the bowel that may occur at any point in the gastrointestinal (GI) tract, from mouth to anus. The inflammation is transmural; it may extend from the intestinal mucosal lining through the serosal layer. In this condition diseased segments of the bowel may border on segments of healthy tissue, which gave the conditions its former name "regional enteritis." The disease most commonly affects the terminal ileum and proximal segments of the colon (50% to 60%); in about 25% of those individuals with Crohn's disease the terminal ileum alone is affected. Diffuse small bowel disease is seen in 15% to 25% of affected individuals, followed more rarely (approximately 10%) by colonic disease alone (Hyams, 1988). Oral, esophageal, and gastric manifestations of Crohn's disease are also seen (Kirschner, Schmidt-Sommerfeld, and Stephens, 1989). Perianal disease is not uncommon in Crohn's disease; affected children may have skin tags, fissures, hemorrhoids, and fistulas. Disease of the rectum, however, is unusual in Crohn's disease.

Ulcerative colitis is an inflammatory disease that affects the colonic and rectal mucosa. Pancolitis is reported in 50% to 60% of those individuals with this disorder. Disease limited to the descending colon occurs less often (22%-35%), whereas rectal disease alone is seen still less frequently (15%) (Hyams, 1988; Kirschner, 1988a).

The etiology of IBD is unclear. Some theories implicate infectious, immunologic, genetic, and environmental causes of these diseases. Psychogenic causes for these illnesses have been disproved but stress may exacerbate a present illness. Current information seems to indicate that environmental trigger (a virus or bacterium) may act as an antigen to induce a cellular reaction in the GI tract of the child. This response is thought to be one that is immunologically mediated and to which the individual may be genetically predisposed (Kirschner, 1988a).

INCIDENCE

The incidence of Crohn's disease has been increasing over the past 20 to 30 years, whereas that of ulcerative colitis appears to have remained stable. Although it is argued that the increase in cases of Crohn's disease may be explained by improved recognition, the figures seem to indicate that the increasing incidence is real (Mendeloff and Calkins, 1988). Incidence rates for Crohn's disease range from 4 to 6 cases per 100,000. Figures for ulcerative colitis range from 3 to 13 cases per 100,000.

Table 18-1. Comparison of Crohn's disease and ulcerative colitis: presenting symptoms

	Crohn's disease	Ulcerative colitis
Alteration in bowel pattern	Diarrhea is common; one may also see constipation, alternating with diarrhea.	Diarrhea is a hallmark; an increase in frequency of bowel movements with urgency is often a component. Constipation may be seen if the disease is obstructive.
Blood in stool	Grossly bloody stools are occasionally seen, most often when colonic disease is present. Occult blood is not uncommon in Crohn's disease.	It is common to see grossly bloody diarrhea; one may also see pus or mucus.
Abdominal pain	Abdominal pain is frequently seen in association with meals; pain is often periumbilical.	Abdominal cramping is often present in association with passage of stool. Pain is often noted in the lower part of the abdomen.
Fever	It is not uncommon to have intermittent, usually low-grade fever.	Fever is sometimes seen.
Onset of disease	Classically the signs of Crohn's disease are more subtle than those of ulcerative colitis, though in a smaller percentage onset may be abrupt.	Onset may be insidious or abrupt.
Weight loss	Weight loss is a common feature of Crohn's disease; it can have occurred for many months to years before diagnosis.	It is not uncommon to see weight loss; typically it will be more abrupt than in Crohn's disease.
Perianal disease	Perianal disease is common.	Perianal disease is rarely seen.

Children make up as much as 30% of all new diagnoses of IBD, with the majority being between the ages of 10 and 18 years. Fewer than 5% of all children with IBD are less than 5 years of age (Hyams, 1988).

CLINICAL MANIFESTATIONS AT TIME OF DIAGNOSIS

Crohn's disease and ulcerative colitis are similar in many presenting symptoms (Table 18-1). These symptoms include abdominal pain, diarrhea, fever, blood in the stool, and weight loss. The symptoms noted are dependent on the location of the disease and its severity.

Classically the child who has ulcerative colitis complains of frequent, watery diarrhea that is grossly bloody. Often pus and mucus are noted as well. The diarrheal stools may be associated with abdominal cramping and, if rectal disease is present, tenesmus (a cramping pain in the rectum accompanied by urgency, most commonly noted after the passage of a bowel movement). Fever, weight loss, and fatigue may also be seen in the child who has ulcerative colitis. The onset of symptoms may be either abrupt or more insidious, occurring over weeks or months. The child may appear essentially well or chronically or acutely ill.

As with ulcerative colitis, the symptoms of Crohn's disease may manifest in an array of fashions. The child may have an acute, severe attack, or, more commonly, the symptoms of the disease are subtle and have been present for months or years before the diagnosis is made (Kanof, Lake, and Bayless, 1988). Symptoms of Crohn's disease affecting the small bowel are commonly obstructive in nature. A diffuse abdominal discomfort that may be associated with meals may be seen along with diarrhea or constipation, and blood may be noted in the stool. Usually the blood is occult, though the stool may be grossly bloody. Fever, anorexia, and weight loss are more commonly seen in these children than in those with ulcerative colitis. Failure to grow or to develop sexually is a presenting symptom in approximately 30% of all children with

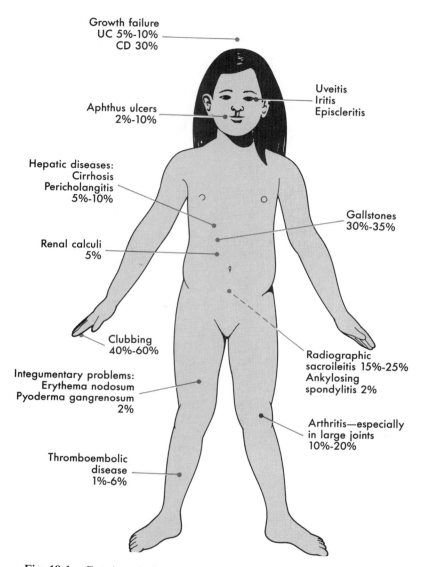

Growth failure
UC 5%-10%
CD 30%

Aphthus ulcers
2%-10%

Hepatic diseases:
Cirrhosis
Pericholangitis
5%-10%

Renal calculi
5%

Clubbing
40%-60%

Integumentary problems:
Erythema nodosum
Pyoderma gangrenosum
2%

Thromboembolic
disease
1%-6%

Uveitis
Iritis
Episcleritis

Gallstones
30%-35%

Radiographic
sacroileitis 15%-25%
Ankylosing
spondylitis 2%

Arthritis—especially
in large joints
10%-20%

Fig. 18-1. Extraintestinal manifestations of inflammatory bowel disease.

Crohn's disease (Hyams, 1988; Kirschner, 1988a) and may have been the original cue for the GI evaluation to commence.

Inflammatory bowel disease may manifest itself as symptoms other than those attributed to the GI tract alone (Fig. 18-1). Children may have or may eventually develop extraintestinal symptoms of their disease. Extraintestinal manifestations of the disease not uncommonly seen at diagnosis include aphthous ulcers of the mouth, arthritic inflammation (especially of large joints) and dermatologic complications such as erythema nodosum and pyoderma gangrenosum. Clubbing is another extraintestinal manifestation seen most commonly in the child with Crohn's disease.

The diagnostic evaluation for IBD most often

includes radiographic examination of the GI tract, endoscopy and biopsy, evaluation of growth parameters, and assessment of laboratory values. Common laboratory findings associated with IBD include an elevated erythrocyte sedimentation rate (ESR), low hematocrit value, and low hemoglobin level. In Crohn's disease affecting the small bowel and in severe ulcerative colitis, hypoalbuminemia and a decreased total protein serum value may also be noted.

The severity of presenting symptoms may not be indicative of the disease course that is to follow for the child. Symptoms seen at diagnosis, such as the extraintestinal manifestations previously noted, may remain with the child, may reappear with exacerbations of the disease, or may never return. Also, new symptoms (GI or extraintestinal) may appear with exacerbations, which can be indicative of disease progression. An exacerbation of Crohn's disease or of ulcerative colitis may sometimes be preceded by an intercurrent illness, a dietary indiscretion, or an emotional stress or may occur for no apparent reason. Quite often children with IBD become adept at anticipating which activities may be most likely to trigger a flare of their disease; for example, an adolescent with IBD may find that during school examinations or around an important social event their symptoms worsen.

TREATMENT

The course of treatment for IBD is based on several modes of drug therapy (Table 18-2), nutritional replenishment, and nutritional supplementation. The specific treatment plan is dependent on the location and severity of the disease, the impact of disease on growth and development, and the degree of debilitation felt by the child. When standard, conservative medical treatment fails to adequately control symptoms, or when complications, such as toxic megacolon, obstruction, or abscesses fail to respond to medical management, surgical intervention is indicated.

Mild cases of ulcerative colitis have generally been found to respond satisfactorily to therapy with sulfasalazine (Azulfidine). Sulfasalazine is partially (20% to 30%) absorbed from the upper intestinal tract. In the colon the remainder is split into two active metabolites of the drug, 5-aminosalicylic acid (5-ASA) and sulfapyridine. 5-Aminosalicylic

acid is believed to be the therapeutic agent. The most common side effects of sulfasalazine are nausea, vomiting, and headache. Less common but more severe reactions are leukopenia, hemolytic anemia, and allergy. These side effects may be alleviated or avoided by gradually increasing the child's dosage to the therapeutic range (50-75 mg/kg/day) over the first few weeks of therapy. During the initiation of therapy, leukopenia and hemolytic anemia should be monitored every few weeks by a complete blood count (CBC). Should either of these occur, the dosage should be decreased until blood values return to normal. The dose may then gradually be returned to the therapeutic range. Sulfasalazine may inhibit folate absorption. For the child taking sulfasalazine who is anemic, folic acid supplementation is recommended.

Retention enemas containing 5-ASA (Rowasa) are now available for children with IBD. They are useful for the child with disease of the rectum or descending colon. The child is able to benefit from the active metabolite of sulfasalazine without the side effects most commonly attributed to its sulfa component. Oral preparations containing only 5-ASA have recently become commercially available for use in individuals with IBD. The completed studies evaluating these drugs have demonstrated fewer side effects than sulfasalazine and comparable efficacy (Martin, 1987).

In moderate disease, as well as during exacerbations, corticosteroids given with sulfasalazine have been found to be very effective in achieving remission. Children are first given a dosage ranging from 1 to 2 mg/kg/day, which is maintained until their symptoms diminish and they achieve their previous level of comfort and activity. The time period often allotted for this is 1 to 2 months (Kirschner, 1988b). The dose is then gradually tapered to an alternate-day therapy while the child's symptoms and laboratory values, particularly the ESR, are monitored. This enables the child to continue to derive benefit from the drug while experiencing fewer side effects. The dose continues to be tapered until the child is able to function normally without its use. Side effects of prednisone include Cushingoid features, weight gain, hypertension, acne, striae, mood swings, calcium depletion, aseptic necrosis of the hip, and cataracts. Another side effect of special significance to children

Table 18-2. Drugs used for treatment of inflammatory bowel disease

Drug/dosage	Uses in IBD	Side effects in use with children with IBD	Special considerations
Sulfasalazine (Azulfidine) 50-75 mg/kg/ day	Treatment of ulcerative colitis Treatment of mild to moderate Crohn's disease, especially when there is colonic involvement	Common Headaches, GI upset, impaired folate absorption, male infertility Less common but significant Allergy (rash, bronchospasm) Leukopenia, worsening of disease	Fewer adverse reactions (allergy, headaches) may be noted if the dose is gradually increased to reach the planned therapeutic dosage. Enteric coated tablets may alleviate GI upset. It is available in suspension form. Adverse reactions are generally noted within the first 3 mo of therapy. It is available as a suspension. Monitor WBC count over first 3 mo of treatment.* It impairs folic acid absorption.
Corticosteroids (prednisone) 1-2 mg/kg/ day	Useful in children who do not respond adequately to sulfasalazine Used in moderate to severe disease Available as foam (Cortifoam) and retention enema (Cortenema) for rectal disease	Common Growth retardation, cushingoid features, weight gain, striae, mood swings, acne, impaired calcium absorption, hypertension Less common but significant, cataracts	Alternate-day therapy at lowest possible dose is frequently used to minimize adverse effects. The child should not discontinue corticosteroid use suddenly; this could result in not only hypocorticism but a flare-up of symptoms. Ophthalmic examination should be done at each visit.
Metronidazole (Flagyl) 15-20 mg/kg/day	Effective adjunct treatment of Crohn's disease May be useful in the management of perineal disease	Common GI upset, metallic taste, urticaria, darkening of the urine Less common but significant, paresthesia	Neurologic assessment should be done at each visit to monitor for any CNS effects.† Paresthesia most commonly is reversible after discontinuation of medication or after reduction of dosage.
6-Mercaptopurine (6-MP; Purinethol) 1.5 mg/kg/day	Used when sulfasalazine and corticosteroid therapy has failed Used when child is unable to be weaned from corticosteroids	Leukopenia Pancreatitis Possible risk of lymphoma in long-term use	If fever develops, drug should be discontinued. It may take 3-6 mo to achieve remission. The WBC count should be monitored throughout therapy.

*WBC, white blood cell.
†CNS, central nervous system.

with IBD is growth retardation. Although the impact of corticosteroids on growth in children is a concern, their contribution to growth failure in children with IBD remains controversial. Alternate-day corticosteroid use has been demonstrated to allow a normal growth rate to occur (Sadeghi-Nejad and Senior, 1969). Alternative corticosteroid preparations such as retention enemas and foams for rectal instillation are also available. Rectal administration of the medication allows for local treatment of disease with fewer systemic side effects. Children with rectal disease, perianal disease, or disease of the descending colon may benefit from this therapy (Hanauer and Kirsner, 1988).

Children with severe ulcerative colitis who are experiencing debilitating symptoms, pronounced abdominal pain or distension, severe electrolyte abnormalities, or anemia and hypoalbuminemia require aggressive medical intervention. They are hospitalized, placed on complete bowel rest, and receive intravenous (IV) hyperalimentation and corticosteroid therapy.

The use of antispasmodic agents for the relief of chronic diarrhea on a daily basis in children with IBD is controversial. Drugs such as loperamide (Imodium) or diphenoxylate (Di-Atro) with atropine may be of use in controlling symptoms during daytime activities (Gitnick, 1989b; Hyams, 1988; Kirschner, 1988b) but may be injudiciously used as a palliative measure. Bowel stasis, dilatation, and subsequently toxic megacolon may result (Barrett and Dharmsathaphorn, 1988; Reddy and Jeejeebhoy, 1988).

Crohn's disease is less responsive to treatment with sulfasalazine than is ulcerative colitis. Although some children, especially those with disease affecting the colon, have some success with this mode of therapy, corticosteroids are more likely to be necessary as a first-line therapy.

Metronidazole has been found to be effective in the care of children with Crohn's disease. Of special interest is its effectiveness in the treatment of perianal disease. However, when the dosage is lowered or the drug is discontinued, it is common for the perianal disease to relapse. The effects of long-term use of metronidazole are not known. There is concern that it may potentially be carcinogenic or mutagenic, because this response has been identified in mice and rats (Brandt et al.,

1982). The recommended pediatric dosage ranges from 15 to 20 mg/kg/day (Frank, Brandt, and Bernstein, 1983; Hyams, 1988). Side effects of metronidazole include GI upset, urticaria, and a metallic taste. A more worrisome side effect of metronidazole is peripheral neuropathy. In one study up to 85% of those adolescents receiving metronidazole had abnormal nerve conduction studies (Duffy et al., 1985). Interestingly, far fewer than this percentage of clients noted any loss of sensation. Several weeks to months after discontinuation of the drug almost all individuals will have reversal of the paresthesia (Duffy et al., 1985; Hyams, 1988).

6-Mercaptopurine (6-MP) is an immunosuppressive agent that is finding increased acceptance in the treatment of IBD. It is currently used as a second-line therapy in children for whom more conservative medical or surgical management has failed. The recommended dosage of 6-MP is 1.5 mg/kg/day. Response to 6-MP is not immediate, averaging 3 months (Korelitz, 1983). The most commonly cited complications of 6-MP are leukopenia and pancreatitis. Some clinicians are concerned about a possible increased risk of lymphoma in individuals treated with 6-MP (Kirschner, 1988b; Korelitz, 1983), though the extent of this risk is unclear. Some investigators have found the risk to be no greater than the background risk for malignancy in IBD (Present et al., 1989). The possibility of long-term teratogenetic effects on the offspring of those who received 6-MP as children is another concern that causes hesitation when this therapy is prescribed for children. Other complications noted include allergy, hepatitis, and infectious complications (Present et al., 1989). For the first several months of therapy a CBC should be checked every 2 weeks to assess for leukopenia. The WBC count should be checked monthly thereafter. The recommendation is to reduce the dosage or to terminate therapy if the WBC count falls to less than 5,000 WBCs/mm^3 (Korelitz, 1983). Therapy may be reinstituted after the values return to normal. The primary care provider, family, and child must be aware that any fever during therapy with 6-MP is an indication for concern and needs to be evaluated. Discontinuing the drug may be necessary.

Cyclosporine (Sandimmune) is an experimental therapy for IBD that has been undergoing its first controlled therapeutic trials in adults. It is hoped that cyclosporine will be another option as a second-line therapy for IBD that is refractory to more conservative treatment. Response to cyclosporin therapy has been inconsistent, and treated individuals have had a significant incidence of relapse while receiving therapy and reoccurrence when discontinuing the drug. Some investigators have been encouraged by the response of perianal disease to cyclosporine (Parrott et al., 1988, Stange et al., 1989). Side effects associated with cyclosporine include nephrotoxicity, hepatotoxicity, tremor, hirsutism, gingival hyperplasia, hypertension, and growth failure.

The elemental diet, or formula providing total nutrition and supplying nitrogen in the form of simple amino acids, as therapy for IBD in children is a new and exciting development. Elemental diet has been successful in attaining remission (Belli et al., 1988; Kleinman et al., 1989) and reversing growth failure in children with Crohn's disease (Belli et al., 1988). In some trials elemental diet has provided superior therapeutic results to the more traditional treatment with sulfasalazine and corticosteroids alone. In one study the intermittent use of elemental diet as the sole source of nutrition over a 1-year period resulted in decreased corticosteroid requirements and lower disease activity for the experimental group than during the year before therapy and lower than that of the controls (Belli et al., 1988). The children receiving elemental diets achieved significantly greater growth, and their height, weight, triceps skinfold, and mid-arm circumference were significantly increased relative to those not treated with elemental feedings. Pubertal change, as measured by Tanner scores, and bone age were not, however, significantly different from their peers in the control group, indicating that there is potential for significant catch-up growth among those children who are treated in this fashion before puberty.

Nutritional therapy with parenteral hyperalimentation has also demonstrated improvement in disease activity and reversal of growth failure (Seidman et al., 1987). However, enteral feedings pose significant advantages over the parenteral route of nutrition because nasogastric feedings are less invasive, less costly, and pose fewer infectious risks than does the parenteral route.

The role of surgical management in the case of growth failure is controversial. Some children display catch-up growth after surgery to resect diseased bowel. Current consensus is that surgery is appropriate only when it is believed the surgery will provide a reasonable period of remission during which growth could occur (Gryboski and Spiro, 1978; Kirschner et al., 1981).

Proctocolectomy is the procedure of choice for the child with ulcerative colitis requiring surgery. Twenty-five percent to thirty percent of children with ulcerative colitis will need proctocolectomy within 5 years of diagnosis (Kirschner, 1988a). Alternatives to the standard external ileostomy are the ileal pouch–anal anastomosis and the Kock pouch. The ileal pouch–anal anastomosis provides relative continence with no need for a stoma. Individual experiences vary from child to child, particularly during the first year following the procedure. Overall acceptability of the ileal pouch–anal anastomosis has been very good. Individuals have reported greater satisfaction in activities of daily living relative to the traditional ileostomy with collecting appliance (Pemberton et al., 1989). Some children report a small amount of soiling during the day; a higher percentage experience soiling during sleep. The Kock pouch provides an abdominal reservoir that is emptied by the child using a catheter drainage appliance. The pouch opening is otherwise covered by a small dressing or bandage. This procedure is an alternative for the individual who as a result of the disease or because of previous surgical resections has anal sphincter control difficulties.

Approximately 70% of individuals diagnosed as having Crohn's disease in childhood will have surgery within the first 7 or 8 years after diagnosis, with the highest frequency occurring among those with ileocolonic disease (95%) (Farmer and Michner, 1979). Most often resection of the diseased portion of the bowel is the approach chosen for the child with Crohn's disease who requires surgery. The likelihood of repeated surgical resections is high (Andrews, Lewis, and Allan, 1989). In addition, the likelihood of recurrence at the site of surgery makes the child with Crohn's disease ineligible for such procedures as the Kock pouch or the ileal pouch–anal anastomosis.

Because stress has been identified as a factor

that may contribute to the exacerbation of IBD symptoms, some children find it helpful to master relaxation and stress management techniques for controlling or preventing flares of their disease. The practitioner may assist the family in finding programs that will promote the development of stress management and problem-solving skills.

PROGNOSIS

The overall life expectancy of individuals with IBD is essentially that of the general population (Harper et al., 1987). There is, however, a significantly greater risk for intestinal malignancies among this group than among those who do not have IBD. It appears that in ulcerative colitis the risk of malignancy increases with the extent and duration of the disease. This fact indicates that those diagnosed with ulcerative colitis during childhood or adolescence have a greater likelihood of developing a related cancer as a result of their greater life expectancy (Feczko, 1987). The prognosis is less clear for children with Crohn's disease. It is agreed that these individuals are also at greater risk for the development of an intestinal malignancy. The extent of that risk is not clear; the risk for colonic cancer may be similar to those with ulcerative colitis. The risk for small bowel malignancies is significantly greater than that of the general population (Feczko, 1987; Gitnick, 1989a).

The information regarding the long-term impact of IBD on quality of life indicates that a significant percentage of adult clients with IBD report that their overall life satisfaction is low or affected negatively by their disease (Joachim and Milne, 1987). In another evaluation of life satisfaction (Farmer and Michner, 1979), only 20% of adults with long-established Crohn's disease felt that they were in good health.

ASSOCIATED PROBLEMS
Growth failure

Growth failure and delayed onset of sexual maturation are common and significant problems for children with IBD. At the time of diagnosis, 5% to 10% of children with ulcerative colitis and up to 30% of children with Crohn's disease have growth retardation (Kirschner, 1988a). A significant percentage of these children (approximately 50%) may have begun to demonstrate a decrease

in height velocity an average of 12 months before the onset of any other symptoms attributable to Crohn's disease (Kanof, Lake, and Bayless, 1988).

Etiologic theories for growth failure have included malabsorption, excessive protein loss, and increased energy needs of children with IBD. The cause for growth failure among children with IBD appears at this time to be multifactorial. To some extent it is believed that malabsorption and the increased metabolic needs that accompany fever may contribute to the problem of growth failure in children with IBD. The primary cause of growth failure in IBD is believed to be malnutrition. In one study the caloric intake of children with Crohn's disease was approximately 56% that of the recommended intake for height for age of the affected child (Kirschner et al., 1981). This caloric insufficiency may in part be the result of anorexia related to the association of pain with meals, to chronic illness, and to iatrogenic causes such as unnecessary dietary restrictions (Seidman et al., 1987).

Musculoskeletal problems

Musculoskeletal problems associated with IBD include peripheral arthritis, ankylosing spondylitis, and sacroileitis. Peripheral arthritis is seen in approximately 10% of those individuals with IBD. Inflammation and discomfort are noted in the large joints, especially those of the hip and the knee. Inflammation does not occur symmetrically. Unlike the other musculoskeletal manifestations of IBD, the arthritic symptoms often fluctuate with the activity of the bowel disease and respond to treatment of the disease. Other therapy for peripheral arthritis in IBD includes treatment with corticosteroids and nonsteroidal antiinflammatory agents. Ankylosing spondylitis may be seen in 2% to 6% of individuals with IBD and more commonly in those individuals with ulcerative colitis (Mayer and Janowitz, 1988). Sacroileitis may be noted on roentgenogram in 10% to 15% of those individuals with IBD, with far fewer than this percentage of individuals noting symptoms (Mayer and Janowitz, 1988) such as low back pain. Although not an extraintestinal manifestation of IBD itself, osteoporosis is a significant risk for children with IBD because of their poor absorption of vitamin D (Vogelsang et al., 1989) and corticosteroid therapy (Rimsza, 1978).

Dermatologic manifestations

Dermatologic manifestations occur in up to 5% of individuals with IBD (Gitnick, 1989). Erythema nodosum is a tender, reddened nodule that commonly appears on the anterior aspect of the lower leg, although it may be seen on the foot, the back of the leg, or on the arm. Erythema nodosum is seen more frequently with Crohn's disease than with ulcerative colitis. Pyoderma gangrenosum is a more serious dermatologic condition that may be found in 1% to 5% of those individuals with ulcerative colitis. Pyoderma gangrenosum is also most frequently noted on the anterior aspect of the lower leg. It appears as one or many bullae bordered by an area of dark red or purple. Pyoderma gangrenosum may continue to penetrate into the tissues below and may result in osteomyelitis (Lewicki and Leeson, 1984). The child with this condition warrants immediate referral to a dermatologist. Treatment must include management of the IBD because pyoderma gangrenosum appears to closely mirror the activity of the underlying disease, and topical or systemic corticosteroid therapy.

Visual changes

Ocular manifestations of IBD include iritis, episcleritis, uveitis, and conjunctivitis. It should also be noted that the child who is being treated with corticosteroids is at increased risk for cataracts (Rimsza, 1978).

Hepatobiliary complications

Other GI manifestations of IBD include hepatobiliary complications such as pericholangitis, cirrhosis, and primary sclerosing cholangitis. The physical examination should be closely monitored for hepatic enlargement or signs of portal hypertension. Gallstones are not infrequently seen in the individual with IBD, particularly in the client with extensive ileal disease or ileal resection. Their occurrence seems to be related to the malabsorption of bile salts with concomitant cholesterol precipitation and calculus formation (Williams and Harned, 1987).

Renal changes

Renal calculi may also be seen in the individual with IBD. They have been noted in 5% of those individuals with ulcerative colitis and in 10% to 25% of those with Crohn's disease. The child with severe ileal disease or resection of the ileum is at risk for the formation of calcium oxalate stones, which are the type seen more frequently in individuals with IBD (Banner, 1987). Hydronephrosis may also be seen in the child with IBD, particularly in those children who have had extensive scarring or inflammation of the small bowel or who have abscesses that may obstruct the ureter. Hydronephrosis associated with IBD is frequently asymptomatic; therefore, the practitioner should be suspicious of this complication in a child with a history of fistulas or abscesses or who has a suspected abdominal mass (Banner, 1987).

Fistulas and abscesses

Fistula and abscess formation are complications of Crohn's disease. Fistulas may form between the bowel and the surface of the skin or between the bowel and other organs or orifices. The clinician should question the child or parent about the passage of air or stool through the vagina or the urethra, because this may indicate a rectovaginal or rectourethral fistula.

Toxic megacolon

Toxic megacolon is a life-threatening complication of IBD. It is most commonly associated with ulcerative colitis, but it may also occur early in the course of Crohn's disease. Toxic megacolon is an acute distension of the colon that may result in perforation, hemorrhage, and peritonitis. Signs of this complication are tachycardia; hypovolemia; fever, abdominal distension; decreased bowel sounds; and continuous, diffuse abdominal pain. The child taking corticosteroids, however, may have their fever supressed. The child with suspected toxic megacolon should have all oral intake withheld and should be referred immediately to the gastroenterology team. Progression from severe disease to toxic megacolon and subsequent perforation may occur rapidly. The clinician should maintain a high index of suspicion for the likelihood of toxic megacolon in the child with worsening or severe disease. The evaluation includes radiologic assessment of the abdomen and clinical assessment. The role of the barium enema in precipitating a toxic megacolon remains controversial, it is recommended that flat plates of the abdomen are sufficient (Reddy et al, 1988). Medical management includes bowel rest with nasogastric suction, parenteral hyperalimentation, and antibiotics given intravenously. If the toxic megacolon does not resolve within 24 to 72 hours, a colectomy is usually performed.

Lactose intolerance

Children with IBD, particularly those with diffuse Crohn's disease of the small bowel, may have some degree of lactose intolerance with resultant cramping, distension, and diarrhea. This may obfuscate the true disease activity or may actually cause or prevent recovery from an exacerbation. It is often suggested that children eliminate lactose-containing products from their diet during their initial period of diagnosis and recovery to decrease confusion regarding the child's response to therapy. A significant number of children with IBD will eventually be able to tolerate some amount of lactose in their diet.

Anemia

As a result of chronic malnutrition, malabsorption, the interference of sulfasalazine in the absorption of folates, and chronic blood loss, children with IBD are at increased risk for vitamin B_{12} deficiency and hypochromic microcytic or iron deficiency anemia. Daily supplementation with folic acid is recommended for them, as well as monitoring of CBC for all children with IBD. Also, iron supplementation is recommended for the symptomatic child.

PRIMARY CARE MANAGEMENT
Growth and development

Children with IBD should have growth parameters measured and graphed on a National Center for Health Statistics chart at each primary care visit. For those children who have been recently diagnosed, it is helpful to go back through previous visits to calculate the child's growth curve in the years before the diagnosis was made. This will help the practitioner assess for any deceleration in growth rate. Often school health or athletic offices may be of assistance in reconstructing the growth curve. Growth parameters of particular importance are both height and weight for age, Tanner stage, and arm anthropometry. Once growth retardation is identified as an actual or potential problem, a bone age should be obtained to identify the child's remaining growth potential. Continued careful measurement and graphing for growth parameters are essential. Catch-up growth is considered to be adequate if the child returns to his or her pre-illness growth percentiles.

Immunizations

No change from the normal immunization schedule is necessary unless the child receives maintenance therapy of corticosteroids or other immunosuppressive agents such as 6-MP or cyclosporine. These children should not receive live virus immunizations until they have been tapered from these drugs. If this is not feasible or exposure is of particular concern, a killed virus vaccine may be given. Children who receive maintenance therapy of immunosuppressive drugs should receive prophylaxis with varicella-zoster immune globulin for varicella exposure.

Screening

Vision. Ophthalmic examinations are necessary at each well child visit because children with IBD are at risk for ocular manifestations of their disease. In the case of iritis, the examiner may note redness of the eye, eye pain, photophobia, or blurred vision. In uveitis, abnormal pupillary reaction may also be assessed. A reddened eye may be noted in episcleritis or conjunctivitis (Danzi, 1988). If the child is receiving prolonged corticosteroid therapy a yearly ophthalmology referral and assessment for cataracts is recommended. Any child with an abnormal ophthalmoscopic examination or who complains of the previously mentioned symptoms should be referred to an ophthalmologist and to the gastroenterology team.

Hearing. Routine screening is recommended.

Dental. Children who are being treated with cyclosporine are at risk for gingival hyperplasia. Proper dental hygiene and yearly dental visits should be reinforced at each well child visit.

Blood pressure. Children who are taking cyclosporine or corticosteroids are at increased risk for hypertension. Their blood pressures should be measured every 6 months.

Hematocrit. Hemoglobin and hematocrit values should be measured yearly for children who are asymptomatic and who have no history of anemia. For any child with a history of anemia or who is experiencing increased symptoms of their disease, a CBC should be checked every 6 months or as needed.

Urinalysis. No change in the usual protocol for screening is necessary unless the history indicates renal involvement or the child is experiencing symptoms indicative of any of the previously mentioned conditions.

Tuberculosis. The child who is receiving immunosuppressive therapy may not respond to testing. Screening may be withheld until immunosuppressive drugs are discontinued. If exposure is suspected, a control may be placed along with the purified protein derivative of the tuberculosis to assess for anergy. Chest radiography may be necessary to screen for active disease.

Condition-specific screening

ERYTHROCYTE SEDIMENTATION RATE. An ESR should be measured yearly for the asymptomatic child. The ESR may be used for some children with IBD as an index of disease activity, though for approximately 15% of individuals with Crohn's disease or 30% of those with ulcerative colitis, this may not be a true measure (Castile et al., 1980; Kirschner, 1988a). The ESR should be normal in the child with inactive disease. A variation from baseline should be followed up with close questioning regarding current disease activity, onset of new symptoms, or any recent dietary indiscretions.

FECAL OCCULT BLOOD TEST. For the child who is asymptomatic, stool should be monitored yearly for the presence of occult blood using a fecal-occult blood reagent (e.g., Hemocult). The results should, in most instances, be negative in the child with inactive disease. Some children with IBD will always carry a trace of blood in their stool. The child whose stool is routinely normal but has a positive occult blood result should be assessed more carefully for indications of increased disease activity.

CHEMISTRIES. The child taking cyclosporine or 6-MP should have renal (blood urea nitrogen and creatinine levels) and liver function studies (fractionated bilirubin, aspartate aminotransferase, alanine aminotransferase, and alkaline phosphatase values) monitored at least every 6 months throughout their therapy. Liver function studies should be assessed every few years in the otherwise asymptomatic child with IBD. The child with Crohn's disease should also have albumin levels checked yearly.

LACTOSE INTOLERANCE. The diagnosis of lactose intolerance may be made empirically by eliminating lactose-containing products from the diet and monitoring for changes in symptoms such as cramping, distension, and diarrhea. The diagnosis may also be made by the breath hydrogen test. The clinician may also cursorily screen for lactose intolerance in the office by testing stool for reducing substances or by testing the pH of the stool. An acidic pH (<6.5) would be indicative of lactose intolerance.

NEUROLOGIC EXAMINATION. Children who are being treated with metronidazole require close neurologic examination at each visit.

Drug interactions

Sulfasalazine, the mainstay of traditional therapy for both ulcerative colitis and Crohn's disease, potentiates the action of both oral-form hypoglycemia agents, resulting in lower than anticipated blood glucose values, and phenytoin (Dilantin), resulting in higher than expected blood values of this drug and increased risk of drug toxicity. Sulfasalazine, metronidazole, and corticosteroids potentiate the action of warfarin (Coumadin). Finally, when administered along with digoxin (Lanoxin), sulfasalazine has been found to inhibit absorption, resulting in decreased blood levels of the drug. Metronidazole has a disulfiram (Antibuse) type of reaction when the individual ingests alcohol or alcohol-containing elixirs during drug therapy. Corticosteroids also diminish the efficacy of hypoglycemic agents taken orally, resulting in higher than desired blood glucose levels (Bradbury and Mehl, 1989).

DIFFERENTIAL DIAGNOSIS

The symptoms of IBD and its associated problems are varied. Symptoms of common childhood illnesses may be difficult to differentiate from exacerbations of the child's underlying disease process. Gastrointestinal symptoms are the ones that will most likely cause concern or alarm to the child, family, and primary care provider. An index of disease activity for some, but not all children, is the ESR. This may from time to time be of assistance in clarifying the child's symptoms.

Intercurrent illnesses, such as a viral or bacterial

gastroenteritis or another illness that must be treated with antibiotic therapy, may contribute to the flare of the child's IBD. This may be a result of the alteration of the normal flora of the bowel, usually a predominance of *Clostridium difficile*, following antibiotic therapy.

Diarrhea

Children with IBD can and do have bouts of gastroenteritis similar to those of their peers and family members. The child's physical examination and history should include an evaluation of any IBD-like symptoms such as the presence of any blood, pus, or mucus in the stool; cramping or urgency associated with bowel movements; weight loss or anorexia, and the occurrence of any symptoms that might be extraintestinal manifestations of the disease. The child's abdomen should be closely examined for any change. Stool cultures should always be obtained because *Yersinia*, *Campylobacter*, *Shigella*, and *C. difficile* may mimic IBD. The child should be treated for any identified pathogen. Any child who has prolonged symptoms, significant hematochezia (with no identified pathogen), or weight loss should be referred to the gastroenterology team.

Abdominal pain

The child with abdominal pain should be examined for any changes that might indicate a progression of their disease, toxic megacolon, or an obstruction. The child should be questioned as to the similarity of the current pain to the pain previously experienced as a part of the IBD. Similarity to previous episodes, location of known disease, and a history of accompanying symptoms that would indicate disease rather than influenza or another acute condition of the abdomen should guide the practitioner. Pain that is acute in an ill-appearing child should be referred immediately to the gastroenterology team; less acute symptoms should be watched carefully, with referral if the symptoms fail to abate within 24 to 48 hours.

Vomiting

Vomiting in a child with Crohn's disease could indicate an obstruction. The history and physical examination should elicit information regarding distension, any associated pain and its relation to meals and nature of the emesis, and accompanying abdominal pain. As always, information should be gathered regarding the child's bowel pattern and the nature of the stools.

Skeletal complaints

Children who are receiving corticosteroid therapy are at increased risk for osteoporosis and aseptic necrosis of the hip. In addition, children with IBD have a greater likelihood of having peripheral arthritis, sacroileitis, and ankylosing spondylitis. The child with IBD who complains of back or hip pain requires radiologic examination to adequately assess the symptoms. When the child with IBD complains of joint pain, he or she should be questioned regarding the presence of erythema or swelling. If joint involvement is a concern, the child should also be assessed for any increased disease activity.

DEVELOPMENTAL ISSUES
Safety

The child with IBD requires no special restriction of activities. The child should be encouraged to participate in all sports he or she feels able to enjoy. Vigorous activities such as lacrosse or tackle football should pose no problem for the child in remission. The child with osteoporosis, however, should refrain from such sports. Because, as in many populations with special needs, there may be a tendency for anxious families to shelter their child from discomfort or tense situations, the care provider can play an integral role in advocating for a normal life-style for the child.

Alcohol consumption by the adolescent with IBD who is in remission is no more of a concern than is alcohol consumption by nonaffected peers. Alcohol ingestion may cause discomfort for some individuals with IBD. If this is the case, this individual should limit intake. Persons taking metronidazole should be informed that concomitant alcohol intake will induce a disulfiram type of reaction.

Child care

Parents of children with IBD should be encouraged to use the same guidelines for choosing child care arrangements for this child as they would their well siblings. Because the onset of IBD in children most commonly occurs in childhood, the increased risk of diarrheal illness secondary to diaper-changing areas and day-care providers handling food does not often need to be addressed by these families. Should the child become infected, the illness should be promptly treated and the child monitored for signs of exacerbation of the disease. The overriding philosophy, however, is to not unduly isolate the child from normal activities of daily living.

Diet

No specific dietary restrictions have been documented to be helpful in controlling symptoms for the individual with IBD. Some individuals may feel most comfortable when they avoid certain foods; the child and family can be assisted in identifying such foods. The fear is that the diet may become overly restricted by the anxious parent who feels able to attribute symptoms to multiple foods. This may result in a diet that is unappealing to the child and so restrictive as to provide too few calories to promote growth and development.

As a part of ongoing assessment of nutritional status, an evaluation of usual dietary intake is essential. If growth is unsatisfactory (i.e., less than 5 cm/year, height less than the third percentile for age, or 2 standard deviations less than chronologic age), a referral should be made for a dietary consultation. The dietician may assess the child's intake and nutritional status and counsel the child and family regarding ways in which caloric intake may be augmented. Commerically available calorically dense nutritional supplements may be a good adjunct to the child's diet in such circumstances.

If growth retardation associated with IBD is to be reversed, adequate nutritional supplementation is necessary. It is generally agreed that given adequate calories, a child or adolescent (before epiphyseal closure) may recover lost growth. As nutritional replenishment begins, a child or an adolescent with IBD may require 70 to 85 kcal/kg/day. These values represent 100% to 150% of the recommended daily allowances for children and adolescents (Hyams, 1988; Kleinman et al., 1989).

During periods of active disease, many children, particularly those with Crohn's disease affecting the small bowel, may feel most comfortable on a low-roughage diet. Children with Crohn's disease of the small bowel are also more likely to experience some degree of lactose intolerance, which may persist even during periods of remission. During periods of inactive disease, these children may drink Lactaid milk or use lactase capsules and tablets which are readily available. For those children who feel especially deprived or set apart from their peers as a result of their dietary restrictions, such products may be of value. Experience has shown that these products are not helpful for all lactose-intolerant individuals, however. Children on milk-restricted diets and those taking corticosteroids should receive calcium supplementation because they are at risk for osteoporosis (Reid and Ibbertson, 1986).

Discipline

Behavioral expectations for the child with IBD are similar to those of their nonaffected peers. One area of concern may be the issue of compliance for those children who are responsible or are assuming the responsibility for their treatment regimen. Those children in whom IBD remains in remission may not perceive the need for their medications because they may be essentially asymptomatic and feeling well. The concept of remission and disease being present but not discernable is a difficult one for the school-aged child or early adolescent to master. Because a large percentage of those children diagnosed with IBD are in their early to middle adolescence, rebellion and testing are normal developmental issues (Erikson, 1963). For adolescents with IBD, medications and treatment regimens become a fertile battleground for testing their independence. The primary care provider can help the family identify ownership of responsibility for the disease management.

Toileting

Incontinence is an experience shared on occasion by many individuals with IBD; for those children who have frequent bowel movements accompanied by urgency, the fear of this occurrence is ever present. Children and families should be assisted in planning to prevent or to handle in a low-key fashion such an eventuality. In the context of an overview of the child's condition and its implications, the possibility of incontinence occurring should be shared with the school nurse and classroom teachers. They may then make plans to ensure that incidents will be handled with sensitivity and that the child may retain as much control and dignity as possible. The classroom teacher should be encouraged to move the child's seat nearer the door and to liberalize bathroom privileges so that he or she may leave the room unobtrusively. The care provider may suggest that an extra change of clothing be kept in the child's locker or in the nurse's office.

Sleep patterns

Children who are taking corticosteroids twice daily may feel agitated or euphoric at bedtime and may have some difficulty sleeping (Lewicki and Leeson, 1984). Dosage times may be shifted somewhat to alleviate this problem. Once the dose is decreased, a single dose may be given in the morning. The child experiencing a flare of disease or whose disease is under poor control may be troubled by the need to use the bathroom many times during the night. This may make it difficult for the child to feel well rested and refreshed in the morning.

School issues

School-related issues pertinent to the child with IBD, such as absences, stigma, and adjustment difficulties during adolescence, are similar to those that affect many children with chronic health problems. The nature of the disease process and their treatment regimen often sets children with IBD apart from their peers in significant ways. These include the Cushingoid faces of the child receiving corticosteroid therapy, the need for embarrassing treatments such as the installation of rectal medications, and the use of nocturnal nasogastric feedings. They may decrease the likelihood of compliance with the treatment regimen or, alternatively, decrease the child's level of social activity. Sensitivity to these issues, creative problem solving, and anticipatory guidance by the care provider will support the child and family in achieving as normal a life-style as possible. An issue frequently faced by the individual with IBD is the common misunderstanding by lay people and some in the medical community that IBD is a psychologic disease. A primary role of the health care provider is that of educating school personnel and other significant adults in the child's life, such as club leaders, coaches, and day-care providers.

Sexuality

Adolescence is a time when concerns regarding body image, interpersonal relationships with members of the opposite sex, and plans for one's future are paramount. It is not unusual then that an adolescent or young adult with IBD would be concerned about the impact this diagnosis might have on their appeal as a sexual partner, their ability to perform sexually, and their fertility. The significant changes in appearance that the adolescent with IBD must withstand include, in many instances, the late onset of puberty, weight gain, and acne, all of which contribute to his or her feelings of self-consciousness and stigma. Individuals with Crohn's disease frequently have stomas or perianal involvement, which often is disfiguring. This, too, may affect one's feelings of sexual attractiveness or acceptability to another person. Positive feelings of self-worth and a sense of acceptance must be conveyed to the adolescent who has IBD. The option of joining a network of other adolescents who share common concerns should be offered whenever possible. Formal organizations or casual social gatherings may provide opportunities for teens and families to obtain support and acceptance.

Sulfasalazine has been demonstrated to cause infertility in men; a decrease in sperm count, dysmotility, and malformation have been documented. These effects have been demonstrated to be reversible, however, when these men stop taking sulfasalazine for 3 months (Hanan and Kirsner, 1985; Korelitz, 1988). No analogous effects of sulfasalazine in women have been reported. Crohn's disease may negatively affect the ability of a woman to become pregnant. Disease activity and possible occlusion of fallopian tubes by inflamed bowel or abscesses have been implicated as causes of diminished fertility (Hanan and Kirsner, 1985). Outcome of pregnancy in women with IBD approximates that of the general population, though some researchers have found a somewhat higher incidence of prematurity in infants born to mothers with Crohn's disease than in the general population (Mayberry and Weterman, 1986). The influence of pregnancy on disease activity seems to correlate rather strongly with the activity of disease at the time of conception (Hanan and Kirsner, 1985).

Surgical resection for Crohn's disease or ulcerative colitis appears to affect neither the fertility nor the outcome of pregnancy. Men who have undergone colectomy with ileostomy or one of the other continent ileostomy procedures have some risks of impaired sexual functioning, though many report that the likelihood of such an outcome is relatively small (Glotzer, 1988).

SPECIAL FAMILY CONCERNS

Families of children with IBD, like families of children with other chronic conditions, may focus on the child's symptoms and treatment regimen. In the case of the family dealing with IBD, however, this often means disclosing such private and potentially embarrassing issues as toileting and personal hygiene. The invasion of privacy felt by the child may become a source of stress for the entire family. As the child enters adolescence, these issues are magnified as he or she seeks increased independence from the family and becomes increasingly self-conscious and concerned about body image and function. This may lead to poor communication and distrust between parent and child regarding disease activity and compliance with treatment regimens. If it is possible for the child to become relatively independent in disease management before this difficult time, the child and family may develop confidence and trust in one another and perhaps alleviate or avoid some of these conflicts. Another battle for control is often fought over the dietary habits of children with IBD who, because of individual sensitivity, disease activity, or parental misconception, use a restrictive diet. The primary care giver should anticipate such issues arising in the family of a young adolescent with IBD and provide anticipatory guidance, ongoing counseling, and advocacy to achieve an individualized and manageable treatment regimen for the child.

SUMMARY OF PRIMARY CARE NEEDS FOR THE CHILD
WITH INFLAMMATORY BOWEL DISEASE

Growth and development

Growth failure is a common problem for children with both Crohn's disease and ulcerative colitis.

Growth parameters are important to measure and graph at each visit.

Cognitive abilities are unimpaired by IBD.

Immunizations

No change in the normal immunization protocol is indicated unless the child is taking maintenance doses of immunosuppressive agents; in this case no live vaccines should be administered.

Screening
Vision

Ophthalmic examination is necessary at each visit. Some centers suggest yearly ophthalmologist visits for the child taking maintenance doses of corticosteroids.

Hearing

Routine screening is recommended.

Dental

Routine care is adequate, but children taking cyclosporine are at increased risk for gingival hyperplasia.

Blood pressure

Routine screening is recommended; if the child is taking cyclosporine or corticosteroids, blood pressure should be measured every 6 months.

Hematocrit

Hematocrit and hemoglobin values should be obtained yearly if the child is asymptomatic and has no history of anemia; otherwise a CBC should be obtained every 6 months or as necessary.

Urinalysis

Routine screening is recommended unless the child has a history of fistulas or abscesses.

Tuberculosis

Routine screening is recommended.

Condition-specific screening

Erythrocyte sedimentation rate
Check annually.
Fecal occult blood test
Check stool yearly and with potential disease flare.
Lactose intolerance
Test as indicated.
Renal and liver function tests
For children taking cyclosporine or 6-MP, test every 6 months.

Drug interactions
Sulfasalazine

Potentiates include orally administered hypoglycemic agents, phenytoin, and warfarin. It causes decreased absorption of digoxin.

Metronidazole

Potentiates include warfarin. It interacts with alcohol and produces a disulfiram type of reaction.

Corticosteroids

Potentiates include warfarin. It diminishes the efficacy of orally administered hypoglycemic agents.

Differential diagnosis
Diarrhea

Rule out flare of disease; obtain stool cultures.

Abdominal pain

Rule out flare of disease, toxic megacolon, and obstruction.

Vomiting

Rule out flare of disease and assess for obstruction.

Skeletal complaints

Rule out arthritic manifestations of the disease (sacroileitis and ankylosing spondylitis).

Developmental issues
Safety

No special safety recommendations are necessary for the child with inactive disease. The child

Continued.

SUMMARY OF PRIMARY CARE NEEDS FOR THE CHILD
WITH INFLAMMATORY BOWEL DISEASE — cont'd

with osteoporosis should not participate in contact sports.

Child care

Standard developmental counseling is advised.

Diet

No special diet is recommended; some children may be lactose intolerant, and some children during active disease may have less pain on a low roughage diet. Adequate caloric intake is essential for growth.

Discipline

Standard developmental counseling is advised.

Toileting

Occasional incontinence may be an issue for some children.

Sleep

Generally these children have no special needs; children receiving an evening dose of corticosteroids may have some difficulty sleeping. The child may also have some nighttime stooling, which interrupts sleep.

School issues

School personnel must be educated regarding special issues related to IBD; any misunderstandings regarding psychologic etiology of IBD should be alleviated.

Sexuality

Sulfasalazine may cause infertility in men while they are taking the drug. Pregnancy outcomes are similar to those of the general population. Self-esteem and body image issues are important to adolescents with IBD.

Special family concerns

Issues regarding compliance with the treatment regimen are commonly an area of concern for these families in light of the fact that the child has typically reached adolescence by the time of diagnosis and is experiencing the developmental problems associated with that stage of growth. Privacy issues regarding toileting are often difficult for children and families to deal with.

RESOURCES
Organizations

Crohn's and Colitis Foundation of America, Inc
444 Park Ave S, 11th Floor
New York, NY 10016-7374
(800) 343-3637
(212) 685-3440
The Crohn's and Colitis Foundation (CCFA) is an organization with many chapters across the country that provides education and support for its members and for members of the community. Individuals with IBD and their families are encouraged to join and attend meetings and educational offerings. Many chapters have subcommittees that specifically deal with issues related to the needs of children with IBD and their families. The NFIC also publishes educational books and pamphlets written for the lay public. Inquiries may be made regarding lists of publications and pamphlets, as well as chapter locations.

REFERENCES

Andrews HA, Lewis P, Allan RN: Prognosis after surgery for colonic Crohn's disease, *Br J Surg* 76:1184-1190, 1989.

Banner MP: Genitourinary complications of inflammatory bowel disease, *Radiol Clin North Am* 25:199-209, 1987.

Barrett KE and Dharmsathaphorn K: Pharmacological aspects of therapy in inflammatory bowel diseases: Antidiarrheal agents, *J Clin Gastroenterol* 10:57-63, 1988.

Belli DC, Seidman E, Bouthillier L, et al: Chronic intermittent elemental diet improves growth failure in children with Crohn's disease, *Gastroenterology* 94:603-610, 1988.

Bradbury K, Mehl B: Pharmacology focus: Drug interactions, *Foundation Focus*, November 1989.

Brandt LJ, Bernstein LH, Boley SJ, et al: Metronidazole therapy for perineal Crohn's disease: A follow-up study, *Gastroenterology* 83:383-387, 1982.

Castile RG, Telonder RL, Cooney DR, et al: Crohn's disease in children: Assessment of the progression of disease, growth, and prognosis, *J Ped Surg* 15, 462-469, 1980.

Danzi JT: Extraintestinal manifestations of idiopathic inflammatory bowel disease, *Arch Intern Med* 148:297-302, 1988.

Duffy LF, Daum F, Fisher SE, et al: Peripheral neuropathy in Crohn's disease patients treated with metronidazole, *Gastroenterology* 88:681-684, 1985.

Erikson EH: *Childhood and society*, ed 2, New York, 1963, WW Norton.

Farmer RG and Michener WM: Prognosis of Crohn's disease with onset in childhood or adolescence: *Dig Dis Sci* 24:752-757, 1979.

Feczko PJ: Malignancy complicating inflammatory bowel disease, *Radiol Clin North Am* 25:157-174, 1987.

Frank MS, Brandt LJ, and Bernstein LH: Pharmacotherapy of inflammatory bowel disease: Part 2. Metronidazole, *Postgrad Med* 74:155-160, 1983.

Gitnick G: Inflammatory bowel diseases: Part 1. Classification and cancer risk, *Am Fam Phys* 39:216-220, 1989a.

Gitnick G: Inflammatory bowel diseases: Part 2. Extraintestinal involvement and management, *Am Fam Phys* 39:225-233, 1989b.

Glotzer DJ: The surgical management of idiopathic inflammatory bowel disease. In Kirsner JB and Shorter RC, eds: *Inflammatory bowel disease*, Philadelphia, 1988, Lea & Febiger 585-644.

Gryboski JD and Spiro HM: Prognosis in children with Crohn's disease, *Gastroenterology* 74:807-817, 1978.

Hanan IM and Kirsner JB: Inflammatory bowel disease in the pregnant woman, *Clin Perinatol* 12:669-682, 1985.

Hanauer SB and Kirsner JB: Medical therapy in ulcerative colitis. In Kirsner JB and Shorter RC, eds: *Inflammatory bowel disease*, Philadelphia, 1988, Lea & Febiger.

Harper RH, Fazio VW, Lavery IC, et al: The long term outcome in Crohn's disease, *Dis Colon Rectum* 30:174-179, 1987.

Hyams JS: Inflammatory bowel disease in children and adolescents. *Endosc Rev* 5:46-60, 1988.

Joachim G and Milne B: Inflammatory bowel disease: Effects on lifestyle, *J Adv Nurs* 12:483-487, 1987.

Kanof ME, Lake AM, and Bayless TM: Decreased height velocity in children and adolescents before the diagnosis of Crohn's disease, *Gastroenterology* 95:1523-1527, 1988.

Kirschner BS: Inflammatory bowel disease in children. *Pediatr Clin North Am* 35:189-208, 1988a.

Kirschner BS: Medical management of inflammatory bowel disease in children. In Kirsner JB and Shorter RC, eds: *Inflammatory bowel disease*, Philadelphia, 1988b, Lea & Febiger, pp 503-512.

Kirschner BS, Klich JR, Kalman SS, et al: Reversal of growth retardation in Crohn's disease with therapy emphasizing oral nutritional restitution, *Gastroenterology* 80:10-15, 1981.

Kirschner BS, Schmidt-Sommerfeld E, and Stephens JK: Gastroduodenal Crohn's disease in childhood, *J Pediatr Gastroenterol Nutr* 9:138-140, 1989.

Kleinman RE, Balistreri WF, Heyman MB, et al: Nutritional support for pediatric patients with inflammatory bowel disease, *J Pediatr Gastroenterol Nutr* 8:8-12, 1989.

Korelitz BI: Pharmacotherapy of inflammatory bowel disease: Part 3. 6-Mercaptopurine, *Postgrad Med* 74:165-172, 1983.

Korelitz BI: Fertility and pregnancy in inflammatory bowel disease. In Kirsner JB and Shorter JC, eds: *Inflammatory bowel disease*, Philadelphia, 1988, Lea & Febiger, 319-326.

Lewicki LJ and Leeson MJ: The multisystem impact on physiologic processes of inflammatory bowel disease, *Nurs Clin North Am* 19:71-80, 1984.

Martin F: Oral 5-aminosalicylic acid preparation in treatment of inflammatory bowel disease, *Dig Dis Sci* 32 (suppl) 57S-63S, 1987.

Mayberry JF and Weterman IT: European survey of fertility and pregnancy in women with Crohn's disease: A case control study by European Collaborative Group, *Gut,* 22, 821-825, 1986.

Mayer L and Janowitz H: Extraintestinal manifestations of inflammatory bowel diseases. In Kirsner JS and Shorter RC, eds: *Inflammatory bowel disease*, Philadelphia, 1988, Lea & Febiger, 299-317.

Mendeloff AI and Calkins BM: The epidemiology of idiopathic inflammatory bowel disease. In Kirsner JS and Shorter RC, eds: *Inflammatory bowel disease*, Philadelphia, 1988, Lea & Febiger, 3-34.

Parrott NR, Taylor RMR, Venables CW, et al: Treatment of Crohn's disease in relapse with cyclosporin A, *Br J Surg* 75:1185-1188, 1988.

Pemberton JH, Phillips SF, Ready RR, et al: Quality of life after Brooke ileostomy and ileal pouch–anal anastomosis, *Ann Surg* 209:620-626, 1989.

Present DH, Meltzer SJ, Krumholz MP, et al: 6-Mercaptopurine in the management of inflammatory bowel disease: Short- and long-term toxicity, *Ann Intern Med* 111:641-649, 1989.

Reddy JB and Jeejeebhoy KN: Acute complications of Crohn's disease, *Crit Care Med* 16:557-561, 1988.

Reid IR and Ibbertson HK: Calcium supplements in the prevention of steroid-induced osteoporosis, *Am J Clin Nutr* 44:287-290, 1986.

Rimsza ME: Complications of corticosteroid therapy, *Am J Dis Child* 132:806-811, 1978.

Sadeghi-Nejad A and Senior B: The treatment of ulcerative colitis in children with alternate-day corticosteroids, *Pediatrics* 43:840-845, 1969.

Seidman EG, Roy CC, Weber AM, et al: Nutritional therapy of Crohn's disease in childhood, *Dig Dis Sci* 32(suppl)82s-88s, December 1987.

Stange EG, Fleig WE, Rehklau E, et al: Cyclosporin A treatment in inflammatory bowel disease, *Dig Dis Sci* 34:1387-1392, 1989.

Vogelsang H, Ferenci P, Woloszczuk W, et al: Bone disease in vitamin-D deficient patients with Crohn's disease, *Dig Dis Sci* 34:1094-1099, 1989.

Williams SM and Harned RK: Hepatobiliary complications of inflammatory bowel disease, *Radiol Clin North Am* 25:175-188, 1987.

19 *Juvenile Rheumatoid Arthritis*

Patricia M. Reilly

ETIOLOGY

The diagnostic term juvenile rheumatoid arthritis (JRA) is the officially designated term used in the United States to describe a form of idiopathic inflammatory peripheral arthritis that differs in many respects from adult rheumatoid arthritis (RA) (Cassidy, 1989). The terms juvenile arthritis and juvenile chronic arthritis reinforce this important distinction between JRA and adult RA and are preferred by many for this reason. Diagnosis of JRA presumes exclusion of more common types of arthritis in children (see the box at right).

The etiology of JRA is unknown. More recent studies focus on the role of infection, autoimmunity, and immunogenetics in the etiology of JRA. Infectious agents are known to cause arthritis in children (Kunnamo, 1987). Several clinical features of systemic-onset JRA, including high fever, rash, pericarditis, adenopathy, and seasonal variation, suggest a viral etiology. However, researchers have been unable to isolate specific infectious agents or to identify the mechanism whereby such agents invoke systemic and local immune responses in children with JRA (Bennett, 1989).

An autoimmune component is suggested by the presence of autoantibodies, such as rheumatoid factor (RF) and antinuclear antibodies (ANAs), in certain JRA subtypes. Elevated levels of circulating immune complexes and aberrations of cellular immunity present in some individuals with JRA further indicate a disease-related challenge to the immune system (Bennett, 1989).

DIAGNOSTIC CRITERIA FOR THE CLASSIFICATION OF JUVENILE RHEUMATOID ARTHRITIS

1. Age at onset less than 16 years
2. Arthritis in one or more joints defined as swelling or effusion, or the presence of two or more of the following signs: limitation of range of motion, tenderness or pain on motion, and increased heat
3. Duration of disease of 6 weeks to 3 months
4. Type of onset of disease during the first 4 to 6 months classified as
   a. Polyarthritis—five joints or more
   b. Oligoarthritis—four joints or fewer
   c. Systemic disease
      (1) Arthritis
      (2) Intermittent fever
      (3) Rheumatoid rash
      (4) Visceral disease (hepatosplenomegaly, lymphadenopathy, etc.)
5. Exclusion of other diseases

From Cassidy JT: Juvenile rheumatoid arthritis. In Kelley WN, Harris ED, Ruddy S, et al, eds: *Textbook of rheumatology,* Philadelphia, 1989, WB Saunders, p 1300. Copyright by WB Saunders. Reprinted by permission.

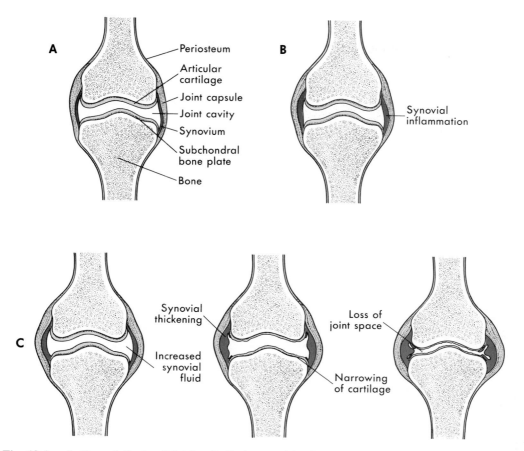

Fig. 19-1. **A,** Normal diarthrodial joint. **B,** Early synovitis. **C,** Progressive destruction of an inflamed joint.

Immunogenetic studies suggest that specific genetic predispositions exist for various subgroups of JRA. Human leukocyte antigen (HLA) is the name of the major histocompatibility complex (MHC) in humans. The MHC is a chromosomal region containing genes that encode cell surface molecules to facilitate immune response (Stastny, 1987). Studies of HLA have demonstrated that clinical subgroups of JRA can be differentiated on the basis of genetic variation and that most subgroups are clearly distinguishable from adult RA (Albert and Ansell, 1987; Lotz and Vaughn, 1988).

INCIDENCE

In the United States, studies have variously estimated the incidence at 9.2 new cases per 100,000 children annually (Sullivan, Cassidy, and Petty, 1975) and 13.9 cases per 100,000 annually (Towner et al., 1983). Prevalence of JRA among American children may be as high as 113.4 cases per 100,000 (Towner et al., 1983).

CLINICAL MANIFESTATIONS AT TIME OF DIAGNOSIS

Juvenile rheumatoid arthritis is a group of conditions characterized by the presence of chronic synovial inflammation (Fig. 19-1). Synovitis may exist for months or years without causing joint destruction or may damage cartilage, subchondral bone, or other joint structures in a relatively short period. Clinical features range from mild synovitis in one joint with no systemic symptoms to severe

Table 19-1. Clinical manifestations of juvenile arthritis

Mode of onset Immunogenetics	Incidence			Findings		Prognosis
	Frequency (% of all cases)	Age	Sex (M:F)	Articular	Extraarticular	
Systemic ANA – RF – HLA –	20	Any age	M > F (1.5:1)	Multiple joint involvement; myalgia, arthralgia, or transient arthritis	High fever, rash, hepatosplenomegaly, pericarditis, pleuritis, abdominal pain (systemic manifestations, typically remit within 6 months), leukocytosis, anemia, thrombocytosis, mildly elevated LFTs, uveitis rare	Severe disabling polyarthritis (20%-50%); all disease mortality in this group (2-4%)
Polyarticular (>5 joints) Rheumatoid factor + ANA + (75%) RF + HLA-DR4	5	Late childhood (> 8 years)	M < F (1:6)	Symmetrical involvement of large and small joints	Mild fever, mild to moderate hepatosplenomegaly and lymphadenopathy, other systemic symptoms generally mild, anemia, rheumatoid nodules, uveitis (5%)	Severe polyarthritis resembling adult RA (50%)
Rheumatoid factor – ANA + 25% RF – HLA	20	Any age	M < F (1:8)	Symmetrical involvement of large and small joints	Low grade fever, mild or absent systemic symptoms, anemia, uveitis rare	Severe polyarthritis (10%)
Pauciarticular (<5 joints) Early onset ANA + (60%) RF – HLA-Dw8 – DRw6, – DR5	40	Early childhood (<5 years)	M < F (1:7)	Asymmetrical large joint involvement, hips and SI joint spared	Chronic uveitis, few systemic symptoms, anemia	Polyarthritis (20%-30%). Loss of vision (33%)
Late onset ANA – RF – HLA – B27	15	Late childhood (>8 years)	M > F (10:1)	Asymmetrical large joint involvement, common hips and SI joint involvement common	Acute uveitis, occasional fever, anemia	Some may develop spondyloarthropathy

disease in many joints with fever, rash, lymphadenopathy, and organomegaly.

Manifestations of JRA at the time of onset suggest three major subtypes: systemic, polyarticular (five or more joints), and pauciarticular or oligoarthritis (fewer than 5 joints). These subtypes are based on variations in patterns and severity of joint disease, extraarticular manifestations, immunogenetic characteristics, age at onset, sex of child, and prognosis (Schaller, 1989) (Table 19-1).

In disease of systemic onset, severe constitutional and systemic involvement may develop concurrently with arthritis or precede overt arthritis by many weeks or months. The most characteristic findings are high intermittent fevers and a morbilliform rash occurring during febrile episodes. Laboratory findings typically show severe anemia, leukocytosis, and elevated erythrocyte sedimentation rate (Cassidy, 1989). In polyarticular JRA, onset is generally gradual and most often associated with symmetric joint involvement. A child may not complain of pain despite obvious swelling. Rheumatoid factor–positive polyarthritis is the only JRA subgroup equivalent to classic adult RA. The arthritis is often severe, with joint destruction occurring rapidly in the first year. Rheumatoid factor–negative arthritis is less aggressive, with little joint destruction despite months or years of synovitis (Schaller, 1989). Arthritis of pauciarticular onset develops in predominantly lower extremity joints. The ANA-positive subgroup is at high risk for developing chronic uveitis, but articular involvement typically follows a mild disease course (Schaller, 1989).

Juvenile rheumatoid arthritis is a disease characterized by exacerbations and remissions. Exacerbations, or flares, may occur during episodes of acute illness or stress, but the frequency and duration of flares are generally unpredictable. Many children have complete remission of the disease without complications. Others have residual problems, such as contractures or visual impairment, despite remission. A small number of children continue to have active disease into adulthood. Although criteria for remission vary among pediatric rheumatology centers, remission is commonly defined as no symptoms of active disease for at least 6 months while the child is taking medications and for an additional 6 months after all medications are discontinued.

TREATMENT

Management of JRA attempts to relieve symptoms, reduce disease activity, maintain musculoskeletal function, anticipate and treat complications, and promote the normal development of the child and family (Alepa, 1984). This is best achieved by a coordinated, multidisciplinary team: pediatric rheumatologist, nurse specialist, primary care provider, occupational and physical therapists, orthopedist, ophthalmologist, and social worker. Treatment progresses in a stepwise fashion beginning with the simplest, safest, and most conservative therapies to suppress inflammation and prevent deformity (Cassidy, 1989).

The pharmacologic agents most frequently used in the treatment of JRA are nonsteroidal antiinflammatory drugs (NSAIDs) and slower-acting antirheumatic drugs (SAARDs). Glucocorticoids, immunosuppressive agents, and cytotoxic agents are used for illness resistant to other forms of therapy (Cassidy, 1989; Fink, 1990). Medications commonly used in JRA treatment are summarized in Table 19-2.

Physical therapy and occupational therapy are critical to the successful management of the child with JRA. To maintain joint function and prevent deformity, therapists develop individualized exercise programs, teach the principles of joint protection and energy conservation, and recommend assistive devices for performance of daily activities (Melvin and Atwood, 1989). The child with arthritis, together with family members or other care givers, must carry out a recommended program of therapies at home. Periodic consultation with therapists is arranged as needed.

Soft tissue release, epiphysiodesis for leg length discrepancy, and total hip and knee replacements are the most frequently required surgical procedures among children with JRA. Less common surgeries include synovectomy for persistent synovitis, osteotomy, and arthrodesis, or bone fusion (Scott and Sledge, 1989; Swann, 1990).

PROGNOSIS

The prognosis for children with JRA is generally good, with 70% to 90% surviving the disease without significant functional disability (Cassidy, 1989). Better prognosis is associated with early diagnosis, treatment by providers experienced in pediatric rheumatology, receptive parental attitudes

Table 19-2. Medications commonly used in treatment of juvenile rheumatoid arthritis*

Drug	Trade name	Daily dose (mg/kg/day)	Side effects	Monitored parameters
NONSTEROIDAL ANTIINFLAMMATORY DRUGS				
Salicylates			GI irritation and blood loss, mild hepatitis, hematuria, proteinuria, salicylism (tinnitus, hyperpnea, behavior change), bleeding, anemia, oral ulcers, dental caries, allergic reaction, peptic ulcers	CBC, platelet count, UA, and AST and ALT levels 2 and 6 wk after initiation of treatment and every 2-3 mo thereafter
Acetylsalicylate acid	Aspirin†	80-100 (<25 kg)		AST and ALT levels; for sustained elevations of enzyme levels or levels 5 times normal, drug must be discontinued temporarily or dose reduced by 20% until levels are normal
Choline salicylate	Arthropan	2.5 g/day (>25 kg)		Occult blood in stools and PTT as required
Choline magnesium trisalicylate	Trilisate			Salicylate levels (to guide correct dosage)
Salicylsalicylic acid	Disalcid	Not determined		Therapeutic range: 20-30 mg/dl 2 hr after dose
Diflunisal	Dolobid	10-20		
Proprionic acid derivatives			Side effects common to all nonsalicylate NSAIDs: GI irritation and blood loss, proteinuria, hematuria, anemia, fluid retention, headache, dizziness, mild hepatitis, peptic ulcer, skin manifestations	CBC, platelet count, AST and ALT levels, and UA 2 and 6 wk after initiation of treatment and every 2-3 mo thereafter; BUN value and serum creatinine every 3-6 mo
Naproxen	Naprosyn†	7-20		Occult blood in stools and PTT as required.
Ibuprofen	Advil, Motrin, Nuprin	20-40		
Fenoprofen	Nalfon	900-1800 mg/m²/day (maximum 3200 mg/day)		
Indoleacetic acids				
Tolmetin sodium	Tolectin†	15-30	As above	As above
Sulindac	Clinoril	50 mg total (<25 kg) 75-100 mg total (>25 kg)		
Fenamates				
Meclofenamate sodium	Meclomen	3-7.5 (maximum 300 mg/day)	As above, with anemia and nonspecific skin rash more frequent	As above
Oxicams				
Piroxicam	Feldene	5-10 mg total (<25 kg) 10-20 mg total (>25 kg)	As above	As above
SLOW-ACTING ANTIRHEUMATIC DRUGS				
Gold sodium thiomalate Aurothioglucose	Myochrysine Solganal	0.5-1.0 mg/kg/wk (after initial test dose) injectable maintenance dose for 20 wk	Nitritoid reaction, hematuria, proteinuria, stomatitis, exfoliative dermatitis, bone marrow suppression, photosensitivity, diarrhea	CBC, platelet count, UA and liver function tests before initial dose, CBC count, platelet count, and UA before each injection or weekly with oral preparation
Auranofin	Ridaura	0.1-0.2 (oral preparation)		

D-Penicillamine	Cuprimine, Depen	Slow increase to maximum 10 mg/kg/day (750 mg/day)	Proteinuria, thrombocytopenia, dermatitis, lupus-like syndrome, iron deficiency anemia, vitamin B_6 deficiency	CBC, platelet count, and UA before initial dose and weekly for 2 mo, every other week for 6 mo, then monthly
Sulfasalazine	Azulfidine	Initial therapy: 40-60 mg/kg/24 hr in 3-6 doses Maintenance therapy: 30 mg/kg/24 hr in 4 divided doses	Anorexia, headache, nausea, vomiting, oligospermia, photosensitivity, blood dyscrasias, hypersensitivity reactions, hematuria crystalluria, folic acid deficiency, orange discoloration of urine and skin	CBC, UA monthly; liver function tests, BUN values, serum creatinine periodically
GLUCOCORTICOID DRUGS				
Systemic corticosteroid Prednisone		0.5-2.0 (lowest possible dose, alternate-day therapy preferred)	Growth retardation, osteoporosis, infection, Cushing's syndrome, hypertension, cataracts, glaucoma, GI symptoms, vertebral collapse	CBC, other monitoring as needed for numerous side effects; ophthalmologic examinations
Ophthalmic corticosteroids Dexamethasone Prenisolone		Doses vary according to degree of inflammation and magnitude of therapeutic response from 1 drop every 2 hr to 1 drop every other day	Cataracts, glaucoma, eye infections, Cushing's syndrome	Ophthalmologic examination every 2-3 wk for several months and every 2-3 mo thereafter
IMMUNOSUPPRESSIVE DRUGS				
Methotrexate	Mexate	0.3-0.6 mg/kg/wk	Bone marrow suppression, infection, hepatic damage, GI symptoms, alopecia, sterility	CBC, platelet count, and UA every week, liver function tests every 2-4 wk

*GI, gastrointestinal; CBC, Complete blood cell count; UA, urinalysis; AST, aspartate aminotransferase; ALT, alanine aminotransferase; PTT, partial thromboplastin time; BUN, blood urea nitrogen; Cr, creatinine.

†Food and Drug Administration approval for use in children.

toward treatment, and the cooperation of the child (Cassidy, 1982; Hull, 1988).

The child at greatest risk for poor functional outcome is one with late-onset polyarthritis, early involvement of hands and feet, rapid appearance of articular erosions, unremitting inflammatory activity or prominent systemic manifestations, RF positivity, and subcutaneous nodules (Cassidy, 1989).

ASSOCIATED PROBLEMS
Skeletal abnormalities

Juvenile rheumatoid arthritis subjects the growing skeleton to unique deformities. Chronic hyperemia in an inflamed joint stimulates accelerated maturation of the epiphyseal plates, resulting in skeletal overgrowth of the extremity. This process is most characteristically seen in children with early-onset pauciarticular disease who have unilateral knee involvement. Significant discrepancies in leg lengths result when overgrowth and subsequent elongation of the arthritic leg occur simultaneously with delayed maturation of the opposite leg (White, 1990).

Micrognathia

Arthritis-induced abnormalities of the temporomandibular joint (TMJ) result in mandibular undergrowth, micrognathia, and malocclusion. The highest percentage of TMJ abnormalities is found in the polyarticular subgroup with severe progression of the disease. Combined orthodontic and surgical procedures may improve function and esthetics in children with this problem (Myall et al., 1988).

Cervical spine involvement

Cervical spine involvement is thought to be characteristic of JRA. Cervical spine abnormalities develop in 70% of children with systemic arthritis and 55% of children with polyarticular arthritis (Brewer, Giannini, and Person, 1982). Apophyseal joint disease, fibrosis, and bony fusion occur most frequently in the upper cervical segments, typically C-2, C-3, and C-4 (Espada et al., 1988). Stiffness of the cervical spine, particularly in extension, is a common early finding. Neck pain and torticollis are infrequent in JRA children. Therefore, additional problems of infection or fracture should be suspected in a child with JRA who has these symptoms (Hensinger, DeVito, and Ragsdale, 1986).

Scoliosis

The incidence of scoliosis in children with JRA may be 10 times higher than that in the general population (Svantesson, Marhaug, and Haeffner, 1981).

Uveitis

Uveitis (also known as iridocyclitis) refers to an inflammation of the uveal tract, the middle vascular layer of the eye, which is composed of the iris, ciliary body, and choroid. Juvenile rheumatoid arthritis–associated uveitis is characterized by an insidious, asymptomatic, typically bilateral onset that often precedes arthritis and by a pattern of remissions and exacerbations that does not parallel articular disease (O'Brien and Albert, 1989).

Risk factors associated with developing uveitis include female sex, young age, ANA positivity, RF seronegativity, and pauciarticular onset. Significant visual loss may develop in as many as 75% of children with JRA. Early and aggressive treatment with mydriatics and topically applied corticosteroids along with frequent ophthalmologic follow-up have been effective in preserving the vision of children who do not have advanced disease. Uncontrolled uveitis results in glaucoma, cataracts, band keratopathy, and posterior synechiae and is much more difficult to treat (O'Brien and Albert, 1989).

Anemia

Microcytic, hypochromic anemia is a common feature of systemic and polyarticular JRA. The severity of anemia parallels the extent of disease activity. Microcytosis is associated with reduced levels of serum iron and serum iron–binding capacity and does not typically respond to iron supplementation (Harvey, Pippard, and Ansell, 1987). Poor nutrition and NSAID-induced GI blood loss must also be considered in the evaluation of anemia.

Problems associated with systemic onset or course

Systemic onset of JRA can be accompanied by significant extraarticular manifestations. Hepatosplenomegaly and generalized lymphadenopathy occur in most children with active systemic disease. Pericarditis is a common cardiac finding among children with systemic onset or course. Clinical manifestations vary from asymptomatic pericarditis with mild pericardial effusions to severe life-threatening cardiac involvement. Renal manifestations unrelated to drug therapy are rare. Hematuria associated with renal glomerulitis and proteinuria may be present before drug therapy is initiated (Cassidy, 1989).

PRIMARY CARE MANAGEMENT
Growth and development

Compared with unaffected children, a significantly greater proportion of children with JRA are below the third percentile in height before the onset of clinical symptoms and signs of the disease (Bernstein et al., 1977). This suggests that latent disease may affect growth before overt symptoms develop.

Differences in growth exist among the three types of JRA. Short stature occurs most frequently in children with polyarticular or systemic JRA. The child with polyarticular disease tends to be low in weight for height, but the child with systemic disease tends to be above average in weight for height. As a group, children with pauciarticular JRA generally fall within normal percentiles for weight and height. (Bacon et al., 1990).

In children with severe JRA, linear growth is retarded during periods of active systemic disease. Final height may be reduced by 25% of predicted height or greater in the most severe cases (Brewer, Giannini, and Person, 1982). Catch-up growth usually occurs during remission or with suppression of disease activity by therapy. Height returns to normal within 2 to 3 years if premature epiphyseal fusion has not occurred (White, 1990).

Corticosteroids suppress growth hormone production. Children with severe JRA who receive large daily doses of corticosteroids exhibit the greatest degree of growth retardation. With cessation of corticosteroids, height and weight return to near normal within 1 to 2 years.

Underweight children must be evaluated. Factors contributing to poor weight gain include systemic disease, increased nutrient requirements because of fever, GI side effects of medications, anorexia, depression, and limitations of TMJ or upper extremity joints. Excessive weight gain should be avoided to minimize stress on involved joints. Depression, poor food choices, and decreased physical activity as a result of pain, stiffness, or deformity contribute to weight increase.

Gross motor delays or temporary regressions are not uncommon in the child with JRA. Fine motor skills are less likely to be delayed as long as the child is provided with toys and activities that encourage manipulation (Atwood, 1989a). Limited mobility and decreased opportunities to actively interact with the environment place a child at risk for cognitive and social delays. Language acquisition is generally unaffected unless a child has significant TMJ arthritis.

Children with severe JRA often fall behind in acquisition of hygiene, toileting, dressing, and feeding skills. Regression in performance of these skills is common during acute illness and may be sustained during remissions because of lowered parental expectations and continued reinforcement of a child's dependent behaviors. Demonstration by the child of personal care skills is preferred to child or parent report during evaluation of functional level. When parents habitually perform such duties for a child, neither parent nor child may have an accurate understanding of the child's abilities (Atwood, 1989a).

Standard infant and early childhood assessment and screening tools, such as the Bayley Scales and Denver Development Screening Test, may be of questionable value in evaluating delay in seriously affected children. However, a verbally based tool may be useful for partial developmental assessment of some children. An occupational-physical therapy team familiar with the impact of JRA on the child's overall development can be a valuable resource for the primary care provider.

Immunizations

Children with JRA who are not taking immunosuppressive medications should receive routine immunizations. In the absence of other symptoms of infection, a child with the classic intermittent fever of JRA can be immunized during febrile episodes.

Children whose immunocompetence is altered by antimetabolites or large doses of corticosteroids should not receive live vaccines for at least 3 months after discontinuation of these drugs (Committee on Infectious Diseases, 1991). Live viral or bacterial vaccinations may be administered to children with JRA whose only exposure to corticosteroids is topically applied ophthalmic medication or intraarticular, bursal, or tendon injections (American Committee on Immunization Practices, 1989).

Children receiving long-term salicylate therapy

and other NSAIDs may be at increased risk for developing Reye's syndrome in the presence of influenza and varicella infections (Forsyth et al., 1989; Rennebohm et al., 1985). Yearly immunizations for types A and B influenza are recommended for children treated with aspirin and other NSAIDs who are older than 6 months of age according to the dosage and schedule set out by the American Academy of Pediatrics (1988). All NSAIDs, including aspirin, should be stopped temporarily if a child develops chickenpox or influenza.

Screening

Vision. Thorough fundoscopic examination and acuity screening should be performed at each office visit. At the time of diagnosis every child must be examined for uveitis by an ophthalmologist. Frequent ophthalmologic examinations are recommended for children at risk for uveitis, glaucoma, and cataracts. Young children with pauciarticular and ANA-positive arthritis are at greatest risk for development of ocular inflammation and require frequent screening for at least 7 to 10 years from disease onset (Kanski, 1989).

The following screening regimen for uveitis has been proposed: ANA positive, every 2 to 3 months; pauciarticular onset, every 2 to 3 months; polyarticular onset, every 6 months; systemic onset, every 6 to 12 months (Kanski, 1989; Rosenberg, 1987). More frequent follow-up is needed for children with active uveitis.

Corticosteroid-induced glaucoma or cataracts can occur at any time during treatment. When children begin using topically applied corticosteroids, their baseline intraocular pressure should be measured and then reexamined frequently during continued therapy (O'Brien and Albert, 1989; Wolf, Lichter, and Ragsdale, 1987).

Hearing. Routine office evaluation of auditory acuity is advised. Decreased acuity in children taking salicylates should be promptly investigated, however, because tinnitus associated with salicylate toxicity may impair hearing.

Dental. Salicylates dissolved in the mouth cause erosion of the occlusal surfaces of the teeth and eruption of white, mildly inflamed oral mucosal lesions (Christensen, 1984). Dental visits every 6 months, or more frequently if erosive signs develop, are recommended (Tanchyk, 1986). Pre-

vention of lesions depends on a child's avoiding overretention of salicylate preparations in the mouth and rinsing after ingestion of medication.

Increased incidence of dental caries occurs in children with JRA, possibly because of poor oral hygiene secondary to TMJ or upper extremity limitations. Malocclusions and crowded mandibular teeth occur as a result of micrognathia (Adair et al., 1981). Frequent dental visits, fluoride application, and sealants are recommended and orthodontic referrals made as needed.

Prophylactic antibiotic coverage for dental work or other surgeries is indicated for children with total hip replacements or those taking corticosteroids (see Chapter 11 for prophylactic schedule). Supplemental doses of corticosteroids are needed to meet the increased stress of dental treatment (Tullman, 1984). Dental work for children taking sulfasalazine who develop thrombocytopenia or leukopenia should be postponed until blood counts have returned to normal (U.S. Pharmacopeial Convention, 1990). Consultation with the pediatric rheumatology team and the dentist in these situations is necessary.

Blood pressure. Routine screening is recommended. Mild hypertension may occur in children taking NSAIDs and SAARDs. Corticosteroid-induced hypertension is also reported (Brewer, Giannini, and Person, 1982).

Hematocrit. Hematologic testing is done routinely by the pediatric rheumatology team, therefore routine screening may be deferred.

Urinalysis. Urinalysis is recommended at the start of treatment and at intervals of 6 to 12 months. Periodic and mild proteinuria and hematuria occur in many children with JRA. Protein greater than $1+$, red blood cell (RBC) counts greater than 5/mm^3 and the presence of casts should be immediately reported to the pediatric rheumatologist.

Tuberculosis. Routine screening is recommended, especially before starting corticosteroid treatment.

Condition-specific screening

LABORATORY SCREENING. Erythrocyte sedimentation rate, CBC with differential, platelet count, urinalysis, and liver function tests are routinely reviewed by the staff of the pediatric rheumatology center to monitor disease activity, response to therapy, drug toxicity, and anemia. Periodic testing of salicylate levels is indicated to evaluate therapeutic levels (20-30 mg/dl).

Drug interactions

There are many potential interactions between medications commonly used to treat JRA and over-the-counter and prescription drugs used to manage other common pediatric conditions. The box at right identifies the major interactions the primary care provider must be aware of in providing care to these children. Because of the complexity of possible drug interactions, the practitioner should work in conjunction with the rheumatology team when recommending any medications.

The primary provider should not discontinue the child's condition-specific medications without consulting the pediatric rheumatologist. Conditions warranting possible temporary cessation of medications include (1) exposure to chickenpox or influenza-like illness; (2) significant bleeding of the nose or gums; (3) dehydration as a result of illness (may result in possible salicylate toxicity); and (4) rapid, deep breathing (until salicylate toxicity is ruled out) (Mahy, 1987).

DIFFERENTIAL DIAGNOSIS AND MANAGEMENT OF COMMON PEDIATRIC CONDITIONS
Fever

Children with JRA may have fevers as a response to an infectious process or as a result of their chronic condition. The classic fever of systemic JRA is characterized by daily or twice daily temperature elevation to 39.5° C or higher, usually in the afternoon or evening, with a rapid return to baseline. Remittent and low-grade fever are less frequently seen patterns. Children often appear very ill during febrile periods and well when afebrile (Brewer, Giannini, and Person, 1982; Cassidy, 1989). Fever occurs typically at disease onset and may recur with arthritis flares. Moderate or mild temperature elevations occur with polyarticular and pauciarticular disease. A careful history and complete physical examination will usually determine the source of the fever.

Dermatologic symptoms

The classic JRA fever is usually accompanied by a rheumatoid rash that consists of 2- to 6-mm eva-

---

POTENTIAL DRUG INTERACTIONS IN CHILDREN TREATED FOR JUVENILE RHEUMATOID ARTHRITIS

Aspirin plus salicylate-containing medications can cause salicylate toxicity.

Antacids may alter the absorption rate of NSAIDs, resulting in subtherapeutic serum levels.

Antacids can alter renal excretion of aspirin, leading to higher serum levels of salicylate with antacid withdrawal or subtherapeutic levels with antacid addition.

Antihistamines may decrease NSAID levels.

Nonsteroidal antiinflammatory drugs may decrease the effectiveness of oral contraceptives.

Salicylates can increase penicillin levels.

Ampicillin may decrease the availability of sulfasalazine, causing loss of therapeutic efficacy.

Corticosteroids decrease plasma concentration of salicylates.

Penicillamine absorption is decreased by antacids.

Penicillamine must be given 2 hours apart from iron supplements and aluminum hydroxide antacids.

Methotrexate concentrations are increased by salicylates.

Sulfonamides may displace or be displaced by other highly protein-bound drugs, such as NSAIDS, salicylates, and methotrexate. Monitor children for increased effects of highly bound drugs when sulfonamides are added.

Reduced efficacy and increased incidence of breakthrough bleeding have been reported in oral contraceptive users treated with sulfonamides, such as sulfasalazine.

Concomitant administration of iron supplements and sulfasalazine results in a decreased blood level of sulfasalazine. It is not known whether the efficacy of either agent is altered.

From US Pharmacopeial Convention: *Drug information for the health care professional*, Rockville, Md; 1990, US Pharmacopeia.

nescent, salmon pink, generally circumscribed macular lesions. The rash may become confluent with larger lesions developing pale centers and pale periphery. It is most commonly seen on the trunk, on the extremities, and over pressure areas; the face, palms, and soles may also be involved. The rash is most prominent during fever spikes and may be visible only after rubbing or scratching the skin. A hot bath or stress may also induce it (Brewer, Giannini, and Person, 1982; Cassidy, 1989).

Otologic symptoms

Temporomandibular joint arthritis may cause referred pain to the ear, and this should be considered when children are evaluated for otitis media.

Respiratory symptoms

Aspirin intolerance, characterized by acute bronchospasm, severe rhinitis, or generalized urticaria and angioedema occurring within 3 hours after ingestion of aspirin or other NSAID, has been reported. Any child with recurrent rhinitis or asthma must be considered at risk for bronchoconstriction when given aspirin or other NSAIDs (Morassut, Yang, and Karsh, 1989).

Tachypnea occurs with aspirin toxicity. A serum salicylate level should be drawn immediately when a child on aspirin therapy has an increased respiratory rate. Salicylates should be withheld pending laboratory results.

Because of the potential risk of Reye's syndrome, differentiation of influenza from cold symptoms is essential for the practitioner and parent of a child on NSAID therapy. Treatment for type A influenza with amantadine (Symmetrel) is indicated for children taking NSAIDs. Temporary discontinuation of NSAID therapy is also indicated. Colds and influenza may cause arthritis flares.

Gastrointestinal symptoms

Nearly one fourth of children with JRA complain of nonspecific abdominal pain. Symptoms may be difficult to evaluate because all NSAIDs cause some degree of nausea, dyspepsia, and pain. The nonspecific pain of JRA is often cramping and may last for minutes to several days. It is usually epigastric or periumbilical, without rebound tenderness or guarding (Brewer, Giannini, and Person,

1982). A careful history and physical examination, as well as consultation with the pediatric rheumatologist as needed, will assist the practitioner in the evaluation of differential diagnoses.

Drug- or stress-induced GI bleeding must also be considered in children receiving NSAIDs or corticosteroids (Barrier and Hirschowitz, 1989). Peptic ulcers may manifest as chronic anemia secondary to occult blood loss or as acute GI hemorrhage. The classic symptom of epigastric pain that improves with eating and worsens with an empty stomach is more common in the adolescent but may be absent in the young child (Steinhorn and Berman, 1987).

Renal symptoms

Children taking aspirin may experience increased urinary urgency and frequency; however, this problem is generally temporary. Urinary tract infection (UTI) must be ruled out first. Hematuria and proteinuria are renal side effects of many JRA medications. Urine cultures are typically the more reliable diagnostic test for infection.

DEVELOPMENTAL ISSUES
Safety

Drug therapy is essential to the successful management of JRA. Subsequently education about medication safety becomes an important responsibility of the primary care provider. All medications must be kept in childproof containers out of reach of young children. This becomes especially important as older children assume responsibility for self-care. Children taking long-term immunosuppressant drugs are encouraged to wear medical alert bracelets or necklaces.

Photosensitive skin reactions occur with naproxen (Naprosyn), injectable gold-gold sodium thiomalate and aurothioglucose, sulfasalazine (Azulfidine), and hydroxychloroquine (Plaquenil). Hypoallergenic sunblock lotion with a minimum sun protection factor of 15 should be used on exposed skin.

Orthotic appliances are often recommended for joint protection. Important safety issues related to splint wearing include care of the splint to maintain integrity, proper skin care, recognition of signs and symptoms of an ill-fitting splint, and proper splint application. The splint should be checked at regular intervals to detect damage to the appliance and to ensure that the child has not outgrown it (Boutaugh and Tehan, 1987).

Superficial heat and cold modalities are frequently recommended to relieve pain and stiffness. Determining the type of applications used by the family and reviewing safety precautions specific to each type of application are important.

Adaptive equipment such as electrical devices, lamp switch extenders, and elevated toilet seats are used by children with JRA to minimize joint stress and increase independence. Safety can often be maximized by such assistive devices. For example, bath safety can be improved by the use of safety strips, rubber mats, wall grab bars, tub chairs, and one-handed hose attachments (Atwood, 1989b). Adaptive equipment should be evaluated for the safety of all family members.

Child care

Parents of children receiving medications may have difficulty locating child care providers who are willing to administer them. For care givers who accept this responsibility, parents should prepare a list that includes the name, dose, time and method of administration, and side effects of each drug. The name and telephone number of the person to contact for questions or problems should be provided.

It is important for care givers to understand that exacerbations and remissions characterize the JRA disease pattern and that a child's functional capacity, energy level, and developmental progress may fluctuate. Education about JRA and about a child's actual or anticipated limitations is likely to decrease anxiety among child care staff and promote appropriate interactions between care givers and a child affected by JRA. Because children who receive corticosteroids and immunosuppressants should avoid persons with communicable diseases, group child care is not recommended.

Diet

As many as 36% of children with JRA are at risk for protein-calorie malnutrition (Henderson and Lovell, 1987). Decreased iron and calcium intake, as well as decreased calorie intake unrelated to disease activity, have been reported (Miller, Chacko, and Young, 1989). Low plasma levels of zinc, vitamins A and C, and proteins (abumin,

prealbumin, and retinol binding protein) have been identified in children with polyarticular and systemic JRA (Bacon et al., 1990). The addition of a daily multivitamin preparation and iron supplements is frequently recommended for children with JRA.

Corticosteroid therapy can cause increased appetite, fluid retention, weight gain, and osteoporosis secondary to calcium depletion. A low-sodium diet may be indicated. Calcium intake should be evaluated and supplementation considered if dietary sources are insufficient (Warady and Shields, 1987). Sulfasalazine increases folic acid requirements in children taking this drug.

Up to 43% of individuals with JRA may use unconventional dietary remedies for arthritis (Southwood et al., 1990). Among the most popular are avoidance of nightshade vegetables such as potatoes and eggplant and acid foods such as tomatoes, diets with increased fish or fish oil, fasting, herbal remedies, and megavitamin therapy. Research has not established a relationship between either active disease or remission of arthritis and diet. Educating families about proper nutrition for a growing child with a chronic condition and evaluating potentially harmful dietary manipulations, especially those involving nutrient restrictions, are important responsibilities of the practitioner.

Discipline

Parents of children with JRA may experience difficulty with discipline. Overly protective parents impose unnecessary limitations on activities or enforce excessive safety precautions. Feelings of guilt, sorrow for a child in pain, or fear that stress will trigger a flare-up cause some parents to adopt an overly permissive discipline style. In addition, overindulgence during periods of active disease alternating with normalization of discipline practices during remissions fosters inconsistent limit setting (Erlandson et al., 1987).

Parent education about every child's need for clear, reasonable, and consistent limits should include a review of alternatives to physical punishment. Guidance regarding age-specific developmental tasks and the effect of JRA on the acquisition and performance of self-care, language, motor, and social skills offers parents a framework for making decisions about discipline (Atwood, 1989a).

Toileting

The acquisition of self-care skills may be delayed in the child with JRA. Toilet training should be postponed during periods of active disease because the child may lack the motivation and physical capability to perform tasks necessary for successful toileting.

Limitations in upper and lower extremities create difficulty in transferring on and off the toilet, managing toilet paper, and dressing and undressing for toileting. Safety bars and elevated toilet seats are reliable assistive devices for children with lower extremity involvement. For children with upper extremity limitations, effective aids for wiping after toileting are difficult to locate. Occupational therapists will be helpful in devising solutions to this problem. A bidet can be attached to a toilet, thereby circumventing the need for paper. Adapted clothing and dressing aids can facilitate toileting (Atwood, 1989b).

Consideration should be given to toilet hygiene in facilities outside the home where assistive devices will not be available. In addition, bedpans and urinals may be required at night if pain and stiffness limit mobility.

Sleep patterns

Research with adults suggests that children with JRA may be at risk for sleep disturbances that affect the extent of daytime fatigue and degree of morning stiffness. Marked sleep fragmentation as a result of sleep apnea, frequent movements of extremities, and frequent arousals occurs in adults with RA and may be related to daytime fatigue experienced by these individuals (Mahowald et al., 1989). Micrognathia occurring as a result of TMJ destruction can cause obstructive sleep apnea and sleep disturbance (Davies and Iber, 1983).

Active disease causes increased wakefulness at night. A child fatigues more readily during flares and requires longer periods of rest during the day. The severity and duration of morning stiffness increase. Recommendations to alleviate morning symptoms include the use of flannel sheets, thermal underwear, joint comforters, warmed clothing, and a sleeping bag. An electric blanket with a timer set to warm the blanket 1 hour before a child is scheduled to awaken can also reduce morning stiffness. Except for children with hip and knee involvement

who are at risk for lower extremity contractures, warm waterbeds may be helpful. Finally, taking medications with food 30 to 60 minutes before rising and exercising in a warm bath before starting daily activities can increase range of motion (Boutaugh, 1987).

School issues

Children with JRA face many potential difficulties in school. The practitioner should periodically question children and parents about school-related problems such as fatigue, mobility, absences, and medications. The practitioner should work with the family, school staff, and pediatric rheumatology team to identify and remedy problems when they occur.

There may be discrepancies between what teachers, parents, and students perceive to be obstacles. Parents and teachers more often identify limitations in activities of daily living and physical health as primary difficulties. Affected children focus on self-concept and peer relations and prefer to solve peer issues by themselves (Taylor, Passo, and Champion, 1987).

Many students will require only minor adjustments in school programs. Surgery or disease flares may necessitate temporary home tutoring and should be planned for in a child's individualized education plan. Public Law 94-142 requires that special services such as occupational therapy, physical therapy, adaptive physical education, and transportation between home and school be available to students with JRA attending federally funded schools.

A student with JRA can participate in modified school athletic programs but should not perform any activity that causes an impact to the body or the joints. Prolonged activity that holds a joint in one place should also be avoided, as should activities such as handstands and chin-ups that place total body weight on non-weight-bearing joints (Brewer, Giannini, and Person, 1982).

Sexuality

Sexual maturation may be delayed in adolescents with JRA, particularly in those with systemic disease. Menarche has been shown to occur later in girls with JRA (mean age 13.2 years) than in unaffected controls (mean age 12.5 years), although no clear etiology for this difference was identified (Fraser et al., 1988). Development of secondary sexual characteristics may be delayed in both boys and girls.

Contraceptive advice should include discussion of interactions among arthritis medications and various oral contraceptives, as well as the effects, if any, of arthritis medications on fertility and fetal development. If mechanical methods of birth control are difficult to use for adolescents with hand or hip involvement, a review of alternative birth control methods and consultation with the occupational therapist on the pediatric rheumatology team are indicated.

SPECIAL FAMILY CONCERNS

Divergent views regarding perceptions and impact of JRA may exist among family members. Areas of potential divergence include perceptions about limitations as a result of physical disability, type of information wanted about JRA, and causes of stress related to an empathy-resentment-guilt cycle of family dynamics (Konkol et al., 1989). Family-based education about JRA will be most effective when such incongruencies can be examined and reconciled.

Between 66% and 70% of children with JRA may use remedies that are not part of generally accepted medical therapy (Southwood et al., 1990). Practitioners should assume that a family will try unconventional therapies, such as copper bracelets, acupuncture, patent medicines, diet manipulation, and skin creams. It is important to foster trust and create an accepting environment where frustrations with conventional treatment can be aired and unproved remedies openly discussed. Practitioners should help families differentiate between harmless and potentially harmful interventions and assist them in evaluating the claimed efficacy of unconventional remedies (Manfred, Boutaugh, and Tehan, 1987).

Growth and development

Linear growth may be retarded during active systemic disease. Catch-up growth occurs with suppression of disease activity or during remission.

Corticosteroids may suppress growth.

Poor weight gain may be the result of systemic disease.

Excessive weight gain may occur as a result of inactivity, depression, or poor nutrition.

Gross motor delays and temporary regressions are not uncommon. Fine motor skills are less likely to be affected.

Language acquisition is affected only with severe TMJ arthritis.

Standard infant development screening tests may be of questionable value in the evaluation of severely affected children.

Immunizations

Routine immunizations may be given to children who are not taking immunosuppressive drugs.

In the absence of neurologic symptoms, a child with classic, intermittent JRA fever can be immunized during febrile episodes.

No live viruses should be given to child receiving antimetabolites or large doses of corticosteroids.

Yearly immunizations for types A and B influenza are recommended for children older than 6 months treated with aspirin and other NSAIDs.

Screening
Vision

Fundoscopic examination and acuity screening should be done at each visit. Ophthalmologic examinations for uveitis is recommended. Children using topically applied or systemic-route corticosteroids require close ophthalmologic follow-up.

Hearing

Routine office screening is recommended. Tinnitus associated with salicylate toxicity should be investigated as a cause for diminished acuity.

Dental

Children taking salicylates require dental visits every 6 months or more frequently if erosive signs develop. Children with micrognathia should have frequent dental visits. Prophylactic antibiotics should be prescribed for dental work in children with total hip replacements or those taking corticosteroids.

Blood pressure

Routine screening is recommended.

Hematocrit

Frequent screening is done by the rheumatology team to rule out anemia.

Urinalysis

Urinalysis should be performed every 6 to 12 months or more frequently with some JRA medications. Report protein greater than $1+$, RBC count more than $5/mm^3$, and the presence of casts to pediatric rheumatologist immediately.

Tuberculosis

Routine screening is recommended.

Condition-specific screening

A CBC, differential, ESR, platelet count, and liver function tests are routinely drawn by pediatric rheumatology staff.

Drug interactions

Aspirin plus salicylate-containing medications can cause salicylate toxicity.

Antacids may alter the absorption rate of NSAIDs, resulting in subtherapeutic serum levels.

Antacids can alter renal excretion of aspirin, leading to higher serum levels of salicylate with antacid withdrawal or subtherapeutic levels with antacid addition.

Antihistamines may decrease NSAID levels.

Nonsteroidal antiinflammatory drugs may decrease the effectiveness of oral contraceptives.

Salicylates can increase penicillin levels.

Ampicillin may decrease the availability of sulfasalizine, causing loss of therapeutic efficacy.

Corticosteroids decrease plasma concentration of salicylates.

Penicillamine absorption is decreased by antacids.

Penicillamine must be given 2 hours apart from iron supplements or aluminum hydroxide antacids.

Methotrexate concentrations are increased by salicylates.

Sulfonamides may displace or be displaced by other highly proteinbound drugs, such as NSAIDs, salicylates, and methotrexate. Monitor for increased effects of highly bound drugs when sulfonamides are added.

Reduced efficacy and increased incidence of breakthrough bleeding have been reported in oral contraceptive users treated with sulfonamides, such as sulfasalazine.

Concomitant administration of iron supplements and sulfasalazine results in a decreased blood level of sulfasalazine. It is not known whether the efficacy of either agent is altered.

Differential diagnosis
Fever

Differentiate classic, intermittent JRA fever from fevers of infectious origin.

Dermatologic symptoms

Rule out rheumatoid rash in systemic JRA; rule out drug-related photosensitivity reactions.

Otologic symptoms

Differentiate TMJ arthritis with referred ear pain from otitis media.

Respiratory symptoms

Rule out salicylate-induced tachypnea or bronchospasm; differentiate cold from influenza symptoms, and treat all type A influenza with amantadine; colds and influenza may cause arthritis flares.

Anemia

Differentiate anemia of chronic disorder from anemia related to NSAID-induced blood loss or poor nutrition.

Gastrointestinal symptoms

Rule out nonspecific pain of JRA-related mesenteric adenopathy, drug-induced peptic ulcer, and drug-related GI symptoms.

Renal symptoms

Increased urinary urgency or frequency in a child receiving aspirin therapy may be temporary drug side effect, but UTI must be ruled out first.

Developmental issues
Safety

Use childproof containers for medications.

Recommend that the child taking immunosuppressive agents wear a medical alert bracelet or necklace.

Review safety issues related to splintwearing, heat and cold applications, and adaptive equipment.

Child care

Care giver must be capable of giving medications, using assistive devices, and applying splints.

Parents should prepare the care giver with information about the child's medications.

Care givers should be educated about the effect of JRA on the child's functional capacity, energy level, and developmental progress.

Home-based, single-provider day-care setting rather than group child care is recommended for the child taking corticosteroids or immunosuppressants.

Most infants and young children with JRA are eligible for Public Law 99-457 educational programs.

Diet

The risk of protein-caloric malnutrition is increased.

Improper nutrition may contribute to problems of underweight or overweight.

Daily vitamin and iron supplements are recommended.

"Arthritis diets" should be evaluated for nutri-

Continued.

SUMMARY OF PRIMARY CARE NEEDS FOR THE CHILD WITH JUVENILE RHEUMATOID ARTHRITIS — cont'd

tional adequacy and the family educated about proper nutrition for a growing child with a chronic disease.

Discipline

Identify overprotection, overindulgence, and inconsistent limit setting.

Give guidance regarding the effect of JRA on age-specific developmental tasks to offer parents a framework for decision making about discipline.

Toileting

Postpone training during periods of active disease.

Utilize assistive devices to compensate for upper and lower extremity limitations.

Anticipate situations in public facilities where assistive devices are not available.

Use bedpans and urinals as necessary if pain and stiffness limit mobility at night.

Sleep patterns

Daytime fatigue and morning stiffness may be related to sleep fragmentation.

Active disease causes increased wakefulness at night, necessitates longer periods of rest during the day, and increases the severity of morning stiffness.

Recommendations to alleviate morning stiffness should be discussed with the family.

School issues

Public Law 94-142 entitles most students with JRA to occupational therapy, physical therapy, adaptive physical education, and transportation between school, home, and facilities where services are provided.

Most students with JRA can participate in modified school athletic programs.

Sexuality

Pubarche may be delayed in children with JRA.

Adolescents should be referred to a physical therapist with a pediatric rheumatology team for difficulties with sexual postures or with problems related to the use of mechanical birth control devices.

Special family concerns

Divergent views regarding perceptions and impact of JRA may exist among family members.

The provider should anticipate the use of nontraditional therapeutic interventions and the need to differentiate between harmless and harmful remedies.

RESOURCES
Organizations

American Juvenile Arthritis Organization
Arthritis Foundation
1314 Spring St NW
Atlanta, GA 30309
(404) 872-7100

The American Juvenile Arthritis Organization (AJAO) is a national membership association of the Arthritis Foundation that serves the special needs of young people with arthritis or rheumatic diseases and their families. Videotapes, quarterly newsletters, educational materials for children, parents, and health professionals, and information about summer camps, pen pal clubs, and family support groups are available through the national office of the AJAO or through local chapters of the Arthritis Foundation.

REFERENCES

Adair SM, Floyd TP, Baum J, et al: Temporomandibular joint involvement in juvenile rheumatoid arthritis: Report of two cases, *Pediatr Dent* 3:271-273, 1981.

Albert E and Ansell BM: Immunogenetics of juvenile chronic arthritis, *Scand J Rheumatol* 66(suppl):85-91, 1987.

Alepa FP: Juvenile rheumatoid arthritis, *Primary Care* 11:243-258, 1984.

American Committee on Immunization Practices: General recommendations on immunization, *MMWR* 38:205-227, 1989.

Atwood M: Developmental assessment and integration. In Melvin JL, ed: *Rheumatic disease in the adult and child: Occupational therapy and rehabilitation*, Philadelphia, 1989a, FA Davis, pp 188-214.

Atwood M: Treatment consideration. In Melvin JL, ed: *Rheumatic disease in the adult and child: Occupational therapy and rehabilitation*, Philadelphia, 1989b, FA Davis, pp 215-234.

Bacon MC, White PH, Raiten DJ, et al: Nutritional status and growth in juvenile rheumatoid arthritis, *Semin Arthritis Rheum* 20:97-106, 1990.

Barrier CH and Hirschowitz BI: Controversies in the detection and management of nonsteroidal antiinflammatory drug-induced side effects of the upper gastrointestinal tract, *Arthritis Rheum* 32:926-932, 1989.

Bennett JC: Etiology of rheumatic diseases. In Kelley WN, Harris ED, Ruddy S, et al (eds): *Textbook of rheumatology*, ed 3, Philadelphia, 1989, WB Saunders, pp 138-147.

Bernstein BH, Stobie D, Singsen BH, et al: Growth retardation in juvenile rheumatoid arthritis, *Arthritis Rheum* 20(suppl):212-216, 1977.

Boutaugh ML: Comfort measures. In Arthritis Foundation, ed: *Understanding juvenile rheumatoid arthritis: A health professional's guide to teaching children and parents,* Atlanta, 1987, The Arthritis Foundation, pp 6-1 to 6-I.

Boutaugh ML and Tehan N: Saving joints and energy. In Arthritis Foundation, ed: *Understanding juvenile rheumatoid arthritis: A health professional's guide to teaching children and parents*, Atlanta, 1987, The Arthritis Foundation, pp 7-1 to 7-D.

Brewer EJ, Giannini EH, and Person DA: *Juvenile rheumatoid arthritis*, Philadelphia, 1982, WB Saunders.

Cassidy JT: *Textbook of pediatric rheumatology*, New York, 1982, John Wiley & Sons.

Cassidy JT: Juvenile rheumatoid arthritis. In Kelley WN, Harris ED, Ruddy S, et al, eds: *Textbook of rheumatology*, ed 3, Philadelphia, 1989, WB Saunders, pp 1289-1311.

Christensen JR: A soft tissue lesion related to salicylate treatment of juvenile rheumatoid arthritis: Clinical report, *Pediatr Dent* 6:159-161, 1984.

Committee on Infectious Diseases: Report of the Committee on Infectious Diseases, ed 22, Elk Grove Village, Il, 1991, The American Academy of Pediatrics.

Davies SF and Iber C: Obstructive sleep apnea associated with adult-acquired micrognathia from rheumatoid arthritis, *Am Rev Respir Dis* 127:245-247, 1983.

Erlandson D, Kovalevsky A, Boutaugh ML, et al: Psychosocial issues and JRA. In Arthritis Foundation, ed: *Understanding juvenile rheumatoid arthritis: A health professional's guide to teaching children and parents*, Atlanta, 1987, Arthritis Foundation, pp 13-1 to 13-E.

Espada G, Babini JC, Maldonado-Cocco JA, et al: Radiologic review: The cervical spine in juvenile rheumatoid arthritis, *Semin Arthritis Rheum* 17:185-195, 1988.

Fink CW: Medical treatment of juvenile arthritis, *Clin Orthop* 259:60-69, 1990.

Forsyth BW, Horwitz RI, Acampora D, et al: New epidemiologic evidence confirming that bias does not explain the aspirin/Reye's syndrome association, *JAMA* 261:2517-2524, 1989.

Fraser PA, Hoch S, Erlandson D, et al: The timing of menarche in juvenile rheumatoid arthritis, *J Adolesc Health Care* 9:483-487, 1988.

Harvey AR, Pippard MJ, and Ansell BM: Microcytic anaemia in juvenile chronic arthritis, *Scand J Rheumatol* 16:53-59, 1987.

Henderson CJ and Lovell DJ: Comprehensive nutritional assessment of children and adolescents with juvenile rheumatoid arthritis, *Arthritis Rheum* 30(suppl):202, 1987.

Hensinger RN, DeVito PD, and Ragsdale CG: Changes in the cervical spine in juvenile rheumatoid arthritis, *J Bone Joint Surg* 68-A:189-197, 1986.

Hull RG: Outcome in juvenile arthritis, *Br J Rheumatol* 27(suppl I):66-71, 1988.

Kanski J: Screening for uveitis in juvenile chronic arthritis, *Br J Ophthalmol* 73:225-228, 1989.

Konkol L, Lineberry J, Gottlieb J, et al: Impact of juvenile arthritis on families: An educational assessment, *Arthritis Care Res* 2:40-48, 1989.

Kunnamo I: Infections and related risk factors of arthritis in children, *Scand J Rheumatol* 16:93-99, 1987.

Lotz M and Vaughn JH: Rheumatoid arthritis. In Samter M, ed: *Immunological diseases*, ed 4, Boston, 1988, Little, Brown, pp 1365-1416.

Mahowald MW, Mahowald ML, Bundlie SR, et al: Sleep fragmentation in rheumatoid arthritis, *Arthritis Rheum* 32:974-983, 1989.

Mahy M: Medications. In Arthritis Foundation, ed: *Understanding juvenile rheumatoid arthritis: A health professional's guide to teaching children and parents*, Atlanta, 1987, The Arthritis Foundation, pp 4-1 to 4-H16.

Manfred SM, Boutaugh ML, and Tehan N: Unproven remedies. In Arthritis Foundation, ed: *Understanding juvenile rheumatoid arthritis: A health professional's guide to teaching children and parents*, Atlanta, 1987, The Arthritis Foundation, pp 9-1 to 9-A.

Melvin JL and Atwood M: Juvenile rheumatoid arthritis. In Melvin JL, ed: *Rheumatic disease in the adult and child: Occupational therapy and rehabilitation*, Philadelphia, 1989, FA Davis, pp 135-187.

Miller ML, Chacko JA, and Young EA: Dietary deficiencies in children with juvenile rheumatoid arthritis, *Arthritis Care Res* 2:22-24, 1989.

Morassut P, Yang W, and Karsh J: Aspirin intolerance, *Semin Arthritis Rheum* 19:22-30, 1989.

Myall RWT, West RA, Horwitz H, et al: Jaw deformity caused by juvenile rheumatoid arthritis and its correction, *Arthritis Rheum* 31:1305-1310, 1988.

O'Brien JM and Albert DM: Therapeutic approaches for ophthalmic problems in juvenile rheumatoid arthritis, *Rheum Dis Clin North Am* 15:413-437, 1989.

Rennebohm RM, Heubi JE, Daugherty CC, et al: Reye syndrome in children receiving salicylate therapy for connective tissue disease, *J Pediatr* 107:877-880, 1985.

Rosenberg AM: Uveitis associated with juvenile rheumatoid arthritis, *Semin Arthritis Rheum* 16:158-173, 1987.

Schaller JG: Rheumatology. In Avery ME and First LR, eds: *Pediatric medicine*, Baltimore, 1989, Williams & Wilkins, pp 1251-1256.

Scott RD and Sledge CB: Surgical management of juvenile rheumatoid arthritis. In Kelley WN, Harris ED, Ruddy S, et al, eds: *Textbook of rheumatology*, ed 3, Philadelphia, 1989, WB Saunders, pp 2083-2090.

Southwood TR, Malleson PN, Roberts-Thomson PJ, et al: Unconventional remedies used for patients with juvenile arthritis, *Pediatrics* 85:150-153, 1990.

Stastny P: HLA and the role of T cells in the predisposition to disease, *Rheum Dis Clin North Am* 13:1-17, 1987.

Steinhorn D and Berman WF: Gastrointestinal hemorrhage. In Hoekelman RA, ed: *Primary pediatric care*, St Louis, 1987, CV Mosby pp 974-978.

Sullivan DB, Cassidy JT, and Petty RE: Pathogenic implications of age of onset in juvenile rheumatoid arthritis, *Arthritis Rheum* 18:251-255, 1975.

Svantesson H, Marhaug G, and Haeffner F: Scoliosis in children with juvenile rheumatoid arthritis, *Scand J Rheumatol* 10:65-68, 1981.

Swann M: The surgery of juvenile chronic arthritis, *Clin Orthop* 259:70-76, 1990.

Tanchyk AP: Prevention of tooth erosion from salicylate therapy in juvenile rheumatoid arthritis, *Gen Dent* 34:479-480, 1986.

Taylor J, Passo MH, and Champion VL: School problems and teacher responsibilities in juvenile rheumatoid arthritis, *J Sch Health* 57:186-190, 1987.

Towner SR, Michet CJ, O'Fallon WM, et al: The epidemiology of juvenile arthritis in Rochester, Minnesota 1960-1979, *Arthritis Rheum* 26:1208-1213, 1983.

Tullman MJ: Coordinating dental-medical care in arthritis, Arlington, Va, 1984, National Arthritis and Musculoskeletal and Skin Diseases Information Clearinghouse, biblio-profile No 5.

US Pharmacopeial Convention: *Drug information for the health care professional*, Rockville, Md, 1990, US Pharmacopeia.

Warady B and Shields C: Nutrition management. In Arthritis Foundation, ed: *Understanding juvenile rheumatoid arthritis: A health professional's guide to teaching children and parents*, Atlanta, 1987, The Arthritis Foundation, pp 8-1 to 8-F.

White PH: Growth abnormalities in children with juvenile rheumatoid arthritis, *Clin Orthop* 259:46-50, 1990.

Wolf MD, Lichter PR, and Ragsdale CG: Prognostic factors in the uveitis of juvenile rheumatoid arthritis, *Ophthalmology* 94:1242-1248, 1987.

20 *Learning Disabilities*

••

Janice Selekman

ETIOLOGY

Although children with learning disabilities (LDs) are commonly seen by primary care providers (Cantwell and Baker, 1987a to c, Wender, 1987), there still is considerable confusion as to what constitutes a learning disability. The current diagnosis of LD has been preceded by multiple other labels. Among these are brain injured, perceptually handicapped, and minimal brain dysfunction (Gearheart, 1985). The term learning disability was introduced in 1963 and defined in 1981. It was amended in 1987 as a generic term that refers to a heterogeneous group of disorders manifested by significant difficulties in the acquisition and use of listening, speaking, reading, writing, reasoning, mathematical abilities, or social skills.

These disorders are intrinsic to the individual and presumed to be the result of central nervous system (CNS) dysfunction. Even though a learning disability may occur concomitantly with other handicapping conditions (e.g., sensory impairment, mental retardation, social and emotional disturbance) or untoward socioenvironmental influences (e.g., cultural differences, insufficient or inappropriate instruction, psychogenic factors), a learning disability is not the direct result of those conditions or influences (Interagency Committee on Learning Disabilities, 1987).

Attention deficits and hyperactivity, although considered components of an LD, actually compromise two separate diagnoses: undifferentiated attention-deficit disorder (UADD) and/or attention-deficit hyperactivity disorder (ADHD) (DSM-III-R, 1987). Either of these often, but not necessarily, occurs concurrently with a learning disability (Fig. 20-1).

Undifferentiated attention-deficit disorder refers to "the persistence of developmentally inappropriate and marked inattention that is not a symptom of another disorder" (DSM-III-R, 1987, p. 95). If a child is mentally retarded, emotionally ill, socioeconomically or culturally disadvantaged, sensory or motor impaired, or comes from an abusive or impoverished environment, a diagnosis of UADD is inappropriate.

Attention-deficit hyperactivity disorder refers to "developmentally inappropriate degrees of inattention, impulsiveness, and hyperactivity" (DSM-III-R, 1987, p. 50). The manifestations of hyperactivity occur in all facets of the child's life and frequently worsen in situations requiring sustained attention.

Before a child may be considered to have ADHD, 8 of the 14 criteria presented in the box on p. 357 must be met. These symptoms should have their onset before the child is 7 years old and must be present for a minimum of 6 months. Although they may be present during the preschool years, they may go unrecognized until after the child enters a structured school environment. The symptoms can be categorized as mild, moderate, or severe. Coleman and Levine (1988) warn that the symptoms may be more subtle in the adolescent

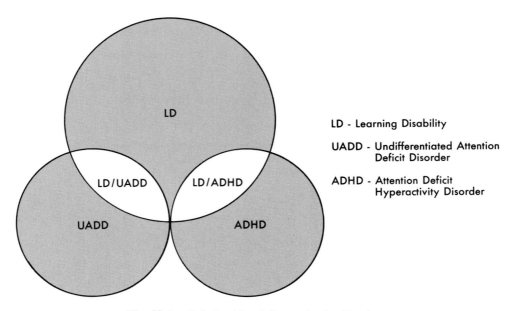

Fig. 20-1. Relationship of diagnostic classifications.

than in the school-aged child and often manifest as poor academic performance, social-behavioral difficulties, or both.

Because of the confusion surrounding these definitions, each state has developed its own criteria of what it will consider a learning disability. Thus, each state has different standards as to who is classified as learning disabled and who receives services. Individual states may or may not separate an LD from ADHD or UADD. Moreover, a learning disability is not considered a separate entity by the American Psychiatric Association. Although steeped in a great deal of controversy, there are areas of the country where the only way comprehensive services and third-party reimbursement can be obtained for these children is to diagnose them according to the *Diagnostic and Statistical Manual of Mental Disorders* (DSM-III-R, 1987) as having ADHD (314.01) or UADD (314.00).

The cause and the exact mechanisms of LD, UADD, and ADHD remain unknown. There are multiple hypotheses ranging from (1) neurobiologic, which focuses on neurotransmitter function, especially catecholamines; (2) neuropsychologic, which seeks a deficit in the response inhibition mechanism of the brain; (3) neuroanatomic, which

attempts to identify structural anomalies of or damage to the brain; to (4) toxic substances, such as foods and chemicals; and (5) allergic responses (Bond, 1987; Munoz-Millan and Casteel, 1989). It should be noted that none of these mechanisms has been empirically supported in replication studies.

Other suggested causes include delayed cerebral maturation as a result of immature neurologic development, endocrine gland imbalances, and genetic predisposition because a significant number of children with LDs, ADHD, UADD, or a combination of these have at least one parent who is learning disabled (Bond, 1987; Gaddes, 1985; Meents, 1989; Rapp and Bamberg, 1986).

Specific groups appear to be at increased risk for developing learning disabilities: (1) very low birth weight infants, some of whom later develop difficulty with spatial relations and visual motor integration (Bauchner, Brown, and Peskin, 1988); (2) children with late effects of cancer treatment from cranial irradiation and intrathecal chemotherapy (see Chapter 8) (Peckham, 1988); (3) adopted children; and (4) children with chronic conditions (Dworkin, 1985).

There has been study of the brain structure as

CRITERIA FOR DETERMINING ATTENTION-DEFICIT HYPERACTIVITY DISORDER

1. Often fidgets with hands or feet or squirms in seat (in adolescents, may be limited to subjective feelings of restlessness)
2. Has difficulty remaining seated when required to do so
3. Is easily distracted by extraneous stimuli
4. Has difficulty awaiting turn in games or group situations
5. Often blurts out answers to questions before they have been completed
6. Has difficulty following through on instructions from others (not due to oppositional behavior or failure of comprehension), e.g., fails to finish chores
7. Has difficulty sustaining attention in tasks or play activities
8. Often shifts from one uncompleted activity to another
9. Has difficulty playing quietly
10. Often talks excessively
11. Often interrupts or intrudes on others, e.g., butts into other children's games
12. Often does not seem to listen to what is being said to him or her
13. Often loses things necessary for tasks or activities at school or at home (e.g., toys, pencils, books, assignments)
14. Often engages in physically dangerous activities without considering possible consequences (not for the purpose of thrill-seeking), e.g., runs into street without looking

From *Diagnostic and statistical manual of mental disorders: DSM-II-R,* ed 3 revised, Washington, DC, 1987, American Psychiatric Association, pp 52-53.

sual-spatial perception and is the site of hand-eye-brain coordination. A defect in the right hemisphere may result in a deficit in drawing or spatial imagery. This would interfere with such activities as math, art, map reading, and sewing (Gaddes, 1985).

If each hemisphere of the brain is responsible for its own set of functions, a defect in a specific area would presumably alter normal function. Thus far, autopsy findings, as well as computerized tomography scans and magnetic resonance images, have not been helpful in identifying these proposed structural defects. Learning disabilities may, in fact, be caused by a multitude of factors rather than a single etiologic determinant.

INCIDENCE

From 1982 to 1983, 1,741,054 American children with LDs received special education or related services for their disability (Dworkin, 1985). This was a larger number than for any other handicapping condition. An estimated 5% to 10% of children and adolescents, or approximately 4 million children, in the United States are learning disabled (Silver, 1988). Moreover, the "single most chronic behavior disorder in the preadolescent group" is said to be ADHD and UADD associated with or without an LD (Copeland and Wolraich, 1987, p. 271). Prevalence rates for attention-deficit disorders range from 1.2% to 20%, with boys being affected 4 to 8 times more frequently than girls (Bond, 1987).

There has been a recent increase in the number of children identified as learning disabled. Whether this increase reflects a true increase or just better diagnostic measures and access to testing cannot be determined at this time. Some states, however, have restricted the maximum percentage of students who can be considered learning disabled for purposes of state reimbursement. Others have attempted to apply a "percentage of deficit" type of limitation (Gearheart, 1985), although this has recently been successfully challenged in several states.

CLINICAL MANIFESTATIONS AT TIME OF DIAGNOSIS

Multiple lists of symptoms have been generated to assist primary care providers in identifying LDs. A more conceptual approach is to view alterations

it relates to the different manifestations of learning disability. Because the left hemisphere is normally responsible for perception of speech and language, lesions or defects on that side of the brain may result in decreased verbal memory and a deficit in reading, writing, and verbal skills. Most teaching is verbal and therefore is directed to the left hemisphere. The right hemisphere is responsible for vi-in the areas of sensory-receptive, integrative, motor, and diffuse abilities (Selekman, 1988).

Alterations in sensory-receptive intake

Alterations in sensory-receptive intake involve deficiencies in using and processing information received via the senses, including visual perceptual, auditory perceptual, and sensation-related deficits.

Visual perceptual deficits involve difficulty in decoding or comprehending (or both) written language because of either reversals of letters or words (dyslexia); difficulty in visual memory and perception of symbols, such as musical notes; or misperception of distance. These children may have difficulty copying and identifying letters or shapes, differentiating right from left, drawing a clock, and reciting multiplication tables. The dyslexic child's eyes may not be able to move evenly across a printed line but instead jump from line to line, causing the child to lose his or her place. This child may also have difficulty with figure-ground visual perception, that is, difficulty differentiating an object from its background.

The child with an auditory perceptual deficit has difficulty with phonetics, recitation from memory (e.g., the alphabet), understanding and following directions (especially multistep instructions), and interpreting one's tone of voice. Because of this they may be erroneously judged to be emotionally disturbed, retarded, or "problem children" who do not do as they are told. This deficit will also manifest as an inability to differentiate similar-sounding words, such as pit and pet.

Children who have difficulty in perceiving tactile or body sensations may be unable to read their own body cues. Sensations such as the need to toilet or the onset of menses may be missed or misread, leading to difficulty in toilet training, resolving enuresis or encopresis and establishing self-care behaviors. Kinesthetic misperception can result in difficulty understanding the body language and facial expressions of others.

Alteration in integrative processing

The child with an alteration in integrative processing can receive stimuli adequately but has difficulty in retrieving and using this information accurately. This manifests itself in difficulty sequencing data or parts of a story; difficulty understanding the con-

cepts of time and space, parts and whole, and cause and effect; disorganization of thought and planning; and difficulty in analysis and abstract thinking. They may become lost easily and have difficulty reading maps. These children are limited in the amount of general knowledge processed from their environment, e.g., knowing the number of days in a week and important dates and holidays and relating seasons of the year to the calendar.

Older school-aged children with integrative difficulties frequently find it difficult to process multiple intake stimuli at the same time. To listen to a lesson plan, observe visual aids, and take notes simultaneously may prove to be confusing, because they may be easily distracted and have difficulty identifying the important points. In addition, these children may find it difficult to understand humor, cliches, and puns, because they interpret language literally. Their limited understanding of concepts may result in their perception being worse than the reality of the problem.

Alteration in motor-expressive performance

Alteration in the motor-expressive aspects of developmental tasks is a third classification of LDs. This ranges from (1) difficulty in performing gross or fine (or both) motor tasks, resulting in the labels of "clumsy," "noncoordinated," or "accident prone"; (2) speech disorders, including dysphasia, stuttering, and poor articulation; to (3) difficulties in skills such as handwriting, spelling, calculating, drawing, and sports activities. These children may try to avoid hobbies and extracurricular activities that require physical activity.

Diffuse alterations

The final category is labeled diffuse. This is a combination of the other three categories. This heterogeneous form is more commonly seen in girls. Frequently this diagnosis is delayed because the signs of dyslexia and hyperactivity are more common in boys and learning disabilities are rarely considered as a differential diagnosis for girls. These children may appear to be daydreaming or may appear to drift off in the middle of an activity. They are highly distractible by activity or noise.

Additional findings. One controversial set of findings is that of "soft neurologic signs." These minor abnormalities are identified during neurologic assessment and history taking. They consist of motor findings (clumsiness, posturing, repetitive finger tapping), mirror movements, poor directionality (especially left-right orientation), and poor gross motor skills. Most of these are seen normally in young children (Trauner, 1986). Because they are so common, they are often correlated with LDs after the diagnosis is made. If a child has soft signs and is happy and doing well, it is recommended that no further intervention be made other than routine follow-up. If a diagnosis of LD has already been made, the presence or absence of soft signs has not been noted to alter the prognosis.

No one test or tool is able to diagnose a child as having LD, ADHD, or UADD. Multiple data sources are used over time to make the diagnosis. These include a family history, perinatal history, developmental history with current developmental assessment, assessment of past and current temperament of the child, health history, assessment of academic performance, comprehensive age-appropriate psychologic and intelligence testing, and a comprehensive physical assessment with an emphasis on neurologic and motor abilities. It is helpful for the health care practitioner to arrange time to observe the child's performance and behavior in school compared with performance and behavior at home or during unstructured activities. Although all of these data are needed to make the diagnosis of LD, ADHD, and UADD, it is important to reevaluate the child on these same parameters every 2 to 3 years to identify changes and new areas for needed intervention.

It is the responsibility of the primary care practitioner to initiate the diagnostic process for the child who has been identified as being at risk. The history and the physical and developmental assessments are within the abilities and responsibilities of the health care provider. Psychologic testing may have to be referred to individuals trained in pediatric psychologic testing. Regardless of the amount of input the health care practitioner makes toward the diagnostic process, they must assume the role of the child's advocate to initiate and collaborate in the diagnostic process.

TREATMENT

Cognitive, behavioral, and psychosocial strategies are used in treating LD, ADHD, and UADD. Phar-

macologic intervention may also be helpful in treating children with ADHD and UADD. Just as no one test can identify a child with LDs, no one approach works for all children. Working with the child and family does, however, require an interdisciplinary team approach. This team may include some or all of the following individuals: (1) the nurse and physician (one of whom is the primary care provider); (2) psychologist; (3) occupational and physical therapists; (4) specialists in vision, hearing, and speech and language; and (5) educators. Different strategies may be needed at different ages. It is important to identify how the child learns best and to use that modality as the initial approach throughout the routine health care teaching and treatment implementation. The primary care practitioner can then recommend these generalized approaches for the home and school environments to meet the specific needs of each child.

For the child with a visual perceptual deficit, it is important to present material verbally in addition to using hands-on experiences. This is an appropriate intervention for the clinician who is trying to provide information for or promote compliance in this child. The child with an auditory perceptual deficit will need health education materials presented in writing and pictorially, as well as tactilely. For this child a short list of directions should be provided with either pictures of a procedure or demonstration on a model.

The child with integrative deficits may need multisensory approaches. Directions can be written down and explained with the child watching; charts can be used if the child can read them. Feedback should constantly be elicited from the child to check his or her understanding. Calendars and lists can be used to help the child organize specific tasks or daily health-related activities.

Interventions for the child with motor deficits are similar to those for the child with cerebral palsy (see Chapter 9). Steps of a particular skill need to be delimited and verbally described. These children will need extra time to perform or verbalize. The meaning of children's comments must be validated, because they may have a limited expressive vocabulary.

Pharmacologic management is effective for approximately 70% to 75% of children with ADHD (Copeland and Wolraich, 1987; Pelham, 1987).

Table 20-1. Medications most commonly used for hyperactivity

Drug	Dosage		Maximum	Onset	Half-life	Duration	Side effects
	Average						
Methylphenidate (Ritalin)	Start with 5 mg twice daily (before breakfast and lunch); increase at gradual increments of 5-10 mg weekly		Daily dosage above 60 mg is not recommended	30 mins	2-4 hrs	3-5 hrs	Nervousness and insomnia are most common adverse reactions Hypersensitivity, anorexia, nausea, dizziness, palpitations, headache, drowsiness, blood pressure and pulse changes (both up and down), tachycardia, and weight loss with prolonged therapy
Dextramephatamine (Dexedrine)	For children 3-5 years: 2.5 mg daily; increased at 2.5-mg increments weekly, until desired response is obtained For children 6 yrs+: 5 mg, 1-2 times daily; increased at 5 mg increments weekly until desired response is obtained		Rare case: 50 mg daily or more	30 mins	4-6 hrs	24 hrs	Restlessness, insomnia, euphoria and headache, diarrhea, constipation, anorexia, dry mouth, and unpleasant taste are most common
Pemoline (Cylert)	Start with 37.5 mg/day. Increased at 18.75 mg weekly until desired response is obtained Effective daily dose for children: 56.25 mg-75 mg		112.5 mg daily	2-4 hrs	8 hrs	Prolonged	Elevated liver functions, hepatitis and jaundice, insomnia, anorexia and weight loss, nausea, suppressed growth in children on long-term therapy

"Of those who do respond, only a minority show sufficient improvement for their behavior to fall within the normal range; the rest are improved but their behavior is not normalized" (Pelham, 1987, p. 102). The drugs of choice are methylphenidate (Ritalin), dextromephatamine (Dexadrine), and pemoline (Cylert) (Table 20-1). These CNS stimulants are short acting, and their effectiveness is measured by behavioral changes such as decreased motor activity and increased attention span and concentration. Behavioral changes can be identified 30 to 90 minutes after ingestion. Their mechanism of action is presumed to be at the CNS transmitter level by increasing the availability of catecholamines at the neural synapse (Pelham, 1987). These drugs do not directly act on the symptoms of hyperactivity; they allow the child to develop self-control and be more available for learning. These drugs also have no effect on problem solving, reasoning, or actual school achievement. Medication is used with treatment, not as treatment.

Methylphenidate is the initial drug of choice and is started with a low dose of 5 mg in the morning and at noon. These times correspond to school hours and the time when attention is most needed. Methylphenidate has a peak plasma concentration 1 to 3 hours after ingestion and a half-life of 2 to 4 hours (Bond, 1987). If there are no adverse side effects and the child continues to be unable to focus on classwork, the dose is increased. Most children with ADHD and UADD require a dosage regimen from 0.2 to 1.0 mg/kg/day; the average dose is 0.3 mg/kg (Copeland and Wolraich, 1987). Doses of 30 to 40 mg/day are considered high and may require alternative drug or behavioral therapy (Trauner, 1986), although doses may go as high as 60 mg/day. A long-acting form of this drug, Ritalin-SR, is also available, thus eliminating the dose required at lunch time.

Dextroamphetamine can be given at any time in relation to meals. Some doses (2.5-5 mg) are given initially twice daily at breakfast and lunch. The dosage is then gradually increased by 5 mg/day at weekly intervals until remission of symptoms is seen. Doses greater than 40 mg/day are rarely indicated. Peak concentrations occur 2 to 4 hours after ingestion, and the half-life can be 4 to 11 hours (Bond, 1987).

Pemoline is less potent than other drugs, and its effects are slightly less. Its half-life is longer than the other two drugs (8 hours in children), requiring only a daily dose. The recommended starting dose is 37.5 mg/day, increasing gradually until a clinical response is demonstrated, usually between 56.75 and 75.0 mg/day. Doses should never exceed 112.0 mg/day, however.

Some of the stimulant medications come in both regular tablet and sustained time-released forms. Time-released forms must be taken only once daily in the morning. A major advantage is that children will not need to take drugs to school. Children should be advised not to chew the sustained time-released forms, because this may result in initial overmedication and gastric distress. Moreover, the long-acting properties of the drug will be destroyed.

This group of children has also used tricyclic antidepressants with results less effective than those of stimulants. Imipramine (Tofranil), the drug of choice in this category, results in a reduced level of activity, decreased impulsivity, and increased attention (Copeland and Wolraich, 1987). Because of the high risk of serious side effects, this form of treatment in children is not recommended.

Dosages may have to be individually adjusted for both the child's school and play activities, as well as during weekends and vacations. School-aged children appear to respond more favorably to these medications than younger children. For this reason methylphenidate is not recommended for children less than 6 years of age, and dextroamphetamine is not recommended for those less than age 3 (Bond, 1987).

The effectiveness of stimulant medication should be evaluated periodically. This may involve prescribing "drug holidays" during which time no medications are taken. Most commonly this is at the beginning and end of each school year. Evaluations by parents, teachers, and health care practitioners are essential to determine whether the medication is still needed. It also gives children a break from dependency on drugs that control their behavior. Although this approach is highly controversial, it has been recommended that children be given drug holidays during summer and school vacations to allow for catch-up growth. Critics of this drug holiday suggest that these children may have a decreased response to future doses of the medications. Moreover, some believe that because learning does not stop outside the classroom, children who need pharmacologic support need it continuously. Reports indicate that children who continue taking medication during vacations have fewer accidents and improved social-emotional growth. Occasionally drug holidays occur accidentally; these provide excellent opportunities for evaluating the child.

Although pharmacotherapy can alter behavior, behavioral intervention is more effective in enhancing academic performance and promoting psychosocial adjustment (Gadow, 1985). These children need assistance in learning the steps involved in problem solving, self-control, and decision making, as well as how to use past learning to process new environmental information. They should be encouraged to be actively involved in the learning process rather than passively receiving new data. Health care professionals, educators, and parents must help these children set appropriate goals and then guide them in organizing and prioritizing strategies to obtain them.

Multimodal, multidisciplinary approaches appear to be most effective. Behaviorally oriented approaches that employ multiple mechanisms of action are superior to any one intervention strategy. Because many members of the interdisciplinary team are working with the child at the same time, it is important for the primary care provider responsible for care to become the case manager, parent educator, and child advocate. Responsible for the child's comprehensive care, this individual ensures that other members of the team are called for assistance when needed.

Controversial therapies

Numerous therapies have been recommended to correct LDs and hyperactive behavior. A number of these have received support from small groups of parents and special interest groups, but none has been empirically supported by controlled research. In addition, none is supported by the American Academy of Pediatrics as treatment. Five of the different controversial approaches include behavioristic approaches, neurophysiologic retraining, megavitamins, diet modification, and allergen avoidance.

Behavioristic approaches are mechanical and focus on what is to be learned rather than the process. Behavior modification results in a change of behavior only as long as rewards are immediately forthcoming (Kronick, 1988); it is better for social rather than academic performance. On the other hand, cognitive behavior training programs are not particularly effective unless they are clearly focused on academic task performance.

Neurophysiologic retraining is based on the premise that "by simulating specific sensory inputs or exercising specific motor patterns one can retrain, recircuit, or in some way improve the functioning of a part of the central nervous system" (Silver, 1986, p. 1047). This approach includes patterning, optometric visual training, or cerebellar-vestibular dysfunction. There are no empirical data to support a relationship between the degree of vestibular responsivity and academic performance (Magrun, 1988).

Patterning, or sensory integration, is based on the concept that individuals follow a set sequence in the development of skills. Failure to pass through these stages in sequential fashion results in poor neurologic organization. This "therapy," performed primarily by occupational therapists, is aimed at stimulating the appropriate motor pathway with a frequency and intensity greater than what is normally experienced.

Optometric visual training is based on a similar premise. Proponents state that vision follows developmental steps and that learning is primarily a visual task. Treatment consists of using ocular skills to improve the child's ability to read. Although no eye defects have been identified as the cause of visual perceptual deficits and claims of success with this treatment are without empirical support, some optometrists have convinced school districts to relinquish control of the LD programs to their specialty. The danger for children is that only one form of LD (visual perceptual deficit) is assessed and addressed.

The use of megavitamins (orthomolecular therapy) or trace element replacement has not been empirically supported, and megavitamin use has been shown to increase liver function test results (Copeland and Wolraich, 1987).

Perhaps the best known "treatment" for hyperactivity is the Feingold diet, also known as the Kaiser-Permanente diet. Approximately 1% to 2% of children placed on this dietary management respond positively (Silver, 1986). The diet is not well received by children and is difficult to follow at school cafeterias or eateries catering to school-aged children. It consists of the following restrictions: (1) omit foods containing natural salicylates (almonds, apples, cherries, cucumbers, grapes [raisins], oranges, peaches, tea, tomatoes); (2) omit foods and medications containing artificial colors and flavors (most types of bacon, margarine, ice cream, chocolate syrup, luncheon meats, soft drinks, catsup, bakery goods, chips); and (3) omit toothpaste, tooth powder, and compounds containing aspirin and food additives, such as BHA and BHT (Gearheart, 1985; Johnston, 1987). The generalized effectiveness of this diet cannot be supported in crossover testing measures. Copeland and Wolraich (1987) state that if the diet is strictly followed, "The child may become deficient in Vitamin C because of the fact that many foods high in Vitamin C are also high in salicylates" (p. 288).

Other diet modifications include the elimination of sorbitol (an artificial sweetener), caffeine, and refined sugars. In repeated studies parents' observations of the reactions of these substances on their children's behavior cannot be supported.

The final controversial therapy is described by Rapp and Bamberg (1986) and proposes that children previously described as "hyperactive" are actually "allergic" to foods, chemicals, and other environmental allergens. This may be true for a small number of children, but a complete assessment should be able to rule this out or provide needed allergy control.

PROGNOSIS

A significant number of children diagnosed as learning disabled continue to be affected into adulthood (Silver, 1988), with 50% to 70% of children with attention deficits diagnosed between 6 and 12 years of age manifesting troublesome symptoms through middle adolescence (Coleman and Levine, 1988). This number decreases to 35% in late adolescence and continues to decrease through early adulthood. However, 25% of children are able to stop treatment after approximately 2 years because of improved self-management (Johnston, 1987).

In those children with hyperactivity, Hechtman (1985) concluded that "stimulant treatment in childhood does not seem to secure a positive adolescent outcome for the hyperactive" (p. 188). Twenty percent to 30% continued to exhibit hyperactivity and antisocial behavior, including poor peer relationships and low self-esteem. These young adults are approximately two grade levels behind their peers in core subjects.

It should be noted that many children with LDs grow up to become very successful adults. A number of them have become members of the health care team by entering such fields as dentistry, psychology, medicine, and nursing. Because section 504 of the Rehabilitation Act (1973) indicates that "if otherwise qualified" these individuals must be provided entrance to jobs and continuing education, their potential is limitless.

ASSOCIATED PROBLEMS
Psychologic sequelae

Children who are misdiagnosed or not diagnosed in grade school may experience many years of academic failure. The psychologic sequelae of multiple failures can result in altered self-esteem and altered social interactions with peers. Problem behaviors such as inability to delay gratification and poor emotional control may develop (Bender, 1987). Although some adopt antisocial behavior as a way to cope with failure, there does not appear to be an increase in delinquency in children with LDs. However, chronic school failure can result in anxiety and depression, leading to school absenteeism or resignation.

A number of children with an LD, ADHD, and UADD have difficulty with peer relationships, especially those who have significant psychomotor dysfunction, whose use of language is restricted, who are in special education classes, or who are singled out and labeled as "different" in a regular classroom. However, a similar number of learning disabled children are quite popular. Some of the social behavior problems may be the result of the child's difficulty in reading nonverbal social cues, resulting in misjudgment of acceptance or rejection.

One of the problems in identifying children who have an LD, ADHD, or UADD is the impact of labeling. The label allows the child to receive services to compensate for deficits and adjust to the consequences, but it also may result in a self-fulfilling prophecy. Educators must be careful not to use the label to separate or identify children in a mainstreamed classroom.

Learning disabled children who do not receive appropriate intervention may develop unrealistic life goals. Because of their difficulty in using and understanding language, they may have stopped being inquisitive early in life. All of these factors can result in children who fail to reach their potential and become undereducated and underemployed.

Physical sequelae

Children with ADHD and UADD have an array of associated problems, among which are increased nutritional needs juxtaposed against anorexia from the stimulant medications. Those children receiving stimulant medication also may suffer from the physical side effects of temporary growth retardation, hypertension, difficulty sleeping, headaches, nausea, or irritability.

Psychosomatic complaints

Children who are frustrated and stressed by their inability to perform in an academic or motor task may develop psychosomatic symptoms. As with any psychosomatic disorder, all other physical causes must be ruled out. However, it is important for the health care practitioner to assess the pattern of development of the symptoms (time of day, subject being taught in class, activity being required). Treatment involves addressing the specific needs and referring to members of the interdisciplinary team to develop a plan for intervention.

Pharmacologic sequelae

Stimulant medication is generally well tolerated. There are some side effects general to all three stimulant drugs, as well as specific effects for each drug. In general these drugs can produce nervousness, insomnia, and decreased appetite, with subsequent weight loss. Additional side effects that completely disappear when the drug is stopped include nausea, stomachache, drowsiness, headaches, increased pulse rate resulting in palpitations, affective changes (being quieter, less talkative, and having decreased social interaction), and emotional lability (moodiness, irritability, tendency to crying) (Bond, 1987; Copeland and Wolraich, 1987; Johnston, 1987). Some of the side effects occur more commonly as the drug is wearing off, usually around the dinner hour. The ability to cope with the side effects must be weighed against the desired positive effects and benefits of the medications.

The dosage of methylphenidate has a direct relationship to behavior changes. As mentioned earlier, it is not recommended for children less than 6 years of age because efficacy in this age group has not been established. It has been commonly recommended that methylphenidate be administered 30 minutes before meals because meals were thought to affect the therapeutic effect of the drug. If the lunchtime dose proves difficult for children to take before meals, new evidence suggests that ingesting the drug with food does not damage the drug's pharmokinetic properties and subsequent therapeutic effect. Methylphenidate does not usually result in growth suppression if the dose is less than 20 mg per day (Copeland and Wolraich, 1987) or if the child is in early adolescence (Vincent, Varley, and Leger, 1990). If growth retardation does occur, weight loss is noted first, followed by a decrease in the height percentage as measured by growth charts.

Dextroamphetamine suppresses growth of those who have maintained treatment for more than 3 years. Growth usually rebounds when drug use is interrupted or discontinued, and adult height should not be affected.

The most serious side effect of pemoline is hepatic dysfunction. Before the child is given pemoline and every few months throughout the course of treatment, liver function tests are performed. If toxicity should occur, its results are usually reversible when the drug is withdrawn. There is some suggestion that this reaction is a hypersensitivity reaction (Copeland and Wolraich, 1987).

Although rare, Gilles de la Tourette's syndrome, or the development of tics, is also associated with the administration of methylphenidate and pemoline. This medication should not be used if there is a positive family history of Gilles de la Tourette syndrome (Johnston, 1987).

Increased drug and alcohol abuse were not found in teens, nor were they found to misuse or abuse their stimulant medication (Munoz-Millan and Casteel, 1989).

PRIMARY CARE MANAGEMENT

Learning disabilities have not routinely been diagnosed until the child begins school. However, with the initiation of Public Law 99-457, the Education of the Handicapped Amendments of 1986, assessment of children at risk for developing LDs must be done in the first 3 years of life if signs and symptoms are evident. This will place more responsibility on health care providers to develop and use tools that can measure cognitive abilities and hyperactivity at an earlier age.

Growth and development

Careful attention to measuring weight and physical growth parameters must be done routinely, approximately every 6 months, if the child is taking stimulant medication for hyperactivity. The effect of stimulant medication on growth is somewhat controversial (Vincent, Varley, and Leger, 1990). Some children may have growth retardation and benefit from drug holidays to allow for catch-up growth. Other children appear unaffected and have normal growth patterns.

Because children learn to compensate for their disability and in some cases the nature of their disability changes as they grow and develop, it is important to reevaluate the child's cognitive, motor, and psychosocial level of development every few years. This provides a baseline for changing the individualized education plan (IEP) and accessing other members of the interdisciplinary team.

Immunizations

No changes in the routine schedule of immunizations are needed.

Screening

Vision. Comprehensive vision testing should be performed, especially if a child is suspected of having a visual perceptual deficit. This may be complicated for the child with letter reversals who has to determine the direction of the letter E. It is also helpful to perform a short reading test (if age appropriate) to assess reading comprehension and whether a child can read across a line without skipping words or losing his or her place.

Hearing. Comprehensive audiometric testing should be performed at diagnosis, especially if a child is suspected of having an auditory perceptual deficit. Children with directionality difficulties and kinesthetic misperception and children who have

impaired ability to follow oral directions may have difficulty signaling from which ear the sound is heard, resulting in false-positive results.

Dental. Routine screening is recommended.

Blood pressure. Routine screening is needed except for children receiving stimulant medication. These children may experience hypertension and should be monitored periodically. These children may also have an increased pulse rate.

Hematocrit. Routine screening is recommended.

Urinalysis. Routine screening is recommended.

Tuberculosis. Routine screening is recommended.

Condition-specific screening

LIVER FUNCTION. Children taking pemoline will need to have liver function tests performed every few months.

Drug interactions

Stimulant medications have a number of interactive effects when given with other drugs. They inhibit the liver's ability to release some drug-metabolizing enzymes. This results in prolonged half-life of many seizure medications (phenytoin [Dilantin], primidone [Mysoline], and phenobarbitol), as well as imipramine.

Methylpenidate (1) delays the onset of action of oral anticoagulants (e.g., dicumarol); (2) impairs the hypotensive effects of guanethidine (Ismelin), possibly resulting in arrhythmias; (3) increases serum phenytoin levels, resulting in an increase in the pharmacologic and toxic effects of phenytoin; (4) enhances the development of hypertensive crisis when given with monoamine oxidase (MAO) inhibitors (isocarboxazid, phenelzine, pargyline, tranylcypromine); and (5) increases the serum concentration of tricyclic antidepressants, resulting in either clinical improvement or adverse effects.

Dextroamphetamine also has a number of specific drug interactive effects. When it is given with furazolidone (Furoxone), the body responds more sensitively to the stimulant drug, thus resulting in amphetamine toxicity. Urinary acidifiers and alkalinizers result in altered renal tubular reabsorption of the stimulant. Acidifiers hasten the elimination of dextroamphetamine, thus decreasing its time of action, whereas alkalinizers prolong the effects of the stimulant by decreasing urinary elimination of the unchanged drug.

Dextroamphetamine can reverse the hypotensive effects of guanethidine. This stimulant drug should not be given with MAO inhibitors or with phenothiazides. Pharmacologic effects of MAO inhibitors are exaggerated, with the possible sequela of death caused by hypertensive crisis and the ensuing cerebral hemorrhage. Phenothiazides and dextroamphetamine together result in decreased action of both (Tatro, 1990).

DIFFERENTIAL DIAGNOSIS AND MANAGEMENT OF COMMON PEDIATRIC CONDITIONS
Effects of stimulant therapy

It is important to differentiate between the clinical manifestations of LD, ADHD, and UADD and other problems of childhood, such as the irritability and inability to attend to a task, that are common when one is ill. Side effects of stimulant medications may mask the symptoms of physical and psychologic illness, such as anorexia, weight loss, and insomnia. Prepubertal children who have been taking stimulant medications for a number of years and who experience growth retardation should be evaluated for other causes of short stature, and the side effects of the stimulants should be considered.

Developmental/behavioral deviations

Numerous developmental deviations, including adjustment disorders, cognitive delay, visual and auditory problems, and global delays, may be mistaken for ADHD or UADD. Children must be evaluated carefully to rule out these conditions before a diagnosis is made.

Psychologic conditions, such as chronic anxiety, fear of failure, and those that develop from being in a dysfunctional family (divorce, illness and death in the family, teen pregnancy, poverty, and malnutrition) may result in difficulty attending to academic tasks but should not be confused with a worsening of the disability (Dworkin, 1985).

Increased injuries

Children with an LD who are frequently seen for mild trauma care and are thought to have possibly experienced abuse need to be reassessed from the perspective of their LD. Children who have difficulty following safety directions and those who lack hand-eye coordination may be more prone to environmental injury.

DEVELOPMENTAL ISSUES
Safety

There are a number of safety issues for children and adolescents with learning disabilities. Because of an increase in impulsive behavior and an alteration in judgment in some children beyond that which is common to most young children, they are at higher risk for acting without thinking and engaging in unsafe activities. Children with learning disabilities may have increased frequency of getting lost because of problems in processing information about their environment. Those children who have difficulty understanding directions may be unable to safely complete tasks or to take appropriate action in an emergency.

The health care practitioner may need to help families and older children to develop plans to structure their environment and their activities. Breaking down activities into their component parts and using checklists may help children be more aware of their behavior.

A significant number of adolescents have impaired judgment of space and distance. This, plus decreased ability to pay attention to such things as conditions of the road and driving speed, results in an increase in motor vehicle accidents in this population (Smith, 1988). Driving is an activity that requires one to perform multiple tasks and decision making simultaneously. Adolescents who have difficulty in these areas are advised to delay driving for a few years.

Although no data support abuse of stimulant medications, medication safety should always be a consideration in teaching. Using containers that mark the pills for each day of the week may be helpful for children who are self-administering their medications. Standard precautions for keeping medications safely secured should be followed.

Child care

If day care is a component of child care, a program that has a small class size, a structured and safe environment, constant adult supervision, and an opportunity to engage in gross motor play outdoors should be selected. Children with hyperactivity will need to develop a medication regimen that fits their needs best.

Diet

There are no dietary restrictions. Children on stimulant medications may have a decreased appetite, but their increased activity level may warrant an increased caloric intake. Therefore, foods high in protein should be encouraged to enhance the quality of their nutritional status.

Discipline

All children act out and misbehave at various intervals in the developmental process. As with other children, discipline should fit the seriousness of the misbehavior. However, children with an LD may not be able to understand cause and effect or verbal directions. Even after they have done something wrong, they may not relate their activity to the punishment and will need frequent clarification from adults.

Behavior modification techniques may help the child to develop self-control. If time-out is used, the child needs to be told when the period of restriction has ended. He or she should be reminded of the reasons for the punishment and consistently helped to differentiate between "the act being wrong or bad" and "the child being bad." For the hyperactive child, parents need assistance in determining to what degree the child's normal behavior requires discipline.

Discipline should be part of the daily routine for these children, and it must be consistent. Limit setting is an important component of their day. Structuring the daily routine of the home environment will help these children establish acceptable patterns of behavior. Parents should be reminded to teach the recommended behavioral approaches to the child's significant others, such as grandparents and baby-sitters.

Toileting

There is no impact on toileting unless the child experiences sensory or tactile deficits. In this case the child needs to be walked through the sensations involved in toileting. Routine toilet breaks should be a part of the daily schedule. Elementary schools should also be sensitive to this need and incorporate toileting into the day's activities.

Sleep patterns

Learning disabilities have no effect on sleep unless emotional problems are present or unless stimulant medication is taken too late in the day. Assessment of the drug administration schedule should be completed. Insomnia is a common side effect of stimulant medication and frequently resolves as a tolerance to the medication develops. If this does not resolve, decreasing the dosage or scheduling administration earlier in the day may help.

School issues

A major issue is that of school readiness. The appropriateness of the kindergarten class at age 5 years needs to be evaluated. A number of children with LDs spend 2 years in kindergarten or first grade, thus giving them time to develop the psychosocial and cognitive skills needed to progress. It is important to assess for prerequisite deficits in knowledge or skills and to plan remediation for these. The primary care provider may play a key role in emotionally supporting parents through the difficult decision of holding their child back. Focusing on the long-term gains will help diminish the parents' initial disappointment and grieving. Making the child feel special and giving attention to his or her accomplishments will be beneficial to the child.

Children with LDs, ADHDs, and UADDs may be mainstreamed into regular classrooms, use the resource room, attend special education classes, be tutored, or a combination thereof. The goal is to mainstream these children into normal classrooms, but special education classrooms and resource rooms are very acceptable therapies for these children. In resource rooms (supplementary help) and special education (self-contained) classrooms, teachers can limit the number of students in the classroom, decrease the amount of distraction, and provide specific interventions based on the child's needs.

According to Public Law 94-142, every child with a learning disability should have an IEP developed specifically for them. It should include the type of classroom and the type and length of services the child will use. The educational objectives and the plan for intervention will be identified in the IEP. The primary care provider should be a key member on the education team and have input into the IEP recommendations.

Parents should participate in the IEP development and be encouraged to meet with each member of the interdisciplinary team who will interface with their child. These meetings should occur throughout the year to update the parents and enhance communication between the parents and teachers. The primary care coordinator functions as health care coordinator, educator, and consultant for the IEP team.

A significant part of the educational plan is to help children learn to compensate for their particular disability. Children need to understand which learning modalities work best for them and then to have material presented (or available) to them in that modality. For children with visual perceptual deficits, tape recording class lectures may be more helpful than manual note taking.

The child with altered coordination and difficulty in motor skills may shy away from participating in age-appropriate activities. Being involved in noncompetitive sports, being given a different role in a group activity so that they continue to be a member of the group, and finding alternative motor activities, such as using a computer rather than being required to use script, will enhance the child's self-concept and make the child less fearful of participation.

Classroom teachers who are unfamiliar with the special needs of these children will require specific information as to their role in education, assessment, and control measures (if necessary). The Conners Teacher Rating Scale (Conners, 1987) provides important information in the periodic assessment of hyperactive children. It assesses behavior in the classroom, group participation, and attitude toward authority. This will prove to be essential to the health care provider in determining whether stimulant medication should be continued or the dosage changed.

Children with LDs, ADHDs, and UADDs may be highly distractible. Educational strategies and environmental modifications that have proved beneficial for these children in a regular classroom include the following:

1. Modifying the classroom environment (using muted wall colors; decreasing the clutter on desks; having the child sit in front of the classroom and face away from windows, doors, and distracting wall decorations) will decrease environmental and peer distraction.

2. These children perform better in a structured environment rather than an open, unstructured one. Lessons should be structured in such a way that the children know what is expected in a step-by-step format. Calendars can help a child organize their approach to a project.

3. Providing for untimed tests, allowing lectures to be tape recorded, making word processors available for written assignments, and selecting activities and assignments that are appropriate for the child's needs and abilities will assist the child in school.

4. If the child is removed from a regular class to receive special assistance, ensure that the child has not missed important classroom content.

5. Instructions must be provided both verbally and in writing.

6. The child's success and effort should be positively reinforced.

7. Dividing projects into smaller steps helps the child accomplish them and make connections among the parts.

8. Predictable daily routines and clear and consistent assignments provide structure.

9. Giving continuous feedback and asking questions help ensure that these children understand the content being presented. There should also be some consistency between the child's home and school treatment modalities.

10. For the child taking stimulant medication, it would be helpful to have the most important and complex material taught early in the day when the medication is at its peak.

The child with an LD and his or her family will need to readjust to this condition at every new developmental stage. The psychologic impact of LDs results in specific psychosocial needs. Building a child's self-esteem and self-confidence, as well as an accurate self-perception, becomes even more important when the child is experiencing chronic academic difficulty.

The child who continues to have academic difficulty resulting in failure will need counseling support and assistance in dealing with the related stress. Children with LDs need to understand that even though they failed a course (or an examination), they are not a failure. It is not appropriate to tell a child to "try harder." Their decreased performance is often not a lack of effort, nor is it anyone's fault. These children need to be reassured that they are not stupid and that requests for repetition of directions and clarification of content are not a nuisance.

It is important to assist the child in developing strategies for coping. These should build on the child's strengths and compensate for his or her weaknesses. In addition, encouraging social interaction with peers is another goal of the health care practitioner. It is very difficult for adolescents to adjust to a chronic condition. This is a time of conformity rather than having to meet special needs. Young people need the opportunity to express their feelings about not only having a disability but also being different, especially if they are taking stimulant medication.

Medication administration during school hours has presented some problems for children. Legal guidelines for school personnel administering drugs and for keeping medications in the school vary with each state. These guidelines should be shared with parents so that they can plan accordingly. In addition, some children "forget" to come for their lunchtime dose because they often have to (1) leave their friends to go to the infirmary or office; (2) are involved in group activities; or (3) may feel guilty or self-conscious about having to take pills, especially if "just say no to drugs" information is being promoted.

The health care practitioner must have communication with members of the IEP team and the family and the child at least twice each year to assess and modify the plan of care. These interactions can be much more frequent (every 2-4 weeks) as the need arises.

Sexuality

Sex education for children and adolescents is an important role for the health care practitioner. Using the learning techniques previously identified, sex education must be individualized to the child's specific learning abilities.

SPECIAL FAMILY CONCERNS

Before a diagnosis of LD, ADHD, or UADD is made, parents are often confused, concerned, and even anxious as to why their child is having difficulties. Once a diagnosis is made, parents will grieve for the wished-for "perfect" child and may respond to the diagnosis with embarrassment, frustration, guilt, self-blame, anger, or even relief that the problem has been identified and isn't "imagined."

Before they can begin to accept this child and work toward resolution of the treatment objectives, parents need to be educated about this diability. In this endeavor the family must be empowered to assume control of the plan developed for their child and for guiding their child's development. Routine anticipatory guidance is also provided. It should be kept in mind that often a child with an LD has a parent with an LD. Therefore, teaching about child care and other developmental issues should use the same approaches as discussed earlier, depending on the parent's specific needs.

Environmental control in the home is similar to that discussed for the classroom. Decreasing clutter, developing routines, and providing clear directions in the format that best meets the child's needs may prove beneficial. These parents typically give more commands, directions, and supervision to their children than do parents for a "normal" child. They are concerned about the child's future potential for schooling and vocational choices, as well as their ability to assume an independent lifestyle. This results in increased parental stress, depression, and marital discord. They, as well as their children, need coping strategies and consistent support.

There can be a significant impact on the siblings of a learning disabled child. They may resent the amount of time and attention paid to the child with special needs. Younger siblings will need to be sensitive to the feelings of the child with an LD as the younger sibling matches and often surpasses the academic level of the child with a learning disability.

A learning disability is not just an academic disability; it pervades every area of the child's life and keeps them from functioning at their optimal level. By accepting their diagnosis, they can begin to take control of their life. A learning disability is really a learning difference. These children can learn; they just learn differently. In essence, a learning disability is a living disability. With appropriate intervention, their goal of growing into adulthood using their full potential can be accomplished.

SUMMARY OF PRIMARY CARE NEEDS FOR THE CHILD WITH A LEARNING DISABILITY

Growth and development

Manifestions of an LD varies with development
Medications for hyperactivity may retard growth and result in anorexia.
Toddlers and preschoolers are eligible for diagnostic and intervention services under RL 99-457.

Immunizations

Routine schedule is recommended.

Screening
Vision

Comprehensive visual testing is done to rule out visual perceptual deficit and acuity problems. Children may have difficulty using standard E charts.

Hearing

Comprehensive audiometric testing is done to rule out auditory perceptual deficit and hearing loss. Children may have difficulty with audiometric testing because of directionality problems.

Dental

Routine screening is recommended.

Blood pressure

Routine screening is recommended. If the child is taking stimulant medication, screening must be done more frequently because of possible hypertension.

Hematocrit

Routine screening is recommended.

Urinalysis

Routine screening is recommended.

Tuberculosis

Routine screening is recommended.

Condition-specific screening

Liver function tests are necessary for children taking pemoline.

Drug interactions

Stimulant medications inhibit liver metabolism of other drugs. Methylphenidate affects anticoagulants, quanethidine, phenytoin, MAO inhibitors, and tricyclic antidepressants. Dextroamphetamine affects furazolidone, quanethidine, and phenothiazides. It should not be given with MAO inhibitors.

Differential diagnosis
Irritability

Rule out change in LD or illness.

Anorexia, weight loss, and insomnia

Rule out change in LD or illness.

Trauma

Rule out motor or expressive LD, hyperactivity, or abuse.

Safety

There is a risk of injury because of impulsive behaviors.
Drivers with LD, ADHD, and UADD may have automobile accidents because of spatial perception difficulties.
Medication should be safely kept out of reach of young children.

Child care

Administration of medication may be necessary in day-care setting.
Children perform better in a small, structured, safe environment with constant adult supervision.

Diet

Children may be poor eaters because of distraction and decreased appetite if they are taking stimulant medication. A nutritious diet with adequate protein for growth is important.

Discipline

Children may have difficulty responding to directions. They may not understand discipline. Consistency is important.

◆ ▬▬▬▬▬▬▬▬ ◆

SUMMARY OF PRIMARY CARE NEEDS FOR THE CHILD WITH A LEARNING DISABILITY — cont'd

Toileting

No impact unless child has sensory tactile deficits

Sleep patterns

Learning disabilities, ADHD, and UADD have no impact on sleep patterns unless the child is taking stimulant medications, which may cause insomnia if given late in the day or in large doses.

School issues

Educational strategies to decrease distraction in a regular classroom plus creative teaching modalities appropriate to the specific learning needs of the child should be implemented.

Building a child's self-esteem and confidence is essential.

Children should be helped to learn to compensate for their disability.

Development of the individualized education plan is a team effort.

Special family concerns

The child and the family need to readjust to this disability at every new developmental stage.

Family counseling can provide information and emotional support.

A learning disability is a living disability.

RESOURCES

Vocational rehabilitation services for individuals with learning disabilities

Although Public Law 94-142 provides educational services for the individual less than 21 years of age, the recognition by the American Psychiatric Association that many of these children become learning disabled adults has led to their being eligible for state and federal vocational rehabilitation services (Hoy and Gregg, 1987).

Organizations

The following associations and support groups provide assistance to individuals with learning disabilities and their families:

Children with Attention Deficit Disorders
1859 N Pine Island Rd
Suite 185
Plantation, FL 33322
(305) 384-6869 or (305) 792-8100

Foundation for Children with Learning Disabilities
99 Park Ave
New York, NY 10016
(212) 687-7211

Association for Children and Adults with Learning Disabilities
4156 Library Rd
Pittsburgh, PA 15234
(412) 341-1515

Books

Nuzum M: *What do teens with learning disabilities want to know?* New York, 1985, New York State Developmental Disabilities Planning Council and the Federation of Jewish Philanthropies (YM-YWHA).

REFERENCES

Bauchner H, Brown E, and Peskin J: Premature graduates of the newborn intensive care unit: A guide to follow up, *Pediatr Clin North Am* 35:1207-1226, 1988.

Bender W: Secondary personality and behavioral problems in adolescents with learning disabilities, *J Learning Disabilities* 20:280-285, 1987.

Bond W: Recognition and treatment of attention deficit disorder, *Clin Pharm* 6:617-624, 1987.

Cantwell DP and Baker L: Attention-deficit disorder in children: The role of the nurse practitioner, *Nurse Pract* 12:38, 43-44, 46-48, 50-51, 54, 1987a.

Cantwell DP and Baker L: Differential diagnosis of hyperactivity, *Dev Behav Pediatr* 8:159-165, 1987b.

Cantwell DP and Baker L: Considerations for the classification of ADDH, *Dev Behav Pediatr* 8:169-170, 1987c (response to commentary).

Coleman W and Levine M: Attention deficits in adolescence: Description, evaluation, and management, *Pediatr Rev* 9:287-297, 1988.

Conners CK: How is a teacher rating scale used in the diagnosis of attention deficit disorder? *J Child Contemp Soc* 19:33-40, 1987.

Copeland L and Wolraich M: Disorders of behavioral development. In Wolraich M, ed: *The practical assessment and management of children with disorders of development and learning,* Chicago, 1987, Year Book Medical Publishers, pp 269-295.

Diagnostic and statistical manual of mental disorders: DSM-III-R, ed 3 revised, Washington, DC, 1987, American Psychiatric Association.

Drug facts and comparisons 1990, Philadelphia, 1990, JB Lippincott.

Dworkin P: *Learning and behavior problems of schoolchildren,* Philadelphia, 1985, WB Saunders.

Gaddes W: *Learning disabilities and brain function,* New York, 1985, Springer-Verlag New York.

Gadow K: Relative efficacy of pharmacological, behavioral, and combination treatments for enhancing academic performance, *Clin Psychol Rev* 5:513-533, 1985.

Gearheart B: *Learning disabilities: Educational strategies,* St Louis, 1985, CV Mosby.

Hechtman L: Adolescent outcome of hyperactive children treated with stimulants in childhood: A review, *Psychopharmacol Bull* 21:178-191, 1985.

Hoy C and Gregg N: Vocational rehabilitation needs of the nonverbal learning disabled adult, *J Rehabil* 53:54-57, 1987.

Interagency Committee on Learning Disabilities: *Learning disabilities: A report to the U.S. Congress,* Washington, DC, 1987, US Department of Health and Human Services.

Johnston R: *Learning disabilities, medicine, and myth,* Boston, 1987, Little, Brown.

Kronick D: *New approaches to learning disabilities,* Orlando, Fla, 1988, Grune & Stratton.

Magrun WM: Clinical decision making in treatment of learning disabled children. In *The occupational therapy manager's survival handbook,* New York, 1988, Haworth Press.

Meents C: Attention deficit disorder: A review of the literature, *Psychol Sch* 26:168-178, 1989.

Munoz-Millan R and Casteel CR: Attention deficit hyperactivity disorder: Recent literature, *Hosp Community Psychiatry* 40:699-706, 1989.

Peckham V: Learning disorders associated with the treatment of cancer in childhood, *J Assoc Pediatr Oncol Nurses* 5(4):10-13, 1988.

Pelham W: What do we know about the use and effects of CNS stimulants in the treatment of ADD? *J Child Contemp Soc* 19:99-110, 1987.

Rapp D and Bamberg D: *The impossible child,* Washington, DC, 1986, Life Sciences Press.

Selekman J: The learning disabled child: Another frontier for nursing, *Holistic Nursing Practice* 2(2):1-10, 1988.

Silver L: Controversial approaches to treating learning disabilities and attention deficit disorder, *Am J Dis Child* 140:1045-1051, 1986.

Silver L: A review of the federal government's interagency committee on learning disabilities report to the U.S. Congress, *Learn Disabilities Focus* 3:73-80, 1988.

Smith S: Preparing the learning disabled adolescent for adulthood, *Child Today* 17:4-9, March 1988.

Tatro D, ed: *Drug interaction facts,* Philadelphia, 1990, JB Lippincott.

Trauner D: Learning disabilities: Your role in diagnosis and management, *Consultant* 26:74-84, 1986.

Vincent J, Varlay CK, and Leger P: Effects of methylphenidate on early adolescent growth, *Am J Psychiatry* 147:501-502, 1990.

Wender EH: Commentary on the differential diagnosis of hyperactivity, *Dev Behav Pediatr* 8:166-168, 1987.

21 *Myelodysplasia*

··

Judith A. Farley and *Mary Jo Dunleavy*

ETIOLOGY

The classification of neural tube defects pertains to the malformation of the central nervous system (CNS) during embryonic development. The embryologic development of the CNS begins early in the third week of gestation. During this time the neural plate invaginates and folds together, forming the neural tube. The process of neurolation produces the functional nervous system, or the future brain and spinal cord. If the neural tube fails to close, the process of neurulation is interrupted, which results in the imperfect formation of the brain or spinal cord at a focal point (McLone and Naidich, 1986; Warkany and Lemire, 1986).

Myelodysplasia is one form of neural tube defect. The term myelodysplasia refers to the defective formation and subsequent development and function of the spinal cord. This defect can occur at any level of the spinal cord; the extent of nerve tissue and spinal cord involvement varies. The malformation results in altered body function at and below the level of the defect (Table 21-1).

The etiology of neural tube defects is unknown. Many potential causes or factors have been considered, but none has been confirmed as an isolated cause. There is a higher incidence of neural tube defects in affected families, as well as an overall increased risk of birth defects with poor prenatal care and maternal nutritional deficiencies. At this time, however, there are insufficient data in the literature to link a specific drug exposure with the development of neural tube defects (Lemire, 1986a; McLone and Naidich 1986; Moore, 1987; Rosa,

1991). Recent studies indicate that ingestion of multivitamins with folic acid before conception or early in the pregnancy may offer protection against the occurrence of neural tube defects (Milunsky et al., 1989).

Table 21-1. Functional alterations in myelodysplasia related to level of lesion

Level of lesion	Functional implications
Thoracic	Flaccid paralysis of lower extremities; variable weakness in abdominal trunk musculature; high thoracic level may mean respiratory compromise; absence of bowel and bladder control
High lumbar	Voluntary hip flexion and adduction; flaccid paralysis of knees, ankles, and feet; may walk with extensive braces and crutches; absence of bowel and bladder control
Midlumbar	Strong hip flexion and adduction; fair knee extension; flaccid paralysis of ankles and feet; absence of bowel and bladder control
Low lumbar	Strong hip flexion, extension and adduction, knee extension; weak ankle and toe mobility; may have limited bowel and bladder function
Sacral	Normal function of lower extremities; normal bowel and bladder function

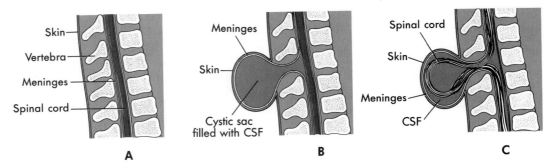

Fig. 21-1. Diagram showing section through **A,** normal spine; **B,** meningocele; **C,** myelomeningocele.

INCIDENCE

The incidence of neural tube defects is approximately 0.7 to 1.0 for every 1000 live births in the United States each year (Badell-Ribera, 1985; Hobbins, 1991; Wallander, Feldman and Varni, 1989). There is a strong association of fetal death with neural tube defects, reducing the actual prevalence of neural tube defects at birth (Lemire, 1986b).

CLINICAL MANIFESTATIONS AT TIME OF DIAGNOSIS

Clinical manifestations at the time of diagnosis will vary depending on the extent of involvement of the spinal cord and surrounding structures of nerve, bone, muscle, and skin. Myelodysplasia is classified based on the pathophysiology of the lesion or defect (Fig. 21-1).

Spina bifida occulta is the failed fusion of the vertebral arches that surround and protect the spinal cord. It may involve a small portion of one vertebra or the complete absence of bone. Absence of the vertebral arch or arches is commonly associated with cutaneous abnormalities such as tufts of hair, hemangiomas, and dermoid cysts located at the area of the defect on the surface of the back. There are usually no neurologic deficits at the time of birth. However, a child with such a defect may develop bowel, bladder, and musculoskeletal difficulties later in life (American Association of Neuroscience Nurses, 1984).

Another type of myelodysplasia is the meningocele in which the neural tube fails to close, resulting in a cystic dilatation of meninges through the vertebral defect and around the malformed tube. This defect does not involve the spinal cord, and hydrocephalus is commonly associated with this diagnosis (AANN, 1984). At birth the infant has a protruding sac on the back at the level of the defect. The sac may be covered by a thin layer of muscle and skin and usually appears as raw, fluid-filled tissue. The child may or may not have abnormal neurologic findings at birth. Manipulation of the sac, surgical closure, and infection may lead to neurologic changes. Functional implications are dependent on the level and severity of the defect (see Table 21-1).

A myelomeningocele is the failure of the neural tube to close, resulting in a cystic dilatation of meninges and protuberance of the spinal cord through the vertebral defect (AANN, 1984). Hydrocephalus is present in virtually all children afflicted with this condition (AANN, 1984). Approximately 80% to 90% of these children will require an internal shunt system to control the hydrocephalus (McLone and Naidich, 1986) (see Chapter 17). The actual involvement of the spinal cord has greater implications for the overall function of the infant throughout childhood (see Table 21-1).

Because the pathophysiology of myelodysplasia is determined early in gestation, prenatal diagnosis is possible. The presence of a neural tube defect may result in an elevated amniotic fluid α-fetoprotein (AFP) level and subsequent elevation in the maternal serum AFP levels. When maternal serum AFP levels are elevated, further testing is indicated for diagnostic purposes (Leonard, 1981). The amniotic fluid is obtained through amniocentesis for evaluation (Macri, Baker, and Baim, 1981). In addition, high-resolution ultrasonography is a noninvasive and efficacious method used to evaluate pregnancies at risk or suspect for neural tube defects (Hogge et al., 1989).

The purpose of antenatal diagnosis is twofold. First, it offers the parents the option to terminate the pregnancy. If they choose to continue the pregnancy, prenatal diagnosis provides the family and health care team with the opportunity to prepare both physically and emotionally for the birth of the child. Delivery by cesarean section may be recommended to minimize trauma to the open cele. Luthy et al. (1991) concluded that "delivery by cesarean section for the fetus with uncomplicated meningomycele before the onset of labor may result in better subsequent motor function than vaginal delivery or delivery by cesarean section after a period of labor" (p. 662).

If prenatal testing is not performed, the infant's clinical manifestation at birth confirms the general diagnosis of neural tube defect. The specific tissue malformation and involvement and the presence of hydrocephalus can be determined only through further diagnostic tests such as ultrasonography, computerized tomography scan, and magnetic resonance imaging. Careful assessment of the infant during the surgical closure often aids in determining the depth and extent of tissue involvement. This information is important for habilitative planning and potential outcome.

TREATMENT

Initial treatment for infants with the diagnosis of meningocele and myelomeningocele is early surgical closure of the defect (Bartoshesky, Young, and Scott, 1986; Charney et al., 1985; Gross et al., 1983; McLaurin, 1986). Often neural tube defects affect several other body systems, creating hydrocephalus, renal and gastrointestinal (GI) disturbances, and musculoskeletal deformities. Because of the multisystem involvement, these infants require a comprehensive multidisciplinary team approach to treatment. The team may include nurses, neurosurgeons, urologists, orthopedists, pediatricians, physical therapists, occupational therapists, and social workers.

PROGNOSIS

Myelodysplasia is a chronic condition. The prognosis is dependent on the success of prophylactic and acute treatment for potential and actual complications that affect each body system. These children are at risk for sudden death because of a shunt malfunction or the Arnold-Chiari II malformation. Improved ventricular shunt systems have helped to minimize infections that may potentially lead to CNS damage. Also, the advent of new urologic interventions such as urodynamic assessment and intermittent catheterization greatly reduce the risk of renal damage. Treatments and interventions will be necessary throughout life. Procedures are individualized to the child's needs and are rendered when indicated by the clinical manifestation, assessment, and evaluation.

ASSOCIATED PROBLEMS
Arnold-Chiari II malformation

One associated problem of myelodysplasia is the Arnold-Chiari II malformation. This deformity involves the downward displacement of the cerebellum, cerebral tonsils, brainstem, and fourth ventricle (Fig. 21-2). The exact pathogenesis of the malformation is not known (Park, Hoffman, and Cail, 1986). The area of the brain involved is referred to as the posterior fossa region, which is responsible primarily for vital functions, including respirations and protective reflexes directed by the 12 cranial nerves (CNs). The downward displacement of this area results in compression and elongation of nerves and tissue, which, in turn, restrict neuronal performance in varying degrees (Lemire, 1986b; McCullough, 1986; Park, Hoffman and Cail, 1986).

Skin integrity

The newborn is at great risk for developing infection secondary to the altered skin integrity over the malformed spine and cord. This is a possible complication until the lesion has completely healed. The risk of skin breakdown continues throughout the individual's life because of the altered sensory function below the level of the lesion.

Hydrocephalus and seizures

Hydrocephalus is a common occurence. Seizures also occur in approximately 15% of those with

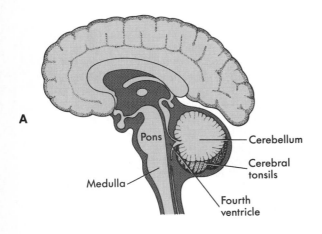 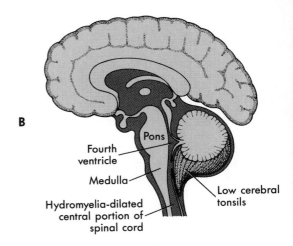

Fig. 21-2. Diagram showing **A,** normal brain; **B,** brain with Chiari malformation.

myelodysplasia (McLaughlin and Shurtleff, 1979) (see Chapters 15 and 17).

Visual and perceptual problems

Visual and perceptual problems, including ocular palsies, astigmatism, and visual perceptual deficits, occur in approximately 80% of these individuals (McLaughlin and Shurtleff, 1979). Pressure on the CNs that control eye movements, namely, CN III (oculomotor), CN IV (trochlear), and CN VI (abducens), may result in a mild disconjugate gaze, or esotropia.

Intelligence

Children born with myelodysplasia without hydrocephalus (10%-20%) are generally reported to have mean IQs in the average range. Children who have shunts because of the associated diagnosis of hydrocephalus have been reported to have IQs generally in the range of low average or less (McLone et al., 1982; Soare and Raimondi, 1977) but may have normal or above-normal intelligence. Hydrocephalus, especially when complicated by frequent shunt revisions, malfunctions, or infections, limits intellectual function in this population (McLone et al., 1982; Shaffer et al., 1985; Soare and Raimondi, 1977) (see Chapter 17). Often these children have strong verbal skills, which may be misinterpreted. Strength in verbal skills and weaknesses in cognitive skills (memory, speed of response, acquired knowledge, integrated functioning, and coordination) must be considered in the intellectual assessment of these children.

Altered motor and sensory function

Invariably motor and sensory functions below the level of the lesions are altered in myelodysplasia. This dysfunction includes weakness, spasticity, or bilateral paralysis of the lower extremities. These associated complications are the result of impaired spinal cord, spinal nerves, and meningeal involvement. Frequently these problems worsen as the child grows and the cord ascends within the vertebral canal, pulling primary scar tissue and tethering the spinal cord (Badell-Ribera, 1985; Humphreys, 1986; Park et al., 1985; Sugar, 1986; Venes and McGuire, 1986). Altered motor and sensory function may also impair peristalsis, leading to constipation, impaction, and incontinence of feces.

Musculoskeletal deformities

Musculoskeletal deformities related to myelomeningocele include club feet, dislocated hip or hips, and improper musculoskeletal alignment from altered embryonic development (Badell-Ribera, 1985). Spinal deformities occur in approximately 90% of individuals with myelomeningocele. Scoliosis is the most common form of spinal deformity (Park et al, 1985).

Urinary dysfunction

Depending on the level of the defect, neurogenic bladder function may occur. Potential complications of the urinary system associated with myelodysplasia include dyssynergy, hydronephrosis, incomplete emptying of the bladder, urinary reflux, urinary tract infections (UTIs), and incontinence. Any of these findings may result in deterioration of urinary function and could lead to renal damage (Bauer, 1989).

Allergic reactions

It has been noted that some children with myelodysplasia have an allergy to rubber products, such as surgical gloves, balloons, catheters, bandages, and breathing bags. This evidence indicates that these children are at risk for anaphylaxis during operations and procedures where this material is used (Slater, 1989). The practitioner should inform the parents of this potential sensitivity, observe for signs, and document the allergy in the child's medical record.

PRIMARY CARE MANAGEMENT
Growth

As with all children, it is crucial to monitor growth and development by obtaining routine heights and weights and plotting them on a standardized growth chart. Obesity is a common problem seen in children with myelodysplasia and is a result of decreased levels of activity. Because this can lead to problems with skin breakdown, brace fittings, and the ability to ambulate, early detection and education is essential (Colgan, 1981). Obtaining heights may be difficult, depending on the child's ability to stand. If necessary, the practitioner should measure the full body length with the child supine. Because of shortening of the spine or muscle atrophy, these children often fall below the tenth percentile in height.

Head circumference should be monitored closely by the practitioner. If a progressive enlargement in size is noted, referral to the neurosurgeon should be made (see Chapter 17).

Development

Motor development may or may not be affected and is directly related to the level of the lesion (see Table 21-1). The degree of weakness, paralysis, and decreased sensation will vary. Early orthopedic and physical therapy assessment and intervention are extremely important to prevent contractures, minimize deformities, and monitor muscle strength and flexibility. This assessment aids in planning for the child's future mobility and independence.

The rate at which cognitive and intellectual skills are acquired depends greatly on the child's interaction with the environment and the severity of the defect. The orthopedist and physical therapist can assist the child by ensuring that the physical developmental sequence proceeds normally (Bunch, 1986). For instance, if the child is not able to stand by age 10 to 18 months, use of a standing frame or a parapodium allows the child to accomplish various developmental tasks and stand with hands free for play (Colgan, 1981; Bunch, 1986).

As the child grows and develops, other adaptive equipment (braces, wheelchairs, etc.) is used to increase mobility and independence. Each child's treatment program will vary because of differences in motivation and variability of social resources. Age-related goals are most important (Shurtleff, 1980).

The deformity, degree of motor impairment, cognitive function, and motivation all influence the growth and development of each child (Feiwell, 1980; Huff and Ramsey, 1978; Tappit-Emas, 1989). Surgical intevention is often recommended and sometimes required to achieve proper muscle balance and body alignment for problems common to this population that would limit the child's potential such as dislocated hips, scoliosis, kyphosis, and clubfeet.

Precocious puberty has been noted in a number of children with myelodysplasia and hydrocephalus. The cause is not known but may be related to early pituitary gonadotropin secretion activated by the hydrocephalic brain (Shaul, Towbin, and Chernausek, 1985).

Immunizations

The recommended schedule for routine immunizations is suggested, although it may be interrupted because of frequent hospitalizations. The primary care provider should attempt to keep the child on schedule with routine immunizations. Alterations in the immunization schedule for children with seizures and hydrocephalus are addressed in Chapters 15 and 17.

Screening

Vision. Screening for visual and perceptual deficits in children with myelodysplasia is extremely important because of the high incidence of associated visual problems.

Hearing. Children with myelodysplasia who have been given shunts for hydrocephalus may be hypersensitive to loud noises. Awareness of this finding may alleviate parental concern. Exposure to the use of aminoglycosides may cause hearing deficits (see Chapter 17).

Dental. Routine dental screening is recommended (see Chapter 17).

Blood pressure. Routine screening is recommended. Children with known renal problems such as urinary reflux or a history of hypertension should have more frequent assessment. Persistent elevated readings should be communicated to the child's urologist.

Hematocrit. Routine screening is recommended.

Urinalysis. Baseline urinalysis and urine cultures are obtained during the newborn period. If at any time a UTI is suspected, a urine culture and sensitivity should be obtained. Because bag specimens have been noted to have a higher incidence of contamination, bladder catheterization is recommended. Routine urine cultures should be obtained every 3 to 4 months provided the child is not symptomatic. Positive urine cultures should be reported to the child's urologist.

Tuberculosis. Routine screening is recommended.

Condition-specific screening

BLOOD TESTS. Frequently children with myelodysplasia are on long-term antibiotic therapy for prevention of UTIs. Those who are taking sulfonamides should have complete blood cell counts checked frequently to monitor changes (Kirulata, Gillingham, and Squires, 1986). Abnormal results should be discussed with the child's urologist so that altered drug therapy can be arranged. Serum creatinine is checked in the newborn period as a baseline study for renal function and should be monitored yearly.

SCOLIOSIS. Screening for scoliosis in children with myelodysplasia should begin during the first year of life and continue throughout adolescence.

Drug interactions

Many of these children are on routine medication therapy. Potential interactions among these and other medications need to be carefully considered when additional pharmotherapeutics are prescribed. Commonly used drug categories are:

1. Antibiotics for treatment of UTIs or prophylaxis. These include amoxicillin (Amoxil), trimethoprim and sulfamethoxazole (Bactrim), sulfisoxazole (Gantrisin), and nitrofurantoin (Furadantin). If a child requires other antibiotic therapy for common childhood illness such as ear infections, the antibiotic for the UTI is discontinued during the needed course of treatment.

2. Anticholinergics to assist in urinary continence and reduce high bladder pressure. These include oxybutynin chloride (Ditropan) and propantheline bromide (Pro-Banthine). Oxybutynin chloride can cause heat prostration in the presence of high environmental temperatures. Anticholinergics may delay absorption of other medications given concomitantly in these children (PDR, 1990).

3. Sympathomimetics to increase urethral resistance. These include ephedrine (Gluco-Fedrin), pseudoephedrine hydrochloride (Sudafed), and phenylpropanolamine. The practitioner should determine if the child is taking any of these drugs before treating cold symptoms.

4. Stool softeners, stimulants, and bulk formers to aid in evacuation of stool. Many products are used for this purpose, and most are over-the-counter drugs. None of these should be administered in the presence of abdominal pain, nausea, vomiting, or diarrhea.

5. Anticonvulsants to control seizure activity. These include phenobarbital, phenytoid sodium (Dilantin), and carbamazepine (Tegretol). Concomitant administration of carbamazepine with erythromycin may result in toxicity (PDR, 1990) (see Chapter 15).

Table 21-2. Implications of cranial nerve dysfunction in myelodysplasia

CN	Functional implications
I Olfactory	Sense of smell
II Optic	Visual acuity, visual fields
III Oculomotor	Raises eyelids
	Constricts pupils
	Moves eyes up, down, and in
IV Trochlear	Moves eyes downward
V Trigeminal	Sensory innervation to face and tongue
	Opens and closes jaw
VI Abducens	Moves eyes laterally (out)
VII Facial	Closes eyelids
	Motor and sensory for facial muscles
	Secretion of lacrimal and salivary glands
VIII Acoustic	Hearing; equilibrium
IX Glossopharyngeal	Gag, swallow
	Taste
X Vagus	Muscles of larynx, pharynx, soft palate
	Parasympathetic innervation
XI Spinal accessory	Shoulder shrug
XII Hypoglossal	Moves tongue

DIFFERENTIAL DIAGNOSIS AND MANAGEMENT OF COMMON PEDIATRIC CONDITIONS
Neurologic symptoms

Arnold-Chiari II malformation is a serious, potentially life-threatening malformation that invariably occurs with myelodysplasia. The Arnold-Chiari II malformation may be a clinically silent phenomenon or may cause the catastrophic events of sudden cardiac or respiratory arrest. Arnold-Chiari II malformation compresses and essentially stretches the posterior region of the cerebellum and brainstem downward through the foramen magnum and into the cervical space. Seldom do children show immediate signs at birth but become symptomatic during the first days to weeks of life. In other children manifestations of the condition may not become obvious until 4 to 5 years of age (Caldarelli, DiRocco, and McLone, 1984; Park, Hoffman, and Cail, 1986). The cerebellum is responsible for coordination and balance. Although pressure is exerted on this region by the Arnold-Chiari II malformation, signs and symptoms of cerebellar dysfunction are uncommon (Caldrelli, DiRocco, and McLone, 1984).

The brainstem houses the 12 CNs (Table 21-2). Pressure on this region results in altered function of these vital nerves or actual palsies. Dysfunction of the lower CNs are common. The infant may have apnea, respiratory difficulties, stridor, and the classic barking cough of croup. The practitioner must be cautious not to dismiss these findings as a simple upper respiratory infection but must consider the possibility that these symptoms result from pressure on CNs IX X, and XII. Pressure on these nerves may result in a depressed or absent gag, feeding difficulties, aspiration pneumonia, or symptoms of failure to thrive.

Pressure on the CNs that control eye movements, CNs III, IV, and VI, may result in a mild disconjugate gaze, or esotropia.

A child's subtle complaints (e.g., headache and weakness), changes in the child's condition reported by the parent, or changes assessed by the practitioner necessitate immediate consultation. Treatment is focused on the symptomatic relief of the presenting problems. For example, a gastrostomy tube and tracheostomy may be placed for an absent gag and cough. Surgical decompression of the cervical region is controversial and to date has not been proved a reliable solution (Park, Hoffman, and Cail, 1986).

Tethering of spinal cord

Tethering of the spinal cord may develop in children with myelodysplasia. Symptoms related to this problem may include scoliosis, altered gait pattern, changes in muscle strength and tone at or below the lesion, disturbance in urinary and bowel patterns, and back pain (Schmidt, Robinson, and Jones, 1990). The practitioner should be alert to these findings and refer the child to the neurosurgeon for further evaluation.

Hydrocephalus

The majority of these children will have an internal shunt system to treat hydrocephalus. The differential diagnosis of shunt malfunction or infection must be considered in the presence of fever, GI distress, and headache (see Chapter 17).

Urinary tract infections

Urinary tract infections are common among children with myelodysplasia. Fever associated with UTIs may be mild or severe. Urine specimens by catheterization should be cultured in the presence of persistent fever. The treatment of positive cultures in this population of children may vary. Some urologists recommend treatment using oral or parenteral antibiotic therapy only in the presence of symptoms or urinary reflux. If the child is free of urinary reflux and requires clean intermittent catheterization, an alternative to systemic therapy is to instill a small amount of antibiotic solution into the bladder at the last catheterization of the day (Bauer, 1989).

Children with urinary reflux must be treated systemically. The usual course of treatment is 7 to 10 days with antibiotics appropriate for the cultured organism. Follow-up cultures should be obtained once during the course of treatment and again approximately 1 week after treatment. Prophylactic antibiotics are discontinued during the treatment course. Additional symptoms of UTIs such as abdominal pain, frequency, and burning may be masked because of decreased sensation. Ongoing consultation with the urologist regarding the child's management is necessary.

Fevers

Fever of unknown origin may be the result of an undetected fracture or burn of an insensate extremity. Osteoporosis associated with paralysis, decreased weight bearing, and inactivity, especially after immobilization in a cast, may contribute to the occurrence of fractures (Badell-Ribera, 1985; Molnar and Taft, 1977). The practitioner should carefully inspect the child's skin for swelling, redness, or skin abrasions. Obtaining a complete history from the parents or the older child may assist the practitioner in determining if there has been recent trauma. Treatment is appropriate to the injury. X-ray studies are obtained if a fracture is suspected, and the child is referred to an orthopedist. A plastic surgeon may be consulted to assist in the treatment of burns.

Differential diagnosis should also include shunt infection, shunt malfunction, or urinary tract infection.

Particular consideration to seizure management must be given in the presence of a fever regardless of origin because it may lower the seizure threshold in these children.

Gastrointestinal symptoms

Nausea, vomiting, and diarrhea are common symptoms in the pediatric population. Urinary tract infections may be a cause of GI distress. A child with a neurogenic bowel may develop an impaction, leading to GI distress. The presence of diarrhea may be misleading because liquid stool passes around the impacted stool. An abdominal and rectal examination will aid in determining the possibility of impaction (Elder and Feetham, 1987). Treatment for this condition may include an enema and manual disimpaction.

For the child with a high lesion, the practitioner should consider the possibility of appendicitis as a cause of nausea and vomiting. Pain may be altered because of the decreased sensation in the right lower quadrant. If no other diagnosis is appropriate, referral to a general surgeon is indicated.

DEVELOPMENTAL ISSUES
Safety

There are many issues regarding safety that are particular to the infant and child with myelodysplasia. Because the neurologic system is the primary system involved, parents must be educated to the changes that may occur and may threaten their child's safety. This includes identification of and interventions for potential symptoms of a shunt malfunction (see Chapter 17 and the earlier discussion of Arnold-Chiari II malformation). Also, in children with seizures, parents should be instructed on how to intervene safely and appropriately during a seizure (see Chapter 15).

There is potential for limited cognitive ability and altered judgment in these children. This is an important concept to discuss with parents when they are considering independence issues. Instructions regarding proper use of equipment for mobility such as wheelchairs, braces, and crutches should be appropriate to the child's developmental and cognitive abilities.

The congenital defect affects nerve function at

and below the level of the spine where it is located, which alters mobility and sensation of bone, muscle, and skin tissue. This decreased sensation puts the child at greater risk for injuries such as burns, fractures, and skin breakdown, leading to decubitus ulcers. This risk can be minimized with proper body positioning, frequent position changes, and assurance that adaptive equipment fits properly and is used correctly. Tepid water should be used for bathing to prevent burns. The condition of the child's skin should be monitored at least twice daily for redness and irritation.

Child care

Because of Public Law 99-457, Early Education for Individuals with Exceptional Needs, and Public Law 94-142, Education for all Handicapped Children Act, children with myelodysplasia have the opportunity to benefit from many services including special daycare programs (U.S. Department of Education, 1984). These two public laws, as well as the Supreme Court decision *Tatro v. Irving Independent School District,* provide for rights of handicapped children, including access to public buildings, education, and nursing services within the school setting (Palfrey, Haynie, and Porter, 1989).

The practitioner should be familiar with resources available for referral because early intervention programs for infants will vary from state to state. The preschooler is eligible for placement in public programs that meet his or her physical and educational needs. It is important that the day care or educational setting be notified in advance about a prospective student to allow for education of day-care staff and to facilitate a smooth transition (Palfrey, Haynie, and Porter, 1989).

The child with myelodysplasia and a ventriculoperitoneal shunt may exhibit signs of shunt malfunction while in the care of someone other than a parent. If so, that individual should be aware of the signs and alert the parent or guardian (see Chapter 17). If the child has a history of seizures, the caretaker or school personnel must be informed. Administration of anticonvulsants may be required during day-care hours. Identification of seizure activity and appropriate first-aid intervention should be taught to the care providers (see Chapter 15). Knowledge of the child's specific bladder and bowel program should be communicated. Any pro-

cedures necessary during day-care hours must be taught to the care provider. This is not usually necessary in the programs for children up to 3 years of age unless the child is also in day care. If so, a trained person should perform the procedure.

Many children with myelodysplasia will have adaptive equipment to aid in mobilization, maintain appropriate body alignment, prevent further deformity, and increase independence. The care provider should be aware of proper application and fit of the equipment. It is also important to communicate the child's actual motor and sensory capacity to help prevent injury.

A list of emergency telephone numbers must accompany the child. If possible, the practitioner should be available to answer questions and concerns from child care staff.

Diet

Poor feeding and prolonged feeding time are common presenting symptoms of the Arnold-Chiari II malformation in affected children (Park et al., 1983). In children with severe symptoms, a gastrostomy tube may be required to avoid malnutrition and aspiration (McLaughlin and Shurtleff, 1979).

Infancy is an excellent time to guide and educate the parents regarding feeding and caloric intake. It is important to teach parents early about the dangers of overfeeding, especially the child who is less mobile and therefore has less caloric needs. Avoidance of obesity is a prime consideration in the nutritional needs of these children. Avoiding the pattern of using food as a reward is very important (Colgan, 1981; Elder and Feetham, 1987).

The child's diet should include plenty of fluids to lessen the chance of constipation and the incidence of UTIs. Dietary management is important in controlling the consistency of stools and in avoiding constipation. A diet high in fiber and low in constipating foods is usually recommended. Early nutritional assessment and guidance are an essential part of the care of the child with myelodysplasia.

Discipline

There is increased risk for a child with such a complex chronic condition to experience psychosocial adjustment problems (Wallander, Feldman and Varni, 1989), which may affect the parents and family members' response to discipline. Parental guidance should be provided early in the child's life. The need for discipline, direction, and encouragement of independence should be addressed with all parents and children. Referral for parent counseling may be necessary to assist with particular needs and challenges that may arise (Kazak and Clark, 1986).

Toileting

Mastery of bowel and bladder continence is crucial to optimal functioning and is of major importance for social acceptance (Colgan, 1981). The child's physical abilities and psychologic readiness for toileting should be assessed. Those who are unable to sit independent of adaptive devices or who are unable to master self-dressing skills will need special consideration when toileting is introduced. A physical or occupational therapist should be consulted regarding the use of bars, adaptive seats, and so forth. Special clothing or underwear may be helpful to make access to the perineum easier.

Because of the personal nature of toileting control evident in our society, it is desirable for the child to master self-care methods before he or she enters school. Urinary and fecal incontinence may partly explain the poor social adjustment experienced by many children with myelodysplasia (Shurtleff, 1980). Usually by age 2 to 3 years the concept of toileting should be introduced to the child.

Bowel management should be monitored from birth to avoid constipation and impaction. The goal of bowel management is to develop a regular schedule to avoid impaction or soiling in between bowel movements. This can be accomplished by sitting on the toilet at regular times, taking advantage of the gastrocolic reflex by toileting after meals, and increasing abdominal pressure by methods such as having the child blow up balloons, tickling the child to make him or her laugh, or by placing the child's legs on a stool to increase pressure by hip flexion (Colgan, 1981). The child should assume responsibility for timed evacuation and good perineal care as physical and cognitive development allows. Some children will not be able to assume all care and will require assistance by parents or caretakers.

The use of medicinal aids may be necessary to control the consistency or to aid in evacuation. A number of agents, including stimulants, bulk agents, softeners, and lubricants, are available. Biofeedback and behavior modification techniques have also been used with some success in this population for treatment of fecal incontinence (Wald, 1981; Whitehead et al., 1981).

Remember that each program of management will vary from child to child. A sympathetic manner in working with the child will help to avoid feelings of guilt and blame for unavoidable accidents. Accidents can be reduced with careful attention to diet and timed defecation (Shurtleff, 1980).

If clean intermittent catheterization has not been started for other reasons, it may be started in the 2- to 3-year age group in an attempt to get the child out of diapers when most other children have achieved this milestone (Bauer, 1989). If the child has used a catheter since birth, the concept of using the toilet for the procedure should be initiated at this time. Ideally the procedure is taught to the parents and other individuals involved in the child's direct care. Often, instituting this procedure causes a resurfacing of emotions in parents related to the child's disabilities. Fear of injuring the child, difficulties with genital touching, and frustration with the mechanics of the procedure are common. Psychologic and emotional concerns are usual and must be addressed before the parent can be expected to understand and comply with the recommendations (Jeter, 1983).

In assisting the child, the practitioner must consider the child's developmental level and perception of the procedure. Often, providing the young child with an anatomically correct doll and catheter will help the child master the skill. The goal is to have this task accomplished by early school age. Children with limited cognitive abilities, or poor manual dexterity, or both may require continued assistance. (Hannigan, 1979).

Noncompliance with self-catheterization may become an issue in adolescence when catheterization is used as a focus in the fight for independence.

Clean intermittent catheterization is the most commonly used method to achieve urinary continence. If continence is not attained by catheterization alone, medications may be used in conjunction with the procedure. Continence may also be achieved successfully through use of bladder stimulation and surgical interventions (e.g., artificial urinary sphincter, bladder augmentation, creation of continent stomas, and sling procedure).

Sleep patterns

An infant or child with respiratory compromise symptomatic of the Arnold-Chiari II malformation may experience sleep apnea, increased stridor, and snoring with sleep. These children are at increased risk for sudden respiratory arrest. It is therefore necessary that they wear a cardiac or apnea monitor during sleep. Parents must also be prepared to perform cardiopulmonary resuscitation in the event of an arrest.

Alteration in the child's normal sleep pattern (longer naps, increased frequency of naps) may indicate increased intracranial pressure from a shunt malfunction (see Chapter 17).

A child may need to wear a diaper during sleep despite a successful continence program during waking hours.

School issues

Cognitive deficits are common in children with myelodysplasia. These need to be addressed early in the educational process so that particular needs may be met and adaptations made to minimize educational problems and frustrations by the child's family, and educators (Shurtleff, 1980). Teachers and other educational professionals need medical information to appropriately place the student and to determine the effect the child's impairment may have on his or her educational program (Elder and Feetham, 1987).

All children by law are entitled to attend a school program by age 5 years. Most states have formalized evaluation before placement to assure that appropriate individualized educational plans (IEPs) will be formulated to take care of each child's specific needs, including educational and physical requirements. It is essential that an educational setting be notified about a student with special health care needs well in advance to assure that all necessary needs will be provided (Palfrey, Haynie, and Porter, 1989). Individualized education plans will assist in reaching this goal. The practitioner must advocate for the family in this planning process. Each child's particular needs,

such as catheterization, timed toileting, administration of medications, physical, occupational, and speech therapy, and individual counseling, must be addressed in the IEP. These particular needs may require assistance from a classroom aide.

One must consider the potential cognitive skill deficits in these individuals when planning for educational and vocational directions (Shaffer et al., 1985; Tew and Lawrence, 1975). Frequent absences because of illnesses and hospitalizations may also affect the child's school performance. Open communication among health care providers and educators will help to minimize related problems.

Adaptive equipment may be necessary and is dependent on the child's degree of disability. School personnel should be aware of what adaptive equipment the child has, how it functions, and what to monitor with regard to fit, skin irritation, and so forth. Elevators are also helpful in assisting the child to get to classes in a timely manner and to minimize fatigue. As children age, they may choose to use a wheelchair for mobilization in the school building. This should be viewed as an increase rather than a decrease in independence. Accessibility is important. The school should be free of structural barriers to enable the child to move freely and to participate in all activities. Occasionally special provisions must be made for safe departure from the building in the event of an emergency (e.g., fire) and for transportation to and from home (e.g., wheelchair van or bus).

Children with chronic conditions and physical disabilities are at risk for experiencing adjustment problems (Breslau, 1985; Cadman et al., 1987; Pless and Roghmann, 1971). Children with myelodysplasia often have low self-concepts, lower levels of general happiness, and higher levels of anxiety (Kazak and Clark, 1986). Awareness of these potential problems will be helpful to those working with the child. Appropriate referrals for further psychologic intervention and support may be advised. The practitioner should encourage the child to be involved in extracurricular activities such as Boy or Girl Scouts and sporting activities to enhance their peer relationships, self-concept, and independence (Elder and Feetham, 1987).

Sexuality

Sexuality is a major area of concern for parents and the child with myelodysplasia. Education, information, and an opportunity to address concerns regarding sexuality and reproductive function should be discussed early in the child's life (Colgan, 1981; Elder and Feetham, 1987). Urodynamic studies in the newborn period may help to determine prognosis regarding sexual function (Bauer, 1989). Maximizing urinary and fecal continence, fostering self-concept, and promoting self-care are beneficial to the child in developing a sexual identity (Colgan, 1981).

The usual sources of sexual information available to adolescents may be restricted because of limited mobility and poor peer relationships (Bunch, 1986). The practitioner should provide anticipatory guidance through sexual education with the child and family. The early onset of menses often seen in these girls necessitates early and appropriate education (Elder and Feetham, 1987). They should be referred for routine gynecologic care. Practitioners must consider the potential for problems secondary to decreased sensation such as a clot formation and pelvic infections when selecting birth control methods.

In general, females are capable of normal sexual function inclusive of orgasm. If a female has severe spinal deformities or complex urologic problems, she may be at risk for complications during pregnancy (McLaughlin and Shurtleff, 1979). Genetic and family planning counseling should be available to these individuals and encouraged by the practitioner.

In males, the level of the lesion will predict the capacity for erection and ejaculation. Because this functional ability will vary among individuals, the reproductive potential is much less predictable than in females (Elder and Feetham, 1987; Shurtleff, 1980). It is difficult to make a definite evaluation before puberty. Males fathering children is a pos-

sibility but is less likely than females achieving pregnancy. A history of erections and ejaculations is an important part of the sexual history in males. Penile implants or collection of sperm by electrical stimulation may be indicated for this population (Elder and Feetham, 1987; Shurtleff, 1980). Technologic advances may offer more possibilities in the future.

SPECIAL FAMILY CONCERNS

These families suffer chronic grief for the "loss of the normal child" at birth. This is expressed repeatedly as the child fails to achieve developmental milestones with growth. Particular to this condition is the profound motor involvement. Their child may never walk or run. Their child may never achieve independence with bowel and bladder control or continence (Elder and Feetham, 1987).

The risk of sudden death because of a shunt malfunction or the Arnold-Chiari II malformation is a chronic and intense stress on the family system. This, in addition to the other complex needs of these children, often results in families becoming overprotective. Families may be hesitant or fearful of allowing others to care for their child because of their special needs. Parents should be encouraged to participate in activities outside the home independent of their children and to seek respite care if other caretakers are not available (Breslau, Staruch, and Mortimer, 1982; Elder and Feetham, 1987).

The multisystem involvement of this condition requires frequent hospitalizations, surgeries, outpatient services, and multidisciplinary care. These factors, in addition to the special equipment, medications, and so forth that may be needed by these children, place a tremendous financial burden on parents. Social service involvement with these families is crucial in providing guidance and support.

SUMMARY OF PRIMARY CARE NEEDS FOR THE CHILD WITH MYELODYSPLASIA

Growth and development

Obesity is common.

Head size may be enlarged if the child has hydrocephalus; the head should be measured at each visit.

Motor delays are common.

Both precocious puberty and short stature are reported.

Immunizations

Repeated hospitalization may interrupt immunization schedule.

Pertussis vaccine may be deferred in infants with seizures.

Measles vaccine may cause seizures in children with seizure disorders but is recommended because of the prevalence of the disease.

Hib vaccination is critical to prevent Haemophilus influenzae type b meningitis.

Screening
Vision

There is a high incidence of visual defects such as ocular palsies, astigmatism, and visual perceptual deficits. Referral to ophthalmologist during infancy is recommended.

Hearing

Routine screening is recommended. The child may have hypersensitivity to loud noises if a shunt has been placed. If the child is exposed to aminoglycosides, hearing should be evaluated by an audiologist.

Dental

Routine screening is recommended. If shunted for hydrocephalus, will need penicillin prophylaxis prior to dental work.

Blood pressure

Routine monitoring is recommended. Children with renal problems may develop hypertension and should be monitored more frequently.

Hematocrit

Routine screening is recommended.

Urinalysis

Baseline urinalysis and cultures should be obtained in the newborn period.

Bladder catheterization is recommended for obtaining cultures.

Tuberculosis

Routine screening is recommended.

Condition-specific screening
  Blood tests

Complete blood cell counts should be obtained frequently if these children are treated with sulfonamides, and serum creatinine clearance should be obtained to monitor renal function. These tests should be done on newborns and then done yearly.
  Scoliosis

Screening for scoliosis should be done yearly from birth through adolescence.

Drug interactions

Medications given routinely include antibiotics, anticholinergics, sympathomimetics, stool softeners, and anticonvulsants. Alterations in drug therapy may be necessary when infections, common colds, and GI symptoms are treated.

Differential diagnosis
Respiratory difficulties, stridor, and croupy cough

Rule out Arnold-Chiari II malformation.

Scoliosis, altered gait pattern, changes in muscular strength and tone, disturbance in urinary and bowel patterns, and back pain

Rule out a tethered cord.

Headaches

Rule out shunt malfunction.

Gastrointestinal symptoms

Rule out increased intracranial pressure with nausea and vomiting. Check for UTI.

Fevers

Rule out shunt or CNS infection, UTI, and fracture or injury of insensate extremity.

Continued.

◆ ▬▬▬▬▬▬▬▬ ◆

SUMMARY OF PRIMARY CARE NEEDS FOR THE CHILD WITH MYELODYSPLASIA — cont'd

Developmental issues

Safety

Recommend education on emergency care with seizures.

These children have an increased risk of injury because of decreased sensation and mobility.

Recommend proper body positioning, frequent position changes, and proper fit of adaptive equipment.

Child care

Special medical needs may be a factor with severe physical involvement.

Early intervention programs for infants and toddlers available through PL 99-451.

Diet

Evaluate regurgitation, vomiting, and difficulties with gag reflex for increased intracranial pressure and Arnold-Chiari II malformation.

Monitor caloric intake to minimize the potential for obesity.

Diet should include increased fluids to lessen the chance of constipation and UTIs.

Discipline

There is an increased risk of psychosocial adjustment problems. Children need discipline and encouragement toward independence.

Toileting

Delayed bowel and bladder training may occur because of neurologic deficit.

Encourage independence when it is developmentally and physically appropriate.

Bowel regimens will vary.

Intermittent catheterization is common; compliance may be an issue during adolescence.

Sleep patterns

Apnea, increased stridor, and snoring may occur in the child with symptomatic Arnold-Chiari II malformation.

Lethargy may indicate increased intracranial pressure.

School issues

Associated problems may be covered by Public Law 94-142.

Assist families in IEP hearings.

Children may have adjustment problems.

Psychometric testing may be needed.

Special provisions for adaptive equipment, transportation, and accessibility may be necessary.

Special physical needs must be tended to during school hours.

Sexuality

Precocious puberty may occur.

Sexual functioning may be altered because of neurologic deficit.

Genetic counseling is necessary.

Special family concerns

Special family concerns include chronic grief for loss of a "normal" child; the possibility of brain damage because of shunt failure or infection; stress related to frequent hospitalizations, surgeries, and the need for multidisciplinary care; and financial burden.

RESOURCES

The health care system can provide an empathetic response to the multiple needs of children with myelodysplasia and their families by offering physical, emotional, and social care, but no one understands or feels the problems these children and families face in their day-to-day lives as well as another child or family with the same disorder. For this reason support groups and efforts to provide a network of support within the community have proved to be a major factor in coping and adaptation for these families (Wallander and Varni, 1989). A list of some of the organizations that offer such support follows. Each region has its own community-based network or local chapter. It is important for the practitioner to be aware of available local resources.

Organizations

Spina Bifida Association of America
1700 Rockville Pike, Suite 540
Rockville, MD 20852
(301) 770-SBAA or (800) 621-3141

Arnold-Chiari Family Network
c/o Kevin and Maureen Walsh
67 Spring St
Weymouth, MA 02188

REFERENCES

American Association of Neuroscience Nurses: *Core curriculum for neuroscience nursing,* ed 2, Park Ridge, Ill, 1984, The Association.

Badell-Ribera A: Myelodysplasia: In Molnar G, ed: *Pediatric rehabilitation,* Baltimore, 1985, Williams & Wilkins, pp 176-206.

Bartoshesky LE, Young GJ, and Scott RM: Outcomes of children with myelomeningocele treated aggressively from birth. In McLaurin RL ed: *Spina bifida. A multidisciplinary approach,* New York, 1986, Praeger, pp 14-20.

Bauer SB: Urologic management of the myelodysplastic child. In Webster G and Galloway N, eds: *Problems in urology,* Philadelphia, 1989, JB Lippincott, pp 86-101.

Breslau N: Psychiatric disorder in children with physical disability, *J Am Acad Child Psychiatry* 24:87-94, 1985.

Breslau N, Staruch KS, and Mortimer EA: Psychological distress in mothers of disabled children, *Am J Disabled Child* 136:682-686, 1982.

Bunch W: Myelomeningocele. In Lovell WW and Winter RB eds: *Pediatric orthopaedics,* ed 2, Philadelphia, 1986, JB Lippincott, vol I, pp 402-403.

Cadman D, Boyle M, Szartmari P, et al: Chronic illness, disability and mental and social well-being: Findings of the Ontario child health study, *Pediatrics* 79:805-813, 1987.

Caldarelli M, DiRocco C, and McLone DG: Chiari II malformation: Clinical manifestations and indications for decompression. In McLaurin RL, ed: *Spina bifida. A multidisciplinary approach.* New York, 1986, Praeger Press, pp 174-181.

Charney EB, Weller SC, Sutton LN, et al: Management of the newborn with myelomeningocele: Time for a decision-making process, *Pediatrics* 75:58-64, 1985.

Colgan MT: The child with spina bifida, *Am J Disabled Child* 135:854-858, 1981.

Elder DS and Feetham SL: Patterns of impairment: Myelomeningocele. In Rose MH and Thomas RB eds: *Children with chronic conditions: Nursing in a family and community context,* Orlando, Fla, 1987, Grune & Stratton.

Feiwell E: Surgery of the hip in myelomeningocele as related to adult goals, *Clin Orthop* 148:87-93, 1980.

Gross RH, Cox A, Tatyrek R, et al: Early management and decision making for the treatment of myelomeningocele, *Pediatrics* 72:450-458, 1983.

Hannigan KF: Teaching intermittent self-catheterization to young children with myelodysplasia, *Dev Med Child Neurol* 21:365-368, 1979.

Hobbins JC: Diagnosis and management of neural-tube defects today, *N Engl J Med* 324 (10):690-691, 1991.

Hogge WA, Thiagarajah S, Ferguson JE, et al: The role of ultrasonography and amniocentesis in the evaluation of pregnancies at risk for neural tube defects, *Am J Obstet Gynecol* 161:520-523, 1989.

Huff CW and Ramsey PW: Myelodysplasia: The influence of the quadriceps and hip abductor muscles on ambulatory function and stability of the hip, *J Bone Joint Surg* 60:432-443, 1978.

Humphreys RP: Tethering: Theories of development and pathophysiology. In McLaurin RL, ed: *Spina bifida. A multidisciplinary approach,* New York, 1986, Praeger, pp 215-220.

Jeter K: Psychosocial issues in cic, urinary diversion and undiversion, *Dialog Pediatr Urol* 6:1-8, 1983.

Kazak AE and Clark MW: Stress in families of children with myelomeningocele, *Dev Med Child Neurol* 28:220-228, 1986.

Kirulata HG, Gillingham D, and Squires D: *Long-term cotrimoxazole prophylaxis in spina bifida: effects on folic acid.* Paper presented at the annual meeting of the Urology Section of the American Academy of Pediatrics, Washington, DC, October 1986.

Lemire RJ: Causes of neural tube defects. In McLaurin RL, ed: *Spina bifida. A multidisciplinary approach.* New York, 1986a, Praeger, pp 2-7.

Lemire RJ: Developmental pathology of meningomyelocele. In McLaurin RL, ed: *Spina bifida. A multidisciplinary approach,* New York, 1986b, Praeger, pp 114-118.

Leonard CO: Serum AFP screening for neural tube defects, *Clin Obstet Gynecol* 24:1121-1132, 1981.

Luthy DA, Wardinsky T, Shurtleff DB, et al: Cesarean section before the onset of labor and subsequent motor function in infants with meningomyelocele diagnosed internally, N Engl J Med 324(10)662-666, 1991.

Macri JN, Baker DA, and Baim RS: Diagnosis of neural tube defects by evaluation of amniotic fluid, *Clin Obstet Gynecol* 24:1089-1102, 1981.

McCullough DC: Theories of development of the Arnold-Chiari malformation. In McLaurin RL, ed: *Spina bifida. A multidisciplinary approach.* New York, 1986, Praeger, pp 159-163.

McLaughlin JF and Shurtleff DB: Management of the newborn with myelodysplasia, *Clin Pediatr* 8:463-480, 1979.

McLaurin RL: Technique of myelomeningocele repair. In

McLaurin RL, ed: *Spina bifida. A multidisciplinary approach,* New York, 1986, Praeger, pp 134-139.

McLone DG, Czyzewski D, Raimondi AJ, et al: Central nervous system infections as a limiting factor in the intelligence of children with myelomeningocele, *Pediatrics* 70:338-342, 1982.

McLone DG and Naidich TP: The embryology of dysraphism. In McLaurin RL, ed: *Spina bifida. A multidisciplinary approach,* New York, 1986, Praeger, pp 101-109.

McLone DG and Naidich TP: Myelomeningocele. In Hoffman HJ and Epstein F, eds: *Disorders of the developing nervous system: Diagnosis and treatment,* Boston, 1986, Blackwell Scientific Publications.

Milunsky A, Jick H, Jick SS, et al: Multivitamin/folic acid supplementation in early pregnancy reduces the prevalence of neural tube defects, *JAMA* 24:2847-2852, 1989.

Molnar GE and Taft LT: Pediatric rehabilitation: II. Spina bifida and limb deficiencies, *Curr Probl Pediatr* 7:3, 1977.

Moore K: *The developing human,* Philadelphia, 1987, JB Lippincott.

Palfrey JS, Haynie M, and Porter SM: *Children assisted by medical technology in educational settings: Guidelines for care,* Boston, 1989, Children's Hospital, pp 13-14.

Park TS, Cail WS, Maggio WM, et al: Progressive spasticity and scoliosis in children with myelomeningocele, *J Neurosurg* 62:367-375, 1985.

Park TS, Hoffman HJ, and Cail WS: Arnold-Chiari malformation, manifestations and management, *Neurosurgery State Art Rev* 1:81-99, 1986.

Park TS, Hoffman HJ, Hendrick B, et al: Experience with surgical decompression of the Arnold Chiari malformation in young infants with myelomeningocele, *Neurosurgery* 13:147-152, 1983.

Physician's Desk Reference, ed 44, Oradell, NJ, 1990, ER Barnhart.

Pless IB and Roghmann KJ: Chronic illness and its consequences: Observations based on three epidemiological surveys, *J Pediatr* 79:351-359, 1971.

Rosa FW: Spina bifida in children of women treated with carbamazepine during pregnancy, *N Engl J Med* 324(10):674-677, 1991.

Shaffer J, Friedrich WN, Shurtleff DB, et al: Cognitive and achievement status of children with myelomeningocele, *J Pediatr Psychol* 10:325-336, 1985.

Shaul PW, Towbin RB, and Chernausek SD: Precocious puberty following severe head trauma, *Am J Dis Child* 139:467-469, 1985.

Shurtleff D: Myelodysplasia: Management and treatment, *Curr Probl Pediatr* X:7-98, 1980.

Slater JE: Rubber anaphylaxis, *N Engl J Med* 320:1126-1129, 1989.

Soare PL and Raimondi AJ: Intellectual and perceptual-motor characteristics of treated myelomeningocele children, *Am J Dis Child* 131:199-204, 1977.

Sugar EC: The neurogenic bladder in the child with myelomeningocele: Neurophysiology and treatment using intermittent catheterization. In McLaurin RL, ed: *Spina bifida. A multidisciplinary approach,* New York, 1986, Praeger, pp 70-83.

Tappit-Emas E: Spina bifida. In Tecklin J, ed: *Pediatric physical therapy,* Philadelphia, 1989, JB Lippincott, pp 106-140.

Tew B and Lawrence KM: The effects of hydrocephalus on intelligence, visual perception and school attainment, *Dev Med Child Neurol* 35:129-134, 1975.

US Department of Education: (1984). *To assure the free appropriate public education for all handicapped children: Seventh annual report to Congress in the implementation of the Education of the Handicapped Act,* Washington DC, 1984, US Government Printing Office.

Venes JL and McGuire: Progressive urological dysfunction in the child with repaired meningomyelocele: A reversible sequelae of cord tethering. In McLaurin RL, ed: *Spina bifida. A multidisciplinary approach,* New York, 1986, Praeger, pp 62-69.

Wald A: Use of biofeedback in treatment of fecal incontinence in patients with meningomyelocele, *Pediatrics* 68:45-49, 1981.

Wallander JL, Feldman WS and Varni JW: Physical status and psychosocial adjustment in children with spina bifida, *J Pediatr Psychol* 14:89-102, 1989.

Wallander JL and Varni JW: Social support and adjustment in chronically ill and handicapped children, *Am J Community Psychol* 17:185-201, 1989.

Warkany J and Lemire RJ: Pathogenesis of neural tube defects. In Hoffman HJ and Epstein F, eds: *Disorders of the developing nervous system: Diagnosis and treatment,* Boston, 1986, Blackwell Scientific Publications, pp 21-33.

Whitehead WE, Parker LH, Masek BJ, et al: Biofeedback treatment of fecal incontinence in patients with myelomeningocele, *Dev Med Child Neurol* 23:313-322, 1981.

22 *Organ Transplants*

Beverly Corbo-Richert and *Karen E. Zamberlan*

ETIOLOGY

Organ transplantation is a complex surgical procedure performed in children with life-threatening conditions as a result of failure of a particular organ. The three most prevalent organ transplant procedures available for children are renal, liver, and heart replacement. A summary of the diseases and conditions that lead to end-stage organ failure in children is listed in Table 22-1.

Graft rejection has been a major obstacle to successful organ transplantation. Conventional regimens for immune suppression relied on azathioprine (Imuran), prednisone (Deltasone), and rabbit antithymocyte globulin (RATG; Atgam) or Minnesota antilymphocyte globulin (MALG). The introduction of the immunosuppressive drug cyclosporine (Sandimmune) in 1978 (Calne et al., 1978) resulted in improved survival rates and consequently increased interest in transplantation. However, complications of the drug have encouraged continued efforts toward discovery of better immunosuppressive agents.

Renal transplants

The first successful pediatric renal transplantations were performed in the early 1960s. The most common diagnosis requiring transplantation was chronic glomerulonephritis (Starzl et al., 1966). The procedure became more prevalent in the late 1960s and early 1970s with the 1-year survival rate for those with live related donor renal transplants of 87% and 42% for those with cadaveric donor transplants (Fine et al., 1970).

Liver transplants

After many years of animal research, experimentation with human liver orthotopic (replacement of an organ in its normal position) transplantation began in the early 1960s with both adults and children. In 1963, the first pediatric liver transplantation was performed on a 3-year-old child with extrahepatic biliary atresia; however, the child died as a result of hemorrhage on the operative day (Starzl et al., 1982). In 1967, the first child who experienced extended survival after a liver transplantation was a 1½-year-old girl with hepatocellular carcinoma who lived for 13 months (Starzl et al., 1982). In the 1960s the 1-year survival rate for children was 34% (Starzl et al., 1979). Research efforts to improve procurement and surgical techniques and preservation of donor organs both were in part responsible for the improved survival currently experienced by recipients in the period between 1980 and 1990.

Heart transplants

Heart transplantation in humans also began in the 1960s. A significant breakthrough was the development of successful orthotopic surgical techniques involving the removal of the recipient's ventricles, leaving the posterior atrial walls and the ridge of the interatrial septum intact (Lower and Shumway,

Table 22-1. Comparative indications for transplantation in children by organ*

Renal	Liver	Heart	Dual transplants
Congenital disease	Cholestatic disease	Cardiomyopathy	Heart and liver
Renal hypoplasia	Biliary atresia	Dilated	Familial hypercholester-
Renal dysplasia	Familial cholestasis	Hypertrophic	olemia with isch-
Obstructive uropathy	Alagille's syndrome	Restrictive	emic cardiomyopa-
Acquired disease	Byler's syndrome	Congenital heart	thy
Glomerulonephritis	Parenchymal disease	defects (se-	Intrahepatic biliary
Hereditary disease	Budd-Chiari syndrome	lect lesions)	atresia and dilated
Alport syndrome	Congenital hepatic fibrosis		cardiomyopathy
Juvenile nephro-	Cystic fibrosis		Liver and kidney
phthisis	Neonatal hepatitis		Cystinosis
Metabolic disorders	Acute fulminant hepatic failure		Oxalosis
Cystinosis	Non-A, Non-B hepatitis		Heart and lung
Oxalosis	Metabolic disorders		Primary pulmonary hy-
	α_1-antitrypsin deficiency		pertension
	Wilson's disease		Congenital heart defects
	Glycogen storage disease, type		with elevated pul-
	IV		monary vascular re-
	Tyrosinemia		sistance

*These are a few of the more common conditions leading to end-stage organ failure; the list is not all inclusive.

1960). The first pediatric heart transplantation was performed on an 18-day-old infant with Ebstein's anomaly who died 6 hours later from complications (Kantrowitz et al., 1968). The 1-year survival rate of people receiving heart transplants improved from 22% in 1968 to 88% in 1982 (Jamieson et al., 1984).

Dual-organ transplants

Dual-organ transplantations involve the replacement of a combination of organs such as heart-liver, heart-lung, or liver-kidney. The first heart-lung transplantation was attempted on a 2-month-old-girl with atrioventricular canal defect whose condition was terminal. Although the child survived the surgery, she died 14 hours later of pulmonary insufficiency (Cooley et al., 1969). The most common indications for heart-lung transplants are primary pulmonary hypertension and congenital heart defects associated with irreversible pulmonary hypertension (Heck, Shumway, and Kaye, 1989). The first successful pediatric heart-liver transplantation was performed in 1983 on a 6-year-old girl with ischemic cardiomyopathy secondary

to familial hypercholesterolemia. This girl subsequently underwent a retransplantation of the liver in 1990 for rejection; however, 9 months later she succumbed to rejection of the heart.

INCIDENCE

The incidence of end-stage renal disease in children is estimated at 3 to 6 children per 1 million total population, with a prevalence of chronic renal failure estimated at 18.5 per 1 million child population (Fine, 1990). Primary glomerular disease is the most prevalent cause of chronic renal failure in children (Fine, Salusky, and Ettenger, 1987).

Approximately 300 children per year await liver transplants in the United States. The incidence varies according to the specific liver disease. The incidence of the most commonly occurring liver diseases are 1 per 10,000 per live births for biliary atresia and 0.02% to 0.06% of newborns for α_1-antitrypsin deficiency (Paradis, Freese, and Sharp, 1988).

The incidence of cardiomyopathy in children less than 15 years of age is approximately 39 per 1 million population in the United States annually

Table 22-2. Comparative clinical manifestations of end-stage renal, liver, and heart disease in children*

Renal	Liver	Heart
Electrolyte abnormalities	Jaundice	Respiratory distress
Sodium retention	Ascites	Tachypnea
Hyperkalemia	Hepatomegaly	Congestive heart failure
Hypokalemia	Splenomegaly	Cardiomegaly
Metabolic acidosis	Portal hypertension	ST- and T-wave abnormalities
Hyperglycemia	Hypercholesterolemia	Cardiac murmurs
Hyperlipidemia	Hyperammonemia	Growth retardation
Anemia	Hypoalbuminemia	Arrhythmias
Congestive heart failure or pericarditis	Hypoglycemia	
Peripheral neuropathy	Prolonged prothrombin time	
Renal osteodystrophy	Hormone imbalance	
Growth retardation	Encephalopathy	

*These are a few of the more common manifestations; they are not all inclusive.

(Gillum, 1986). Congenital heart disease occurs in approximately 1% of all newborns (Fyler and Nadas, 1989); however, only a small percentage of these children would be potential candidates for heart or heart-lung transplants (Penkoske et al., 1984).

According to the United Network for Organ Sharing (UNOS), the number of children 16 years of age or less on the waiting list as of April 1991 were (1) 514 children awaiting renal transplants, (2) 240 children awaiting liver transplants, and (3) 74 children awaiting heart transplants, 11 awaiting heart-lung transplants, and 14 awaiting lung transplants (Benenson, 1991). Because children's organs are so scarce, approximately 20% of children listed for organ transplants die before a suitable donor organ has been obtained.

CLINICAL MANIFESTATIONS

The presenting symptoms of children experiencing end-stage organ failure vary according to the affected organ and to the specific disease. The severity of the symptoms is contingent on the particular disease, the age of the child at the time of diagnosis, medical management, and the individual response of the child to treatment. Table 22-2 presents the comparative clinical manifestations of end-stage organ disease in children.

Renal disease

Children who have undergone transplantation for any of the indications listed in the renal column of Table 22-1 may have experienced many of the clinical manifestations of chronic renal failure. However, because of the availability of dialysis, the urgent need for transplantation may be delayed and the child sustained until a donor kidney becomes available. Manifestations of chronic renal failure are discussed in Chapter 27.

Liver disease

Children with liver disease may have serious clinical manifestations. The condition can be acute or chronic, and depending on the specific disease etiology, the symptoms will vary. The more common manifestations of a failing liver for children with congenital biliary atresia are jaundice, hepatomegaly, splenomegaly, ascites, recurrent spontaneous bacterial peritonitis, cutaneous xanthomas with pruritus, and a history of variceal bleeding (Altman and Levy, 1985) (Fig. 22-1). Other chronic congenital or hereditary liver disease in children can result in delayed growth, malnutrition, rickets or fractures, coagulopathies, and encephalopathy.

Acute end-stage liver disease caused by fulminant failure or acute hepatitis may be insidious in onset, with rapid progression of the clinical course in children over a few days to a few months.

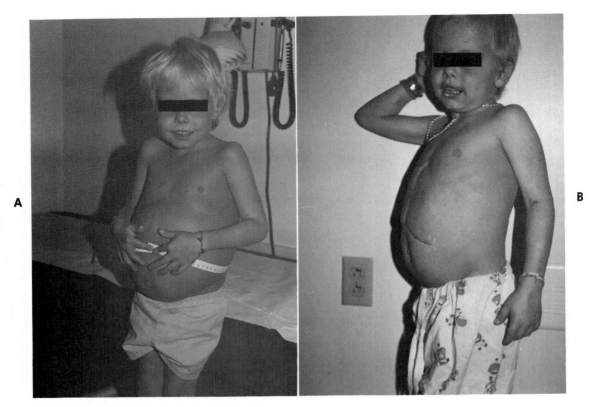

Fig. 22-1. **A,** Boy, four and a half years old, with biliary cirrhosis of unknown etiology at clinic evaluation for liver transplant. **B,** Same boy, follow-up clinic visit, 3 months after liver transplant.

It is characterized by rapidly increased jaundice, shrinkage of the liver, fetor hepaticus, coagulopathy, renal failure, hepatic encephalopathy, and eventual coma or death (Iwatsuki et al., 1989). Chronic liver disease may progress more slowly, with symptoms appearing gradually over a period of several months. Transplantation is clearly indicated if the child has demonstrated any life-threatening complications such as bleeding, recurrent encephalopathy, coagulopathy, malnutrition, deep jaundice, profound growth and development retardation, or metabolic bone disease (Shaw et al., 1988). Liver transplantation may also be indicated for children who have primary unresectable tumors of the liver without metastases.

Heart disease

Clinical manifestations of cardiac disease resulting from congenital heart defects, including the signs and symptoms of congestive heart failure, are addressed in Chapter 11. The clinical manifestations and long-term outcome of children with cardiomyopathies have been described in several retrospective studies (Greenwood, Nadas, and Fyler, 1976; Griffin et al., 1988; Maron and Roberts, 1981; Taliercio et al., 1985). Of a total of 235 children with dilated cardiomyopathy or "primary myocardial disease" described in the previous studies, the most common manifestations included symptoms of congestive heart failure, specifically respiratory distress (Greenwood, Nadas, and Fyler,

1976; Griffin et al., 1988). Other common clinical signs included cardiomegaly on chest radiograph, cardiac murmurs up to grade 3/6 intensity, and ST- and T-wave changes on electrocardiograph. In one study (Taliercio et al., 1985), about one half the children had symptoms of congestive heart failure within 3 months of experiencing a nonspecific febrile illness (thought to be viral). Of the 235 children, nearly one half died, about one third had chronic symptoms, and about one fourth recovered.

The clinical manifestation of hypertrophic cardiomyopathy varies somewhat from the dilated cardiomyopathies. One retrospective study (Maron and Roberts, 1981) of 7 infants and 35 children with hypertrophic cardiomyopathy revealed that all infants and most children had signs of congestive heart failure, often with systolic ejection murmurs and electrocardiographic abnormalities; however, all infants had cardiomegaly, whereas only about one third of the children had cardiomegaly. Initially one half of the children had symptoms only with excessive exertion, a few had symptoms with minimal exertion, and one third were asymptomatic. During follow-up, nearly one half of the children improved or remained stable, one fourth deteriorated, and about one third died; however, all of the infants died. The authors concluded that premature sudden death may occur at any age, in either sex and regardless of whether or not symptoms of cardiac dysfunction have been present (Maron and Roberts, 1981). The majority of children discovered to have hypertrophic cardiomyopathy outside of infancy do not have prominent cardiac symptoms. Despite this they are at considerable risk for sudden death, with a 50% 10-year survival in one extensive study (McKenna et al., 1988).

TREATMENT
Medical management

In chronic renal failure the use of continuous ambulatory peritoneal dialysis or hemodialysis should be considered if the glomerular filtration rate approaches 5 ml/min per 1.73 m^2 (Fine, 1990). The indications for initiating dialysis in an infant, child, or adolescent with chronic renal failure vary and are contingent on the clinical status of the child (see Chapter 27). Dialysis is an expedient therapy

to maintain life until successful transplantation can be accomplished.

Children with chronic liver disease may be managed at home with attention to liver enzymes, supplemental nutrition support from hyperalimentation or enteral feedings, and medical management of complications of the liver disease (e.g., hemorrhage, ascites, rickets, and malabsorption of fat-soluble vitamins). If the child's condition worsens, stabilization may be achieved by hospitalization, followed by urgent transplantation of an available organ.

Portal hypertension, which often develops with biliary atresia, may require sclerotherapy or vasopressors to control bleeding from esophageal varices and hypersplenism. If there is a sudden decrease in the hematocrit level, the child should be hospitalized and an endoscopy performed to rule out gastrointestinal (GI) bleeding. Esophageal endosclerosis is accomplished by the injection of a sclerosant, usually 5% sodium morrhuate, into the distal esophageal varices. Some centers are presently investigating the use of elastic ligature of varices with reportedly good results (Wanek et al, 1989). If endoscopy is not possible, the careful introduction of a Sengstaken-Blakemore tube to decompress varices may be used. Vasopressin (Pitressin) administered intravenously may aid in prevention of hemorrhage by reducing the portal and mesenteric blood flow. The Kasai operation for biliary atresia establishes biliary drainage and may offer an option before liver transplantation.

Cholangitis caused by biliary stasis and bacterial contamination is a frequent complication for children with biliary atresia. Any fever (temperature >38° C), elevation of white blood cell count, increase in serum bilirubin concentration, and positive blood cultures may indicate its presence. Wanek and colleagues (1989) suggest the use of third-generation cephalosporins and aminoglycosides intravenously because of the difficulty in identifying the causative organism of cholangitis.

Children with cardiomyopathy may be managed medically. Therapy ranges from pharmacological treatment of heart failure to cardiac transplantation when drug therapy is no longer effective (Stevenson and Perloff, 1988). Digoxin (Lanoxin) and diuretics continue to be the hallmarks of treatment for the dilated cardiomyopathies (Greenwood et al., 1976; Stevenson and Perloff, 1988; Taliercio et al., 1985).

Treatment for hypertrophic cardiomyopathy includes surgery for severe left ventricular outflow tract obstruction and medication such as β-blockers, calcium channel blockers, and occasionally antiarrhythmics. However, although symptomatic relief may be obtained, it has not been shown to prevent sudden death.

Evaluation for transplantation

Evaluation for organ transplantation involves a multidisciplinary approach. Many institutions involve members from nursing, neurology, psychiatry, physical therapy, dentistry, and social service in the evaluation process, as well as the specialty medical services. Whenever possible, the evaluation is completed on an outpatient basis over a 2 to 3-day period (Corbo-Richert and Zamberlan, 1988). In children who have more advanced disease, hospitalization may be indicated for the evaluation and continued until a donor can be found.

The primary care provider has an important role in the evaluation process. Continuity of care encompassing psychosocial aspects and family preparation for the evaluation can be facilitated by the referring primary care provider. The provider's awareness of the phases of adjustment to the possible transplant will afford anticipation of the family's reactions (Corbo and Dunn, 1987; Watts et al., 1984). The provider is in an optimal position to assess the child and family's previous illness and hospital experiences, life stressors, coping abilities, and level of knowledge and communicate such information to the transplant center staff. This knowledge equips the hospital staff to best explain the transplant process to the child on an appropriate developmental level and to the family in the context of their life experiences. The provider might encourage both parents or parent and significant other to attend the evaluation session so that two adults may hear the information together. If it is not possible for at least two adults to attend, one parent may tape record the sessions for the absent partner, thus including them and also allowing for further reflection on the information. Regardless, parents are encouraged to bring note pads and pencils to take notes and record their own thoughts and questions.

When children are evaluated as transplant candidates, there are almost no exclusion criteria (Lum, Wassner, and Martin, 1985; Staschak and Zamberlan, 1990; Zuberbuhler, Fricker, and Griffith, 1989). Each child is evaluated on an individual basis, and the child's suitability for the particular organ is weighed against the presence of other ongoing problems. Multiple diagnostic tests, cultures (blood, urine, and secretions), blood work evaluation, and radiologic examinations may assist in the evaluation of the child for transplant candidacy.

All children who are transplant candidates should be screened for prior exposure to cytomegalovirus (CMV), *Toxoplasma,* and Epstein-Barr virus (Addonizio and Rose, 1987; Fricker et al., 1987). Screening for tuberculosis and varicella has also been advocated (Addonizio and Rose, 1987). Epstein-Barr screening is performed because it has been associated with the development of lymphoma after transplantation (Hanto et al., 1981). Hepatitis and HIV screens are completed before the transplantation. In certain circumstances attempts may be made to match donors and recipients according to CMV and *Toxoplasma* status. Without such matching these organisms could seriously infect recipients who have not been previously exposed (Addonizio and Rose, 1987).

Donor matching for heart and liver transplantation is primarily by ABO blood type and body size; time constraints and limited donor viability preclude human leukocyte antigen (HLA) matching with the donor except for renal transplants. However, pretransplant screening of all child candidates includes HLA tissue typing, cytotoxic antibody cross-match compatibility, and ABO blood typing, in addition to percent panel reactive antibody (PRA). Percent panel reactive antibody is determined by having the recipient's serum react with normal human lymphocytes and reveals whether a recipient has developed antibody to histocompatible antigens. A PRA of 0% indicates that the recipient has not been previously sensitized, the ideal situation for transplantation (Fricker et al., 1987).

PROGNOSIS
Survival statistics

Although the overall prognosis varies depending on the particular organ that is transplanted, the survival outcomes have improved dramatically for children needing renal, liver, or heart transplants.

Improvements in pediatric renal transplantation and dialysis procedures are contributing factors to the excellent physical survival for children with end-stage renal disease. Current 1-year survival rates reported by one major program parallels national trends, with survival of cadaveric kidney transplants at 75% to 85% and living-related donor transplants at 90% to 95% (So et al., 1986).

In one of the major centers for pediatric liver transplantation, there have been approximately 700 primary transplantations performed from May 1981 through December 1990, with the overall 5-year survival rate ranging from 65% to 80% (Gordon et al., 1991). With the recent development of the experimental immunosuppressive agent FK 506 (see discussion on pp. 395-397), the 6-month survival rate for 40 children after liver transplantation is 94.7% (Reyes, 1991).

Prognosis for children with cardiomyopathy is uncertain; the 1-year survival range is 40% to 80% and the 5-year range is 20% to 70% in varied populations (Griffin et al., 1988). Thus, many of these children are candidates for heart transplants. From 1980 to 1989, The International Heart Registry reported that more than 900 children up to age 19 years received heart transplants. The 5-year actuarial survival for all (orthotopic) heart transplant patients is 72%, while the 5-year survival in pediatric recipients is 62%. One-year survival for children older than 1 year is 76% and for children less than 1 year is 66% (Kriett and Kaye, 1990).

One center, where cardiac transplantation in infancy is the specialty, recently reported that 21 of 25 infants (84%) who had transplantations in the past 3 years are alive (Boucek et al., 1990). The most common diagnosis in this group was hypoplastic left heart syndrome.

As survival statistics and prognosis improve for children undergoing organ trasnplantation, the quality of the survival is coming under closer scrutiny by health care providers. Children who have undergone renal transplantation have experienced improvement in growth, development, and lifestyle (Ildstad et al., 1990; Potter et al., 1986; So et al., 1985).

The majority of children with heart transplants

attend school, participate in sports (Pennington, Sarafin, and Swartz, 1985) and have improved peer and family relationships, self-care, and exercise tolerance (Lawrence and Fricker, 1987). Preliminary reports of 21 children who received heart transplants in infancy revealed normal developmental and neurologic status in nearly all infants (Boucek et al., 1990).

Several quality of life studies of children who have had liver transplantations have been conducted (Kosmach, 1990; Zamberlan, 1989; Zitelli et al., 1988). As many as 5 years later, Zitelli and coworkers (1988) documented objective life-style changes in 65 children who had improved from pretransplant status. Zamberlan assessed 20 school-aged children 3 to 6 years after liver transplantation. Although the children perceived their quality of life to be good to excellent, they related negative changes and feelings about physical appearance, expressed feelings of insecurity, loneliness, and difficulties in peer relations, and had higher anxiety levels than the norm group. In a related descriptive study, seven adolescents who had survived liver transplantation for 1 to 4 years reported a satisfactory quality of life but desired to make changes, perceived limitations, and were concerned about physical appearance and rejection (Kosmach, 1990). Overall, many of the issues expressed by transplant recipients are similar to those of children with chronic conditions and relate to developmental tasks.

ASSOCIATED PROBLEMS AFTER TRANSPLANTATION
Immunosuppression

The routine primary immunosuppressive regimen for children with renal, liver, and heart transplants currently in use at the University of Pittsburgh is presented in the box on p. 396. The major maintenance immunosuppressive agents used solely or in combination therapy to prevent rejection of transplanted organs are cyclosporine, FK 506 (experimental), azathioprine, and prednisone. As mentioned earlier, the newest and most recent development in transplant immunology is the drug FK 506, a macrolide produced from a strain of soil fungus, *Streptomyces tsukubaensis*. FK 506 is currently under clinical investigation and has dem-

---

MAINTENANCE ROUTINE IMMUNOSUPPRESSIVE REGIMENS FOR CHILDREN WITH ORGAN TRANSPLANTS*

Renal transplants

Azathioprine 2-3 mg/kg/day
Cyclosporine 17.5 mg/kg/day twice daily (cadaveric)
        5 mg/kg/day twice daily (living related)
Prednisone 20 mg/day (cadaveric)
        0.5 mg/kg/day (living related)
FK 506 0.15 mg/kg twice daily†

Liver transplants

Azathioprine 1-3 mg/kg/day
Cyclosporine 17.5 mg/kg/day or twice daily
Prednisone 2.5-10 mg/day or every other day
FK 506 0.15 mg/kg twice daily†

Heart transplants

Azathioprine 1-2 mg/kg/day
Cyclosporine 4-20 mg/kg/day
Prednisone 0.1-0.3 mg/kg/day
FK 506 0.15 mg/kg twice daily†

*All medications taken orally. Dosages vary widely depending on the individual's blood levels. For cyclosporine, TDx levels of less than 400 ng/ml of whole blood is desirable.
†Because of the synergistic effect of cyclosporine and FK 506, children receive only one of the two drugs. FK 506 blood levels are measured by enzyme-linked immunosorbent assay (ELIZA), and normal levels are 0.5 to 2.5 ng/ml.

---

onstrated tremendous promise for individuals who undergo renal, liver, and heart transplants (Jain et al., 1990).

Cyclosporine has been the primary immunosuppressant drug used since 1981 to prevent rejection of transplanted organs. Generally the children take maintenance doses of cyclosporine orally every 12 hours. Because predicting absorption of the drug is difficult, the level of drug metabolites in the blood should be measured every 2 weeks based on 12-hour trough levels until an effective maintenance dose is established; blood levels are then monitored monthly.

Careful monitoring of side effects of cyclosporine or FK 506 is required to maintain adequate immunosuppression, as well as to prevent toxicities. These two immunosuppressants are not used in combination because of their synergistic effects (McCauley et al., 1990; Shapiro et al., 1990). Children may require therapy of cyclosporine and prednisone; triple-drug therapy consisting of cyclosporine, azathioprine, and prednisone; or FK 506 either alone or in combination with corticosteroids to maintain their functioning graft. Long-term maintenance may consist of cyclosporine alone in some children. Recently some children who have experienced chronic rejection taking cyclosporine and prednisone have had their immunosuppression therapy changed to FK 506 and have had positive early results. Long-term outcomes have yet to be determined. Recent results of newborns after heart transplantation suggest that they tolerate an immunosuppressive regimen without corticosteroids (Boucek et al., 1990). These newborns were treated with cyclosporine and azathioprine for the first year and then treated with only cyclosporine. Corticosteroids were used only in the immediate postoperative period unless a diagnosis of graft rejection was made.

Some of the more common side effects of cyclosporine are hypertension, renal dysfunction, gum hyperplasia, hirsutism, diarrhea, seizures, and tremors (Sandimmune product monograph, 1989). Side effects experienced after taking FK 506 orally include headache, insomnia, tremors, sensation of racing, hair loss or increased hair growth, nausea, vomiting, diarrhea, and anorexia; however, 74% to 87% of 62 individuals experienced no short-term side effects when they took FK 506 orally (Shapiro et al., 1990). The use of FK 506 is limited in children and side effects are still being assessed.

Other complications of immunosuppressive therapy include hypertension, lymphoproliferative disease, coronary vascular disease, and corticosteroid-induced diabetes. The complication of corticosteroid-induced diabetes is uncommon and usually transient (Addonizio and Rose, 1987; Lum et al., 1985).

In general, transplant recipients who are given cyclosporine maintenance therapy have experienced hypertension, whereas those receiving azathioprine rather than cyclosporine are not affected

(Fricker et al., 1987; Trento et al., 1989). The exception has been with infants from one center treated with cyclosporine after heart transplantations with no evidence of hypertension (Boucek et al., 1990). High-dose corticosteroids are also implicated as a cause of hypertension (Lum et al., 1985).

Hypertension has been controlled with β-adrenergic blockade or calcium channel blockers (Addonizio and Rose, 1987). Usually children are treated initially with diuretics and vasodilating agents such as hydralazine (Apresoline) and prazosin (Minipress). Calcium channel blockers, captopril (Capoten), and α-adrenergic and β-adrenergic blocking agents may also be administered (Fricker et al., 1987). However, captopril as treatment for children with renal artery stenosis after renal transplantation should be used with extreme caution because ischemic damage to the kidney may result (Lum et al., 1985).

Renal dysfunction secondary to cyclosporine therapy, with transient or chronic increases in blood urea nitrogen and creatinine levels, has been reported (Addonizio and Rose, 1987). Renal function has been found to improve with a decrease in cyclosporine dose and with improvement in graft function (Fricker et al., 1987). Serum creatinine level usually returns to baseline about 1 month after transplantation and then increases slowly to reach a plateau at about 1 year. There are concerns that long-term cyclosporine therapy may cause progressive and irreversible renal dysfunction (Trento et al., 1989). More sophisticated measures of renal function may need to be done to determine long-term impairment.

Initial clinical trials with adults receiving FK 506 revealed some renal dysfunction associated with the drug, although it seemed to be mild, with a pattern different from that of cyclosporine. Although cyclosporine-induced acute renal failure is usually associated with toxic drug levels, there appears to be a poor correlation between FK 506 drug levels and renal function (McCauley et al., 1990). Preliminary results after liver transplantation suggest that the degree of renal insufficiency seen with FK 506 is similar to that of cyclosporine (Green, 1990).

Early postoperative seizures, thought to be secondary to high cyclosporine levels, have been reported (Addonizio and Rose, 1987). Major motor seizures have been observed after heart transplantation at one center, with a single seizure occurring 10 days to 4 months after transplantation. Approximately 1% to 5% of 892 renal, heart, and liver transplant patients involved in clinical trials experienced seizures (Sandimmune product monograph, 1989). Effective therapy consisted of standard anticonvulsant doses of phenobarbital (Luminal) and phenytoin (Dilantin) (Fricker et al., 1987). Seizures were absent in infants, possibly because of differing immunosuppressive regimens (Boucek et al., 1990) (see Chapter 15).

Lymphoproliferative disease has occurred in immunosuppressed children who test positively for Epstein-Barr virus infection. It has been seen in children taking azathioprine and prednisone, as well as cyclosporine. The frequency of occurrence in pediatric transplant recipients has been estimated at 4% (Ho et al., 1988); however, the cumulative incidences may be as high as 20% in children taking cyclosporine who had transplantations 7 years earlier (Malatack, 1990). The usual manifestations in children have been enlarged tonsils, enlarged cervical lymph nodes, and GI bleeding. The diagnosis is confirmed by biopsy of the lymph nodes or the mass. The usual treatment is to reduce or discontinue immunosuppressive therapy. Others have suggested the additional use of acyclovir (Zovirax) given intravenously for 14 days. This combined therapy results in a cure in about one half of the individuals (Green, 1990).

Rejection

Despite successful transplantation, rejection of the new organ is a leading cause of graft failure (Heck et al., 1989; Potter et al., 1986) and can occur at any time. Meticulous monitoring of laboratory blood values for elevations in serum transaminases, bilirubin, alkaline phosphatase, and creatinine, as well as the child's physical status, can detect any problems with functioning of the liver or renal graft. Signs and symptoms of rejection include fever, swollen graft, abdominal pain, and irritability (Lum et al., 1985). Rejection of a transplanted kidney is usually determined by decreased blood flow on renal flow scan, whereas rejection of the liver is usually confirmed by biopsy. Fluid retention, ascites, and oliguria may be other accompanying signs of rejection. Rejection is treated with an increased corticosteroid dose (often given intravenously) or increased immunosuppressant drugs. Treatment with one of the antirejection drugs such as MALG, RATG, orthoclone OKT-3, or FK 506 as rescue therapy may also be used to combat the rejection episode.

Monitoring for rejection following cardiac transplantation is complicated by the fact that clinical signs and symptoms occur late and generally indicate moderate to severe rejection is in progress. These manifestations include congestive heart failure, cardiomegaly on chest x-ray film, fever, arrhythmias, ventricular dysfunction, and pericardial effusion. Because of the importance of detecting early subclinical rejection, monitoring is accomplished by endomyocardial biopsy (Beerman, 1990). Biopsies are performed weekly at first, then at 1- to 2-month periods for the first year on an outpatient basis (Addonizio and Rose, 1987; Fricker et al., 1987). Because of the risk of performing repeated endomyocardial biopsies on infants, close clinical follow-up with history, physical examination, chest radiography, electrocardiography, and echocardiography has been used to detect rejection episodes (Boucek et al., 1990).

Approximately 20% of children require retransplantation of the kidney or liver (So et al., 1985) with the majority necessary because of graft rejection (Fung et al., 1990). With improvements in immunosuppressive management and diagnostic testing, rejection episodes are better controlled, thus reducing the need for retransplantation.

Infection

Infection is a major cause of graft failure and death in children who have undergone transplantation. Bacterial, fungal, viral, and protozoan infections leading to renal, heart, and liver dysfunction are well documented (Green et al., 1989; Koneru et al., 1989; Potter et al., 1986). Bacterial infections have occurred early after transplantation and tend to be associated with the site of organ transplantation (Ho et al., 1988). Viral infections have been caused primarily by CMV, with a significant incidence of graft loss and death. More recently the use of ganciclovir (Cytovene) has improved the outcome in these children (Green, 1990). Other important causes of viral infections include adenovirus and Epstein-Barr virus. Fungal infections, primarily *Candida* species, have also significantly contributed to morbidity and mortality.

The difficulty in diagnosis is complicated by the use of immunosuppressive therapy, which may mask infections. Any child who has a fever and other generalized signs suggestive of infection should undergo physical and laboratory examination to determine any obvious source. Cultures for bacteria, fungi, and viruses obtained from blood, oral secretions, and urine should be performed when possible.

In general, medications are prescribed to all children for approximately 6 months to 1 year after transplantation to prevent viral, fungal, and protozoan infections. Since this protocol has been instituted, the incidence of serious infection from these organisms has decreased.

PRIMARY CARE MANAGEMENT
Growth and development

The majority of children who experience organ transplantation are small for their age because of the effects of their chronic conditions (see Chapters 11 and 27) and long-term effects of corticosteroids after transplantation. Therefore, all children with organ transplants should have height and weight documented at each clinic visit. Growth measures should be plotted on growth charts to monitor the rate and consistency of the child's growth and compared with normal percentile curves. Linear growth, anthropometrics of skin fold thickness, and nutritional measurements are important.

The use of cyclosporine in combination with lower-dose corticosteroids has lessened the concerns about limited growth (Pennington et al., 1985). Also, it is recognized from the renal transplant experience in children that severe growth retardation from chronic renal failure could be prevented by transplantation at an earlier age (Fine et al., 1977). Growth-retarding effects of current drugs may not be as severe as the actual growth failure caused by the disease itself (Pennington et al., 1985).

Recent research efforts are focused on growth and development outcomes of children after transplantation. After renal transplantation, children experience improvements in growth and development (Ildstad et al., 1990; Potter et al., 1986; So et al.,

1985). Accelerations in physical growth after liver transplantation have been reported in children who receive cyclosporine and low-dose corticosteroid maintenance therapy. The majority of children who were studied had attained normal physical growth 2 to 4.5 years after transplantation; only a small number experienced growth retardation (Urbach et al., 1987). Linear growth in children after heart transplantation was maintained in most children surviving more than 1 year, and most children experienced a marked increase in weight (Trento et al., 1989).

Research on cognitive functioning and development of children after transplantation are new areas of investigation. Cognitive functioning appears to be minimally affected after a child receives a liver transplant. There were no significant differences in IQs of 29 children tested before and after liver transplantation; about 20% of the children improved to the normal range, and 10% decreased from superior to normal (Zitelli et al., 1988). However, one study (Zamberlan, 1989) revealed deficits in school-aged children who tended to forget and were slow to finish school work. After heart transplantation, infants were achieving normal developmental milestones more than 1 year after surgery (Bailey et al., 1988).

Immunizations

It is not clear whether immunosuppressed children can respond adequately to routine vaccinations (Addonizio and Rose, 1987). Therefore, whenever possible, all required immunizations should be given before the transplant surgery. Live vaccines are ordinarily contraindicated in immunocompromised children because the immunodeficient state may permit viral replication, leading to adverse reactions (McLaughlin et al., 1988). The experiences in children with human immunodeficiency virus (HIV) have led to a change in this practice (Thomas, 1988). Infants and children who are immunosuppressed and their siblings should receive the inactivated poliomyelitis vaccine (IPV, developed by Salk) as recommended both before or after transplantation (Addonizio and Rose, 1987). The disadvantage to the child is that the Salk vaccine must be administered by subcutaneous injection and may require multiple boosters to assure immunity. The measles, mumps, and rubella vaccine is cur-

rently being administered to children with HIV without consequences (Immunization Practices Advisory Committee, 1988); it has also been given to children who have received solid organ transplants when they reside in endemic areas. Serologic confirmation of immunogenicity has not yet been established (Green, 1990).

The new *Haemophilus influenzae* type b (Hib) vaccine is a synthetic vaccine that promotes active immunity and is safe for children who have received transplants. Because *H. influenzae* is one of the major causes of serious infection in infants and young children, infants starting at 2 months of age should routinely receive the vaccine (Committee on Infectious Diseases, 1991).

Children who have had diphtheria, pertussis, and tetanus (DPT), IPV, or Hib immunization schedules disrupted because of chronic conditions can resume a schedule of treatment after the transplantation. Usually the child should be able to resume the immunization schedule within 3 months following the transplantation once minimal immunosuppressant therapy has been achieved.

Hepatitis B is an infrequent but important cause of decreased graft survival, morbidity, and mortality after transplantation. Children waiting for transplants should be vaccinated. Pretransplantation vaccination may be achieved by administration of the inactivated Hib vaccine Heptavax-B, Recombivax, or Engerix-B.

Children who are exposed to chickenpox must receive human varicella-zoster immune globulin (VZIG) within 72 hours following contact exposure if they do not have a positive history of varicella. If children are hospitalized at the time of exposure, they are placed in isolation from day 10 to day 28 after exposure to chickenpox and treatment with VZIG. Children who develop lesions despite VZIG should also receive acyclovir intravenously within 24 hours of eruption of the skin rash and continued for 7 to 10 days (McGregor et al., 1989).

Screening

Vision. Routine screening is recommended. Children taking prednisone should be seen by an ophthalmologist yearly for eye examinations because prednisone may cause changes in eyesight, blurry vision, cataracts, or glaucoma.

Hearing. Children should have routine yearly

audiograms for evaluation of hearing before and after transplantations. During their postoperative recovery, children receive many ototoxic drugs to treat infections. The cumulative effects of the drug therapies should be monitored monthly during the immediate postoperative period and then yearly to evaluate any hearing loss.

Dental. Routine dental visits (twice yearly) are recommended for children after transplantation. It is a usual practice for prophylactic antibiotics to be administered before dental care to prevent infection (see the box on p. 196 in Chapter 11). In addition, children taking cyclosporine may develop gum hyperplasia requiring gingivectomy. Also, bonding of the teeth has been successful in restoring a natural finish to permanent teeth stained in utero for children with biliary atresia.

Blood pressure. Home blood pressure readings are taken and recorded twice daily by parents if their child had hypertension caused by cyclosporine therapy while hospitalized. The primary care provider should carefully evaluate home results and a current blood pressure reading at the clinic visit. Such children usually take nifedipine (Procardia) or captopril for hypertension; however, antihypertensives are most often discontinued by 6 months after transplantation. Preliminary results with FK 506 immunosuppression suggest that children do not require long-term anti-hypertensive medication.

Hematocrit. Hematocrit screening is deferred because of condition-specific screening.

Urinalysis. Routine urinalysis is performed yearly and more often only if fever or related signs and symptoms of infection are detected. Most children take trimethoprim-sulfamethoxazole (Bactrim) prophylactically for *Pneumocystis carinii* for several months; thus, urinary tract infections are uncommon. The color of the urine is assessed because dark orange suggests the presence of conjugated bilirubin.

Tuberculosis. Before transplantation all children should receive the purified protein derivative (PPD) 5 U/0.1 ml test dose intradermally with anergy control to evaluate exposure. A positive skin test reaction is followed by chest radiograph before treatment. Children who are chronically ill are at greatest risk for tuberculosis pneumonia. Children with a history of tuberculosis who are PPD positive

or who demonstrate other symptoms should take isonizid (INH) maintenance therapy for life.

Condition-specific screening

BLOOD WORK. Blood work is drawn at every clinic visit. Most of the following tests are performed: complete blood cell count with differential and platelets, serum potassium, prothrombin time, partial prothromboplastin time, glucose levels, enzymes levels (aspartate aminotransferase [AST], alanine aminotransferase [ALT], phosphate, lactic dehydrogenase [LDH], creatine phosphokinase [CPK], and gamma-glutamyl transpeptidase), uric acid concentration, ammonia level, BUN level, and serum creatinine. Patterns and trends are evaluated for each child. Children taking FK506 may develop anemia requiring iron supplements.

Drug levels of cyclosporine or FK 506 are obtained each time the child has blood work done. The tubes with blood samples are packaged and mailed to the transplant center for consistent monitoring of the child's response to the immunosuppressant drug. Adjustments in immunosuppressant management are made by the transplant center staff.

GRAFT EVALUATION. Children return to the transplant center usually on a yearly basis for follow-up care by the transplant team. A complete history and physical examination is performed. Organ-specific tests such as abdominal ultrasound of the liver, echocardiography, renal flow scan, computerized tomography scan of the abdomen, or biopsy (renal, liver or endomyocardial) are performed if needed. With any invasive procedure (e.g., cardiac catheterization) the child may require overnight admission to monitor for any complications following the procedure.

Drug interactions

Cyclosporine absorption can be affected by phenytoin, phenobarbital, ketoconazole (Nizoral), and erythromycin (Erythrocin) (Venkataramanan, Burckart, and Ptachcinski, 1985). Children who have required anticonvulsant drug therapy for seizure control may need higher doses of cyclosporine because some anticonvulsants accelerate cyclosporine metabolism (Burckart, Venkataramanan, and Ptachcinski, 1985). FK506 absorption may be affected by some of these same drugs (Venkataramanan, 1990). In general, over-the-counter medications are to be avoided without the approval of a transplant team professional because they may interact with the immunosuppressant therapy. Acetaminophen (Tylenol) rather than aspirin is recommended for fever or headache.

DIFFERENTIAL DIAGNOSIS
Fever

Within 3 months of transplantation, children who have fevers are at increased risk for bacterial infections related to surgery or recurrence of viral illness. Fever occurring after that time should be evaluated for routine childhood illness. Once the source of the fever is determined, appropriate treatment is instituted. The occurrence of fever may be upsetting to the child and family who fear potential loss of the organ as a result of rejection because fever accompanies rejection. Support, comfort, and explanations of other possible causes should be discussed with the child and family.

Abdominal symptoms

It is important for the primary care provider to be aware that children who have renal or liver transplants have not usually had incidental appendectomies along with the transplant surgery. Thus, appendicitis cannot be automatically ruled out when symptoms of such occur. Also, children who receive liver transplants have their native gallbladder removed and a cholecystectomy is performed on the donor organ. However, it is possible for children to develop stones that can obstruct the common bile duct, resulting in abdominal pain, jaundice, or fever. Children with abdominal pain should also be screened for complications caused by rejection, ulcers, possible small bowel obstruction, or infection from spontaneous bacterial peritonitis.

Viral illnesses that cause vomiting and diarrhea may result in poor absorption of the immunosuppressant medications, leading to nontherapeutic blood levels. Hydration of the child should be maintained through fluids given orally or intravenously, and intravenous drug therapy considered if the child is unable to orally take and retain their immunosuppressant medication or medications.

Metabolic derangements

It is unusual for children to experience metabolic derangements when a transplanted graft is func-

tioning properly. If electrolyte imbalances occur, they may be related to hyperkalemia from FK 506 (Fung et al., 1990) or increased dietary intake of potassium-enriched foods following discontinuance of diuretic therapy. Long-term corticosteroid therapy may precipitate hyperglycemia.

DEVELOPMENTAL ISSUES
Safety

Even though children are immunosuppressed after transplantation, routine hand washing and general cleanliness are all that are required. Most parents and children are sensitized to good hand-washing techniques during hospitalization, and such techniques should be continued in the home. Families who own cats as pets should avoid having the transplant recipient change the cat's litter box because of the possibility of being infected with the *Toxoplasma* organism found in the animal's feces.

Children taking prednisone may have more photosensitive skin. Use of sunscreen with sun protection factor of at least 15 is recommended.

Exercise is encouraged, but there are some limitations. Recipients should avoid lifting heavy objects for at least 6 months. Push-ups or sit-ups, as well as activities that stretch or put pressure on the abdomen and incision, are to be avoided after liver or renal transplantation. Contact sports and downhill sledding are not recommened. Children are encouraged to resume previous activities; however, it is recommended that they progress slowly.

When children or families are planning to travel, certain precautions should be taken. The transplant team should be notified before departure. They can inform the family of the transplant center nearest to their destiny. Transplant recipients should always take all medications with them on trips and carry them onto airplanes rather than checking medications with luggage. Also, children should wear their Medic-Alert bracelet and carry an identification card that identifies them as a transplant recipient and has the name and telephone number of the transplant physician.

Child care

In general, children who receive transplants are not restricted from day care. However, during the first 2 months after the transplant, children are taking the highest doses of immunosuppressants and are the most susceptible to infections. Accordingly, children should be kept away from people with measles, mumps, varicella, shingles, herpes stomatitis, or influenza. Crowded areas such as airports, movie theaters, or public transportation terminals should be avoided when possible.

Children receiving maintenance doses of immunosuppressants should have adequate immunity to fight the common cold. Thus, exposure to other children is of minimal risk. However, parents should be kept informed by the child care provider of any outbreaks of common childhood illnesses, particularly measles or varicella, because contraction of these illnesses places the child at serious risk. When outbreaks occur, home care is advised during the incubation period.

Diet

Many children experience excessive weight gain after transplantation. Prednisone increases the appetite and causes the body to make fat and lose muscle. Also, children may overeat because most dietary restrictions are now lifted. Before discharge from the hospital, parents and children meet with a dietician to discuss a well-balanced meal plan that includes the basic food groups. Children who take maintenance doses of cyclosporine and are hypertensive may require a low-sodium diet. Children with heart transplants should be on a low-cholesterol and low–saturated fat diet because of the increased incidence of graft atherosclerosis. The child should be assessed for any nutritional problems at each primary care visit and identified problems managed or referred as with other children.

Discipline

For many children who were chronically ill for long periods during the pretransplant phase, certain family role patterns are established. Once the transplant restores children to "health," it is sometimes difficult for families to make the transition from parenting a sick child to parenting a well child. Many parents tend to continue patterns of overprotectiveness. They may have difficulty allowing the child more freedom and insist on setting tight limits that may no longer be warranted.

Noncompliance with immunosuppressive medications resulting in graft loss has been described in both male and female adolescents and preado-

lescents as well as in young adults (Cooper, Lanza, and Barnard, 1984; Fine et al., 1977). Efforts should be made to identify and provide counseling for the child, adolescent, and family who may be at high risk for noncompliance.

Toileting

Some children have experienced nocturnal enuresis after liver transplantation (Zitelli et al., 1988). Once evaluation of enuresis by a urologist demonstrates no physiologic problem, psychologic counseling and behavioral interventions should be considered. The initiation of urine flow in the child with a kidney transplant is often a time of great excitement for the family. The establishment of urinary continence will require support and time for the child to learn to identify the body cues needed for continence. Episodes of incontinence and enuresis are to be expected.

Sleep patterns

Some children have experienced long hospitalizations before and after the transplantation and may have developed erratic sleep patterns and fears. In addition, nightmares may be precipitated by certain drugs such as FK 506, corticosteroids, the stresses of hospitalization, or separation from parents. Corticosteroids have been implicated in impaired sleep, including the decreased need for sleep (Watts et al., 1984). Parents may need to reinstitute familiar home routines and rituals and provide continued emotional support and reassurance until normal patterns return. Professional counseling sessions may be necessary to assist the child to assimilate his or her experiences. Occasionally, medications to help the child relax before sleep can be prescribed.

School issues

It is important for children of school age to return to school as soon as possible. Because of lengthy hospitalization, children often need to repeat a grade in school, attend summer classes, or both. Once in the school setting, they are confronted by peers who tease them about their appearance (Kosmach, 1990; Zamberlan, 1989) at an age when peer acceptance and uniformity are critical to self-esteem.

Although most children are receiving maintenance corticosteroid doses by the time of school reentry, corticosteroid-induced mood changes are possible, particularly if the child is being treated with corticosteroid boluses for organ rejection (Watts et al., 1984). A school-based practitioner is in an optimal position to meet with these children to assess their current treatment needs and to provide emotional support and reassurance. The nurse's knowledge of the transplant process and the routine medications children are taking may help to develop the child's confidence in the nurse. In addition, such children may benefit from individualized or family counseling to assist them in understanding and coping with the stresses they face.

Sexuality

As older school-aged children and adolescents recover after transplantation, their bodies undergo often dramatic changes because of the surgery and medications that may result in lifelong alterations in body image. Transplant surgery usually results in extensive incisional scars. In addition, physical appearance is altered by medication side effects, including hirsutism, obesity, Cushingoid faces, and discoloration of teeth. Thus, it is not surprising that some adolescents who have organ transplants infrequently engage in dating and display a cautious attitude toward sexuality (Kosmach, 1990). Such adolescents may be at risk for psychosocial and emotional difficulties (Kosmach, 1990) and may benefit from professional counseling. Remedies such as electrolysis and cosmetic surgery, though costly, may be helpful to improve self-esteem.

As more pediatric transplant recipients survive to reach childbearing age, concerns about contraception and childbearing become more prominent. For contraceptive management barrier methods of birth control are recommended because oral contraceptives may precipitate thrombus formation. The effects of long-term use of immunosuppressive agents by transplant recipients on the unborn child are not well known. Women have had successful pregnancies after renal transplantation (Potter et al., 1986), and recent reports suggest that women who have undergone liver transplantation and immunosuppressive therapy are able to safely have children, although with an increased risk of premature and cesarean births. The majority of the offspring have had normal physical and mental development thus far (Scantlebury et al., 1990).

SPECIAL FAMILY CONCERNS

Parents are often concerned about the effect of the transplant process on the entire family and wonder how to reestablish a normal home life after transplantation. Fears of organ rejection and the possibility of an unsuccessful search for another donor organ, leading to the child's death, are paramount (Weichler, 1990). Also, the psychologic incorporation of the donor organ into the self-image may be a difficult task for the recipient. Another concern for families is the financial impact of the transplant process. Hospitalization, surgery, immunosuppressive and other medications, housing near the transplant center, and day-to-day living expenses amass to a major financial burden for many families. Financial support can come from third-party health insurance payers, community fund raising, state funding, or self-pay through the family's own resources. Families are in need of information and emotional support from the transplant team and primary care providers to cope with their fears, future milestones, and financial aspects of organ transplantation.

SUMMARY OF PRIMARY CARE NEEDS FOR THE CHILD WITH AN ORGAN TRANSPLANT

Growth and development

Height and weight should be measured each visit.
Linear growth may be affected by long-term corticosteroid use.
Catch-up growth may be attained after transplantation.
Improved physical development after transplantation has a positive effect on psychosocial development.
Cognitive functioning should be monitored.

Immunizations

Immunodeficient children should receive DPT and IPV immunizations.
The MMR vaccine is safe for children after transplantations.
Haemophilus influenzae type b vaccine is recommended for children starting at 2 months.
Varicella-zoster immune globulin must be administered within 72 hours of exposure to varicella for seronegative children
Pretransplant immunization against hepatitis B is recommended.

Screening
Vision

Yearly examinations should be given for changes in eyesight, blurry vision, cataracts, or glaucoma from corticosteroids.

Hearing

Audiograms should be done yearly to evaluate hearing loss from ototoxic drugs.

Dental

Dental screening should be done at minimum every 6 months, with prophylactic antibiotics used. Cyclosporine may cause gingival hyperplasia.

Blood pressure

Blood pressure should be checked at each visit; the effectiveness of antihypertensive medication should be evaluated.

Hematocrit

Routine screening is deferred because of post-transplant blood tests.

Urinalysis

Routine screening is recommended.

Tuberculosis

Routine screening is recommended.

Condition-specific screening
Blood work

At each follow-up transplant clinic visit multiple blood tests are done and assessed for patterns and trends. Serum drug levels are also tested.
Graft evaluation

Diagnostic testing is done yearly to evaluate graft function.

Drug interactions

Cyclosporine and FK506 absorption is altered by phenytoin, phenobarbital, ketoconazole, and erythromycin.
Higher doses of cyclosporine may be needed to achieve therapeutic range when it is administered with anticonvulsants.

Differential diagnosis
Fever

Normal childhood illnesses should be ruled out; fever may indicate organ rejection.

Abdominal symptoms

Abdominal pain should be investigated to rule out appendicitis or intestinal obstruction, ulcers, and peritonitis; vomiting and diarrhea may lower therapeutic blood levels of immunosuppressant drugs.

Metabolic derangement

Hyperkalemia can result from drug therapy; hyperglycemia may result from corticosteroid use.

Developmental issues
Safety

Precautions with animals are recommended to prevent transmission of disease to immunosuppressed children.
Prednisone predisposes to sunburn.
No contact sports or downhill sledding is allowed.
Medic-alert bracelets are recommended.

SUMMARY OF PRIMARY CARE NEEDS FOR THE CHILD WITH AN ORGAN TRANSPLANT — cont'd

Child care

The children may attend day care; precautions should be taken to limit exposure to communicable diseases.

Diet

Prednisone may cause overeating, leading to weight gain; dietary planning is needed for well-balanced meals and possibly sodium-restricted diets.

Children with heart transplants should reduce cholesterol and saturated fats.

Discipline

Parental overprotectiveness is likely; parents may need help to promote independence in their children.

Noncompliance with medications may occur with adolescents.

Toileting

Nocturnal enuresis has occurred after liver transplantation.

Sleep patterns

Hospitalization or drugs may alter sleep patterns.

School issues

Normal schooling should be resumed after transplantation.

Alterations in body image may negatively affect peer interactions.

Sexuality

The transplant experience may effect body image and self-esteem.

Barrier methods of birth control are recommended.

Childbearing after transplantation has produced normal children.

Special family concerns

Special family concerns include fear of rejection, search for a new organ, organ donor issues, and finances.

RESOURCES
Organizations

American Liver Foundation
998 Pompton Ave
Cedar Grove, NJ 07009
(800) 223-0179

Children's Liver Foundation
76 South Orange Ave, No 202
South Orange, NJ 07079
(201) 761-1111

Children's Transplant Association
PO Box 2106
Laurinburg, NC 28352
(919) 276-7171

National Heart Assist and Transplant Fund
PO Box 163
Haverford, PA 19041
(215) 527-5056

American Kidney Fund
6110 Executive Blvd, No 1010
Rockville, MD 20852
(301) 881-3052

American Nephrology Nurses' Association
North Woodbury Rd, Box 56
Pitman, NJ 08071
(609) 589-2187

National Association of Patients on Hemodialysis
and Transplantation
211 E 43rd St, No 301
New York, NY 10017
(212) 867-4486

National Disease Research Interchange
2401 Walnut Street, No 408
Philadelphia, PA 19103
(215) 222-6374

National Kidney Foundation
2 Park Ave
New York, NY 10016
(212) 889-2210

Renal Physicians' Association
1101 Vermont Ave, NW, No 500
Washington, DC 20005-3547
(202) 289-1700

United Network for Organ Sharing
3001 Hungary Spring Rd
PO Box 28010
Richmond, VA 23228
(804) 289-5380

Transplant Recipients' International organization
244 N Bellefield Ave
Pittsburgh, PA 15213
(412) 687-2210

REFERENCES

Addonizio L and Rose E: Cardiac transplantation in children and adolescents, *J Pediatr* 111:1034-1038, 1987.

Altman RP and Levy J: Biliary atresia, *Pediatr Ann* 14:481-482, 484-485, 1985.

Bailey L, Assaad A, Trimm R, et al: Orthotopic transplantation during early infancy as therapy for incurable congenital heart disease, *Ann Surg* 208:279-286, 1988.

Beerman L: Personal communication, July 9, 1990.

Benenson, E: Personal communication, April 11, 1991.

Boucek M, Kanakriyeh M, Mathis C, et al: Cardiac transplantation in infancy: Donors and recipients, *J Pediatr* 116:171-176, 1990.

Burckart G, Venkataramanan R, and Ptachcinski R: Cyclosporine monitoring, *Am Assoc Clin Chem* 6(9):1-11, 1985.

Calne R, Thiru S, McMaster P, et al: Cyclosporin A in patients receiving allografts from cadaver donors, *Lancet* 2:1323-1327, 1978.

Committee on Infectious Disease: Report of the Committee on Infectious Diseases, ed 22, Elk Grove Village, Ill, The American Academy of Pediatrics, 1991.

Cooley D, Bloodwell R, Hallman G, et al: Organ transplantation for advanced cardiopulmonary disease, *Ann Thorac Surg* 8:30-46, 1969.

Cooper D, Lanza R, and Barnard C: Noncompliance in heart transplant recipients: The Cape Town experience, *Heart Transplant* 3:248-253, 1984.

Corbo BH and Dunn MJ: Nursing care of children with heart or liver transplants: Acute phase. In Barnes CM, ed: *Recent advances in nursing,* New York, Churchill-Livingstone, vol 16, pp 117-148, 1987.

Corbo-Richert B and Zamberlan K: Surgical nursing care of children with liver transplants, *Operat Room Nurs Forum* 2:1-3, 6-8, 1988.

Fine R: Recent advances in the management of the infant, child, and adolescent with chronic renal failure, *Pediatr Rev* 11:277-283, 1990.

Fine R, Korsch B, Stiles Q, et al: Renal homotransplantation in children, *J Pediatr* 76:347-357, 1970.

Fine R, Malekzadeh M, Pennisi A, et al: Cadaver renal transplantation in children, *Transplant Proc* 9:133-136, 1977.

Fine RN, Salusky I, and Ettenger R: The therapeutic approach to the infant, child, and adolescent with end-stage renal disease, *Pediatr Clin North Am* 34:789-801, 1987.

Fricker FJ, Griffith B, Hardesty R, et al: Experience with heart transplantation in children, *Pediatrics* 79:138-146, 1987.

Fung J, Todo S, Jain A, et al: Conversion from cyclosporine to FK 506 in liver allograft recipients with cyclosporine-related complications, *Transplant Proc* 22(suppl 1):6-12, 1990.

Fyler D and Nadas A: Congenital heart disease. In Avery ME and First LR eds: *Pediatric medicine,* Baltimore, 1989, Williams & Wilkins, pp 316-386.

Gillum R: Idiopathic cardiomyopathy in the United States, 1970-1982, *Am Heart J* 111:752-755, 1986.

Gordon RD, Todo S, Tzakis A, et al: Liver transplantation under cyclosporine: A decade of experience, *Transplant Proceedings,* 23:1393-1396, 1991.

Green M: Personal communication, June 29, 1990.

Green M, Wald E, Fricker FJ, et al: Infections in pediatric orthotopic heart transplant recipients, *Pediatr Infect Dis J* 8:87-93, 1989.

Greenwood R, Nadas A, and Fyler D: The clinical course of primary myocardial disease in infants and children, *Am Heart J* 92:549-560, 1976.

Griffin M, Hernandez A, Martin T, et al: Dilated cardiomyopathy in infants and children, *J Am Coll Cardiol* 11:139-144, 1988.

Hanto D, Sakamoto K, Purtilo D, et al: The Epstein-Barr virus in the pathogenesis of posttransplant lymphoproliferative disorders, *Surgery* 90:204-213, 1981.

Ho M, Jaffe R, Miller G et al: The frequency of Epstein-Barr virus infection and associated lymphoproliferative syndrome after transplantation and its manifestations in children, *Transplantation* 45:719-727, 1988.

Ildstad S, Tollerud D, Noseworthy J, et al: The influence of donor age on graft survival in renal transplantation, *J Pediatr Surg* 25:134-139, 1990.

Immunization Practices Advisory Committee: Immunization of children infected with human immunodeficiency virus—supplementary ACIP statement, *MMWR* 37:181-183, 1988.

Iwatsuki S, Stieber A, Marsh JW, et al: Liver transplantation for fulminant hepatic failure, *Transplant Proc* 21:2431-2434, 1989.

Jain AB, Fung J, Venkataramanan R, et al: FK 506 dosage in human organ transplantation, *Transplant Proc* 22(suppl 1):23-24, 1990.

Jamieson S, Billingham M, Oyer P, et al: Heart transplantation for end-stage ischemic heart disease: The Stanford experience, *Heart Transplant* 3:224-227, 1984.

Kantrowitz A, Haller J, Jaas H, et al: Transplantation of the heart in an infant and an adult, *Am J Cardiol* 22:782-790, 1968.

Koneru B, Scantlebury V, Makowka L, et al: Infections in pediatric liver recipients treated for acute rejection, *Transplant Proc* 21:2251-2252, 1989.

Kosmach B: *Adolescents' responses to quality of life issues following liver transplantation,* master's thesis, Pittsburgh, 1990, University of Pittsburgh.

Kriett JM and Kaye MP: The registry of the international society for heart transplantation: Seventh official report—1990, *J Heart Transplant* 9:323-330, 1990.

Lawrence KS and Fricker FJ: Pediatric heart transplantation: Quality of life, *J Heart Transplant* 6:329-333, 1987.

Lower RR and Shumway NE: Studies on orthotopic transplantation of the canine heart, *Surg Forum* 11:18-19, 1960.

Lum C, Wassner S, and Martin D: Current thinking in transplantation in infants and children, *Pediatr Clin North Am* 32:1203-1232, 1985.

Malatack J: Personal communication, June 29, 1990.

Maron B and Roberts W: Cardiomyopathies in the first two decades of life. In Engle MA, ed: *Pediatric cardiovascular disease—cardiovascular clinics,* Philadelphia, 1981, Davis, vol II, pp 35-78.

McCauley J, Fung J, Jain A, et al: The effects of FK 506 on renal function after liver transplantation, *Transplant Proc* 22,(suppl 1):17-20, 1990.

McGregor RS, Zitelli BJ, Urbach AH, et al: Varicella in pediatric orthotopic liver transplant recipients, *Pediatrics* 83:256-260, 1989.

McKenna WJ, Franklin RC, Nihoyannopoulos P, et al: Arrhythmia and prognosis in infants, children and adolescents with hypertrophic cardiomyopathy, *J Am Coll Cardiol* 11:147-153, 1988.

McLaughlin M, Thomas P, Onorato I, et al: Live virus vaccines in human immunodeficiency virus-infected children: A retrospective survey, *Pediatrics* 82:229-233, 1988.

Paradis K, Freese D, and Sharp H: A pediatric perspective on liver transplantation, *Pediatr Clin North Am* 35:409-433, 1988.

Penkoske P, Freedom R, Rowe R, et al: The future of heart and heart-lung transplantation in children, *Heart Transplant* 3:233-238, 1984.

Pennington DG, Sarafian J, and Swartz M: Heart transplantation in children, *Heart Transplant* 4:441-445, 1985.

Potter D, Feduska N, Melzer J, et al: Twenty years of renal transplantation in children, *Pediatrics* 77:465-470, 1986.

Reyes JD: The use of FK506 in pediatric hepatic transplantation. Presented at conference: *Organ transplants in children,* Philadelphia, PA, April 8, 1990.

Sandimmune (cyclosporine) product monograph, East Hanover, NJ, Sept 1, 1989, Sandoz Pharmaceutical.

Scantlebury V, Gordon R, Tzakis A, et al: Childbearing after liver transplantation, *Transplantation* 49:317-321, 1990.

Shapiro R, Fung J, Jain A, et al: The side effects of FK 506 in humans, *Transplant Proc* 22(suppl 1):35-36, 1990.

Shaw B, Wood R, Kaufman S, et al: Liver transplantation therapy for children: Part I, *J Pediatr Gastroenterol Nutr* 7:157-166, 1988.

So S, Mauer SM, Nevins T, et al: Current results in pediatric renal transplantation at the University of Minnesota, *Kidney Int* 30:525-530, 1986.

So S, Simmons R, Fryd D, et al: Improved results of multiple renal transplantation in children, *Surgery* 98:729-737, 1985.

Starzl T, Iwatsuki S, Van Thiel D, et al: Evolution of liver transplantation, *Hepatology* 2:614-636, 1982.

Starzl T, Koep L, Halgrimson C, et al: Fifteen years of clinical liver transplantation, *Gastroenterology* 77:375-388, 1979.

Starzl T, Marchioro R, Porter K, et al: The role of organ transplantation in pediatrics, *Pediatr Clin North Am* 13:381-420, 1966.

Staschak S and Zamberlan K: (1990). Liver transplantation: Nursing diagnoses and management. In Sigardson-Poor K and Haggerty L, eds: *Nursing care of the transplant recipient,* Philadelphia, 1990, WB Saunders, pp 140-179.

Stevenson L and Perloff J: The dilated cardiomyopathies: Clinical aspects, *Cardiol Clin* 6:187-218, 1988.

Taliercio C, Seward J, Driscoll D, et al: Idiopathic dilated cardiomyopathy in the young: Clinical profile and natural history, *J Am Coll Cardiol* 6:1126-1131, 1985.

Thomas R: Immunization of children infected with HIV: A public health perspective, *Pediatr Ann* 17:347-351, 1988.

Trento A, Griffith BP, Fricker FJ, et al: Lessons learned in pediatric heart transplantation, *Ann Thorac Surg* 48:617-623, 1989.

Urbach AH, Gartner JC, Malatack JJ, et al: Linear growth following pediatric liver transplantation, *Am J Dis Child* 141:547-549, 1987.

Venkataramanan, R: Personal communication, June 18, 1990.

Venkataramanan R, Burckart G, Ptachcinski R: Pharmacokinetics and monitoring of cyclosporine following orthotopic liver transplantation, *Semin Liver Dis* 5:357-367, 1985.

Wanek EA, Karrer FM, Brandt CT, et al: Biliary atresia, *Pediatr Rev* 11:57-62, 1989.

Watts D, Freeman A, McGiffin D, et al: Psychiatric aspects of cardiac transplantation, *Heart Transplant* 3:243-247, 1984.

Weichler N: Information needs of mothers of children who have liver transplants, *J Pediatr Nurs* 5:88-96, 1990.

Zamberlan K: Quality of life in school-age children following liver transplantation, *Diss Abstr Int* 50:150-05b, 1988.

Zitelli B, Miller J, Gartner J, et al: Changes in life-style after liver transplantation, *Pediatrics* 82:173-180, 1988.

Zuberbuhler J, Fricker F, and Griffith B: Cardiac transplantation in children, *Cardiol Clin* 7:411-418, 1989.

23 Pediatric HIV Infection and AIDS

Rita Fahrner

ETIOLOGY

The human immunodeficiency virus (HIV) causes a continuum of infection to occur, and the end stage of that infectious process is called acquired immune deficiency syndrome (AIDS). The HIV type 1 (HIV-1) belongs to the family of retroviruses, which means that its viral RNA is copied into DNA using the enzyme reverse transcriptase. This virus selectively infects the T-helper (T4 or CD4) subset of T-cell lymphocytes. Other cells that express CD4, such as monocytes, macrophages, and glial cells, are capable of becoming infected, as are some cells without detectable cell surface CD4. Through a process of replication, HIV perpetuates and integrates itself into the genetic material of the organism it infects (Demmler and Taber, 1990). The primary pathologic condition of HIV causes specific immunodeficiency that destroys the host's ability to withstand infection. In addition, the HIV directly invades other major organ systems, including the peripheral and central nervous system (CNS), lungs, heart, kidneys, and gastrointestinal (GI) tract.

Although HIV infections in children and adults share common pathologic conditions, an infant with HIV infection, particularly one who is infected perinatally, represents a distinctive immunologic host with a developing, immature immune system. The fetus and neonate have a well-developed T-cell or cell-mediated immune system, whereas their B-cell, or humoral immune system, is physiologically immature (Wishon and Gee, 1988). Although the function of both B and T cells is altered in HIV-infected children, the consequences of B-cell dysfunction, including hypergammaglobulinemia and failure to form functional antibodies, often become problematic early in the course of disease. For this reason children with HIV disease are more susceptible to bacterial infections than their adult counterparts. T-cell defects, allowing for opportunistic infections (OIs) such as *Pneumocystis carinii* pneumonia (PCP), are also frequently seen in young infants. In addition, the degree of lymphopenia, percentage of T4 (CD4) cells, absolute T4 (CD4) count, and degree of reversal of the helper/suppressor (T4/T8) ratio are more variable in infants. In general, depletion of T-cell numbers and inversion of the helper/suppressor ratio occurs at a later stage of disease than in adults (Onorato, Markowitz, and Oxtoby, 1988). Another major difference between adults and children with HIV infection is that the time period from infection to development of signs and symptoms appears to be shorter in children (Pizzo, 1990).

The HIV is transmitted to children by a variety of modes (Table 23-1). Perinatal transmission is the most common (84%) mode of transmission. Perinatal transmission is believed to occur transplacentally in utero (vertical), during delivery by exposure to infected maternal blood and vaginal secretions, and by postpartum ingestion of infected breast milk. Current prospective

Table 23-1. U.S. pediatric AIDS cases
by route of transmission*

Mode of transmission	%
Mother has or is at risk for HIV infection	84
Recipient of blood, blood product, or tissue	9
Hemophilia or coagulation disorder	5
Undetermined	2
TOTAL	100

Adapted from Centers for Disease Control: HIV/AIDS surveillance report, March, 1991.
*N = 2315.

studies estimate the risk of perinatal transmission to be 25% to 35% (Pizzo, 1990). Some researchers believe that there is an increase in the risk of perinatal transmission when the mother has a T4 cell count of less than 300, indicating long-standing infection (Minkoff, 1989). However, there have been well-documented cases of discordantly infected monozygotic twins.

Children have become infected with HIV from contaminated blood and blood products, tissues, and factor concentrates received between the years of 1978 and 1985. The risk of infection through this route has been extremely high, with infection estimated to occur in up to 95% of those receiving contaminated products. Because of new safeguards in blood and tissue collection and heat treatment of factor concentrates, there have been few new cases of infection by this route.

A small number of children have become HIV infected as a result of sexual abuse. Practitioners caring for children who have experienced abuse must include HIV infection in their differential diagnosis of sexually transmitted diseases.

Teenagers have not been included in the pediatric HIV-AIDS statistics; rather, they have been placed in the adolescent-adult categories because they follow similar patterns regarding progression of disease as do adults. It is important to consider adolescents separately from both children and adults. The differences between infected children and adolescents include the route of transmission; the shorter mean survival time in young children; and their special needs for day care, respite care, and foster care. Some of the differences between

infected teenagers and adults include a higher incidence of heterosexual transmission among adolescents; a larger percentage of infected minority youth than adults; ethical and legal issues concerning consent, testing, and partner and parental notification for underage youth; cognitive, coping, and risk-taking differences of adolescents; and special medical and psychosocial implications of infected teenage parents with infected infants (Hein, 1989).

INCIDENCE

Although pediatric and adolescent AIDS is a reportable condition, the actual incidence/prevalence is probably unknown because of significant underreporting of AIDS cases both in the United States and worldwide. The actual incidence/prevalence of HIV infection in children is unknown because no national statistics have been compiled. The occurrence of AIDS in children was established as early as 1982; 20 children less than 13 years of age had been diagnosed by the end of 1981. By the spring of 1991, more than 2900 cases of AIDS in children had been reported to the Centers for Disease Control (CDC), comprising 1.7% of the total number of reported AIDS cases in the United States (CDC, 1991). Estimates from the CDC suggest that currently there are 10,000 to 20,000 infants and children in this country who are infected with HIV. The incidence of pediatric HIV disease is rapidly increasing as HIV infection continues to increase in the injection drug–using and heterosexual communities. All states in the United States have now reported at least one case of pediatric AIDS.

Because most children with AIDS have been perinatally infected, the demographics of this group closely parallels that of women with AIDS (Table 23-2). In this population HIV is a disease primarily associated with primarily poverty and drug use and is clustered in inner cities and ethnic minority communities. The parenteral cases, on the other hand, represent a broader geographic distribution and a wider ethnic apportionment.

Adolescent AIDS cases account for less than 1% of the total reported to the CDC. However, because the mean time from infection to symptom development is estimated to be 8 years, most in-

Table 23-2. Pediatric AIDS cases ($N = 2433$) by maternal exposure category and race or ethnicity*

Exposure	White (%)	Black (%)	Latino (%)	Asian/ Pac Is (%)	Am Ind/ Alaskan (%)	Total (%)
IV drug use	50	50	51	33	33	50
Sex with IVDU	21	16	31	17	17	21
Born in pattern-11 country	<1	15	1	0	0	9
Sex with other at risk person	13	7	7	17	17	8
Recipient of blood, blood products, or tissue	5	1	2	0	0	2
Risk unspecified	11	11	8	33	33	10
TOTAL						100

Adapted from Centers for Disease Control: HIV/AIDS surveillance report, March, 1991.

*Pac Is, Pacific Islander; Am Ind, American Indian; IV, intravenous; IVDU, intravenous drug user.

fected teens will not become ill until early adulthood. The number of AIDS cases diagnosed in persons aged 20 to 29 years account for 21% of the total (Hein, 1989).

Human immunodeficiency virus is frequently diagnosed late in children because few pediatric providers are alert to the presenting signs and symptoms of HIV infection. Early diagnosis and treatment of HIV-infected infants is believed to enrich and prolong their lives. Currently there are no accurate methods of prenatal diagnosis for HIV infection. However, there are now national clinical trials that involve antiviral therapy during pregnancy and at the time of delivery. Some trials using antivirals in neonates have been completed, and other protocols are being finalized.

CLINICAL MANIFESTATIONS AT TIME OF DIAGNOSIS

Developing a clinical definition of HIV infection and AIDS in children has proved to be a complex task. The prior pediatric AIDS definition provided direction for surveillance but did not describe the spectrum of infection; therefore, in 1987 the CDC developed a classification system for HIV infection in children (see box on p. 411). Although HIV infection is ideally identified by viral culture from blood or tissue, it is generally diagnosed by the presence of specific antibodies to the virus. However, the presence of passive maternal antibody limits the use of HIV antibody testing in infants

suspected of perinatal infection up to the age of 15 months. For this reason two definitions of infection in children are necessary: one for perinatally exposed infants up to 15 months of age and one for older children.

Many pediatric HIV-AIDS centers now use more specific laboratory tests to determine infectivity in perinatally exposed infants as young as 2 weeks of age. Human immunodeficiency virus blood culturing, available for many years, is expensive and labor intensive but becoming more standardized. Polymerase chain reaction (PCR) is a method of gene amplification that directly detects proviral sequences of HIV within DNA using small amounts of blood (Rogers et al., 1989). This method is proving to be superior to viral culture and antigen assays. It may also be useful in determining timing of transmission. A third test that may also be helpful in determining true infection in infants more than 6 months of age is the P24 antigen. Used concurrently, these three specific tests can be highly predictive of HIV infection in infants. Because these tests are not yet widely available community clinicians caring for these children may not have direct access to them but will need to contact the National Institute of Allergy and Infectious Diseases or the Maternal-Child Health Bureau for the nearest participating research group.

For those children meeting the definition of HIV exposure or infection, they may be further grouped

---

CDC CLASSIFICATION FOR HIV INFECTION IN CHILDREN LESS THAN 13 YEARS OLD

CLASS P-0 INDETERMINATE INFECTION

Perinatal exposure up to 15 months of age that cannot be classified definitively, due to presence of maternal antibody

CLASS P-1 ASYMPTOMATIC INFECTION
Subclass A: Normal immune function

Without abnormalities in quantitative immunoglobulins, complete blood cell count with differential, T-lymphocyte subsets

Subclass B: Abnormal immune function

One or more common abnormalities, including hypergammaglobulinemia, decreased T4/T8 ratio, decreased T4 count, and absolute lymphopenia

Subclass C: Immune function not tested

CLASS P-2 SYMPTOMATIC INFECTION
Subclass A: Nonspecific findings

Two or more of the following persisting for more than 2 months: fever, failure to thrive, or weight loss greater than 10%, hepatosplenomegaly, lymphadenopathy, parotitis, or diarrhea

Subclass B: Progressive neurologic disease

Loss of milestones or intellectual ability, impaired brain growth, or progressive motor deficits

Subclass C: Lymphoid interstitial pneumonitis

Subclass D: Secondary infectious diseases
    Category D-1
Specified secondary infectious diseases listed in the CDC surveillance definition for AIDS
    Category D-2
Recurrent serious bacterial infections: sepsis, meningitis, pneumonia, abscess, or bone or joint infections
    Category D-3
Other specified secondary infectious diseases: oral *Candida* persisting 2 months or more, two or more episodes of herpes stomatitis, or disseminated herpes zoster virus (HZV)

Subclass E: Secondary cancers
    Category E-1
Specified secondary cancers listed in the CDC surveillance definition for AIDS
    Category E-2
Other malignancies possibly associated with HIV

Subclass F: Other diseases

Conditions possibly caused by HIV such as hepatitis, cardiopathy, nephropathy, hematologic disorders, and dermatologic diseases

Adapted from Centers for Disease Control: *MMWR* 36:225-236, 1987.

---

into one of three mutually exclusive classes based on the presence or absence of clinical signs and symptoms (see the box on p. 412). This classification system is similar in design to the adult classification system and is helpful for health care planning and epidemiologic purposes.

Because HIV infection is clearly a multisystem disease process, infected infants and children may have a wide range of signs and symptoms. Often the clinical manifestations that occur early in infection are nonspecific and may be seen in healthy children and children with other conditions (see the box on p. 412). However, children with HIV infection generally experience more chronic and severe signs and symptoms and often fail to respond to appropriate therapy. Some children have acute opportunistic infections (OIs) with the same protozoal, viral, fungal, and bacterial pathogens as do adults, which are indicator diseases for an AIDS diagnosis. Others may have nephropathy, hepatitis, cardiomyopathy, and hematologic abnormalities.

Some children are diagnosed with HIV infection before they exhibit any signs or symptoms of illness. Infants and children born to mothers known

---

CLINICAL FEATURES ASSOCIATED WITH EARLY HIV INFECTION IN INFANCY AND CHILDHOOD

Failure to thrive	Thrombocytopenia
Diarrhea, chronic or recurrent	Hepatosplenomegaly
Fever of unknown origin	Parotitis
Atopic dermatitis	Frequent infections
Persistent or recurrent fungal infections such as thrush or diaper dermatitis	Developmental delay; loss of milestones

---

to be HIV infected may be tested to determine if they are also infected. Retrospective transfusion programs have recently identified many infected children. Boys with hemophilia who received factor concentrate or other blood products before 1985 are counseled about HIV testing (see Chapter 6).

TREATMENT

Human immunodeficiency virus infection is gradually becoming a chronic, treatable, life-threatening disease. The most significant treatments are those aimed at killing HIV in an attempt to eradicate the virus. Currently the only antiretroviral agent approved by the Food and Drug Administration is zidovudine (AZT; Retrovir). Studies using zidovudine in children have established safety and efficacy, particularly with benefit to neurodevelopmental status (Pizzo, 1990).

There are a growing number of investigational treatment protocols for children. Many questions regarding the use of antiretrovirals in children are yet unanswered, including when to start, how long to continue, and when and how to modify dosage. Efforts are underway to test new drugs simultaneously in adults and children rather than to prove efficacy in adults before allowing children access to them. Unfortunately few clinical trials have been open to adolescents 13 to 17 years of age other than hemophilia-specific protocols. Therefore, little information is known about the specific needs and issues of teens. A chemotherapy model utilizing combination therapy and synergism, such as in the treatment of cancer, will be increasingly available in treating HIV infection as new effective agents are developed.

A national placebo-controlled study examining

the efficacy of reconstitution of the immune system with IV gamma globulin (IVIG) in pediatric HIV disease has demonstrated that it reduces the number of bacterial infections in some children, increases the time children are free of infection, and reduces the number of hospitalizations (Marwick, 1991). Despite these findings, however, there was no effect on mortality.

In the absence of a definitive cure, the treatment for children with HIV infection is comprehensive, multidisciplinary care, with prompt diagnosis and aggressive therapy of concurrent infections and other clinical manifestations of disease. The most frequent problems in children with HIV infection are recurrent and severe systemic bacterial infections, which can progress to pneumonia, meningitis, and sepsis. Most often these infections are caused by encapsulated bacteria, such as *Haemophilus influenzae* or *Streptococcus pneumoniae*, reflecting the B-cell abnormality that occurs early in pediatric infection and is distinguished by dysfunctional hypergammaglobulinemia (Pizzo, Eddy, and Falloon, 1988). Although many children seem to have chronic bacterial infections that often require prolonged treatment, the role of prophylactic antibiotic therapy is unknown and not generally recommended (Falloon et al., 1989).

Most children with HIV infection, even those with symptomatic disease, are active, playful, functional children who see themselves as healthy. They may take medications and spend time in the hospital, but they also attend day care and school. It is important for the practitioner to remember that these children will develop common childhood illnesses and that all symptoms are not related to their underlying immunodeficiency. However, children with HIV disease need to be quickly assessed and aggressively managed when the possibility of intercurrent illness occurs. A wait and see attitude is rarely appropriate. These children and their families need to develop a strong partnership with their primary care practitioner so that prompt evaluation and treatment is assured. Children with HIV infection need to be linked with a comprehensive pediatric HIV-AIDS treatment center whenever possible. Centers ensure access to clinical trials, the most up-to-date information and expertise, and other children and families who are living with this disease. Clear lines of access to and responsibility of the primary provider and the center team need to be developed for each family.

PROGNOSIS

Acquired immune deficiency syndrome is among the 10 leading causes of death in children. It exceeds other infectious causes and will most likely be among the top five causes of death within the next few years (Pizzo, 1990). More than 50% of the children diagnosed with AIDS have died, but the actual mortality rate may be changing as treatment advances are made. Two distinct disease courses of perinatally infected children seem to exist: Those who have a shorter median survival time appear to develop symptoms by 4 to 6 months of age, qualify for an AIDS diagnosis by 1 year, and often die by the age of 2 years; Those with a longer median survival time seem to develop symptoms after the first year of life and often procure an AIDS diagnosis on the basis of lymphoid interstitial pneumonitis (LIP) around the age of 5 years (Falloon et al., 1989). Children who are infected during or after birth tend to run a course similar to adults, with the time from infection to development of symptoms in excess of 5 years. Still others will not become symptomatic until the middle school years. The age at diagnosis of AIDS may serve as a surrogate marker for the aggressiveness of the disease process (Scott et al., 1989).

ASSOCIATED PROBLEMS
Failure to thrive

Nutrition can be a significant problem in children with HIV disease, particularly those with chronic diarrhea and *Candida* esophagitis. Many infants and children with symptomatic disease demonstrate poor weight gain and frequently fall below the fifth percentile for weight on the National Center for Health Statistics growth curves.

Specific etiologies of chronic diarrheas, such as *Cryptosporidium, Giardia,* and *Mycobacterium avium-intracellulare* (MAI) are rarely found, even after exhaustive GI and stool examinations. Some children thrive better on lactose-free diets, whereas others experience cyclical diarrhea unresponsive to dietary manipulations. Many clinicians believe that these problems are caused by changes in the gastrointestinal (GI) tract secondary to direct invasion by HIV.

Encephalopathy and developmental delay

The brain is a target site for HIV infection in infants and children (Epstein et al., 1987). Fortunately, many children function well or with minimal delay for years. However, by end stage of their disease, the majority develop characteristic progressive encephalopathy. This results in developmental delays, deterioration of motor skills and cognitive functioning, and possibly behavioral abnormalities. The course may be static or progressive but most often is episodic, with plateaus of relative stability lasting months, alternating with intervals of marked deterioration occurring over weeks. The degree of neurologic deficit usually parallels the degree of immunodeficiency, and the onset of progressive encephalopathy is a prognostic sign that correlates with poor outcome (Epstein, Sharer, and Goudsmit, 1988).

Acquired microcephaly is frequently observed in infants and young children with HIV disease. Computerized tomographic scanning and magnetic resonance imaging often demonstrate diffuse cortical atrophy and basal ganglia calcifications in severely affected infants (Falloon et al., 1989). Cerebrospinal fluid (CSF), even if HIV culture positive, usually shows normal glucose and protein levels and cell count.

These children may demonstrate gradual apathy, progressive motor deficits resulting in generalized weakness and gait disturbances, and difficulties with expressive language. It is often perplexing to differentiate the impact of HIV infection from the effects of prenatal and perinatal drug exposure, prematurity, chronic disease, and chaotic social environments (Wishon and Gee, 1988).

Opportunistic infections

OIs are the major cause of death. Data on treatment of OIs are available only for adults, although there are some important differences between children and adults that may affect treatment. Opportunistic infections in adults are believed to be reactivations of latent infections acquired at an earlier time, whereas in children OIs may develop from primary infections. *Pneumocystis carinii* pneumonia (PCP) is the most frequent OI in pediatric AIDS, cited in more than 50% of the cases of AIDS in children reported to the CDC (Rubenstein, Morecki, and Goldman, 1988). The mortality rate for children with PCP is as high as 85% compared with about 20% in adults (Nicholas et al., 1989).

Pulmonary disease

One of the most characteristic manifestations of HIV infection in children is LIP, accounting for the AIDS diagnosis in more than one half of the children (Barrett, 1988). It is as yet unclear whether this entity is caused by opportunistic infection or infiltration of the lungs by HIV-infected lymphocytes. Lymphoid interstitial pneumonitis is a chronic interstitial process of diffuse bilateral infiltration that may be diagnosed presumptively by clinical and radiographic means and definitively by bronchoscopy and open lung biopsy. Other symptoms include generalized lymphadenopathy, digital clubbing, and salivary gland enlargement (Falloon et al., 1989). Treatment is symptomatic. Children who have LIP rather than OIs tend to have a more gradual disease course and a longer median survival time. The onset is often insidious, with slowly progressive hypoxia and resultant respiratory failure (Rubenstein, Morecki, and Goldman, 1988).

Pneumocystis carinii is the most frequent OI seen in pediatric AIDS. The initial manifestation of the child with PCP is likely to be acute with fever, dyspnea, dry cough, cyanosis, and hypoxemia (Falloon et al., 1989). Diagnosis is made by the same methods as for LIP. Prophylaxis using the oral form of trimethoprim-sulfamethoxazole (TMP-SMX; Bactrim, Septra) 3 days weekly has become standard therapy in children. Those who are unable to tolerate this sulfa combination may be given pentamidine (Pentam, NebuPent) either intravenously or aerosolized monthly. The same drugs are used for treatment of acute PCP but in different dosages and routes of administration.

Other pathogens causing pulmonary disease include cytomegalovirus (CMV), respiratory syncytial virus, *Mycobacterium tuberculosis,* MAI, rubeola, varicella, and a variety of bacteria.

Pancytopenia

Hematologic abnormalities are common in children with HIV infection, occurring as a result of HIV infection itself or as an adverse effect of treatment. Some children have thrombocytopenia, which is usually an immune response to circulating platelets, because their bone marrow produces megakaryocytes, which break down into platelets in the peripheral blood. Intravenous immunoglobulin (IVIG) is sometimes effective in raising the platelet count, and platelet transfusions are rarely required. Anemias of chronic disease or iron deficiency are common among this population and often require iron supplementation. Red blood cell (RBC) transfusions are sometimes indicated, particularly in AZT-induced anemia. Cytomegalovirus-negative, washed, irradiated RBCs and irradiated platelets are used to avoid introducing new infection and to protect against graft-versus-host disease. Abnormalities of the white blood cell line, including neutropenia, lymphopenia, and leukopenia, are also frequently observed.

Fungal infections

Candidiasis occurs frequently and may be manifested as either oral thrush or diaper dermatitis. The usual first-line treatments for oral thrush include topical nystatin (Mycostatin) and clotrimazole (Mycelex) oral troches. However, clotrimazole vaginal suppositories (100 mg) used orally are often more efficacious because they are 10 times more potent than the oral suspensions or troches. Infants can be treated either by placing the suppository into the nipple of a bottle, allowing the infant to suck formula through it, or by dissolving the suppository in warm water and swabbing the mouth. Older children can suck the suppositories. Both nystatin and clotrimazole creams are available for skin infections. Refractory cases of mucous membrane and dermatologic infections may be treated systemically with oral ketaconazole (Nizoral) or the newer fluconazole (Difucan).

Prenatal and perinatal drug exposure

Children with HIV who have been born to drug and alcohol-using, HIV-infected mothers are frequently premature, small for gestational age, and have very immature immune systems. Their development is often delayed, and learning and behavioral difficulties are common (see Chapter 26).

PRIMARY CARE MANAGEMENT
Growth and development

The poor growth of children with symptomatic HIV disease appears to be more related to the general failure to thrive associated with the underlying HIV infection rather than to specific problems with caloric intake or GI losses. Height and weight should be measured carefully by a practitioner or a skilled assistant and plotted on the child's individual National Center for Health Statistics growth chart at least monthly. The same scale should be used each visit if at all possible. Nutritionists need to be part of the multidisciplinary primary care team, taking dietary histories and performing nutritional assessments to guide clinical decisions.

As previously noted, cortical atrophy and acquired microcephaly are common findings in the more severely affected infants. All children up to age 3 years require serial head circumference measurements at least every 3 months, with results plotted on the child's growth chart and carefully evaluated. Symptomatic children need careful measurements by the practitioner.

Standard developmental screening tests used by primary care clinicians, such as the Denver Developmental Screening Test, are of little value in assessing the child with HIV disease. Developmental delay is a hallmark of pediatric HIV infection, and early intervention appears to produce significant results; therefore, it is imperative that these children be assessed regularly by a skilled clinical psychologist as part of the comprehensive team approach. It is important for the practitioner and the psychologist to discuss their developmental assessments and to formulate a plan of action together.

Intervention strategies must begin as early as possible in an attempt to maximize the child's capabilities. Infant stimulation programs that focus on motor and language skills and add specialties such as physical, occupational, and speech therapy can be provided at home, in the hospital, or in clinic or group settings. Preschool and school-aged children who have the physical stamina necessary can best be mainstreamed into regular programs, with special services added.

Immunizations

There has been much discussion regarding immunization practices in children with HIV infection. Historically, live-virus vaccines have not been recommended for children with congenital or drug-induced immunodeficiencies because of the concern that administration of live, attenuated vaccine viruses has the potential to produce infection in an immunocompromised host (Onorato, Markowitz, and Oxtoby, 1988). However, a retrospective study of more than 300 children with HIV infection in New York City who received live-virus vaccines demonstrated no serious adverse effects (Onorato, Markowitz, and Oxtoby, 1988). Current prospective studies have also failed to disclose problems (Falloon et al., 1989).

In addition, the dysfunction of the B-cell system typical of infants with HIV disease, which includes markedly elevated immunoglobulin levels, reflects nonspecific stimulation suggestive of poor immune response to antigens and therefore to vaccines. Because of this immunologic dysfunction, immunogenicity and vaccine efficacy may be lower than in immunocompetent children. Symptomatic children have demonstrated lower serum concentrations of diphtheria and tetanus (DT) antibodies and responded less well to pneumococcal and DT boosters. Nonetheless, many developed sufficient antibodies to be considered protected (Onorato, Markowitz, and Oxtoby, 1988). Because live-virus, attenuated immunizations may be ineffective if given to children who have received IVIG during the previous 3 months, the general practice is to administer these vaccinations at the midpoint between monthly IVIG infusions.

Polio. Human immunodeficiency virus exposed and infected children should receive the injectable inactivated poliomyelitis vaccine (IPV) rather than oral poliomyelitis vaccine (OPV). Inactivated poliomyelitis vaccine should be used by all household members and contacts because there is a theoretical risk for vaccine-associated poliomyelitis; polio virus can be excreted in the stool up to 4 weeks after the primary immunization (Onorato, Markowitz, and Oxtoby, 1988).

Measles, mumps, and rubella. The measles, mumps, and rubella (MMR) vaccination should be administered at the standard age of 15 months unless there is an increased risk of measles or rubeola exposure. Monovalent measles vaccine can be used for infants 6 to 11 months old, with revaccination with MMR at 12 months of age or older. It is now recommended that all children be revaccinated with MMR at school entry or at 5 years of age (Immunization Practices Advisory Committee, 1989). Immune globulin (IG) may be helpful in preventing or minimizing measles if it is administered within 6 days of exposure. It is also indicated for measles-susceptible household contacts of children with asymptomatic HIV disease, especially for infants less than 12 months of age. Immune globulin prophylaxis is explicitly recommended for exposed children with symptomatic HIV infection; however, it may be unnecessary if the child is receiving regular IVIG infusions and the last dose was within 3 weeks of exposure (Immunization Practices Advisory Committee, 1988).

Haemophilus influenzae type b. Conjugated polysaccharide-diphtheria *Haemophilus influenzae* type b vaccine is recommended for all children starting at 2 months of age (Committee on Infectious Diseases, 1991). As previously noted, *H. influenzae* is a common and serious pathogen in children with HIV infection, increasing the importance of immunization. Even children who have had one or more episodes of documented infection with *H. influenzae* before the age of 2 years may not produce enough antibody to prevent subsequent infections, making vaccination imperative. Prophylaxis with rifampin (Rifadin) is required even after vaccination if there is a known contact with Hib (Committee on Infectious Diseases, 1991).

Pneumococcus. Polyvalent pneumococcal vaccine (Pneumovax) should be administered to children with HIV disease at 2 years of age because of their underlying immunosuppression and the fact that pneumococcus is a prevalent pathogen in this population (Committee on Infectious Diseases, 1991).

Influenza. Yearly influenza vaccination with the subvirion (split-virus) bivalent vaccine is recommended for children more than 6 months of age

with HIV exposure or infection and their household contacts (Committee on Infectious Diseases, 1991).

Varicella. Varicella (HZV) poses significant risks for dissemination, encephalitis, and pneumonia in immunosuppressed children. Unfortunately the varicella vaccine is not yet licensed or recommended. Children with HIV infection need to receive varicella-zoster immune globulin (VZIG) intramuscularly within 72 hours of exposure if they have not received IVIG within the past 3 weeks.

Screening

Vision. Because of the incidence of CMV retinitis in adults with HIV disease and therefore the theoretical risk of a similar process affecting children, the practitioner must elicit a thorough visual history and provide a careful visual and fundoscopic examination. Comprehensive pediatric HIV centers may recommend that all children with HIV infection be referred to a knowledgeable pediatric ophthalmologist for baseline screening. If the findings are normal, the practitioner can then continue to provide regular follow-up.

Hearing. Because of the frequent acute suppurative otitis media (OM) in children with HIV infection and the possibility of hearing loss, periodic audiometry and tympanometry should be performed. Children who require myringotomy tube placement require special precautions for swimming and showers, such as regular use of well-fitting earplugs.

Children with severe neurologic disease, some children with chronic OM, and those on maintenance aminoglycoside therapy need baseline brainstem auditory evoked response hearing testing if routine acuity testing cannot be done or is abnormal.

Dental. Early screening beginning at 2 to 3 years of age is strongly recommended because dental caries can create a focus of infection. Fluoride treatments are recommended if the community water supply does not contain adequate amounts to protect enamel. Severe dental caries and gingivitis, as well as dental abscesses, are being reported in some infected children. The clinician must educate families regarding appropriate oral hygiene and encourage regular dental care.

Blood pressure. Blood pressure measurements

should be taken every 3 to 6 months unless changes warrant more frequent measurements.

Hematocrit. Screening is deferred because of the need for frequent CBC assessment.

Urinalysis. Children with HIV disease require urinalysis with microscopic examination at least every 3 months because urine abnormalities can be the first sign of illness. Findings can include hematuria and proteinuria and can result in azotemia and nephrotic syndrome (Falloon et al., 1989).

Tuberculosis. Yearly screening is strongly advised. As more tuberculosis is being diagnosed in adults with HIV infection, more children in infected households are at risk. Because many HIV-infected individuals demonstrate anergy to skin testing, close surveillance of families may include regular chest x-rays studies. *Mycobacterium avium-intracellulare* (MAI) is a common bacterium of the same family as *M. tuberculosis* that is prevalent in the population of HIV-infected persons. Unlike *M. tuberculosis,* MAI is not contagious by the respiratory route but may be transmitted through infected GI secretions. Because it can invade many organ systems, including the bone marrow and the GI system, MAI may be responsible for much morbidity.

Condition-specific screening

VITAL SIGNS. Vital signs should be assessed and documented at each visit. Children can be asymptomatic yet febrile, needing a work-up. Elevations in heart and respiratory rate can indicate pulmonary or cardiac dysfunction. Increased blood pressure can indicate renal disease.

COMPLETE BLOOD COUNT. Because of bone marrow suppression caused by HIV and some OIs, as well as by many of the drugs used in treatment, children with HIV disease require regular determinations of CBCs with differential and platelet counts. Asymptomatic children should have a CBC done every 3 to 6 months; symptomatic children usually need them done at least monthly. This blood work can be performed by the primary care provider or at the pediatric HIV center.

Anemia should be investigated as to the cause, because children with iron deficiency anemia will usually benefit from oral iron supplementation. Often no specific cause is discovered. Children taking AZT need CBC and reticulocyte counts assessed frequently because anemia is a common adverse effect. Complete blood counts with reticulocyte

counts are usually completed every 2 weeks for the first 2 months and then done monthly as long as the counts are stable. Dosage is modified based on the degrees of anemia. Some children taking AZT require RBC transfusions. Neutropenia and thrombocytopenia are also common side effects of AZT, and dose reductions may be indicated.

IMMUNOLOGIC MARKERS. Baseline T- and B-cell counts and quantitative immunoglobulin (QUIG) determinations are necessary to assess immunologic status. T-cell subset values and T4/T8 ratios are usually checked every 3 to 6 months. T4 counts less than $500/mm^3$ are generally an indication for prescribing antivirals, such as AZT. Children receiving monthly IVIG infusions do not have serial QUIG assessments because they would reflect the infused rather than endogenous immunoglobulins.

CHEMISTRY PANEL. Routine serum chemistry panels should be obtained every 3 to 6 months and more frequently for symptomatic children or those taking medications that might affect liver or kidney function. Many HIV-infected children have elevated baseline liver function test results, with both aspartate aminotransferase (AST) and alanine aminotransferase (ALT) enzyme levels frequently 2 to 3 times normal.

PULMONARY FUNCTION. Children with chronic lung disease need baseline pulmonary function testing with oxygen saturation and regular serial testing based on disease severity. Pulse oximetry, a noninvasive technique, is used in place of arterial blood gas sampling when available. A baseline radiograph is useful as a comparison study for pulmonary complaints. Often the child with either acute infection or chronic pneumonitis has no adventitial sounds. Pulmonary consultation is a useful adjunct for the practitioner in following these children.

Drug interactions

The main toxicity of AZT in children is bone marrow suppression—anemia and neutropenia (Pizzo, Eddy, and Falloon, 1988). Drug interactions with AZT are currently being analyzed but have not yet been promulgated.

Major toxicities of TMP-SMX are neutropenia and thrombocytopenia. Children may develop side effects when it is taken alone or in combination with AZT. When these toxicities persist, the drug must be discontinued. Because allergic reactions to sulfa are not uncommon, practitioners need to teach families how to recognize the symptoms of skin rash and hives as part of the reaction complex. The child who shows allergy to one form of sulfa should not be prescribed other antibiotics containing sulfa.

DIFFERENTIAL DIAGNOSIS AND MANAGEMENT OF COMMON PEDIATRIC CONDITIONS

Fever

Fever is a frequent sign in children with HIV disease. It can be caused by HIV disease itself or can indicate a separate infectious process. Practitioners must ensure that families have a thermometer, are able to use it accurately, and have clear guidelines about when to contact their primary care provider. Generally whenever a child's temperature measures 38.5° C or greater, the child needs to be examined and a treatment plan initiated based on the objective and subjective findings.

A thorough interval history and complete physical examination are the most important part of the work-up of a febrile child with HIV infection. Some of these children will have OM, sinusitis, pneumonia, or sepsis; others will have common colds and other viral infections that can be traced to school or household contacts.

In consultation with the infectious disease specialist or the HIV center, the primary care clinician can order cultures of blood and other body fluid as indicated for aerobic, anaerobic, and fungal organisms. Cultures are essential in an attempt to identify the infectious process. Frequently the cultures are negative, even in seriously ill children, but positive cultures will determine specific antibiotic therapy. Chest x-ray studies may be an important part of the work-up of a febrile child with HIV infection.

Respiratory distress

A variety of respiratory complaints may plague children with HIV disease. Again, the history and physical examination are of paramount importance in the differential diagnosis. A dry hacking cough is a common complaint of children with LIP but can also be a sign of PCP. Children with acute onset of respiratory distress need speedy evalua-

tion, because the condition can progress extremely rapidly, sometimes over hours. Pulmonary consultation is often necessary. Occasionally children with cardiac disease have respiratory complaints. These children need cardiology consultation and diagnosis.

Children with known reactive airway disease may benefit from having equipment and medications for aerosol delivery at home. The practitioner must evaluate the family's ability to provide such sophisticated assessment and treatment, and if they are capable, they can be taught the necessary skills.

Otitis media

Otitis media is one of the most common infectious diseases seen in children with HIV disease. Frequently it is diagnosed on routine physical examination when no pain or fever is present, even at times when the tympanic membrane may be ruptured with pus filling the external canal. Follow-up must be done after treatment is completed because the OM may not resolve and complications may occur. Children who have persistent and refractory OM should be referred to an ear, nose, and throat specialist for evaluation of myringotomy tube placement.

Sinusitis

Although sinusitis is rare in children, it is seen commonly in children with HIV disease, often occurring after a viral respiratory tract infection. The practitioner can teach the family to report changes in the color of nasal mucus from clear or white to yellow or green, which may indicate infection. Sinusitis, if not appropriately treated, can lead to mastoiditis and can directly extend into the brain, causing meningitis.

Varicella

Because of the risk of dissemination as a result of immunocompromise, varicella in the child with HIV disease is potentially life-threatening. Because there is no licensed immunization as yet, HZV continues to cause chickenpox as a primary manifestation and zoster as a secondary manifestation of infection in most children. If primary prevention with VZIG fails, or if the child was not known to be exposed until the rash occurs, the usual practice at most centers is to hospitalize and treat with acyclovir intravenously as soon as the disease is diagnosed. With this treatment few children progress to disseminated disease, and most go home within 5 days of starting therapy, continuing with oral therapy to complete a 7- to 10-day course.

DEVELOPMENTAL ISSUES
Safety

The practitioner must teach the family safety precautions for children with neutropenia and thrombocytopenia and how to evaluate the neutropenic child for signs and symptoms of infection (see Chapter 8).

Caretakers may benefit from education on infectious disease transmission and control, such as the need for frequent handwashing and avoiding crowds. Children with HIV infection and their household contacts need to learn universal blood and body substance precautions. Because there is such concern in the community regarding casual contagion, families need to be well educated and able to withstand the apprehension of others. Several prospective studies of family and school contacts have found no evidence of HIV infection spread within these settings (Rogers et al., 1990). Although HIV has been isolated in a variety of body fluids, including blood, CSF, pleural fluid, breast milk, semen, cervical secretions, saliva, and urine, only blood, semen, cervical secretions, and human milk have been implicated in its transmission (American Academy of Pediatrics Task Force, 1988).

It is important to counsel the child's caretaker concerning safe storage of medications and equipment in the home. HIV-infected parents may also have many potentially hazardous medications at home. Children with HIV infection may be developmentally delayed or exhibit neurologic regression as the infection progresses. Safety precautions must be adjusted accordingly. If the child is cared for by a parent with HIV infection, the parent's ability to safely care for the child must be frequently assessed because of the symptom of dementia often associated with adult HIV infection.

Child care

Child care, respite care, and preschool placement are difficult issues for families of children with HIV infection. The practitioner must advise parents that children who are in group settings have an increased risk of exposure to infectious diseases and common childhood illnesses compared with children who remain at home. The particular setting for each child must be individualized, based on the child and family's needs and resources. Practitioners can provide education regarding universal infection control and infectious disease guidelines for these agencies.

Child care and respite care are important resources for families who are caring for children with chronic conditions. Some foster families have access to respite hours through their social services division, whereas others have none. In some areas there are few, if any, child care or respite workers who are willing to care for infants and children with HIV infection. This is an enormous problem for infected families who need time to care for their own HIV disease, as well as for their infected and noninfected children. The regular availability of respite care and other support services may allow many infected mothers to continue to care for their children.

Public Law 99-457, Early Education for Individuals with Exceptional Needs, may offer valuable services for children with HIV (see Chapter 4). Head Start, a federal preschool program that provides preschool for economically deprived children, is specifically mandated to enroll children with HIV infection.

Because day care and preschool are not a legal requirement for children, individual day-care providers may develop their own policies in accordance with local, state, and federal regulations. Many private day-care centers and preschools refuse to accept children with HIV infection, probably because of their fears of casual contagion, litigation, and disenrollment if other families discover the diagnosis. Some areas of the country with high prevalence of pediatric HIV disease have developed day-care programs specifically for these children. Such services are directed toward children who are too ill to attend regular day-care programs. It is optimal to educate day-care and preschool personnel and families before a child with HIV disease is enrolled. It may be useful for the practitioner to call preschools, stating that a family is interested in enrolling their HIV-infected child. The school is notified that there is no "duty to inform" and that the child will not be identified. Feelings regarding children with HIV infection are explored, and an offer is made to provide in-service training about pediatric HIV disease and general infection control.

Some families choose to conceal the fact of HIV in their family; other families discuss it openly. As more children take antiviral medications such as AZT that need to be administered frequently, it is becoming harder to conceal HIV infection from day-care providers. However, many families schedule dosing around school hours and create unusual stories about why they need to know immediately about chickenpox or other contagious illnesses in the classroom. The clinician has a large role to play in helping families to decide how, when, and to whom information about HIV disease should be disclosed.

Diet

Children with HIV infection need a well-balanced diet with emphasis on adequate calories to maintain and increase weight with growth. There are no special dietary recommendations or restrictions based on HIV infection. Because failure to thrive is common in this population, early nutritional intervention before wasting occurs is important. Dietary supplementation and special formulas (e.g., Instant Breakfast for those who can tolerate dairy products and Pediasure for infants and younger children and Ensure for older children and adolescents who are lactose intolerant) are often beneficial for weight stabilization and potential weight gain. Enteral feedings and IV alimentation may be used acutely, intermittently, or chronically for children with severe anorexia, vomiting, diarrhea, and other GI problems. Consultation between the family and practitioner regarding the child's particular needs should take place on a regular basis.

Discipline

Discipline is often difficult for the family of a child with a life-threatening illness. Some parents are unable to set age-appropriate and necessary limits and need guidance and information from their provider. Other factors such as homelessness, chaotic life-style, and parental illness can make consistent discipline difficult. Practitioners may be helpful in assisting families to understand the child's needs for safety and limits.

Toileting

Nontoilet-trained children with HIV infection may experience profound diaper dermatitis. this is frequently associated with candidiasis, as well as with chronic and/or cyclical diarrhea. Impeccable perineal care including frequent diaper changes, exposure of the perineum to air, and the use of topical medications can significantly reduce morbidity. When the perineum is bloody or the child has hematuria or diarrhea, the caretakers should wear gloves to protect themselves during diapering.

Sleep patterns

Children taking AZT or other medications that interrupt normal sleeping hours may experience difficulty in returning to sleep. Parents may need to try a variety of schedules to find one that works best for them and their child. The practitioner must be sure that the family has access to a reliable alarm clock so that doses are not missed.

School issues

The major school issues faced by young children with HIV infection have little to do with their educational needs and much to do with concerns regarding confidentiality, information sharing, and infection control. This issue has created strife in many communities nationwide. As these children age, however, their needs for special education programs will undoubtedly increase. The practitioner can help the family secure the appropriate services (see Chapter 4).

Because AIDS is recognized as a handicap, attendance in public schools is supported by Public Law 94-142. In some areas of the country, public school attendance is decided by committees composed of educators, public health officials, and the child's primary care provider. If the decision is made to ban the child from attending school, the school district then must provide home teaching. Children benefit greatly from attending school, and this option should be strongly encouraged. When children are too ill to attend, home teaching is a viable alternative for that time period only.

There is no legal duty to inform school officials about a child's diagnosis, although this will vary from state to state. However, as more children become aware of their own HIV infection, there will be more discussion among the children themselves.

This will lead to greater awareness in the school and larger community that a child with HIV infection is in attendance. It is important for the provider to be available to the school — students, faculty, and parents — for educational discussion sessions.

Teenagers with HIV infection often have difficulty in school. Rumors that circulate about HIV infection and students who are believed to be infected can cause tremendous anxiety for an infected adolescent regardless of the route of infection. Primary care providers can support their teen-aged clients, helping them gain more knowledge and differentiate whom they might trust with this sensitive information. Referral to the school nurse or counselor may be appropriate.

Sexuality

Children and adolescents with HIV disease need to learn about sexual and perinatal transmission of this condition. Adolescence is the time for sexual experimentation and the emergence of sexual identity. Sexual activity increases steadily throughout these years. Teens who are infected with HIV face much difficulty in attaining a healthy, integrated sexual identity because of the risks of oral and genital sexual transmission. Some teens deny the reality of their HIV infection, refusing to practice safer sex, and sometimes choosing pregnancy. The practitioner needs to be comfortable discussing transmission and sexual risk reduction strategies, as well as demonstrating the proper use of condoms and dental dams.

SPECIAL FAMILY CONCERNS

Human immunodeficiency virus infection is a family disease, and when a child is diagnosed, a family crisis results. The majority of children with HIV disease have infected mothers who are ill, dying, or deceased; there may be an infected father and siblings in the family as well. Most infected mothers who transmit HIV to their children experience tremendous guilt. The physical and emotional bur-

den of caring for a child who requires frequent medical and supportive treatments, may have developmental delay, and will probably die as a result of the illness is enormous.

The most significant psychosocial issue facing children with HIV infection and their families is the social stigmatization associated with the disease. Initially many families feel isolated and unable to call on their normal support systems for fear of rejection and retaliation. In addition, these families may lack other resources; they are primarily poor, of minority heritage, undereducated, and burdened by the social ills of inner-city life. With support the family may reach out to utilize extended family, friends, and community agencies.

Some children are placed in foster or adoptive care after birth if the mother is unable to care for the infant. Others are placed out of the home at a later date when resources are insufficient to support the parents' ability to care for the child. Foster and adoptive parents need considerable support to provide optimal care for these children. They need ongoing education, financial support, respite care, emotional support and counseling, and social and legal counseling (American Academy of Pediatric News, 1989). Because children in foster care are wards of the juvenile court, decisions regarding consent for investigational drugs and experimental protocols, as well as do-not-resuscitate orders, must be court ordered. Working relationships need to be developed between the primary care provider, HIV center, and social services to ensure that children with HIV disease in the child welfare system receive optimal care.

Helping a child and family face a chronic, life-threatening illness that ultimately leads to death is a pivotal role for the primary care provider. Counseling about the physical and emotional issues of the death and dying process, options for hospital or home death, hospice services, funeral plans, and bereavement is imperative as an integral part of the clinician's role.

SUMMARY OF PRIMARY CARE NEEDS FOR THE CHILD WITH HIV INFECTION

Growth and development

Growth in both weight and height may be poor; measure and plot monthly.

Cortical atrophy and acquired microcephaly are common in severely affected infants.

Measure and plot head circumference monthly until the child is 3 years of age.

Standard developmental screening tests are not useful; serial screening by a psychologist if available is recommended.

Early intervention programs are recommended.

Immunizations

Use IPV for exposed/infected child, all household members, and close contacts.

Give immune globulin within 6 days of measles exposure to prevent or modify course unless child received IVIG within previous 3 weeks.

Haemophilus influenzae type b and polyvalent pneumococcal vaccines are recommended.

Yearly influenza vaccine is recommended.

Varicella-zoster immune globulin is recommended within 72 hours of varicella exposure.

Screening
Vision

Ophthalmologist should do baseline fundoscopic examination; practitioner follow-up every 3 to 6 months.

Hearing

Periodic audiometry and tympanometry screening is recommended.

A BSER hearing test should be given to those with chronic OM or abnormal screening.

Dental

Early screening is recommended to prevent dental infections.

Blood pressure

Measurements should be taken every 3 to 6 months.

Hematocrit

Routine screening is deferred because of the need for frequent CBC tests.

Urinalysis

Urinalysis with microscopic examination should be done at least every 3 months.

Tuberculosis

Yearly screening is recommended. Chest x-ray studies may be needed if the child is anergic.

Condition-specific screening
Vital signs

Temperature, heart rate, and respiratory rate should be checked at each visit.

Complete blood count

The CBC should be assessed every 3 to 6 months if the child is asymptomatic; every 2 to 4 weeks if the child is taking AZT or another myelosuppressive agent.

Immunologic markers

Baseline T- and B-cell counts, QUIG values, repeat T-cell subset levels, and T4/T8 ratios should be checked every 3 to 6 months.

Chemistry panel

Serum chemistry panels should be obtained every 3 to 6 months if the child is asymptomatic; more frequently if child is symptomatic or is taking liver or kidney toxic agents.

Pulmonary function

Baseline pulmonary function testing, including pulse oximetry if available, is recommended for children with lung disease.

Drug interactions
Zidovudine

Bone marrow suppression may occur.

Trimethoprim-sulfamethoxazole

Bone marrow suppression (neutropenia, thrombocytopenia) and allergic reactions may occur.

Differential diagnosis
Fever

Rule out bacterial infection and OI.

Respiratory distress

Rule out LIP, PCP, and cardiac disease.

Otitis media

Rule out tympanic membrane perforation.

SUMMARY OF PRIMARY CARE NEEDS FOR THE CHILD WITH HIV INFECTION — cont'd

Sinusitis

Rule out bacterial sinusitis, mastoiditis, and meningitis.

Varicella

Use VZIG as primary prevention and acyclovir as secondary prevention.

Developmental issues

Safety

The risk of infection because of immunocompromise is increased.

The risk of bleeding because of thrombocytopenia is increased.

Universal blood and body substance precautions should be taught to the family and community.

Safe storage of medication in the home is important. Developmental delay or regression may alter safety requirements.

Parents with HIV infection must be evaluated for safe care practices because of symptom of dementia.

Child care

The child care program should be individualized to meet the child's and family's needs.

Public Law 99-457 covers early intervention services.

Diet

Emphasize a balanced, high-calorie diet.

Use nutritional supplements.

Discipline

Discipline is often difficult for the family; lifestyle issues can exacerbate problems.

Toileting

Impeccable perineal care needed to reduce morbidity of diaper dermatitis. Caretaker to use gloves for blood or diarrhea.

Sleep patterns

Sleep patterns may be disturbed because of medications needed around the clock.

School issues

Public school attendance is aided by Public Law 94-142.

There is no duty to inform school officials of a child's HIV status.

The school community may benefit from education.

Teens may need extra support from the school nurse or counselor.

Sexuality

Discuss sexual and perinatal transmission.

Demonstrate safer sex techniques and the use of condoms and dental dams.

Special family concerns

Human immunodeficiency virus is a family disease.

Many families lack resources.

The disease is an enormous physical and emotional burden.

Stigmatization is a major issue.

Many of these children are placed in foster or adoptive homes.

Counseling on death and dying, and during bereavement is helpful.

RESOURCES

Support groups are invaluable resources for networking, keeping current, and decreasing social isolation. Most pediatric HIV-AIDS comprehensive treatment centers offer such groups on an ongoing basis. The primary care provider should become familiar with the local, national, and international organizations (see the list that follows).

Organizations

AIDS Resource Foundation for Children
182 Roseville Ave
Newark, NJ 07107
(201) 483-4250

Camp Sunburst National AIDS Project
148 Wilson Hill Rd
Petaluma, CA 94952
(707) 769-0169

Children and Youth AIDS Hotline
(212) 430-3333

Children with AIDS Care Program
Northern Lights Alternatives
78 W 85th St, Suite 5E
New York, NY 10024
(212) 337-8747

National AIDS Hotline
(800) 342-AIDS

National AIDS Information Clearinghouse
PO Box 6003
Rockville, MD 20850
(800) 458-5231

National Center for Youth Law
114 Sansome St, Suite 900
San Francisco, CA 94104-3820
(415) 543-3307

NIAID Intramural Trials for HIV Infection and AIDS
(800) AIDS-NIH (800-243-7644)

Pediatric AIDS Foster Care Network
Leake and Watts Children's Home
487 S Broadway, Suite 207
Yonkers, NY 10705

Pediatric AIDS Foundation
2407 Wilshire Blvd, Suite 613
Santa Monica, CA 90403
(213) 395-9051

Foundation for Children with AIDS, Inc
77B Warren St
Brighton, MA 02135
(617) 783-7300

Local and state resources

County health department
State health department
AIDS task forces
AIDS hotlines

REFERENCES

American Academy of Pediatrics Task Force on Pediatric AIDS: Pediatric guidelines for infection control of human immunodeficiency virus (acquired immunodeficiency virus) in hospitals, medical offices, schools, and other settings, *Pediatrics* 82:801-807, 1988.

American Academy of Pediatrics Task Force on Pediatric AIDS: Infants and children with acquired immunodeficiency syndrome: Placement in adoption and foster care, *Am Acad Pediatr News,* April 1989, pp 8-9.

Barrett DJ: The clinician's guide to pediatric AIDS, *Contemp Pediatr* 5:24-47, 1988.

Berkman SA, Lee ML, and Gale RP: Clinical uses of intravenous immunoglobulins, *Semin Hematol* 25:140-152, 1988.

Centers for Disease Control: Classification system for human immunodeficiency virus (HIV) infection in children under 13 years of age, *MMWR* 36:225-236, 1987.

Centers for Disease Control: *HIV/AIDS surveillance report,* March, 1991.

Centers for Disease Control: *HIV/AIDS surveillance report,* March, 1991.

Committee on Infectious Diseases: *Report of the committee on infectious diseases,* ed 22, Elk Grove Village, Ill, 1991, American Academy of Pediatrics.

Connor E, Bagarazzi M, McSherry G, et al: Clinical and laboratory correlates of *Pneumocystis carinii* pneumonia in children infected with HIV, *JAMA* 265:1693-1697, 1991.

Demmler GJ and Taber LH: Virology of HIV-1, *Semin Pediatr Infect Dis* 1:17-20, 1990.

Epstein LG, Goudsmit J, Paul DA, et al: Expression of human immunodeficiency virus in cerebrospinal fluid of children with progressive encephalopathy, *Ann Neurol* 21:397-401, 1987.

Epstein LG, Sharer LR, Goudsmit J: Neurological and neuropathological features of human immunodeficiency virus infection in children, *Ann Neurol J* 23(suppl):s19-s23, 1988.

Falloon J, Eddy J, Wiener L, et al: Human immunodeficiency virus infection in children, *J Pediatr* 114:1-30, 1989.

Hein K: Commentary on adolescent acquired immunodeficiency syndrome: The next wave of the human immunodeficiency virus epidemic? *J Pediatr* 114:144-149, 1989.

Kovacs A, Frederick T, Church J, et al: CD4 t-lymphocyte counts and *Pneumocystis carinii* pneumonia in pediatric HIV infection, *JAMA* 265:1698-1703, 1991.

Marwick C: Example of prepublication data release: Immunoglobulin for concomitant infections, *JAMA* 265:953, 1991.

Minkoff H: Personal communication, 1989.

Nicholas SW, Sondheimer DL, Willoughby AD, et al: Human immunodeficiency virus infection in childhood, adolescence, and pregnancy: A status report and national research agenda, *Pediatrics* 83:293-308, 1989.

Onorato IM, Markowitz LE, and Oxtoby MJ: Childhood immunization, vaccine-preventable diseases, and infection with human immunodeficiency virus, *Pediatr Infect Dis J* 7:588-595, 1988.

Pizzo PA: Pediatric AIDS: Problems within problems, *J Infect Dis* 161:316-325, 1990.

Pizzo PA: Therapeutic considerations for children with HIV infection, *AIDS Updates* 2:1-9, 1989.

Pizzo PA, Eddy J, and Falloon J: Effect of continuous intravenous infusion of zidovudine (AZT) in children with symptomatic HIV infection, *N Engl J Med* 319:889-896, 1988.

Rogers MF, Ou CY, Rayfield M, et al: Use of polymerase chain reaction for early detection of the proviral equences of human immunodeficiency virus in infants born to seropositive mothers, *N Engl J Med* 320:1649-1654, 1989.

Rogers MF, White CR, Sanders R, et al: Lack of transmission of human immunodeficiency virus from infected children to their household contacts, *Pediatrics* 85:210-214, 1990.

Rubenstein A, Morecki R, and Goldman H: Pulmonary disease in infants and children, *Clin Chest Med* 9:507-517, 1988.

Scott GB: HIV infection in children: Clinical features and management, *J Acq Immun Defic Synd* 4:109-115, 1990.

Scott GB, Hutto C, Makuch RW, et al: Survival in children with perinatally acquired human immunodeficiency virus type 1 infection, *N Engl J Med* 321:1791-1796, 1989.

US Department of Health and Human Services: *Report of the Surgeon General's workshop on children with HIV infection and their families,* Washington, DC, 1987 USDHHS.

US Department of Health and Human Services: *Final Report: Secretary's work group on pediatric HIV infection and disease,* Washington, DC, 1988 USDHHS.

Wishon SL and Gee G: Children and HIV infection. In Gee G and Moran T, eds: *AIDS: Concepts in nursing practice,* Baltimore, Williams & Wilkins, pp 41-61.

24 *Phenylketonuria*

•••

Kathleen Ann Schmidt

ETIOLOGY

Phenylketonuria (PKU) is an inherited metabolic disorder that causes plasma phenylalanine (phe) levels to rise to more than 1.2 mM (>20 mg/dl).* Phenylketonuria is caused by phenylalanine hydroxylase (PAH) deficiency. Although not as severe as PKU, mild hyperphenylalaninemia (HPA) is a related disorder in which plasma phe levels are less than 1.2 mM but greater than 0.12 mM. Mild HPA may have the same effects as PKU when plasma phe levels exceed 1 mM (16.5 mg/dl) (Scriver, Kaufman, and Woo, 1989).

The metabolic pathway for phe is in the liver: PAH enzyme converts phe by hydroxylation to tyrosine (tyr) in the hepatocyte for use in the biosynthesis of (1) protein, (2) melanin, (3) thyroxine, and (4) the catecholamines in the brain and adrenal medulla. Loss of PAH enzyme activity causes an accumulation of phe in the serum, resulting in an accumulation of phenylpyruvic acid and derivatives (phenylketones) in the serum and urine. High levels of phe inhibit large neutral amino acids' entry into the brain, contributing to the neuropathology of PKU (Kaufman, 1989).

In a growing child the recommended daily allowance (RDA) for phe is utilized by the body in two major ways: (1) 60% is used for new tissue protein synthesis, and (2) 40% is hydroxylated to form tyr. Homeostasis of phe in the body reflects the interaction among (1) dietary intake of phe; (2)

turnover of the body's tissue protein pool; and (3) outflow by means of hydroxylation (to form tyr), transamination (to form phenylpyruvic acid and derivatives), and conversion to other minor metabolites (Scriver, Kaufman, and Woo, 1989).

The phe hydroxylation system is a complex biochemical reaction that requires the presence of tetrahydrobiopterin (BH4), oxygen, and phe for the hydroxylation of phe. Enzymes responsible for the synthesis of BH4 are also necessary for the hydroxylation of phe and, when deficient, cause atypical PKU. Atypical PKU is characterized by HPA and progressive neurologic deterioration related to impaired neurotransmitter synthesis. Atypical PKU is genotypically distinct from the PAH-deficient forms of PKU and mild HPA. All children with PKU are screened for atypical PKU. Atypical PKU is a different disorder from PKU, requiring different methods of diagnosis, having different modes of therapy, and having a different prognosis.

Phenylketonuria is caused by many different molecular mutations on chromosome 12 that change the DNA code for PAH protein, creating an unstable PAH enzyme with varying degrees of activity. The PAH alleles that encode for the abnormal production of little or no functional PAH enzyme are mutant PKU alleles that cause the variable degree of HPA associated with both PKU and mild HPA (DiLella and Woo, 1987; Woo, 1989).

All individuals have normal variations in the DNA surrounding the PAH locus on chromosome 12 called restriction fragment length polymorphisms (RFLPs). A constellation of RFLPs that

---

*1 mM/1000 ml = 165.2 mg/1000 ml = 16.52mg/dl or

(x) mM − 16.52 × mg/dl (molecular weight of phe) = 165.2.

426

segregate with the PKU mutation on the PAH gene, called PKU haplotypes, act as markers for the PKU alleles on chromosome 12. More than 50 different PKU haplotypes have been identified and assigned a PKU haplotype number (Woo, 1990). Because PKU follows the mendelian autosomal recessive pattern of inheritance, PKU haplotype analysis can trace the segregation pattern of the PKU alleles in a family at risk for PKU. Two identical PKU haplotypes can segregate within a family, resulting in an individual receiving the same type of PKU from each parent. An individual who is homozygous for PKU inherits the same two identical PKU alleles. Or, different PKU haplotypes can segregate within a family, resulting in an individual with two different types of PKU, one from each parent. Clinically this explains why individuals with PKU, mild HPA, and even affected siblings have different degrees of hyperphenylalaninemia (Fig. 24-1).

Molecular study of individuals with PKU is useful not only for prenatal diagnosis and carrier testing of families at risk but also for prediction of the clinical severity and the prognosis for newborns diagnosed with PKU. Individuals who are homozygous or compound heterozygous for PKU haplotypes 2 and 3 have PKU. Individuals who are homozygous or compound heterozygous for haplotypes 1 and 4 usually have mild HPA (Okano et al., 1990a, 1990b).

The study of molecular genetics has provided insight into the population genetics of PKU. Approximately 90% of all PKU alleles are associated with only four PKU haplotypes (haplotypes 1-4). Two mutations (haplotypes 2 and 3) account for as many as 50% of all PKU cases seen in individuals of Northern European origin. One mutation (haplotype 4) accounts for 90% of PKU cases observed in individuals of Asian ancestry. Yet the same PKU mutation (haplotype 38) has been found in both the Danish population and North African population (Okano et al., 1990a). Selective advantage for the carrier may account for why the PKU gene is so prevalent in some populations (Kidd, 1987; Woo, 1989; Woolf, 1986).

INCIDENCE

Based on a worldwide incidence for PKU of 1:10,000, approximately 1 out of 50 individuals in the general population carries the PKU gene (Scriver, Kaufman, and Woo, 1989). The PKU gene frequency remains constant in the population from generation to generation, regardless of whether the incidence of PKU can be altered by prenatal diagnosis or carrier testing of the general

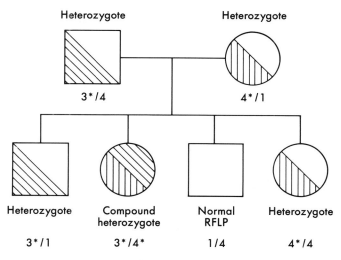

Fig. 24-1. Theoretical segregation of PKU allelles* and the RFLP haplotypes for each family member based on leukocyte DNA analysis.

population when available. Because PKU is heterogeneous, there is great geographic and ethnic variation in the incidence of PKU ranging from 5 to 190 cases per 1 million live births. The overall incidence of HPA from all causes is 100 cases per 1 million live births. Mild HPA accounts for approximately 15 to 75 cases per 1 million births (Table 24-1).

The concurrence of PKU or mild HPA with other genetic multifactorial disorders is not unheard of, particularly when the second disorder is relatively common in the general population, such as PKU in a child with Down syndrome (author's experience). However, when PKU occurs with another mendelian inherited disorder, there is the remote chance that proximity of loci on chromosome 12q is the explanation and should be further investigated at a medical genetics clinic (Scriver, Kaufman, and Woo, 1989).

Both PKU and mild HPA are currently screened for using nonselective newborn screening (NBS) in all 50 of the United States and in more than 30 countries. The NBS programs are the greatest source of referrals of HPA cases, but there will continue to be individuals of all ages who may or may not know whether they were previously diagnosed and treated for PKU or even that they have mild HPA.

Women with PKU are a clinically significant group because their offspring are at risk for maternal PKU (MPKU) syndrome. At least 3000 women with PKU between the ages of 16 and 26 years are residing in North America. More than one half of the women with PKU and mild HPA who were born before newborn screening for PKU (1965) are undiagnosed. Therefore, more than 1000 additional fetuses will be at risk from undiagnosed MPKU over the next 20 years. Mothers of newborns with transient HPA, as well as mothers who have delivered infants with any of the features of MPKU syndrome, should be tested for PKU (Hanley, 1988).

Case finding for PKU, mild HPA, and MPKU syndrome should always be uppermost in the primary care practitioner's mind when (1) a "presumptive positive" PKU NBS test result is reported; (2) a child has unexplained microcephaly, intrauterine or postnatal growth delay, dysmorphic facial features, and/or a history of a congenital heart defect (MPKU syndrome); and (3) an infant has unexplained developmental delay or a child (or parent) has any degree of mental retardation.

The NBS program coordinator for the given region should be consulted for the false-positive rate for a given NBS program and its causes, for the follow-up protocol of a presumptive positive NBS test result for PKU in a newborn, and whenever there is a question regarding any newborn's condition or treatment that might affect the NBS test result (Schmidt, 1989). Knowledge concerning the false-positive rate for a given PKU test and the biologic variables present in the individual that cause false-positive and false-negative results are necessary for the accurate interpretation of any test result for phe.

Table 24-1. Incidences of hyperphenylalaninemia variants by phenotype, religion, and ethnic group

Variant	Geographic region or ethnic group	Incidence (per 10^6 births)
PKU	Yemenite Jews	190
	Scotland	190
	Eire	190
	Czechoslovakia	150
	Poland	130
	Hungary	90
	France	75
	Scandinavia	
	Denmark	85
	Norway	70
	Sweden	25
	Finland	5
	England (London region)	70
	Italy	60
	China	50
	Canada	45
	Japan	5
	Ashkenazi Jews	5
Mild HPA (all regions except Finland)		15-75
BH4-deficient (panethnic and panregional)		1-2

Adapted from Scriver CR, Kaufman S, and Woo SLC: The hyperphenylalaninemias. In Scriver CR, Beaudet A, Sly DW, et al., eds: *The metabolic basis of inherited disease*, New York, 1989, McGraw-Hill, pp 495-546.

CLINICAL MANIFESTATIONS AT TIME OF DIAGNOSIS

The NBS test alone does not establish the diagnosis of PKU: a positive PKU test result does not constitute the diagnosis of PKU; nor does a negative PKU test result dismiss the possibility of PKU. Further investigation for PKU is warranted in a child with manifestations of untreated PKU. Berg (1984) states:

Affected infants usually appear normal at birth, but within several months become irritable and may have recurring vomiting. Though milestones may be reached at a normal time, they are usually delayed in both motor and intellectual skills. Acquisition of speech and language is delayed. Seizures occur in at least 25% of untreated PKU patients and in early life are typically infantile spasms. As the patients become older, the convulsions assume other forms of generalized epilepsies. Microcephaly is common and increased muscle tone with hyperreflexia is generally present. Patients often assume an unusual seated position, "schneidersitz" (tailor's position) and many children have a fine, rapid and irregular tremor at rest as well as with outstretched arms. The plantar responses are variable. Electroencephalograms are usually abnormal and hypsarrhythmia is commonly found, sometimes when no clinical convulsive activity has been noted.

If untreated, the toxic effects of phe in a child with PKU causes a drop in developmental quotient to 50 points by 1 year of age and to 30 points by 3 years of age (Koch and Wenz, 1987). Since the advent of NBS and earlier diagnosis and treatment, it has been demonstrated that an average of 10 intelligence quotient (IQ) points are lost if phe homeostasis is not achieved during the first month of life and an additional 10 points is lost if it is not achieved by the second month (Fishler et al., 1987).

Boys with untreated PKU have measurements for height that are consistently 2 SDs less than the mean when compared with boys without PKU. In contrast, mean height and weight measurements for girls with untreated PKU are consistently 2 SDs more than the mean when compared with girls without PKU (Fisch, Gravem, and Feinberg, 1966). Characteristic bone changes have been radiographically observed in children with untreated PKU less than 1 year of age during the period of rapid growth (Fisch, Gravem, and Feinberg, 1966). Approximately 25% of children with untreated PKU have eczema. A lingering musty odor sometimes described as mousey, barnlike, or old urine is commonly present and is secondary to the urinary excretion of phenylacetic acid, which accumulates over the first month of life. The results of complete blood cell count, routine urinalysis, and liver, renal, and endocrine function tests are normal in children with untreated PKU (Koch and Wenz, 1987).

Typically the child with PKU has a fairer complexion than the composite coloring of other family members, which is related to inhibitions of tyr metabolism and reduced melanin production. In ethnic backgrounds where black hair is expected, this feature will be expressed as hair that is brown or even reddish. Whites will typically have blonde hair and blue eyes. Because these manifestations are not pronounced at birth, their expression may not be evident until irreversible brain damage has already occurred.

TREATMENT

Treatment for PKU is simple in theory but difficult in practice. It involves restricting phe in the diet to maintain a nontoxic level of plasma phe between 2 and 10 mg/dl while allowing optimum growth and brain development by supplementing the diet with adequate sources of energy, protein, and other nutrients. Tyrosine is supplemented when plasma tyr levels are less than 0.33 mg/dl. Optimal management is a phe-restricted diet initiated within the first 2 weeks of life and continued throughout childhood, adolescence, and adulthood, especially before conception and throughout pregnancy for the benefit of the offspring.

Clinical tolerance of phe distinguishes PKU from mild HPA. The phe requirement for infants and young children is between 250 and 500 mg/day and not more than 1.5 times greater than this level in the older child. Children with PKU have a narrower tolerance between the lower and upper limits of required phe than individuals with greater PAH activity. An individual with HPA requiring dietary restriction of phe to maintain a plasma phe level of less than 10 mg/dl needs treatment regardless of the distinction made between PKU and mild HPA. Tolerance of phe is observed over time and can change within weeks, months, or even years. Rarely, PKU and mild HPA can be transient, and a child's tolerance for phe can increase to normal levels because of either a regulatory defect affecting PAH activity or a transient disorder of biopterin metabolism. Careful and continuous monitoring of individuals whose phe intake is restricted is necessary to avoid phe deficiency when tolerance changes because of these rare cases or because of changes related to growth rate.

Dietary restriction of phe is accomplished by the use of commercially available elemental medical foods (EMFs). These products are modified protein hydrolysates in which phe is removed or are mixtures of free amino acids that do not contain phe. They provide the essential amino acids in suitable proportions for the given age of the individual (Table 24-2). Because natural protein contains 2.4% to 9% of phe by weight, adequate protein cannot be obtained from natural foods without ingesting excess phe. Therefore, phe-restricted diets are usually designed so that EMF products provide the majority of the essential nutrients with the exception of the caloric requirement, which is derived from no- or low-protein, high-calorie natural sources. Nutrient intakes must be sufficient to meet the anabolic requirements of the individual and maintain essential conversion reactions (Acosta, 1989).

Phenylalanine-restricted diets are prescribed by the medical genetics PKU treatment center team who continually monitor the child's phe tolerance. Individuals' phe requirements depend on PAH activity, age, growth rate, adequacy of energy and protein intakes, and state of health (Tables 24-3 and 24-4).

The greatest benefit of continuing the diet are in those areas of cognitive functioning measured by IQ tests and by the reading and spelling subtests of the Wide Range Achievement Test. There is a strong relationship between the IQ of the child and the age at which dietary control is lost (blood phe level consistently more than 15 mg/dl) (Table 24-5). The best predictor of IQ in a child with PKU and of the deficit in IQ between the child and unaffected siblings or parents is the age when dietary control is lost. The IQ deficit is greatest when phe control is lost before 6 years of age. If phe control continues past 8 years of age to at least 12 years of age, IQ remains at the national average; there is virtually no change in IQ between 6 and 12 years of age (Fishler et al., 1987).

Children with late-diagnosed PKU should also be placed on the phe restricted diet no matter how late they are identified as having PKU. Improvement in behavior and cognitive functioning has been seen in severely retarded individuals who had untreated PKU (Clarke, Gates, Hogan et al., 1987; Koch and Wenz, 1987).

Other modes of therapy currently under investigation hold promise for the treatment of PKU (Danks and Cotton, 1987). Nutrient supplementation of the large neutral amino acids and micronutrients is another dietary modality being explored. Enzyme therapy is the substitution of bacterial phe ammonia lyase (PAL) for PAH. It converts phe to ammonia and *trans*-cinnamic acid, a nontoxic metabolite. Given orally in an enteric coated gelatin capsule, PAL has a beneficial effect

Table 24-2. Elemental medical foods used in the treatment of PKU according to developmental stage

Developmental stage	Elemental medical food
Infant	Lofenalac*
	PKU 1*
	Analog XP†
	PK Aid 1‡
	Albumaid XP‡
	Albumaid XP Concentrate‡
Child	Phenyl-Free*
	PKU 2*
	Maxamaid XP Powder‡
	Unflavored
	Orange flavored
	Maxamaid XP Bar‡
Adult	PKU 2*
	Analog XP†
	Maxamum XP‡
Maternal PKU	Phenyl-Free*
	PKU 3*
	Maxamum XP‡
	Unflavored
	Orange flavored

*Mead Johnson, Evansville, Indiana.
†Ross Laboratories, Columbus, Ohio.
‡Scientific Hospitals, Limited, Ross Laboratories.

Table 24-3. Recommended daily nutrient intakes (average and range) for infants with PKU

	Nutrients			
Age in (mo)	Phe (mg/kg)	Protein (g/kg)	Energy (kcal/kg)	Fluid (ml/kg)
0<3	55 (70-25)	3.00-2.50	120 (145-95)	150-125
3<6	35 (55-20)	3.00-2.50	115 (145-95)	160-130
6<9	30 (50-15)	2.50-2.25	110 (135-80)	145-125
9<12	25 (45-15)	2.50-2.25	105 (135-80)	135-120

From Acosta PB: *Ross metabolic formula system nutrition support protocols*, Columbus, Ohio, 1989, Abbott Laboratories.

Table 24-4. Recommended daily nutrient intakes (average and range) for children, adolescents, and adults with PKU

	Nutrients					
Age (yr)	Phe (mg/day)	Tyr (g/day)	Protein (g/day)	Fat (% energy)	Energy (kcal/day)	Fluid (ml/day)
Female and male						
1<4	325 (200-450)	2.80 (1.40-4.20)	25	45-40	1300 (900-1800)	900-1800
4<7	425 (225-625)	3.15 (1.75-4.55)	35	40-35	1700 (1300-2300)	1300-2300
7<11	450 (250-650)	3.50 (2.10-4.90)	40	35-30	2400 (1650-3300)	1650-3300
Female						
11<15	500 (300-700)	3.85 (2.45-5.25)	55	35-30	2200 (1500-3000)	1500-3000
15<19	475 (275-675)	3.50 (1.40-5.60)	55	35-30	2100 (1200-3000)	1200-3000
≥19	475 (275-675)	3.50 (1.58-5.40)	50	30-25	2100 (1400-2500)	1400-2500
Male						
11<15	550 (350-750)	4.55 (2.45-6.55)	50	35-30	2700 (2000-3700)	2000-3700
15<19	550 (350-750)	4.20 (2.10-8.10)	65	35-30	2800 (2100-3900)	2100-3900
≤19	500 (300-700)	3.85 (2.10-5.60)	65	30-25	2900 (2000-3300)	2000-3300

From Acosta PB: *Ross metabolic formula system nutrition support protocols*, Columbus, Ohio, 1989, Abbott Laboratories.

on lowering blood phe level in trials with individuals who had PKU, without overt side effects. Somatic gene therapy in the animal model indicates that primary hepatocytes can be successfully cultured and transformed with recombinant genes using retroviral vectors. Preliminary results provide a model for future somatic gene therapy in which functional genes can be introduced into human hepatocytes by viral-mediated gene transfer (Woo, 1990).

Table 24-5. Summary of 12-year PKU collaborative study IQ data*

Age (yr)	Test	Age (mo) at loss of dietary control		
		≤71 (N = 23)	72-95 (N = 42)	≥96 (N = 30)
6	Stanford-Binet	91 ± 15	100 ± 14	102 ± 14
7	Stanford-Binet	93 ± 12	98 ± 13	103 ± 14
8	WISC†			
	Verbal	92 ± 12	98 ± 14	103 ± 12
	Performance	93 ± 15	100 ± 14	103 ± 12
	Full scale	92 ± 13	99 ± 14	103 ± 12
10	WISC			
	Verbal	91 ± 12	98 ± 12	103 ± 12
	Performance	96 ± 16	100 ± 13	105 ± 12
	Full scale	92 ± 14	99 ± 13	105 ± 12
12	WISC			
	Verbal	85 ± 15	94 ± 14	100 ± 10
	Performance	92 ± 15	98 ± 13	101 ± 11
	Full scale	87 ± 14	95 ± 14	101 ± 10

From Fishler K, Azen CG, Henderson R, *Am J Ment Defic* 92:65-73, 1987.
*Mean ± SD by age at loss of dietary control.
†WISC, Wechsler Intelligence Scale for Children.

PROGNOSIS

Individuals with mild HPA whose blood phe levels remain less than 1 mM have no symptoms (Scriver, Kaufman, and Woo, 1989). Optimal long-term intellectual development is dependent on early diagnosis and careful diet therapy that maintains phe homeostasis. Imperfections in the dietary treatment of PKU as it is currently known, delays in treatment, and possible undetectable prenatal damage are evidenced by neuropsychologic and cognitive functions that are slightly less than the average in individuals with PKU.

ASSOCIATED PROBLEMS
Neurologic changes

Abnormal findings in the cerebral white matter have been demonstrated on cranial magnetic resonance imaging (MRI) studies of children with treated PKU. The extent of MRI changes does not correlate with the start, duration, or quality of dietary treatment. Intelligence quotients tend to be lower in children with PKU who have severe MRI changes. The described changes are consistent with altered myelin composition, demyelinization, or both.

There is no correlation between electroencephalogram examination and the MRI in the respective anatomic region (Bick et al., 1990).

Electroencephalographic abnormalities increase with advancing age independent of IQ development and show no relation to either age at onset or quality of dietary treatment. The genesis of brain electricity and cognitive function observed during periods of elevated blood phe levels is attributed to a disturbed synthesis of neurotransmitters (dopamine and serotonin) (Pietz et al., 1990).

Cognitive deficits. Deficits in cognitive function relative to mathematical conceptualizations is a troubling finding in children with PKU who have maintained good blood phe control since birth. When tested at 12 years of age, children with well-controlled PKU scored 17 points lower on the Wide Range Achievement Test for Arithmetic than previous baseline levels. This does not indicate gross deficits in the intellectual status of treated children with PKU but is evidence of subtle deficits that become more pronounced over time.

Children with PKU who have maintained good phe control often have difficulty with visual perception and linguistic development (Brunner, Berch, and Berry, 1987). Neither the age at which treatment was initiated nor the phe level during the early years of life correlate with a discrepancy in skills of children with PKU compared with their siblings at 5 years of age on tests of visual perception and at 7 years of age on tests of psycholinguistic abilities (Fishler, Azen, and Henderson, 1987). Behavioral and emotional factors noted in children with chronic disorders further compound these problems. The lifelong outcome for children with well-treated PKU is yet to be observed because the history of treated PKU is relatively short (Danks and Cotton, 1987).

Pyloric stenosis

Pyloric stenosis has been observed more frequently in males with PKU than in the general male newborn population (male/female ratio is 5:0). Children of either sex identified with pyloric stenosis should be retested for PKU (Koch and Wenz, 1987).

Peptic ulcer

Peptic ulcer, with the uncommon complication of bleeding or perforation, has been documented in both sexes of individuals (11-25 years of age) with PKU. The relationship of peptic ulcer to PKU is not clear. Elevated blood phe concentrations secondary to PAH deficiency may lead to increased gastric secretion, which in some individuals results in peptic ulceration; vomiting which was formerly a common presenting symptom in untreated children with PKU, could possibly be explained by this same mechanism (Scriver, Kaufman, and Woo, 1989). Peptic ulcer could be related to the dietary treatment; L-amino acid supplements can stimulate gastric acid secretion (Greeves, Carson, and Dodge, 1988).

PRIMARY CARE MANAGEMENT
Growth and development

Growth and development are normal for children with PKU on a controlled, phe-restricted diet. Head circumference, weight, and length are measured at scheduled monthly intervals for the first year, then every 3 months until after the prepubertal growth spurt, and then every 6 months throughout adolescence to monitor adequacy of diet. There is a tendency toward obesity in children with PKU, which is related to the high caloric density of natural food sources necessary to meet the child's RDA for calories, the free sugar in the EMF product, and the free foods high in carbohydrates.

Children with PKU are at risk for having low self-esteem. The fact that they require a special diet and the fact that they are different from others are obvious causes. The possible consequences of being taken off the diet and the effect that high blood phe levels has on their behavior contribute to this risk (Moen, Wilcox, and Burns, 1977). Children with PKU older than age 4 years are at risk for having immature social interaction and interpersonal skills (Kazak, Reber, and Snitzer, 1988). Continuing the phe-restricted diet, becoming involved in PKU peer support groups, promoting self-control of the diet at an early age, and deemphasing that children with PKU are "different" are easier said than done. Art therapy with younger children and role playing for older children are only some of the creative ways to elicit the child's attitudes about having PKU. As children approach school age, parents need to be encouraged to enhance their child's social development by allowing them to spend increasing amounts of time outside the immediate family.

Affective disorders and acting out behaviors are not the norm for well-managed children with PKU; the psychologist on the medical genetics PKU treatment team is a resource for dealing with these issues and knowing when professional intervention is required.

Immunizations

The immunization schedule for children with PKU is the same as it is for any child. The child with PKU needs to be closely observed for a reaction to the immunization. A febrile reaction can lead to a catabolic state, increasing plasma phe levels. Any illness should be supported with adequate hydration and calories.

Screening

Vision. Routine screening is recommended.
Hearing. Routine screening is recommended.
Dental. The diet for PKU contains sufficient

carbohydrate to present more than the usual potential for dental decay. The phe-restricted diet relies on frequent intake of carbohydrates to meet the daily requirement for calories. Explanations to parents about the role frequency of carbohydrate consumption has and the effects of extremes such as nursing bottle caries or uncontrolled access to candy helps focus their efforts. Practical goals include weaning the child with PKU to a glass as soon as possible, starting with sips at 6 months of age; retentive foods should be followed by fibrous ones to effect food removal; liquid forms of carbohydrate should be used when possible to promote oral clearance; free foods such as fruits should be offered in place of more retentive forms of refined sugars; and dental hygiene and screening should be initiated at the eruption of the first tooth with close follow-up thereafter (Casamassimo et al., 1984).

Blood pressure. Routine screening is recommended.

Hematocrit. Iron status is monitored by plasma ferritin levels at 6, 9 and 12 months of age and then every 6 months thereafter. Hemoglobin and hematocrit values are evaluated at 6 and 12 months of age and annually thereafter. The child with anemia will have a falsely low phe level, and the newborn with polycythemia can have a falsely high phe level.

Breast-fed infants with PKU have exaggerated physiologic anemia of infancy, requiring iron supplementation when the hematocrit value approaches 30% (McCabe et al., 1989).

Urinalysis. Routine screening is recommended.

Tuberculosis. Routine screening is recommended.

Condition-specific screening

URINE SCREENING FOR PHENYLKETONURIA. The urine pterin excretion test is done on all individuals with persistent HPA to differentiate PKU and mild HPA from atypical PKU disorders. This selective screening test is best collected by the primary care practitioner and analyzed by a metabolic geneticist at a recognized medical genetics PKU treatment center (see the list of resources on pp. 442-444).

The qualitative urine test for PKU (ferric chloride reaction, or Phenistix) measures phenylpyruvic

acid, which is not excreted in the urine until blood phe levels exceed 12 to 20 mg/dl (Kaufman, 1989). Care must be taken in the interpretation of a ferric chloride reaction because of false positive and false negative test results caused by instability of urine specimens and interfering metabolites (Nystaform-HC ointment or iodochlorhydroxyquin, salicylates, phenothiazine derivates, isoniazid, and L-dopa metabolites).

BLOOD PHE MONITORING. The blood test for phe (newborn, child, and adult), whether for screening or diet monitoring, is a capillary blood sample obtained from a free-flowing puncture wound (using a 2.45-mm disposable lancet) collected directly onto filter paper (Schleicher & Schuell) 2 to 4 hours postprandially. The phe content of the blood can be directly measured by different laboratory techniques. Only a blood specimen is reliable in detecting quantitative or semiquantitative levels of phe. Serum phe values are slightly less than filter paper values; however, either method can be used (Jew, Koch, and Cunningham, 1986).

Normal blood phe levels in newborns (birth weights >2500 g) gradually rise after birth, peak between 7 and 12 hours of age (Cunningham, Kan, and Mourdant, 1987), and thereafter subside to near-adult levels (phe upper limit of normal is <120 mM for infants, 62 mM $\pm$ 18 for children, 60 mM $\pm$ 13 for adolescents, and 58 mM $\pm$ 15 for adults) (Scriver, Kaufman, and Woo, 1990).

Plasma phe and tyr levels are evaluated twice weekly by quantitative methods in the newborn until concentrations are stabilized and approximate dietary phe and tyr requirements are known. Thereafter, blood phe is evaluated twice weekly with dietary changes or weekly without dietary changes in both the infant and child. The plasma phe and tyr levels are evaluated by the medical genetics PKU treatment center team.

PHENYLALANINE TOLERANCE TESTING. The benefit of phe challenges performed at approximately 3 years of age by some medical genetics PKU treatment centers to establish the degree of HPA present in a child remains ethically controversial. An alternative would be the molecular analysis of blood specimens obtained from the family to determine the child's PKU haplotype number (genotype). Molecular analysis is still a research endeavor, but most results prove to be informative and can provide practical clinical information regarding prognosis (Woo, 1990).

NUTRITIONAL INDICES SCREENING. Nutrient intake is recorded for 3 days before each blood phe test on forms provided by the medical genetics PKU treatment center and evaluated by the genetic nutritionist for phe, tyr, protein, and energy intake. Protein status is evaluated by plasma albumin or prealbumin levels (or both) every 3 months in the infant and every 6 months in the child and adolescent. Individuals on semisynthetic diets are at high risk for deficiencies in the trace elements. Insufficient intake of iron, zinc, and selenium and the interaction of iron with copper and zinc at the intestinal level can cause deficiencies. Safe ranges of fluoride, selenium, and molybdenum are also monitored by the medical genetics PKU treatment center team. Overall balance of nutrients is critical in the child with PKU.

Drug interactions

Aspartame. Aspartame is a food additive marketed under the brand name Nutrasweet. Aspartame is a white, odorless, crystalline powder and consists of two amino acids, L-aspartic acid and L-phenylalanine. The Food and Drug Administration (FDA) has approved its use as an additive to numerous foods, beverages, multivitamins, and breath mints (see the list of resources on pp. 442-444). The acceptable daily intake of aspartame in the individual who does not have PKU or mild HPA is 40 mg/kg of body weight (Garriga and Metcalf, 1988).

The FDA requires the statement "PHENYL-KETONURICS: CONTAINS PHENYLALA-NINE" on labels of food products containing aspartame. Individuals with PKU should avoid the consumption of aspartame. For the child with PKU, ingesting 34 mg of aspartame per kg of body weight will elevate the plasma phe level to approximately 850 mM. For individuals with mild HPA who tolerate 50 to 100 mg of phe/kg of body weight per day, ingestion of aspartame is also not recommended.

Given the 1:2 concentration gradient for phe between the maternal and fetal blood, the use of aspartame during pregnancy for women who are known to carry the PKU gene or who themselves have PKU is not recommended.

Monoamine oxidase inhibitors. Individuals with PKU who receive monoamine oxidase (MAO) inhibitors will have elevated levels of phenylethylamine, a phenylketone, in the urine and tissues without a detectable level in the cerebrospinal fluid and without signs of clinical deterioration. Use of MAO inhibitors for the treatment of a psychiatric disorder in an individual with PKU is controversial because of conflicting reports of the neurotoxicity of phenylethylamine (Kaufman, 1989).

Oral contraceptives. Fluctuations can occur in plasma amino acids during the menstrual cycle. Plasma phe and tyr levels should be monitored when women with PKU are using oral contraceptives.

DIFFERENTIAL DIAGNOSIS AND MANAGEMENT OF COMMON PEDIATRIC CONDITIONS
Management during illness

If a child with PKU has a negative nitrogen balance for any reason, the blood phe content can be elevated because body tissue protein catabolism occurs, releasing phe. The paradox of phe-restricted diets is in the transient elevations of plasma phe when phe is overrestricted; protein synthesis is blocked by nutrient deficiency (negative nitrogen balance), resulting in impaired flow of phe to anabolic nitrogen pools. An elevated temperature is just one of many reasons for a negative nitrogen balance. An accurate history of the child's illness and dietary intake before the illness may help distinguish the cause of a catabolic reaction.

During common childhood illnesses the blood phe level is not tested until the child is well as long as the illness is less than 3 weeks' duration. During the illness supportive measures should be undertaken to limit protein catabolism. In the infant or adolescent energy intake should be enhanced by allowing (1) as much fruit juice as tolerated; (2) liquid flavored gelatin; (3) polycose glucose polymers (liquid or powder) added to the fruit juices; and (4) caffeine-free, nondiet soft drinks. With close consultation with the medical genetics PKU treatment team, the child with PKU is returned to the EMF and preillness diet plan as rapidly as tolerated; usually the EMF product is initiated at one-half original strength, then full strength as tolerated (Acosta, 1989).

Management during minor surgery

Minor uncomplicated surgery (tonsillectomy, hernia repair, cystoscopy, etc.) with the child under general anesthesia does not cause major alteration in the blood phe level. Maximum blood phe levels (≤ 17 mg/dl) occur approximately on the second postoperative day and decline on the fourth postoperative day (≤ 10 mg/dl). Because the elevation in phe level is transient, no special dietary measures are needed (Fiedler et al., 1982).

Skin lesions

Localized or generalized eczema and peeling of the soles of the feet and the palms of the hands occur after a long-term catabolic state. Skin lesions related to an amino acid imbalance and disturbed phe/tyr ratio need to be distinguished from other rashes by accurate history of the lesion and diet. Establishing phe homeostasis will resolve eczema and peeling that are not responsive to topical medications.

Children with skin lesions suggestive of scleroderma, severe localized induration of the skin, subcutaneous tissue, and muscle, should be tested for PKU. Scleroderma, a rare, often familial, connective tissue disorder and untreated PKU both have a common secondary biochemical deficiency of tryptophan. Tryptophan is an immediate precursor of serotonin and the catecholamines in the tyrosine metabolic pathway. An increased concentration of phe decreases the availability of tyr and tryptophan. The skin lesions soften when individuals with PKU adhere to a phe-restricted diet.

Pigmented lesions, melanin spots that are light brown to black, occur in individuals with PKU. The oculocutaneous pigmentary dilution observed even in children with PKU who adhere to a phe-restricted diet is a systemic mechanism related to the disturbed phe/tyr ratio in the circulation. The pigmentary activity of the epidermal melanocytes is unimpaired in individuals with PKU and is normal at the skin level peripherally. Erythema response and ability to tan after exposure to artificial or natural light for individuals with PKU have been

demonstrated to be no different than for individuals without PKU who are blond (Bolognia and Pawelek, 1988; Hassel and Brunsting, 1959). Limiting exposure to the sun and using sunblocks are recommended for the child with PKU as they are for any child.

DEVELOPMENTAL ISSUES
Safety

Children with PKU are not at an increased risk of acute safety hazards. Chronic ingestion of excess dietary phe is more deleterious to the health of the child than the accidental intake of a product containing aspartame. A Medic-Alert bracelet or necklace that indicates "special PKU diet" is added assurance that a child with PKU will receive proper care in case of an emergency.

Because chronic ingestion of EMF products can lead to nutritional deficiencies, they are contraindicated for any individual not diagnosed as needing a phe-restricted diet.

Child care

It is important that more than one individual in the child's home environment be knowledgable about the phe-restricted diet and the preparation of EMF products. Materials about PKU written specifically for baby-sitters, grandparents, and teachers, as well as creative ideas on how to deal with these issues, can be found in the National PKU Foundation newsletter (see the list of resources on pp. 442-444).

Diet

Dietary support at all developmental stages of the individual with PKU is an important component of therapy. Monitoring of phe concentrations with weight and diet changes will need to occur throughout the individual's life. It is important to initiate self-management of the phe-restricted diet early in childhood. Some reasons for failure to achieve long-term adherence to the phe-restricted diet include poor family coping skills, increasing independence of children, limited food choices, and unpalatable EMF products.

In the infant, protein is initially prescribed in an amount greater than the RDA. When the EMF is the primary source of protein, the requirement for protein increases because of rapid absorption, early and high peak of plasma amino acids, and rapid catabolism of amino acids. Mature human breast milk ($>$15 days' lactation) is an ideal source of whole protein for the infant with PKU. Breast milk, compared with cow's milk, contains an amino acid composition that supports adequate growth at a lower protein intake (0.9-1.0 versus 3.3 g/dl) and enhances bioavailability of minerals and trace elements (especially zinc) because of the greater percentage of protein (70% versus 20%) from the predominant whey fraction. Breast milk has a lower phe content per ounce compared with other formulas.*

Infants with PKU should be given a variety of foods at the appropriate ages so that these foods become part of their diet later in life. A system of food exchanges where the phe content is used as the basis for providing specific amounts of foods by food group is employed. Foods of similar phe content are grouped together and are exchanged, one for another, within the list to give variety to the diet (see pp. 442-444).

Elemental medical food products are sensitive to heat and a prolonged shelf life. These products should not be heated beyond 54.5° C because of the Maillard reaction; amino acids, peptides and proteins condense with sugars, forming bonds for which no digestive enzymes are available. The reaction is characterized by initially a light brown color, followed by buff yellow and then dark brown; caramellike and roasted aromas develop. Any amino acid preparation should be inspected for these changes and the expiration date checked before use. The shelf life of Analog is 1 year; for other EMF products it is generally 2 years. The vitamin C content diminishes initially, followed by the vitamin A and D content, which can decrease to as much as 30% below labeled values after the expiration date. In addition, the fats in EMF products become rancid after the expiration date. Products containing L-amino acids taste best when they are served cold (frozen to a slush) to disguise the sulfurous bitter taste. There is no contraindication for freezing EMF products or warming them to less than 54.5° C. Terminal sterilization of an infant's

EMF formula is contraindicated (Acosta, 1989).

Activities other than those that revolve around food can be promoted with peers. It is quality peer relationships that are important, not that an individual has to eat the same things to be accepted. Food is a social instrument for a child of any age, and every effort should be made to use the available tips from an experienced nutritionist to approximate the visual, textural, and taste appeal of the unrestricted diet (see pp. 442-444).

Discipline

Consistent discipline for children with PKU is as, if not more, important, as it is for any child. Food is a very major social component in any child's life, and how it is managed from the very beginning by parents can determine the success of the only current therapy for PKU, dietary restriction of phe. A major pitfall in disciplining children with PKU is to use food as a reward system and to use the need for blood tests as punishment. Strategies helping children to adhere to special diets are available (see pp. 442-444).

Toileting

Infants with PKU who are prone to eczema may experience more problems with diaper dermatitis. Careful, explicit instructions on standard management techniques should be given and follow-up appointments made for evaluation of treatment success. Toileting habits become an issue when phe control is lost. When the blood phe level is elevated for any reason, phenylketones are present in the urine and sweat, causing the characteristic musty odor of PKU. Attention to and training of the child in his or her hygiene needs at all ages will avoid unnecessary embarrassment.

Sleep patterns

There are diurnal variations of phe and tyr levels in children who have and do not have PKU. The difference in children with PKU is an elevation of the tyr level in the evening, like children without PKU, but a decrease in the phe level at night, unlike nonaffected children. The implications of this variation in the phe/tyr ratio is in their relationship to tryptophan, the precursor of serotonin. In the presence of low phe levels, the tryptophan level is elevated. Elevation of tryptophan markedly reduces

---

*Breast milk = 12.3 mg of phe/oz; Enfamil = 17 mg of phe/oz; Similac[20] = 22 mg of phe/oz; SMA = 24 mg of phe/oz; Isomil and Prosobee = 29 mg of phe/oz; and cow's milk = 104 mg of phe/oz.

the total time in rapid eye movement (REM) sleep to 3% (normal REM time in children is 29.5% ± 4.8%). During lower levels of tryptophan, REM sleep is increased to 8% to 11%. Children with PKU are more susceptible to sleep disturbances, which can be expressed as insomnia or hyperactivity at night. Children who have elevated levels of phe can often have disturbed sleep patterns with nightmares. Any alteration in the ratios of phe, tyr, and tryptophan can cause sleep disturbances; a phe-restricted diet balanced throughout the 24-hour time period optimizes sleep patterns in the child with PKU (Guttler, Olesen, and Wamberg, 1969; Herrero et al., 1983; Wyatt et al., 1971).

School issues

Children with treated PKU experience difficulties in school more frequently than nonaffected children; 33% of children with PKU are 1 or more years below grade level compared with 14% of children in the general white population. For grades 1 through 4, 38% of girls with PKU are 1 or more years below compared with 29% of boys with PKU (Fishler et al., 1987).

Children with PKU need comprehensive integrated psychodiagnostic and neuropsychologic assessments. Developmental testing is performed ideally at the medical genetics PKU treatment center at scheduled intervals starting at 6 months of age and every 6 months until 2 years of age, then annually thereafter. It is important for optimal performance that the child's blood phe level be in maintenance range on the day of testing.

Anticipatory guidance in the development of visual-spatial skills may be required. Computer games and software programs that train and stimulate the development of visual spatial skills and hand to eye coordination are ideal. Special education in math and language acquisition may also be necessary. Teacher involvement at all stages of the child's schooling is important.

Sexuality

Sexual development and curiosity are no different for the child with PKU than for any other child. Genetic counseling specifically for the child with PKU is individualized to the child's understanding of PKU and assessment of readiness. The medical genetics PKU treatment team works closely with families on this issue, and often PKU peer support groups and videos specific to the developmental stage of the child or adolescent with PKU are beneficial (see pp. 442-444).

For the female adolescent with PKU, the onset of menses can cause fluctuations in the plasma amino acid pattern, specifically the tyr level. Monitoring the quantitative plasma amino acid levels is important to assure that excesses or deficiencies can be alleviated by dietary intervention. Discussions of contraception and the implications of being a female with PKU should be individualized and approached with sensitivity. Again, PKU peer support groups and written materials and videos designed specifically for female adolescents with PKU are available.

Women with PKU who do not maintain blood phe levels between 2 and 4 mg/dl before and throughout an entire pregnancy may have infants without PKU but with other birth defects. The fetus is at great risk for the teratologic affects of phe exposure because of a positive transplacental gradient of phe approximately 1.13 to 2.19 times higher than the maternal blood phe level. The results of high maternal blood phe levels in the fetus, especially in the first trimester, are mental retardation, microcephaly, intrauterine and postnatal growth delay, and a constellation of facial dysmorphic features (MPKU syndrome). All offspring ($N = 22$) of pregnant women with PKU whose blood phe level during pregnancy was consistently greater than 20 mg/dl have some abnormality: 86% microcephaly, 73% postnatal growth delay, and 18% intrauterine growth delay (Rouse et al., 1990).

Facial dysmorphology in MPKU syndrome (Fig. 24-2) is similar to the facies described in fetal alcohol syndrome: abnormal ears (large, low set, or ear pits), long philtrum, anteverted nares, high arched palate, wide inner canthal distance, wide outer canthal distance, small or wide palpebral fissures, epicanthal folds, telecanthus, slanted eyes, ptosis, and micrognathia. Congenital cardiac anomalies are seen in offspring from pregnancies during which phe level was not under control during the first trimester: ventricular septal defects, coarctation of the aorta, tetralogy of Fallot, severe arrhythmia, and harsh heart murmur (Rouse et al., 1990).

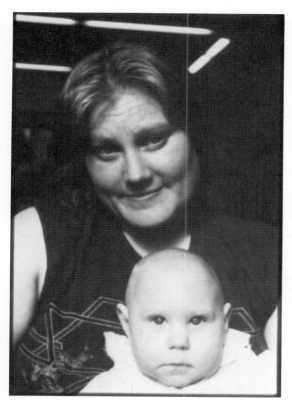

Fig. 24-2. Mother with 8-month-old daughter with MPKU syndrome.

Pregnancy in the teenager with PKU is a medical challenge. The goals of diet are similar to pregnant teenagers without PKU with respect to normal and appropriate weight gain based on height, prepregnancy weight, and gestational age, with indices of nutritional status in the normal range. Concentration of blood phe and tyr is between 2 and 4 and 1.65 mg/dl, respectively. The phe requirements vary in the same woman throughout pregnancy depending on age, weight gain, trimester of pregnancy, adequacy of energy and protein intakes, and state of maternal health. At 20 weeks of gestation the phe requirements increase dramatically. Magnesium, copper, and cholesterol levels are significantly lower in MPKU (Acosta, 1989), and special EMF products (see Table 24-2) have been developed to meet these needs.

Fertility does not appear to be affected in men with PKU. However, an inverse correlation between plasma phe level and semen volume and between plasma phe level and sperm count has been observed (Brown, 1986; Fisch, Tsai, and Clark, 1981). Investigation of paternal PKU is ongoing as part of the nationwide Maternal PKU Collaborative Project (see pp. 442-444).

SPECIAL FAMILY CONCERNS

Parents must live with the knowledge that their child's intellectual development depends on how well the diet is managed. Outcome is directly related to the effectiveness of dietary control. Families with children who have PKU perceive themselves to be less adaptable and cohesive than other families. Mothers of children with PKU particularly feel separated rather than connected within the family structure and feel rigid rather than structured. More rigid family systems may be an adaptive response to children whose daily routine is less flexible than most children. Helping the family discover ways in which to provide a flexible, yet structured organization of the child's management of PKU would be supportive, allowing them to let go of their perceived need for rigidity. On other measures of family stress, parents of children with PKU did not report significantly greater degrees of parental psychologic distress, marital dissatisfaction, or parenting stress than other parents, although the tendency for stress in these areas was present (Fehrenbach and Peterson, 1989; Kazak, Reber, and Snitzer, 1988).

Reproductive patterns in families after birth of a child with PKU is affected by the birth order of that child, the age of the parents at the time of the birth of the child with PKU and the expressed intentions of the parents whether to have additional children (Burns et al., 1984). Having a child with PKU does not appear to limit parental reproductive plans. Since the advent of prenatal diagnosis for PKU, another factor that contributes to the reproductive decision-making process includes the parents' perception of the progress of the child with PKU. For families with at least one child with PKU who decided not to have more children, family size was the primary limiting factor (35%), followed by concern about PKU (25%) and finances (20%) (Jew, Williams, and Koch, 1988).

Information about nonselective newborn screening is optimally given to all expectant parents prenatally (Holzman et al., 1983). Information should be given to the newborn's parents at least before discharge from the birth facility, assuming the newborn is less than 1 week of age. If information about the significance of NBS for the child's health and the NBS testing process is not sufficient, parents experience a greater degree of anxiety and depression about their child's health than about the fact that their child needs to be tested again for a presumptive positive NBS test result (Sorenson et al., 1984). If the child is diagnosed with PKU, the parents' guilt over their genetic contribution to the illness is accentuated by not having received information about the immediate need for re-screening.

SUMMARY OF PRIMARY CARE NEEDS FOR THE CHILD WITH PHENYLKETONURIA

Growth and development

Growth and development are normal if the child adheres to a controlled phe-restricted diet.

Caloric intake of high-carbohydrate free foods should be controlled to avoid obesity.

Children with PKU may have underdeveloped social skills.

Immunizations

Routine immunizations are recommended.

Any catabolic reaction should be supported with hydration and calories.

Screening
Vision

Routine screening is recommended.

Hearing

Routine screening is recommended.

Dental

Screening should be initiated at the eruption of the first tooth and closely followed thereafter. Frequent carbohydrate intake increases the risk of caries.

Blood pressure

Routine screening is recommended.

Hematocrit

Plasma ferritin levels are checked at 6, 9, and 12 months of age and every 6 months thereafter. Hemoglobin and hematocrit values are assessed at 6 and 12 months of age and then annually. Breast-fed infants have exaggerated physiologic anemia of infancy and require iron supplementation.

Urinalysis

Routine screening is recommended.

Tuberculosis

Routine screening is recommended.

Condition-specific screening

All children with persistent HPA require a urine pterin screening test.

Blood phe should be monitored with weight and dietary changes for phe tolerance.

Nutritional indices that should be monitored include tyr, vitamins, prealbumin, albumin, trace elements, and metals.

Drug interactions

Aspartame ingestion is contraindicated.

Monoamine oxidase inhibitors are contraindicated.

Plasma tyr levels of women taking oral contraceptives should be monitored.

Differential diagnosis

Differentiate elevated blood phe level from illness or intake of too little or too much dietary phe by accurate history.

Prevent catabolic state related to common childhood illness with adequate hydration and caloric intake.

Minor surgery results in only transient elevation of phe.

Differentiate skin lesions from eczema, peeling, and scleroderma related to imbalance of blood phe, tyr, or tryptophan.

Limit sun exposure and use sun blocks as for any child.

Developmental issues
Safety

Children need sun protection.

Medic-Alert bracelet or necklace indicating special diet is advisable.

Elemental medical food products should be ingested only as prescribed, and only individuals with confirmed diagnosis of PKU should use them.

Child care

Providers should be aware of the need for special diet and hydration and calories during illness and trauma.

Diet

Controlled phe-restricted diet must be used indefinitely.

Blood phe monitoring with weight and diet changes must be done indefinitely.

Continued.

Self-management of phe-restricted diet should be initiated early in childhood.

For optimum bioavailability of nutrients, EMF products should be prepared and delivered as prescribed.

Sensitivity toward the social and cultural importance of food at each developmental level is needed.

Discipline

Avoid use of food as a reward system and blood tests as punishment.

Expectations are normal based on age and developmental level.

Toileting

Infants may be more prone to diaper dermatitis.

Daily hygiene is important, especially for musty odor related to uncontrolled phe homeostasis during illnesses and changes in dietary and activity levels.

Sleep patterns

Disturbed sleep patterns or nightmares may occur during uncontrolled phe homeostasis.

School issues

Visual spatial skills should be promoted.

Special education in math and language skills may be necessary. Annual development testing is recommended.

School personnel may be made aware of a child's special dietary needs at the discretion of parents.

Sexuality

Women with PKU should be educated about the importance of dietary compliance during childbearing years.

Fertility is not affected in men with PKU who maintain phe homeostasis.

Genetic counseling should be offered to the individual with PKU at the appropriate age.

Special family concerns

Special family concerns include the delay in diagnosis after initial newborn screen presumptive positive result for PKU, the vigilant supervision of the child's diet throughout many years, the potential parental guilt at having passed a "hidden gene" on to their child, genetic counseling of immediate and extended family members, family planning and prenatal diagnosis options, and financial support of the lifelong need for EMF products and medical care.

RESOURCES
Informational materials
Audiovisual materials

Helmore JD, producer: *A message to PKU parents,* Berkeley, Calif, 1989, Genetic Disease Branch, California State Department of Health.

The purpose of this program is to help parents of children newly diagnosed as having PKU understand some of the practical sides of the condition and to show that children with PKU can grow to healthy adulthood, leading normal lives. Running time is 21 minutes and 23 seconds. It was produced in cooperation with the Children's Hospital of Los Angeles, Division of Medical Genetics, Kathy Jew, and Julian C. Williams. To order call (415) 540-2534.

Husain M, producer: *Teenagers and PKU,* Chicago, 1987, Center for Educational Development, University of Illinois at Chicago.

The purpose of this program is to help teenagers diagnosed with PKU understand the disorder, learn how to communicate with their friends about PKU, and learn how to integrate PKU into their lives. Running time is 13 minutes. Content authors are Kimberlee Michals, Lynn Hurtt, Linda Gleason, and Grace Racster.

Messer S, producer: *Ethan and Elizabeth have PKU . . . and so do you,* Vienna, Va, 1989.

Included are a videotape, workbook, and evaluation tool prepared by a nurse who is the mother of a child with PKU. It is geared for ages 3 to 9 years and features several children with PKU. It teaches diet management concepts and deals with feelings of being different. Running time is 15 minutes. It may be ordered from Shirley Messer, 2809 Knollside Lane, Vienna, VA 22180. The cost is $34 for families and $49 for organizations.

PKU and you: Young women share their thoughts, Berkeley, Calif, 1988, Maternal PKU Project, Genetic Disease Branch, California State Department of Health.

The purpose of this program is to (1) give young women (≥13 years) with PKU an opportunity to hear about the experiences of other women like themselves and how they have dealt with various situations related to growing up with PKU, (2) reaffirm some of the thoughts and feelings that young women have about PKU and the diet, (3) motivate young women with PKU to stay on the diet or return to the diet before pregnancy and continue it throughout pregnancy, and (4) introduce viewers to California's Maternal PKU Camp as an educational resource for diet self-management and coping with PKU. Running time is 20 minutes. To order call (415) 540-2534.

Written materials for adults

Andrews LB: *State laws and regulations governing newborn screening,* monogr 85-071872, Washington, DC, 1985, US Department of Health and Human Services.

It may be ordered from the National Center for Education in Maternal and Child Health, 3520 Prospect St, NW, Washington, DC 20057, or call (202) 625-8400.

Griesemer P, Schaefer AM, Prochaska G, et al: *Monitoring blood levels at home: For infants, children and adults with PKU and other disorders,* Ann Arbor, Mich, 1986, University Hospital.

It may be ordered from the Pediatric Neurology Metabolic Clinic, C7123 Outpatient Bldg, Box 0800, University Hospital, Ann Arbor, MI 48109.

Henderson RA, Trahms CM, and Berlow S: *PKU and the schools: Information for teachers, administrators and other school personnel,* publication No (HSA) 80-5233, Washington, DC, 1980, US Department of Health and Human Services.

It may be ordered from the National Center for Education in Maternal and Child Health, 3520 Prospect St, NW, Washington, DC 20057, or call (202) 625-8400.

Kaufman M and Nardella M: *A teachers guide to PKU,* Phoenix, Ariz, 1985, Arizona Department of Health Services.

It may be ordered from the Office of Nutrition Services, Arizona Department of Health Services, 1740 W Adams St, Phoenix, AZ 85007.

NutraSweet® in foods and beverages: Information about PKU and diet, No US 005-982, Skokie, Ill, Searle Food Services. This is a booklet provided as a public service.

It may be obtained from Searle Food Resources, Inc, subsidiary of GD Searle & Co, PO Box 1111, Skokie, IL 60077.

Schuett V: *Low protein cookery: For phenylketonuria,* ed 2, Madison, Wis, 1988, University of Wisconsin Press.

Schuett V: *The low protein food list,* Madison, Wis, 1988, Waisman Center.

Schuett V: *State treatment centers for metabolic disorders,* Washington, DC, 1988, US Department of Health and Human Services.

It may be ordered from the National Center for Education in Maternal and Child Health, 3520 Prospect St, NW, Washington, DC 20057, or call (202) 625-8400.

Taylor JF and Latta S: *Special diets and kids: How to keep your child on any prescribed diet,* New York, 1989, Dodd Mead.

This sample spot contains enough information to save a life: Follow these eight important steps for proper neonatal blood sample collection. Keene, NH, Schleicher & Schuell. This is a brochure provided as a public service. To order call (800) 245-4024.

Written materials for children

All About PKU. This is an 18-page coloring book for ages 4 years and up. A Spanish version, *Todo Acerca PKU,* is also available. This booklet is designed to help children better understand their diet. It is filled with simple drawings and is easy for a school-aged child to read.

It may be ordered from Melanie Hunt, Children's Hospital Research Foundation, Elland and Bethesda Ave, Cincinnati, OH 45229. A single copy costs $1.50; 10 or more are $1.00 each.

Chef Lophe's Phe-Nominal Cookbook. This cookbook contains 16 quick and easy recipes for children. The phe amounts (≤40 mg) for all ingredients are given for most recipes. Some of the recipes rely on other recipes from *Low Protein Cookery for PKU.* It has cute illustrations.

It may be ordered from the National MCH Warehouse, 38 and R Sts, NW, Washington, DC 20057.

Games that teach. It contains nine games and activities for ages 2 to 6 years. This is a 1987 revision and expansion of a booklet developed 10 years earlier. The games were tested in a model preschool for children with PKU. It is appropriate for parents and clinic staff.

It may be ordered from the National MCH Warehouse, 38 and R Sts, NW, Washington, DC 20057. A single copy is free.

I can do it. It contains 12 lesson plans in a looseleaf binder for ages 3 years through adolescence. It was developed by a nutritionist and tested by children with PKU. It teaches about the PKU diet and emphasizes learning to make correct food choices for greater independence in self-management. Clinic staff may use it with individual children or in small groups, or motivated parents may use it at home.

It may be ordered from Iris Crump, 9360 Monona Dr, La Mesa, CA 92042. It costs $18.

Why is Mary On a Diet? This is a 14-page booklet on colorful construction paper for children ages 3 to 6 years. The story is about a little girl with PKU. Young children will enjoy having it read at home and taking it to school to share with the whole class.

It may be ordered from the Children's Memorial Hospital, PKU Clinic, 2300 Children's Plaza, Chicago, IL 60614. A single copy is free.

You and PKU. This is a 43-page spiral-bound notebook for children ages 3 to 8 years. It contains information about PKU, diet, blood drawing, and clinic visits and is presented in storybook fashion with appealing illustrations. Older children may be able to read it on their own. It includes helpful suggestions for parents to teach their child about the diet.

It may be ordered from the University of Wisconsin Press, 114 North Murray Street, Madison, WI 53715. It costs $6.

Organizations

*Helping Hand**
Mead-Johnson
Nutritional Sales Representative
Evansville, IN 47721

Maternal PKU Collaborative Study Coordinating Center
Children's Hospital of Los Angeles
4650 Sunset Blvd
Los Angeles, CA 90027
(213) 669-2152

National PKU Foundation
PO Box 5129
Pasadena, TX 77508
(713) 487-4802

Products

Dietary Specialties
PO Box 227
Rochester, NY 14601
(716) 263-2787

Ener-G Foods, Inc
6901 Fox Ave, S
PO Box 24723
Seattle, WA 98124
(206) 767-6660

Mead Johnson Nutritionals
A Bristol-Myers Company
Evansville, IN 47721

*This program is available to members of the medical profession for their patients by request only. It helps needy families by finding financial assistance for obtaining Mead-Johnson special formulas.

Ross Laboratories
Division of Abbott Laboratories
Columbus, OH 43216

Scientific Hospital Supplies, Ltd
Distributed by Ross Laboratories

REFERENCES

Acosta PB: *Ross metabolic formula system nutrition support protocols,* Columbus, Ohio, 1989, Abbott Laboratories.

Berg BO: *Child neurology,* Greenbrae, Calif, 1984, Jones Medical Publications.

Bick U, Fahrendorf G, Ludolf A, et al: *Alterations of myelin in treated patients with hyperphenylalaninemia.* In *Proceedings of the Fifth International Congress of Inborn Errors of Metabolism,* Asilomar, Calif, 1990.

Bolognia JL and Pawelek JM: Biology of hypopigmentation, *J Am Acad Dermatol* 19:217-254, 1988.

Brown ES: Paternal hyperphenylalaninemea, *Pediatrics* 70:201-205, 1986.

Brunner RL, Berch DB, and Berry H: P.K.U. and complex spatial visualization: An analysis of information processing, *Dev Med Child Neurol* 29:460-468, 1987.

Burns JK, Azen CG, Rouse B, et al: Impact of PKU on the reproductive patterns in collaborative study families, *Am J Med Genet* 19:515-524, 1984.

Casamassimo PS, Entwistle B, Ernest A, et al: *Dental health in children with phenylketonuria and other inborn errors of amino acid metabolism managed by diet,* Publication No HRS-D-MC 84-1, Rockville, Md, 1984, US Department of Health and Human Services.

Clarke JTR, Gates RD, Hogan SE, et al: Neuropsychological studies on adolescents with phenylketonuria returned to phenylalanine-restricted diets, *Am J Ment Retard* 92:255-262, 1987.

Cunningham GC, Kan K, and Mordaunt VL: Phenylalanine level of newborns in their first few days of life. In Therrell BL, ed: *Advances in neonatal screening,* New York, 1987, Elsevier North Holland.

Danks DM and Cotton RGH: Future developments in phenylketonuria, *Enzyme* 38:296-301, 1987.

DiLella AG and Woo SL: Molecular basis of P.K.U. and its clinical applications, *Molec Biol Med* 4:183-192, 1987.

Fehrenbach AM and Peterson L: Parental problem solving skills, stress and dietary compliance in P.K.U., *J Consult Clin Psychol* 57:237-241, 1989.

Fiedler AE, Miller MJ, Bickel H, et al: Phenylalanine levels in PKU following minor surgery, *Am J Med Genet* 11:411-414, 1982.

Fisch RO, Gravem HJ, and Feinberg SB: Growth and bone characteristics of phenylketonurics: Comparative analysis of treated and untreated phenylketonuric children, *Am J Dis Child* 112:3-10, 1966.

Fisch RO, Tsai MY, and Clark BA: Semen studies on phenylketonuria, *Biochem Med* 26:427-434, 1981.

Fishler K, Azen CG, Henderson R, et al: Psychoeducational findings among children treated for phenylketonuria, *Am J Ment Defic* 92:65-73, 1987.

Garriga MM and Metcalf DD: Aspartame intolerance, *Ann Allergy* 61:63-69, 1988.

Greeves LG, Carson DJ, and Dodge JA: Peptic ulceration and phenylketonuria: A possible link? *Gut* 29:691-692, 1988.

Guttler F, Olesen ES, and Wamberg E: Diurnal variations of serum phenylalanine in phenylketonuric children on low phenylalanine diet, *Am J Clin Nutr* 22:1568-1570, 1969.

Hanley W: Undiagnosed PKU in adult females—'newborn screening before conception'. In Skeels MR, Buist NRM, and Tuerck JM, eds: *Proceedings of the 6th National Neonatal Screening Symposium,* Portland, Ore, 1988.

Hassel CW and Brunsting LA: Phenylpyruvic oligophrenia: An elevation of the light-sensitive and pigmentary characteristics of seventeen patients, *AMA Arch Dermatol* 79:458-465, 1959.

Herrero E, Aragon MC, Gimenez C, et al: Inhibition by L-phenylalanine of trytophan transport by synaptosomal plasma membrane vesicles: Implications in the pathogenesis of phenylketonuria, *J Inherited Metab Dis* 6:32-35, 1983.

Holtzman NA, Faden R, Chwalow AJ, et al: Effect of informed parental consent on mothers' knowledge of newborn screening, *Pediatrics* 72:807-812, 1983.

Jew K, Koch R, and Cunningham G: Can PKU be predicted in early discharged infants? In *Proceedings of the Sixth International Neonatal Screening Symposium and Fifth National Neonatal Screening Symposium,* Austin, Tex, 1986, Texas Department of Health, Association of State and Territorial Public Health Laboratory Directors.

Jew K, Williams JC, and Koch R: *Reproductive decision making in PKU families.* In Proceedings of the Sixth National Neonatal Screening Symposium, Portland, Ore, 1988.

Kaufman S: An evaluation of the possible neurotoxicity of metabolites of phenylalanine, *J Pediatr* 114:895-900, 1989.

Kazak AE, Reber M, and Snitzer L: Childhood chronic disease and family functioning: A study of phenylketonuria, *Pediatrics* 81:224-230, 1988.

Kidd KK: P.K.U., population genetics of a disease, *Nature* 327:282-283, 1987.

Koch R and Wenz E: Phenylketonuria, *Ann Rev Nutr* 7:117-135, 1987.

McCabe L, Ernest AE, Neifert MR, et al: The management of breast feeding among infants with phenylketonuria, *J Inherited Metab Dis* 23:467-474, 1989.

Moen JL, Wilcox RD, and Burns JK: PKU as a factor in the development of self-esteem, *J Pediatr* 90:1027-1029, 1977.

Okano Y, Eisensmith RC, Guttler F, et al: Recurrent mutation in the human phenylalanine hydroxylase gene, *Am J Hum Genet* 46:919-924, 1990a.

Okano Y, Wang T, Eisensmith RC, et al: Correlation of mutant genotypes and clinical phenotypes of PKU in Caucasians. In Proceedings of the Fifth International Congress of Inborn Errors of Metabolism, Asilomar, Calif, 1990b.

Pietz J, Benninger C, Schmidt H, et al: Long-term development of intelligence (IQ) and EEG in 34 children with phenylketonuria treated early, *Eur J Pediatr* 147:361-367, 1990.

Rouse B, Lockhart L, Azen C, et al: Maternal PKU collaborative study (MPKUCS): A report of major and minor anomalies related to maternal blood phenylalanine levels during pregnancy. In Proceeding of the Fifth International Congress of Inborn Errors of Metabolism, Asilomar, Calif, 1990.

Schmidt K: Primer to the inborn errors of metabolism for perinatal and neonatal nurses, *J Perinat Neonatal Nurs* 2:60-71, 1989.

Scriver CR, Kaufman S and Woo SLC: The hyperphenylalaninemias. In Scriver CR, Beaudet A, Sly DW, et al, eds: *The metabolic basis of inherited disease,* New York, 1989, McGraw-Hill, pp 495-546.

Sorenson JR, Levy HL, Mangione TW, et al: Parental response to repeat testing of infants with 'false-positive' results in a newborn screening program, *Pediatrics* 73:183-187, 1984.

Woo SLC: Molecular basis and population genetics of phenylketonuria, *Biochemistry* 28:1-7, 1989.

Woo SLC: Molecular genetics and somatic gene therapy for phenylketonuria. In Proceedings of the Fifth International Congress of Inborn Errors of Metabolism, Asilomar, Calif, 1990.

Woolf LI: The heterozygote advantage in phenylketonuria, *Am J Med Genet* 38:773-774, 1986 (letter to the editor).

Wyatt RJ, Zarcone V, Engelman K, et al: Effects of 5-hydroxytryptophan on the sleep of normal human subjects, *Electroencephalogr Clin Neurophysiol* 30:505-509, 1971.

25 *Prematurity*

••

Diane J. Goldman and *Steven L. Goldman*

ETIOLOGY

The population of premature, low birth weight (LBW) infants represents a heterogeneous group. At one end of the spectrum are infants who spend their first weeks of life critically ill and, if they survive, require lifelong chronic care. At the other end, are those infants who have little or no problems during the perinatal period and require no special long-term care.

The terminology used to describe premature or LBW infants is not uniformly applied. This can result in confusing overlap. Premature, or preterm, generally refers to infants born before 38 weeks' gestation. However, the World Health Organization uses birth at less than 37 weeks as the definition of prematurity. Low birth weight refers to infants whose birth weight is less than 2500 g, very low birth weight (VLBW) refers to infants less than 1500 g, and very very low birth weight (VVLBW) refers to infants less than 1000 g. Historically the term low birth weight has been used almost synonymously with the term premature. This usage can be misleading. For example, some term infants have birth weights less than 2500 g (these infants are small for gestational age, or SGA), and some premature infants have birth weights greater than 2500 g (these infants are large for gestational age, or LGA). Appropriate for gestational age infants (AGA) have a birth weight within the normal range for their gestational age. Many of the references cited in this chapter vary in the terminology used. The term premature will be used preferentially in this chapter. However, where the use of this term is not consistent with a reference, some of the other terms will need to be used as well.

The causes of prematurity are varied, and many are interrelated. In simplest terms infants are born prematurely for one of two reasons: either the delivery was iatrogenically caused (pharmacologic induction or cesarean section) or could not be stopped (spontaneous preterm delivery). Some of the known causes or risk factors are listed in the box on p. 447. It must be noted that there is no known cause for at least 25% of premature births (Arias and Tomich, 1982).

INCIDENCE

The incidence of LBW infants in the United States is approximately 7%, a rate higher than 28 of the other Western industrialized countries (Children's Defense Fund, 1990). Between 1985 and 1987, there has been an increase in low birth weight infants, mainly in black infants, suggesting a worsening of a persistent disparity (Centers for Disease Control, 1990).

CLINICAL MANIFESTATIONS

The "condition" of prematurity is definitively diagnosed at the time of birth. The degree of prematurity is most accurately assessed using reliable

---

CAUSES OF PRETERM BIRTH

Iatrogenic preterm delivery
Maternal indications

Severe preeclampsia
Infection placing mother or infant at risk
Bleeding (previa, abruption)
Cardiovascular instability
Uncontrolled diabetes

Spontaneous preterm delivery
Maternal risk factors

Prior premature birth
Pariety = 0 or >4
Incompetent cervix
Abnormal placentation
Infection
Drug use (alcohol, cocaine, tobacco, etc.)
Preterm rupture of membranes
Short interval since last live born
Previous cesarean section

Fetal indications

Death of an identical twin
Poor growth
Unstable biophysical profile
Hydrops

Fetal risk factors

Multiple gestation
Fetal anomalies

---

maternal history. Occasionally when the date of the last menstrual period is uncertain, the gestational age can be confirmed using the measurements obtained at an early ultrasound examination. In the absence of reliable dates or if there are conflicting data, the objective assessment of physical and neurologic findings in the neonate can estimate the gestational age to within ±2 weeks (Ballard, Novak, and Driver, 1979; Constantine et al., 1987; Dubowitz, Dubowitz, and Goldberg, 1970).

Instruments that have been developed for the clinical assessment of gestational age take advantage of the profound physical and neurologic changes that occur in the fetus during the last trimester. For example, an infant of 24 weeks' gestation is extremely hypotonic, with fragile, thin, gelatinous skin. The skin breaks down and the subcutaneous tissue bleeds with minimal trauma. Because the chest wall is so flexible at this gestational age, respiratory effort results in substernal retractions. As the fetus matures, there is a global increase in resting tone, a flexed posture develops, the skin thickens, and bone and cartilage become firmer.

TREATMENT

The most desirable treatment for prematurity is prevention, but if the preterm birth is inevitable, treatment should begin in utero. Corticosteroids given to the mother before delivery will accelerate fetal lung maturation and decrease the risk of respiratory distress syndrome (RDS). If time permits, the mother and fetus should be transferred to a center with expertise in the management of high-risk deliveries and in caring for high-risk infants.

After the infant is born, treatment is tailored to existing or anticipated problems. Often, prophylactic treatment modalities are used in infants at highest risk. For example, exogenous surfactant can be given at birth to prevent or lessen the severity of RDS (Corbet et al., 1991), indomethacin (Indocin) may be given before signs of a patent ductus arteriosus are clinically apparent, and respiratory stimulants such as caffeine or theophylline may be given before apnea occurs.

PROGNOSIS

Probably in no other area is the question of survival and quality of life so important. The "morality of drastic intervention" (Avery, 1987) can be discussed at length without a uniform consensus being reached. Because centers (and individuals) differ in what is considered to be appropriate therapy, the published reports of outcome in terms of morbidity and mortality are not easily compared. However, some generalities can be made. First, prematurity, LBW, and their associated problems are responsible for approximately 18% of infant deaths in the United States, second only to birth defects (CDC, 1989). Infectious disease–related deaths are a major component of postneonatal (1 month through 1 year of age) mortality in LBW infants. Rates of infectious disease–related deaths were 1.6 per 1000 LBW live-born infants in 1982. Rates for black infants were consistently higher than those for white infants. Noninfectious disease–associated LBW postneonatal mortality rates increased from 1.4 per 1000 LBW live-born infants in 1968 to 3.0 per 1000 in 1982, with deaths coded as "sudden death," including sudden infant death syndrome, constituting a large proportion of this increase (Jason, 1989).

Overall, survival is related directly to gestational age or birth weight, and there has been improved survival over the past 15 years. The reason for the improved survival in the smaller infants is, in part, the result of scientific and technologic improvements in many areas such as ventilatory and nutritional support. In addition, however, the application of available technology to infants previously thought to be nonviable has been an important reason for improved survival rates.

With increasing survival there are increasing numbers of infants with significant morbidity. Poor outcome is related to the associated complications of prematurity. Because the smallest infants are those with the most complications, the worst outcome is in the smallest infants.

One measure of the increased morbidity is the higher use of medical resources by LBW infants during the first year of life. Low birth weight infants are twice as likely and VLBW infants 4.5 times as likely to be hospitalized during the first year of life compared with normal birth weight infants (McCormick, 1985; McCormick, Shapiro, and Starfield, 1980). At 5 years of age, VLBW children have an increased number of hospital admissions and days in the hospital as compared with normal birth weight children. Respiratory tract problems and ear, nose, and throat surgery are the most common reasons for readmission (Kitchen et al., 1990).

ASSOCIATED PROBLEMS

As outlined in Table 25-1, the potential clinical problems associated with prematurity are many. Any, all, or none of these clinical problems can develop, and many of these represent risk factors for the development of other problems. For example, an infant with severe RDS is more apt to develop a periventricular-intraventricular hemorrhage (PIVH) than an infant without respiratory disease; an infant with prolonged feeding intolerance or necrotizing enterocolitis (NEC) is more likely to develop rickets. Recognizing that these problems are possible allows the clinician to anticipate the long-term implications.

Periventricular-intraventricular hemorrhage

Periventricular-intraventricular hemorrhage (PIVH) often begins with bleeding into the subependymal germinal matrix. The bleeding can extend into the ventricular system or into the nearby brain parenchyma. PIVH has been classified into four grades according to Papile, Munsick-Bruno, and Schaefer (1983): grade I, subependymal hemorrhage; grade II, intraventricular hemorrhage; grade III, intraventricular hemorrhage with ventricular dilation; and grade IV, intraventricular hemorrhage with parenchymal hemorrhage.

The germinal matrix is a metabolically active, highly vascularized area that persists until term and is predisposed to hemorrhage for several reasons. Because there is poor autoregulation of blood flow to this area in premature infants, the delicate capillaries of the germinal matrix are vulnerable to damage from acute changes in systemic arterial or venous pressure. Perinatal asphyxia, metabolic problems, or respiratory problems can also damage the capillary bed and further predispose toward hemorrhage.

The reported incidence of PIVH varies considerably depending in part on the population studied and method of diagnosis. It is clear that the risk of PIVH increases with decreasing gestational age and

Table 25-1. Associated problems

	Metabolic	Infection	Respiratory	Neurologic	Hematologic	Cardiovascular	GI*
Early onset (≤2 wk)	Decreased calcium level Decrease or increase in glucose level Poor temperature regulation	Perinatally acquired (e.g., group B *Streptococcus*)	RDS TTN† Meconium aspiration Apnea	PIVH‡	Anemia (usually iatrogenic)	Patent ductus	Nonspecific feeding intolerance Necrotizing enterocolitis
Late onset (>2 wk)	Rickets	Hospital acquired (e.g., *Staphylococcus*, gram-negative rods)	BPD§ Apnea	Posthemorrhagic hydrocephalus Periventricular leukomalacia	Exaggerated anemia of prematurity		Postparenteral nutrition cholestasis

*GI, gastrointestinal.
†TTN, transient tachypnea of the newborn.
‡PIVH, periventricular-intraventricular hemorrhage.
§BPD, bronchopulmonary dysplasia.

with a host of risk factors, most of which are a reflection of how ill the infant is. Periventricular or intraventricular hemorrhage of any grade occurs in approximately 40% of infants with birth weight less than 1500 g (Volpe, 1987).

Treatment is supportive, and risk factors thought to contribute to further hemorrhage are minimized. Serial ultrasound examinations are necessary to document the resolution of the hemorrhage and to detect the development of hydrocephalus. If hydrocephalus develops, treatment must be instituted to minimize brain damage (see Chapter 17).

Mortality from PIVH is related to severity. Whereas there is no mortality associated with minimal hemorrhage, as many as 50% of infants with the most extensive hemorrhage do not survive (Volpe, 1987). In most reports of those who do survive, infants with the higher grades of PIVH have the worst outcome. In the series of VLBW infants by Papile, Munsick-Bruno, and Schaefer (1983), the incidence of major disability at 1 to 2 years of age was approximately 8% for infants with no, grade I, or grade II PIVH. However, 25% of those with grade III PIVH and 60% of those with grade IV PIVH had major disabilities. In many reports, infants with posthemorrhagic hydrocephalus tend to have the worst outcome (Krishnamoorthy, 1990). More recently, Papile, Munsick-Bruno, and Lowe (1988) have reported improvement over time in this group of infants, suggesting that the outcome for infants with larger hemorrhages is not as dismal as once thought.

Retinopathy of prematurity

Retinopathy of prematurity (ROP), also known as retrolental fibroplasia, affects the retina of the premature infant. Vascularization of the retina may not be complete until after approximately 42 to 44 weeks' postconceptual age. For reasons that are not clear, in some premature infants, abnormal vascularization of the retina develops. In most cases the retinopathy resolves without sequelae. However, in a few infants a proliferative neovascularization can develop, accompanied by fibrosis and retinal detachment. This leads to total or partial blindness.

The following stages of ROP have been described: stage 1, demarcation line between vascularized and avascular retina; stage 2, ridge (raised demarcation line); stage 3, ridge with extraretinal fibrovascular proliferation; stage 4, partial retinal detachment; stage 5, total retinal detachment (International Committee, 1987).

With increasing survival of infants with birth weight less than 1000 g, there are increasing numbers of infants with ROP. Risk factors for the development of ROP have been identified (Purohit et al., 1985), but clear cause and effect relationships remain to be confirmed. The most important risk factors appear to be prematurity and length of time in supplemental oxygen. The risk of ROP increases with decreasing gestational age, but the precise risk varies considerably from center to center. Infants with birth weight greater than 1500 g have an approximate 0.6% to 3% risk, whereas in some series those infants with birth weight less than 1000 g have as high as a 50% risk. A small proportion of affected infants progress to the most severe stages (Porat, 1984). Other factors that may increase risk are sepsis, apnea, and blood transfusion with adult blood. Most infants with stage 1 or 2 ROP experience regression and have no significant visual sequelae. Infants with ROP stages 3 and higher are likely to have vision problems ranging from myopia to retinal detachment and blindness.

Historically treatment results had been uniformly poor. Vitamin E remains a controversial treatment (Porat, 1984). Recently, however, the role of cryotherapy (localized hypothermia) was evaluated in a nationwide randomized trial. Enrollment was halted in 1988 after preliminary results demonstrated definite benefit, underscoring the importance of making a timely diagnosis (Multicenter Trial, 1988).

Anemia

There is not a single specific definition for anemia in this population. The hemoglobin level or hematocrit value must be assessed in light of the infant's age. For example, a hematocrit value of less than 40% at birth would be considered anemia. It is normal, however, for the hematocrit value to decrease to less than 40% over the weeks after birth. Anemia of prematurity is an exaggeration of the normal newborn's "physiologic" anemia.

Infants with anemia documented soon after birth should be evaluated for hemolysis, chronic blood loss in utero, or acute perinatal blood loss. Common causes of anemia that develop after the immediate perinatal period in the premature infant are iatrogenic blood loss and anemia of prematurity. The blood volume of an infant is only 80 to 100 ml/kg. Even with microtechniques, laboratory tests in a sick infant can easily deplete this blood volume. Anemia of prematurity results from a failure of the erythropoietin feedback system. When the tissues sense inadequate oxygen delivery, the kidney should manufacture erythropoietin. In the newborn and especially the premature newborn, the set point is temporarily too low, probably reflecting the normal hypoxemia of the environment in utero. Early iatrogenic anemia in very small, very sick premature infants is virtually universal. Most such infants will require at least one blood transfusion.

The decision to treat a premature infant for anemia is not based on absolute hematocrit values. Tachycardia, tachypnea, poor weight gain, and acidosis are nonspecific symptoms of anemia. Presence of any of these symptoms in the face of a low hematocrit value may indicate the need for a transfusion of packed red blood cells (Sacher, Luban, and Strauss, 1989). Treatment is not without risk. Transfusion reactions are rare but can occur in neonates. Despite screening, infectious complications include cytomegalovirus, hepatitis, and human immunodeficiency virus (HIV). The risk of HIV virus exposure decreased significantly after 1985 when screening became common (see Chapter 23).

Genetic engineering has made human erythropoietin readily available. Clinical trials are ongoing to determine if erythropoietin is a safe, effective treatment for anemia in premature infants. Anemia of prematurity is a self-resolving condition; however, many premature infants are discharged from the hospital with hematocrit values much lower than those of term infants. This distinction makes follow-up and screening more important in the premature infant.

Nutrition

Nutrition remains a major problem for the smallest premature infants. Generally infants with birth weight greater than 1250 g without significant medical problems tolerate enteral feedings easily. For those with acute problems and for smaller infants, however, enteral feedings are often delayed for days or weeks.

Parenteral nutrition consisting of dextrose, emulsified fat, and amino acids can provide infants with adequate calories for growth. Early complications of parenteral nutrition include hyperglycemia, protein intolerance reflected by hyperammonemia or acidosis, and difficulties related to prolonged intravenous access such as infiltrates and infection. Occasionally these complications prevent the infant from receiving adequate nutrition for long periods. Late complications of parenteral nutrition include cholestatic jaundice, often with elevated liver enzymes, which affects 30% to 40% of infants who weigh less than 1500 g who receive parenteral nutrition for more than 2 weeks (Beale et al., 1979).

Enteral feeding practices have changed over the past decade (American Academy of Pediatrics, 1985). Because premature infants have special nutritional needs (increased need for protein, calcium, phosphate, and sodium), formulas have undergone many changes to meet as many of these needs as possible while maintaining an acceptably high caloric density and an acceptably low osmolality and solute load. Preterm mother's milk supplemented with human milk fortifiers has been shown to be highly suited to the infant's nutritional needs. Despite the availability of parenteral nutrition, fortified breast milk, and premature formulas, most small premature infants do not receive adequate calcium and phosphorous intake. Hence, the incidence of rickets in VLBW infants may be as high as 32% (Callenbach et al., 1981; AAP, 1985).

The process of weaning parenteral nutrition and slowly introducing breast milk or formula can be frustrating. Feedings are often "not tolerated," a catchall phrase that includes vomiting, abdominal distension, and large gastric residuals. Because these nonspecific symptoms may be early signs of NEC, feeding is often temporarily discontinued. This on again–off again phase of enteral feeding results in a period of poor nutrition.

Necrotizing enterocolitis is a condition most common in premature infants and is characterized by ischemic damage to the submucosal layer of the bowel. This condition accounts for approximately 2% of deaths in premature infants. It probably has many etiologies. The large list of risk factors include asphyxia, hypertonic feedings, umbilical vessel catheterization, exchange transfusion, and polycythemia. In severe cases of NEC, intestinal perforation, an absolute indication for surgery, can occur. Whether or not perforation occurs, stricture and obstruction, along with symptoms of abdominal distension and vomiting, occur weeks later in approximately 15% of affected infants. Lifelong problems may develop in those infants with postoperative short bowel syndrome (Kliegman and Fanaroff, 1984).

Respiratory problems

Lung damage. Respiratory distress occurs in approximately 10% of all neonates. Of those, 60% to 70% of the infants have transient respiratory problems. Approximately 10% each will have RDS, aspiration of meconium, blood, or amniotic fluid, or congenital pneumonia (Klaus, Fanaroff, and Martin, 1986).

A wide range of treatment modalities is available, and treatments are tailored to the infants' needs. Most infants require little supportive therapy, such as supplemental oxygen given through a hood. Others require positive pressure as continuous positive airway pressure or mechanical ventilation through an endotracheal tube. Treatment with positive pressure and supplemental oxygen, though lifesaving, may damage the lungs and airways. This damage must be viewed as a continuum. The extreme example of this is bronchopulmonary dysplasia (BPD) (see Chapter 7). Premature infants who require mechanical ventilation but do not develop BPD have evidence of lung and airway damage (Coates et al., 1977). This damage may be subclinical, demonstrated only with pulmonary function testing, or may be reflected in increased airway reactivity or increased pulmonary infections in the first years of life.

Apnea. Twenty-five percent to 30% of LBW infants have apnea, most of which is attributable to respiratory center immaturity (apnea of prematurity). The incidence increases with decreasing gestational age. In most cases, apnea resolves by the time the infant is ready for discharge from the hospital. There is no evidence that apnea of prematurity increases the risk for sudden infant death syndrome (SIDS). However, graduates of intensive care nurseries (ICNs) are statistically at much higher risk for SIDS, a risk that appears to be magnified by other factors such as BPD, maternal drug abuse (especially cocaine), and VLBW. Unfortunately there is no way to predict which infant will go on to develop SIDS. Nevertheless, many centers perform pneumograms on LBW infants as a diagnostic tool to decide which infants should be sent home with a cardiorespiratory monitor.

The premature infant who continues to have apnea when, in all other respects, he or she is ready for discharge, presents a management problem. There appears to be no consensus on treatment. Some care providers keep the infant in the hospital indefinitely, whereas others send the infant home with a cardiorespiratory monitor with or without theophylline or caffeine therapy. Parents of infants at higher risk for apnea or SIDS should be taught infant cardiopulmonary resuscitation (CPR) before the infant is discharged from the hospital.

Gastrointestinal problems

The incidence of inguinal hernias is higher in LBW newborns than in term neonates. Inguinal hernias occur more frequently in those infants born at less than 32 weeks' gestation or who weigh less than 1250 g; for SGA male infants born at less than 32 weeks' gestation, the risk is even higher. Preterm infants requiring inguinal hernia repair may have increased risk of incarceration, recurrent apnea, anesthesia morbidity, and postoperative complications (Peevy, Speed, and Hoff, 1986). Surgical repair should be accomplished as soon as possible by a qualified pediatric surgeon (DeLorimer, 1988).

Genitourinary problems

Low birth weight and premature infants have a higher rate of undescended testes than full-term newborns. Nearly 100% of infants weighing approximately 900 g exhibit bilateral undescended testes. In most of these tiny infants, the testes descend during the first year of life. Medical and surgical intervention is indicated soon after 1 year of age for those children with undescended testes

because there is evidence of decreased spermatogonia if the testes remain in the abdomen (Hawtrey, 1990).

PRIMARY CARE MANAGEMENT
Growth and development

The growth pattern of the majority of preterm AGA infants when plotted by corrected age rather than chronologic age follows the same pattern as full-term infants (Brandt, 1978; Fitzhardinge, 1975). Corrected age is the postnatal age less the number of weeks the infant was premature. Moderately premature infants without serious medical illness show maximal catch-up growth earlier than extremely premature infants or those with serious medical problems. "Healthy" premature infants exhibit catch-up growth within the first year, whereas small or sicker infants may not reach their growth potential until 3 or more years of age (Hack and Fanaroff, 1988; Hirata et al., 1983).

Several studies have shown that LBW and VLBW infants demonstrated lower growth patterns during the first 12 months and remain smaller as a group than normal children at 3 years of age, even when corrected age is used (Casey et al., 1990; Kimble et al., 1982). However, a recent study by Ross, Lipper, and Auld (1990), showed that a group of VLBW premature children who had been smaller than full-term peers at the first and third years of life, had caught up to the normal population by 8 years of age.

Premature SGA infants tend to have poor neonatal growth, with the period of rapid catch-up growth occurring between 40 weeks' corrected age and 8 months of age (Hack et al., 1984). However, approximately one half of these infants have subnormal weights at 8 months of age with no further catch-up growth during the second or third year. Approximately one fourth of SGA premature infants born with subnormal head circumference at birth continue to have small head circumferences at 33 months of age. The SGA infants with normal head circumference at birth tend to have normal weights at 33 months (Hack et al., 1984).

Head circumference of the LBW infant must be followed closely. Catch-up growth, usually occurring in the first 6 weeks after birth and continuing until 6 to 8 months, will result in disproportionately high head circumference percentiles, especially in the first 3 months after term. The primary care provider must be aware of those infants with intracranial hemorrhage during the neonatal course to differentiate catch-up growth from developing hydrocephalus (see Chapter 17). Cranial ultrasound or computerized tomography of the head is indicated when the signs of hydrocephalus are present (see Chapter 17) (Bernbaum et al., 1989).

Early postnatal head growth is an indicator of positive neurodevelopmental outcome. Lack of catch-up growth or initial catch-up growth followed by slow head growth are ominous signs (Hack and Fanaroff, 1988).

The parameters of growth must be followed closely to determine that the infant is thriving. Corrected age should be used until 2 to 3 years of age when measurements are plotted on standard growth charts. The length for weight graph on the National Center for Health Statistics growth chart is helpful in determining proportional growth in those infants with weights and lengths below the fifth percentile. Infants who fail to grow within their established growth curves should be investigated for failure to thrive.

Infants with birth weights of less than 1500 g are at greatest risk for high morbidity. Reports differ as to whether outcomes have improved over time in these infants. Reasons for these varied reports are differences in definitions of abnormalities, diagnostic categories, ages at which examinations are done, and in the measures used in neuropsychiatric evaluation (Knobloch et al., 1982).

Bauchner, Brown, and Peskin (1988) in summarizing the developmental literature, report that for infants with birth weights less than 1000 g approximately 50% will demonstrate normal-range cognitive (developmental quotient $\geq$ 85) and motor development at 2 years of age. For infants with birth weights between 1000 and 1500 g, 75% can be expected to be within the normal range at 2 years of age. For infants weighing more than 1500 g, approximately 90% will be normal (Bauchner, Brown, and Peskin, 1988).

Perinatal risk factors for poor developmental outcome include LBW, outborn, low gestational age, use of mechanical ventilation, asphyxia, intraventricular hemorrhage, and infection (Bauchner,

Brown, and Peskin, 1988). Research suggests that premature infants are also more vulnerable to environmental deprivation, resulting in abnormal developmental outcomes (Escalona, 1982).

The types of developmental disabilities associated with being VLBW include mental retardation, low-average intelligence, static motor disorders (spectrum ranging from incapacitating cerebral palsy to motor clumsiness and incoordination), seizure disorders, behavior disorders, learning disabilities, and peripheral or central visual and auditory impairments. Many children have multiple problems, with the most pervasive and global disabilities becoming evident early (Desmond et al., 1980).

Neuromuscular abnormalities. Low birth weight infants often show signs of neuromuscular abnormalities that resolve during the second year of life and therefore do not carry the same prognostic importance as in the full-term infant. The most common neurologic abnormalities include increased extensor tone of the lower extremities, shoulder retractions caused by hypertonicity of the shoulder girdle and trapezius muscles, mild or transient asymmetry in tone, mild to moderate hypotonicity, and hypertonicity of the upper or lower extremities or trunk (Bernbaum et al., 1989; Dubowitz, 1988). It is essential that the primary care provider perform thorough neurologic assessments during the first 2 years of life to determine the presence and progress of abnormalities.

A child with extreme tone abnormalities and delays must be identified so that intervention can be initiated, but one must be cautious about labeling a child as having cerebral palsy before 18 months' corrected age (see Chapter 9). Experts differ about recommendations for physical therapy during the first 2 years of life. Bernbaum and colleagues (1989) suggest that formal physical therapy is necessary when an abnormality is sufficient enough to adversely affect the infant's functional status or delay the achievement of key developmental milestones.

An essential component of primary care of the premature infant is developmental assessment and anticipatory guidance concerning developmental expectations. Although it is often difficult to do formal testing in an office setting, the Denver Developmental Screening Test can help the clinician effectively screen and formulate a clinical impression of the infant's developmental capabilities. When premature infants are tested, corrected age is commonly used until 2 to 3 years of age. Allen and Alexander (1990) suggest that using chronologic age in assessing gross motor abilities will lead to overdiagnosis of motor delay in most extremely preterm infants. But others advise that chronologic age be used for more accurate referral and follow-up decisions and that corrected age be used to allay undue parental anxiety (Elliman et al., 1985).

Further evaluation is necessary when a delay is evident or the parents are extremely worried about mental development. Referrals can be made to high-risk follow-up clinics, child development centers, regional developmental services, Easter Seal centers, or developmental pediatricians with training in assessment of premature infants.

Recent data suggest that combining early child development and family support services with pediatric follow-up shows substantive promise of decreasing the number of LBW premature infants at risk for later developmental disabilities (Infant Health and Development Program, 1990; Resnick et al., 1987). Public Law 99-457 offers states the option to provide services to handicapped, developmentally delayed, or at-risk children from birth to 3 years of age. The primary care practitioner must be familiar with local early intervention programs and criteria and processes for admission, so that appropriate referrals can be initiated.

Immunizations

Studies have demonstrated that preterm infants immunized with diphtheria, pertussis, and tetanus (DPT) at routine intervals (2, 4, and 6 months after birth) are capable of producing a protective serologic response with fewer side effects than are full-term infants (Bernbaum et al., 1985). Therefore, the American Academy of Pediatrics (AAP) recommends that full doses of DPT be administered to premature infants at the same chronologic ages as recommended for full-term infants (Committee on Infectious Diseases, 1991). The same contraindications for pertussis vaccine in the term infant apply to the premature infant.

Polio vaccine should be administered orally to premature infants at the same chronologic ages as recommended for full-term infants. If the infant remains hospitalized, this vaccine should be withheld until discharge to prevent cross-infection or, alternatively, inactivated polio vaccine (IPV) can be given (Committee on Infectious Diseases, 1991). Measles, mumps, rubella, and *Haemophilus influenzae* type b (Hib) vaccine should be administered at the chronologic ages recommended by the AAP.

Hepatitis B vaccine. The AAP recommends that all infants born to mothers with positive hepatitis B (HB) surface antigen be given HB immunoglobulin (HBIG) at birth and HB vaccine within 7 days after birth and at 1 and 6 months. These same recommendations apply to preterm infants, although data on the effectiveness of HB vaccine are not available for infants with birth weights of less than 2000 g. The administration of the HB vaccine may be delayed if necessary (not HBIG) but should be given within 1 month if possible. If administration of the vaccine is delayed for as long as 3 months, a second dose of HBIG (0.5 ml) should be given (Committee on Infectious Diseases, 1991).

Varicella-zoster immune globulin. Because of the poor transfer of antibodies across the placenta early in pregnancy, the AAP recommends that all infants born before 28 weeks' gestation (or who weigh <1000 g) who still require hospitalization for treatment of prematurity and related conditions and are exposed to varicella should receive varicella-zoster immune globulin (125 U). The recommendation also applies to premature infants born after 28 weeks' gestation whose mothers have a negative history of past infection (Committee on Infectious Diseases, 1991).

Screening

Vision. Ophthalmologic problems, including ROP, myopia, and strabismus, occur with increased frequency among premature infants (Bull et al., 1986). According to AAP recommendations, all oxygen-exposed infants with birth weights less than 1800 g (or <35 weeks' gestation) and all infants weighing less than 1300 g at birth (or born at <30 weeks' gestation) regardless of oxygen exposure should have an ophthalmologic examination before discharge or at 5 to 7 weeks after birth to assess for ROP (AAP, 1988). Because of the significant risk of early and late sequelae, infants who have ROP and, by virtue of their immature retinae, those who are still at risk for ROP should receive close ophthalmologic follow-up after discharge (Bernbaum et al., 1989; Gardner and Hagedorn, 1990).

The eye examination of the LBW infant by the primary care practitioner should include assessment of the vision, the fundus (red reflex), and the alignment of the eyes. Visual assessment includes the infant's ability to fixate and follow objects. This response should be present by 6 weeks' corrected age (Day, 1988). Continued yearly assessment of visual acuity in this population is important to identify more subtle refractive errors that may affect scholastic achievement.

Hearing. The incidence of sensorineural hearing loss in preterm infants is usually reported to be 1% to 3%. Factors associated with prematurity such as hypoxia, hyperbilirubinemia, environmental noise levels, concomitant antibiotic and diuretic therapy, and congenital infections place LBW infants at particular risk for hearing problems (Bernbaum et al., 1989).

All VLBW infants or infants with any other risk factors should be screened for hearing loss preferably under the supervision of an audiologist. Optimally screening should be performed before discharge from the newborn nursery but no later than 3 months of age. Initial screening should include auditory brainstem response (ABR) (American Speech-Language-Hearing Association, 1989). If the results of an initial screening are equivocal, the infant should be referred for general medical, otologic, and audiologic follow-up. Ongoing testing is necessary when there are conditions which increase the probability of progressive hearing loss, such as family history of delayed onset of hearing loss, degenerative disease, meningitis, or intrauterine infections (Joint Committee on Infant Hearing, 1991).

Health care providers should be alerted to those children who have delays in speech development, poor attentiveness, and absent or abnormal responses to sound. It is possible that these findings indicate hearing loss and require more thorough investigation.

Dental. Prolonged orotracheal intubation affects the palate and possibly the dentition; very high arched palates and deep palatal grooves have been observed. In mild cases these deformities usually resolve within the first year of life. Abnormally shaped teeth with notching have been observed in some infants. Dental eruption is usually mildly delayed in premature infants (even allowing for corrected age), with greater delays seen in chronically ill infants (Piecuch, 1988). Specific guidelines for fluoride use in premature infants do not exist. Routine fluoride supplementation is recommended if fluoride in the water supply is less than 0.3 ppm.

Blood pressure. Premature infants may be at risk for developing hypertension. Several studies attribute the hypertension to complications of umbilical arterial catheters. Hypertension screening should be done at 1, 2, 6, 12, and 24 months of age and then routinely in childhood (Cohen and Taeusch, 1987). Infants with a blood pressure greater than the 95th percentile for age on three separate visits should be considered hypertensive and evaluation of etiology should be initiated (Sheftel, Hustead, and Friedman, 1983).

Hematocrit. The hematocrit values of the preterm infant should be checked monthly until the infant is 6 months of age and then every 2 months throughout the first year of life (Koerper, 1988). As in the immediate neonatal period, there is no one hematocrit value that indicates anemia during the months following birth. Between 2 and 3 months of age the hematocrit value can fall as low as 21% and still be considered nonpathologic. The drop in hematocrit value is an exaggerated physiologic anemia and is rarely related to iron deficiency (Committee on Nutrition, 1985). As in term infants, if the drop in hematocrit value is more extreme or fails to increase over time, other causes for anemia must be considered and treated as needed (Chow et al., 1984).

Urinalysis. Routine screening is recommended.

Tuberculosis. Routine screening is recommended.

Condition-specific screening

HERNIA AND TESTICULAR SCREENING. At each primary care visit the infant's caretaker must be asked about the presence of inguinal swelling that increases in size with coughing or crying. The inguinal area and canal must be palpated for any swelling or masses. Because of the increased incidence of undescended testicles in premature male infants, a thorough testicular examination is warranted.

Drug interactions

There are no specific drug interactions.

DIFFERENTIAL DIAGNOSIS
Infection

Respiratory viruses such as respiratory syncytial virus (RSV), parainfluenza viruses, and influenza viruses are a major cause of morbidity for the ICN graduate. Although the clinical symptoms of RSV infection in the term infant may be the expected ones of pneumonia or bronchiolitis, the symptoms in the premature infant may be nonspecific, with apnea being a prominent finding (Arvin, 1988).

Viral respiratory disease is particularly dangerous for infants with residual lung disease, and those infants must be monitored closely by the primary care practitioner for signs of respiratory distress (see Chapter 7). The risk of acquiring lower respiratory tract disease secondary to infection is related to the age at acquisition of the primary infection, with reduced morbidity in the second and third years of life. Since older siblings and adults usually bring viral pathogens into the home, direct contact with the infant by symptomatic individuals should be minimized when symptoms are present, especially during the first year of life (Arvin, 1988).

Herpes simplex virus (HSV) and late-onset group B streptococcal infection are two examples of pathogens that infants are exposed to in the perinatal period that cause rapidly progressive illness in an infant who was considered to be doing well. The incubation period for infants with perinatal exposure to HSV is variable, ranging from 2 days to 6 weeks. Because the attack rate for HSV is increased with prematurity, the diagnosis of HSV should be considered in the high-risk premature infant who has any symptoms compatible with HSV, including lethargy, poor feeding, herpetic lesions, and transient low-grade fever. Because the effects of HSV type 1 can be as devastating to the high-risk infant as HSV type 2, it is necessary to advise parents to avoid exposing the infant to individuals with fever blisters or cold sores (Arvin, 1988).

Organisms such as *Chlamydia,* group B *Streptococcus, Staphylococcus aureus,* or *Escherichia coli* can colonize in an infant during birth or hospitalization and become invasive, causing serious infection after discharge. In addition, premature infants may be at special risk from organisms such as *Streptococcus pneumoniae* (pneumococcus) and Hemophilus influenza type b (Hib). The major sites of infection are the central nervous system, bones, joints, and respiratory system.

Healthy premature infants who have unexplained fever should be assessed according to their corrected ages. The work-up is the same as that of term infants. Antibiotic selection must take into account possible neonatal sources of infection. Parents need to be instructed about signs and symptoms of infection, which include lethargy, poor feeding, irritability, fever, respiratory distress, and bowel changes. Because some of these symptoms may be characteristics of the well premature infant's "baseline" behavior, awareness of changes in this baseline may help to identify illness.

DEVELOPMENTAL ISSUES
Safety

Anticipatory guidance about safety must be adjusted to the child's developmental level rather than to chronologic age. Because many parents continue to consider their children weak or vulnerable, they must be encouraged not to restrict activities but to allow exploration and social interaction within a safe setting.

Recommendations (Committee on Injury and Poison Prevention and Committee on Fetus and Newborn, 1991) for the safe tranportation of premature infants include the following: (1) Place the infant in the car seat in a location that allows for observation by an adult during travel. All infants weighing less than 17 to 20 lb must ride facing the rear. (2) Use blanket rolls inside the car seat to improve head and trunk control. Blanket rolls can be placed on both sides of the infant's trunk for lateral support and between the crotch strap and the infant to reduce slouching. (3) If the infant's head drops forward, tilt the seat back and/or wedge a cloth roll under the safety seat base so that the baby reclines at a 45-degree angle. (4) Avoid using convertible car seats with a shield, abdominal pad, or arm rest if the infant's face or neck could directly

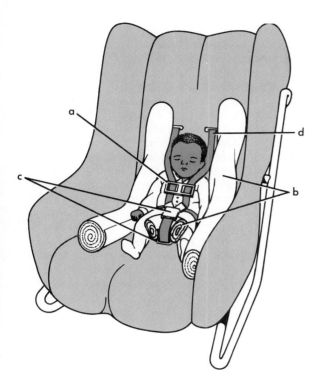

Fig. 25-1. Positioning of premature infant in car seat: *a,* retainer clip positioned on child's chest; *b,* blanket rolls on both sides of trunk, and between crotch strap and infant; *c,* distance of 5½ inches or less from crotch strap to seat back; *d,* distance of 10 inches or less from lower harness strap to seat bottom.

contact these objects during impact. Position the car seat's retainer clip on the infant's chest (See Fig. 25-1).

Specific recommendations regarding travel for infants at possible risk of respiratory problems include (1) counseling families to minimize travel for infants at risk for respiratory compromise, (2) having an appropriate hospital staff person conduct a period of observation of the infant in a car seat before discharge to monitor for possible apnea, bradycardia, or oxygen desaturation on infants of less than 37 weeks' gestation, (3) having infants with prescribed home cardiac and apnea monitors use this monitoring equipment during travel with portable, self-contained power for twice the ex-

pected transport duration, (4) restraining all portable medical equipment with adjacent seat belts, wedged on the floor, or under the seats, and (5) using alternative child restraint devices for infants who must ride prone, supine, or in a less upright position (Committee on Injury and Poison Prevention and Committee on Fetus and Newborn, 1991).

Child care

Many studies have demonstrated the increased incidence of infectious diseases such as diarrhea and respiratory illnesses in infants and children attending day-care centers compared with children cared for in the home. Because LBW infants have greater and more prolonged immune deficiencies, the transmission of infectious diseases within day-care centers may affect the morbidity of the LBW infant attending these facilities. Based on these considerations, home child care would be preferable to other day-care situations. Unfortunately many of the women who have LBW infants are least likely to be able to afford child care in the home (Jason, 1989). For those families unable to afford a one-to-one situation, a small home care program would be more desirable than a large day-care center. Parents must also consider their role in educating the day care provider about the special needs of the LBW infant (e.g., nutrition, stimulation, sleep habits).

Diet

Breast- and bottle-feeding. The use of an electric pump every 3 hours on each breast helps mothers to maintain an adequate milk supply while their infants are hospitalized. Premature infants are now often given the opportunity to suckle as early as age 32 weeks' gestation, with positive effects for both mother and infant (Meier and Anderson, 1987). It is essential for the practitioner to determine the mother's breast-feeding desires. Anxiety, fatigue, and emotional stress may inhibit lactation, and mothers need support, guidance, and breast-feeding education while in the hospital, as well as after discharge, to ensure adequate nutritional intake and a healthy feeding environment for the infant-mother dyad (Fig. 25-2). Many communities and hospitals have lactation counselors who are able to work with mothers to establish a successful breast-feeding regimen.

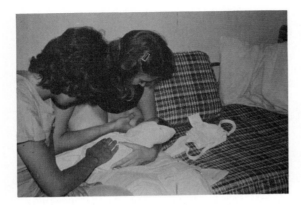

Fig. 25-2. Nurse assisting mother with breast-feeding her preterm infant.

Feeding the premature infant can be difficult because the mouth is small, oral musculature is weak, and the sucking mechanism is disorganized. Certain premature infants may benefit from any or all of the following interventions: frequent, small-volume feedings; soft bottle nipples; support of head, neck, and hips in slight flexion; minimal talking during eye contact, and a quiet, slightly darkened room (Gorski, 1988).

Abnormal feeding behaviors such as tonic bite reflex, tongue thrust, hyperactive gag reflex, or oral hypersensitivity can also be seen. Hypersensitivity secondary to intubation, repeated suctioning, or use of nasogastric or orogastric tubes can make the infant resistant to any type of oral stimulation, including nipples, spoons, and cups (Bernbaum et al., 1989). It is important for the primary care practitioner to continually assess the infant's feeding capabilities and parental concerns about feeding. Referral to a therapist (speech, physical, or occupational) familiar with feeding disorders is warranted when a significant or prolonged problem is identified.

Gastroesophageal reflux is a common problem in preterm infants with characteristics and therapy similar to those described for full-term infants. Treatment is dependent on the clinical findings and degree of severity (Bernbaum et al., 1989).

The AAP dietary guidelines for full-term infants are usually appropriate for healthy preterm infants after discharge if the corrected age is used (Bernbaum et al., 1989). By the time of discharge, mature breast milk is usually nutritionally adequate for the preterm infant. The use of regular commercial formula (20 kcal/30 ml) is also appropriate for the healthy premature infant, and recommended amounts can be based on corrected age. Increasing the caloric density of formula for infants who fail to exhibit catch-up growth can be achieved by adding medium-chain triglycerides, by adding glucose polymers or milk enhancers, or by adding less water to the concentrate or powder. Increasing the caloric density should be considered only after consultation with a neonatologist or pediatric dietician (Bernbaum et al., 1989; Peterson and Frank, 1987).

Solid foods can be introduced to the premature infant when any one of the following criteria is met: (1) the infant consistently consumes more than 32 oz of formula per day for 1 week, (2) the infant weighs 6 to 7 kg, or (3) the infant's corrected age is 6 months. The AAP does not recommend feeding solids before 4 months' chronologic age (Bernbaum et al., 1989).

A multivitamin supplement is often used until the infant is consuming more than 300 kcal/day or when the body weight exceeds 2.5 kg. Infants with poor growth because of recurrent or chronic illness or poor caloric intake should continue to receive a multivitamin supplement until they are consuming a well balanced diet (Bernbaum et al., 1989).

The AAP Committee on Nutrition recommends that LBW infants receive supplemental iron (2 mg/kg/day to a maximum of 15 mg/day) starting at 2 months' chronologic age (Committee on Nutrition, 1985). Infants' vitamin E status must be considered because use of iron in vitamin E–deficient infants can result in a hemolytic anemia (Committee on Nutrition, 1985). Sufficient iron can be supplied by iron-fortified formulas (12 mg/L), multivitamin preparations containing iron, or ferrous sulfate drops. Most authors agree that iron supplementation should continue for 6 to 12 months until the child is eating iron-rich solid foods on a regular basis (Bernbaum et al., 1989; Hagedorn and Gardner, 1991; Koerper, 1988).

If iron deficiency is suspected by history or documented by laboratory testing, the LBW infant may require increased supplementation (3-4 mg/kg/day). Higher doses may be poorly tolerated and do not result in a more rapid response (Dallman, 1988).

Discipline

The stress of having an infant in the ICN leaves many parents prone to what Green and Solnit (1964) have called "the vulnerable child syndrome." These attitudes about the child may result in overindulgence and overpermissiveness. Families often have difficulties setting limits, which can interfere with normal development; the child may exhibit dependent, demanding, or uncontrolled behavior (Bernbaum et al., 1989).

Premature infants are often more difficult to care for than full-term infants. Their sleep-wake cycle is disturbed by their long hospital stays. Many become agitated or nonresponsive to what is considered average stimulation. These infants are often difficult to soothe, have trouble eating, have delayed milestones, and require more care and patience from their parents (Medoff-Cooper and Schraeder, 1982).

It has been suggested that families try to normalize the caretaking and daily activities of their premature infant. This normalization process is seen as critical to the development of a healthy relationship between parents and child. Families should also be encouraged to set disciplinary limits and schedules that enable them to be in control (Bernbaum and Hoffman-Williamson, 1986).

Toileting

Signs of toileting readiness are more likely to appear at the appropriate corrected rather than chronologic age. Abnormal neurologic findings such as increased muscle tone may have a negative effect on the toilet training process, and training may be more effectively done when muscle tone has decreased.

Sleep patterns

The sleep patterns of the premature infant differ from those of the full-term infant. Premature infants can wake up as frequently as every 2 hours until 4 months' corrected age and may not be able to sustain an 8-hour sleep period at night until 8 months' corrected age. This immature sleep organization may be the result of neurologic immaturity, nutritional demands, and metabolic differences (Gorski, 1988).

Whereas full-term infants may be able to sleep through any distraction, many premature infants appear to be hypersensitive to sights and sounds (Gorski, 1988). Conversely, many premature children become habituated to the noise and lights of the ICN and have difficulty adjusting to the quiet and dark of the home environment. The use of a night light or radio is often recommended for these infants to ease their transition to the home.

An infant's ability to sleep through the night is also determined by many factors, such as age, nutritional status, temperament, and previous sleep patterning. Premature infants should not be expected to sleep through the night earlier than 2-4 months of corrected age. Parents must be supported during this period and provided with realistic guidelines for sleep patterning of the premature infant (Ferber, 1985).

School issues

Many studies have documented an increased frequency of educational problems in children who have received ICN care. Some investigators have found premature infants more likely to have lower school achievement and greater need for special class placements. Often these problems manifest as subtle visual-motor, perceptual, language, reading difficulties or hyperactive behavior (Hunt, Tooley, and Halvin, 1982; McCormick, Gortmaker, and Sobol, 1990; Nickel, Bennett, and Lamson, 1982; Vohr and Coll, 1985). The prevalence of learning problems in preterm infants of normal intelligence emphasizes the need for early identification and implementation of individual intervention programs (Hunt, Cooper, and Tooley, 1988; Klein et al., 1985; Sell et al., 1985). Ideally these children should be longitudinally followed in high-risk clinics into the school years. If these services are not available, the practitioner should assess the neurodevelopmental progress of the child, including the presence of soft signs that may be an indication of poor academic performance (Blondis, Snow, and Accardo, 1990). School performance and progress should be discussed with parents and school personnel; referral for educational testing should be initiated if a problem is suspected.

Sexuality

Women who were born SGA have been found to be at increased risk for giving birth to both growth retarded and preterm infants (Klebanoff, Meirik, and Berendes, 1989). Appropriate counseling and early prenatal referral to parents and adolescents is necessary with regard to these findings.

SPECIAL FAMILY CONCERNS

Families with premature infants have multiple issues to address. Parents must deal with the grief of delivering a preterm infant while going through the attachment process. The transition from hospital to home is a period of extreme anxiety; parents are faced with caring for their infant without the support of hospital staff. Parents have financial issues, as well as concerns involving the health and developmental outcome of the infant. It is often difficult for parents to appreciate the progress of their premature infant while friends, relatives, and strangers continually make comparisons to full-term infants. Education and support from primary care providers will enable parents to create an environment that will encourage infants to attain their full potential.

SUMMARY OF PRIMARY CARE NEEDS FOR THE PREMATURE OR LOW BIRTH WEIGHT INFANT

Growth and development

Use corrected age to plot height, weight, and head circumference.

Preterm infants who are AGA follow similar growth patterns as full-term infants.

Infants who are SGA tend to be smaller children.

Catch-up growth occurs within the first year to after 3 years of age.

Monitor head circumference for abnormal growth.

The incidence of abnormal development increases with decreased birth weight.

Transient neuromuscular abnormalities can be present in the first year.

Immunizations

All immunizations should be administered at chronologic ages recommended by the AAP.

Infants may be given OPV after discharge.

Screening
Vision

Assessment of fixation, following alignment and fundoscopic examination are recommended. Ophthalmologic follow-up is necessary for infants with ROP or positive visual finding.

Hearing

Screening is necessary for infants with identified risk factors within 3 months of age.

Dental

Prolonged intubation affects palate and dentition.

Tooth eruptions may be delayed.

Routine fluoride supplementation is recommended.

Hematocrit

Hematocrit values should be checked monthly until 6 months, then every 2 months through 1 year of age.

Urinalysis

Routine screening is recommended.

Tuberculosis

Routine screening is recommended.

Condition-specific screening

Hernia and testicular screening

Infants should be screened for inguinal hernia and undescended testicles.

Drug interactions

No routine medications are given.

Differential diagnosis

These infants have an increased risk of infection.

Herpes simplex virus, *Chlamydia,* group B *streptococcus, Staphylococcus aureus,* and *Escherichia coli* must all be considered possible pathogens.

Developmental issues
Safety

Anticipatory guidance is based on developmental age.

Recommendations for car seat use include using blanket rolls for support, observing while driving, and avoiding models with lap pads or shields.

Child care

Home care or small day-care programs are recommended.

Diet

Breast-feeding or iron-fortified formula is recommended.

Use of multivitamins should be encouraged for infants who weigh less than 2.5 kg or infants who have chronic illness or poor growth. Beginning at 2 months of age, infants should receive 2 mg of iron/kg/day.

Feeding problems such as oral hypersensitivity, and gastroesophageal reflux are common.

Discipline

Children should be assessed for vulnerable child syndrome.

Toileting

Toileting readiness is based on developmental age.

Increased muscle tone may impede toilet training.

Continued.

SUMMARY OF PRIMARY CARE NEEDS FOR THE PREMATURE OR LOW BIRTH WEIGHT INFANT — cont'd

Sleep

Children may have disorganized sleep patterns.

School issues

These children have an increased incidence of educational problems. Psychometric testing is indicated for poor school performance.

Sexuality

Standard developmental counseling is advised. There is an increased incidence of SGA and prematurity in offspring of women who where SGA at birth.

Special family concerns

Special family concerns include grief, attachment issues as a result of prolonged hospitalization, financial considerations, and concerns about developmental outcomes.

RESOURCES

Resources are available for families with premature infants. Many hospitals have parent support groups that work with the family during hospitalization and after discharge. Many ICNs have a follow-up clinic that employs an interdisciplinary team for ongoing evaluation of infants identified as high risk for physical and developmental problems.

Informational materials

Harrison H: *The premature baby book,* 1983, New York, St Martin's Press.

Jason J and Van der Meer A: *Parenting your premature baby,* 1989, New York, H Holt.

Lieberman A and Sheagren T: *The premie parents' handbook,* 1984, New York, EP Dutton.

Organizations

Parent care, Inc
National Headquarters
101½ S Union
Alexandria, VA 22314-3323
(703) 836-4678

Local parent-to-parent groups

REFERENCES

Allen M and Alexander G: Gross motor milestones in preterm infants: Correction for degree of prematurity, *Pediatrics* 116:955-959, 1990.

American Academy of Pediatrics: *Guidelines for perinatal care,* ed 2, Elk Grove Village, Ill, 1988, American Academy of Pediatrics.

American Speech-Language-Hearing Association: Guidelines for audiologic screening of newborn infants who are at-risk for hearing impairment, ASHA 31:89-92, 1989.

Arias F and Tomich P: Etiology and outcome of low birth weight and preterm infants, *Obstet Gynecol* 60:277-281, 1982.

Arvin A: Infectious disease issues in the care of the ICN graduate. In Ballard R, ed: *Pediatric care of the ICN graduate,* Philadelphia, 1988, WB Saunders, pp 216-225.

Avery GB: The mortality of drastic intervention in the ICN. In Avery GB, ed: *Neonatology,* Philadelphia, 1987, JB Lippincott, pp 9-12.

Ballard JL, Novak KK, and Driver M: A simplified score for assessment of fetal maturation of newly born infants, *J Pediatr* 95:769-774, 1979.

Bauchner H, Brown E, and Peskin J: Premature graduates of the newborn intensive care unit: A guide to followup, *Pediatr Clin North Am* 35:1207-1226, 1988.

Beale EF, Nelson RM, Bucciareci RL, et al: Intrahepatic cholestasis associated with parental nutrition in premature infants, *Pediatrics* 64:342-347, 1979.

Bernbaum JC, Daft A, Anolik R, et al: Response of preterm infants to diphtheria-tetanus-pertussis immunizations, *J Pediatr* 107:184-188, 1985.

Bernbaum JC, Friedman S, Hoffman-Williamson M, et al: Preterm infant care after hospital discharge, *Pediatr Rev* 10:195-206, 1989.

Bernbaum J and Hoffman-Williamson M: Following the NICU graduate, *Contemp Pediatr* 3:22-37, 1986.

Blondis T, Snow J, and Accardo P: Integration of soft signs in academically normal and academically at-risk children, *Pediatrics* 85(suppl):421-425, 1990.

Brandt I: Growth dynamics of low birth weight infants with emphasis on the perinatal period. In Falkner F and Tanner JM, eds: *Human Growth,* vol 2, *Postnatal growth,* New York, 1978, Plenum Press, pp 557-617.

Bull MJ, Bryson CQ, Schreiner RL, et al: Follow-up of infants after intensive care, *Perinatol Neonatol* 23-28, 1986.

Callenbach JC, Sheehan MB, Abramson SJ, et al: Etiologic factors in rickets of very low-birth-weight infants, *J Pediatr* 98:800-805, 1981.

Casey PH, Kraemer HC, Bernbaum J, et al: Growth patterns of low birth weight preterm infants: a longitudinal analysis of a large, varied sample, *J Pediatr* 117:298-307, 1990.

Centers for Disease Control: National infant mortality surveillance (NIMs), *MMWR* 38(SS-3):1-46, 1989.

Centers for Disease Control: Contribution of birth defects to infant mortality—United States 1986, *MMWR* 38:633-635, 1989.

Centers for Disease Control: Low birth weight—United States, 1975-1987, *MMWR* 39:148-151, 1990.

Children's Defense Fund: *S.O.S. America! A children's defense fund budget,* Washington, DC, 1990, Children's Fund.

Chow M, Durand B, Feldman M, et al: *Handbook of pediatric primary care,* ed 2, New York, 1984, John Wiley & Sons, pp 759-775.

Coates AL, Bergsteinsson H, Desmond K, et al: Long term pulmonary sequelae of premature birth with and without idiopathic respiratory distress syndrome, *J Pediatr* 90:611-616, 1977.

Cohen M and Taeusch HW: Primary care for the neonatal intensive care unit graduate. In Taeusch HW and Yogman MW, eds: *Follow-up management of the high-risk infant,* Boston, 1987, Little, Brown, p 70.

Committee on Infectious Disease: Report of the Committee on Infectious Disease, ed 22, Elk Grove Village, Ill, 1991, The American Academy of Pediatrics.

Committee on Nutrition: Nutritional needs of low-birth-weight infants, *Pediatrics* 75:976-986, 1985.

Constantine NA, Kraemer HC, Kendall-Tackett KA, et al: Use of physical and neurologic observations in assessment of gestational age in low birth weight infants, *J Pediatr* 110:921-928, 1987.

Corbet A, Bucciarelli R, Goldman S, et al: Decreased mortality rate among small premature infants treated at birth with a single dose of synthetic surfactant: a multicenter controlled trial, *J Pediatr* 118:277-84, 1991.

Dallman PR: Nutritional anemia of infancy: Iron, folic acid, and vitamin B12. In Tsang RC and Nichols BL, eds: *Nutrition during infancy,* Philadelphia, 1988, Hanley & Belfus, pp 216-235.

Day S: The eyes of the ICN graduate. In Ballard R, ed: *Pediatric care of the ICN graduate,* Philadelphia, 1988, WB Saunders, pp 121-126.

DeLorimier AA: Care of ICN graduates after neonatal surgery. In Ballard R, ed: *Pediatric care of the ICN graduate,* Philadelphia, 1988, WB Saunders, pp 187-195.

Desmond M, Wilson G, Alt E, et al: The very low birth infant after discharge from intensive care: Anticipatory health care and developmental course, *Curr Probl Pediatr* 10:1-59, 1980.

Dubowitz LMS: Neurologic assessment. In Ballard R, ed: *Pediatric care of the ICN graduate,* Philadelphia, 1988, WB Saunders, p 84.

Dubowitz LMS, Dubowitz V, Goldberg C: Clinical assessment of gestational age in the newborn, *J Pediatr* 77:1-10, 1970.

Elliman A, Bryan E, Elliman A, et al: Denver developmental screening test and preterm infants, *Arch Dis Child* 60:20-24, 1985.

Escalona S: Babies at double hazard: Early development of infants at biologic and social risk, *Pediatrics* 70:670-676, 1982.

Ferber R: *Solving your child's sleep problems,* New York, 1985, Simon & Schuster.

Gardner SL, and Hagedorn MI: Physiologic sequelae of prematurity: The nurse practitioner's role. Part II. Retinopathy of prematurity, *J Pediat Health Care* 4:72-76, 1990.

Gorski PA: Fostering family development after preterm hospitalization. In Ballard R, ed: *Pediatric care of the ICN graduate,* Philadelphia, 1988, WB Saunders, pp 27-32.

Green M and Solnit A: Reactions to the threatened loss of a child: A vulnerable child syndrome. *Pediatrics* 34:58-66, 1964.

Hack M and Fanaroff A: Growth patterns in the ICN graduate. In Ballard R, ed: *Pediatric care of the ICN graduate,* Philadelphia, WB Saunders, pp 33-39.

Hack M, Merkatz I, McGrath S, et al: Catch-up growth in very-low-birth weight infants, *Am J Dis Child* 138:370-375, 1984.

Hagedorn MI and Gardner SL: Physiologic sequelae of prematurity: The nurse practitioner's role. Part IV. Anemia, *J Pediat Health Care* 5:3-10, 1991.

Hawtrey C: Undescended testis and orchiopexy: Recent observations, *Pediatr Rev* 11:305-308, 1990.

Hirata T, Epcar JT, Walsh A, et al: Survival and outcome of infants 501 to 750 gm: A six-year experience, *J Pediatr* 102:741-748, 1983.

Hunt JV, Cooper BAB, and Tooley WH: Very low birth weight infants at 8 and 11 years of age: Role of neonatal illness and family status, *Pediatrics* 82:596-603, 1988.

Hunt JV, Tooley WH, and Harvin D: Learning disabilities in children with birth weight <1500 gms, *Semin Perinatol* 6:280-287, 1982.

Infant Health and Development Program: Enhancing the outcomes of low-birth-weight, premature infants, A multisite, randomized trial, *JAMA* 263:3035-3042, 1990.

International Committee for the Classification of the Late Stages of Retinopathy of Prematurity: An international classification of retinopathy of prematurity II. The classification of retinal detachment. *Arch Ophthalmol* 105:906-912, 1987.

Jason JM: Infectious disease-related deaths of low birth weights infants, United States, 1968 to 1982, *Pediatrics* 84:296-303, 1989.

Joint Committee on Infant Hearing (1991). 1990 Position statement, ASHA 33 (suppl 5), 3-6, 1991.

Kimble KJ, Ariagno RL, Stevenson DK, et al: Growth to age 3 years among very low-birth-weight sequelae-free survivors of modern neonatal intensive care, *J Pediatr,* 100:622-624, 1982.

Kitchen WH, Ford GW, Doyle LW, et al: Health and hospital readmissions of very-low-birth-weight and normal-birth-weight children, *Am J Dis Child* 144:213-218, 1990.

Klaus M, Fanaroff A, and Martin RJ: Respiratory problems. In Klaus M and Fanaroff A, eds: *Care of the high-risk neonate,* Philadelphia, 1986, WB Saunders, pp 171-178.

Klebanoff M, Meirik O, and Berendes H: Second generation consequences of small-for-dates birth, *Pediatrics* 84:343-347, 1989.

Klein N, Hack M, Gallagher J, et al: Preschool performance of children with normal intelligence who were very low-birth-weight infants, *Pediatrics* 75:531-537, 1985.

Kliegman RM and Fanaroff AA: Necrotizing enterocolitis, *N Engl J Med* 310:1093-1102, 1984.

Knobloch H, Malone A, Ellison P, et al: Considerations in evaluating changes in outcome for infants weighing less than 1501 gms, *Pediatrics* 69:285-295, 1982.

Koerper M: Anemia in the ICN graduate. In Ballard R, ed: *Pediatric care of the ICN graduate,* Philadelphia, 1988, WB Saunders, pp 46-47.

Krishnamoorthy KS, Kuban KCK, Leviton A, et al: Periventricular-intraventricular hemorrhage sonographic localization, phenobarbital, and motor abnormalities in low birth weight infants, *Pediatrics* 85:1027-1033, 1990.

McCormick MC, Gortmaker SL, and Sobol AM: Very low birth weight children: behavior problems and school difficulty in a national sample, *J Pediatr* 117:687-93, 1990.

McCormick MC: The contribution of low birth weight to infant mortality and childhood morbidity, *N Engl J Med* 312:82-90, 1985.

McCormick MC, Shapiro S, Starfield B: Rehospitalization in the first year of life for high-risk survivors, *Pediatrics* 66:991-999, 1980.

Medoff-Cooper B and Schraeder B: Developmental trends and behavioral styles in very low birth weight infants, *Nurs Res* 31:68-72, 1982.

Meier P and Anderson GC: Responses of small preterm infants to bottle- and breast-feeding, *Matern Child Nurs J* 12:97-105, 1987.

Multicenter Trial of Cryotherapy for Retinopathy of Prematurity:

Preliminary results: Cryotherapy for retinopathy of prematurity cooperative groups, *Arch Ophthalmol* 106:471-479, 1988.

Nickel R, Bennett F, and Larison F: School performance of children with birth weights of 1000 g or less, *Am J Dis Child* 136:105-110, 1982.

Papile LA, Munsick-Bruno G, and Lowe J: Grade III and IV periventricular, intraventricular hemorrhage (PIVH): Longitudinal neurodevelopment outcome, *Pediatr Res* 23:4 (part 2):453A, 1988.

Papile LA, Munsick-Bruno G, and Schaefer A: Relationship of cerebral intraventricular hemorrhage and early childhood neurologic handicaps, *J Pedatr* 103:273-277, 1983.

Peevy KJ, Speed FA, Hoff CJ: Epidemiology of inguinal hernia in preterm neonates, *Pediatrics* 77:246-247, 1986.

Peterson K and Frank D: Feeding and growth of premature and small-for-gestational age infants. In Taeusch HW and Yogman MW, eds: *Follow-up management of the high-risk infant,* Boston, 1987, Little, Brown, pp 187-204.

Piecuch R: Cosmetics, skin, scars, and residual traces of the ICN. In Ballard R, ed: *Pediatric care of the ICN graduate,* Philadelphia, 1988, WB Saunders, pp 50-56.

Porat R: Care of the infant with retinopathy of prematurity, *Clin Perinatol* 11:123-151, 1984.

Purohit DM, Ellison RC, Zierler S, et al: Risk factors for retrolental fibroplasia: Experience with 3,025 premature infants, *Pediatrics* 76:339-344, 1985.

Resnick MB, Eyler FD, Nelson RM, et al: Developmental intervention for low birth weight infants: Improved early developmental outcome, *Pediatrics* 80:68-74, 1987.

Ross G, Lipper EG, and Auld PAM: Growth achievement of very low birth weight premature children at school age, *J Pediatr* 117:307-309, 1990.

Sacher RA, Luban NLC, and Strauss RG: Current practice and guidelines for the transfusion of cellular blood components in the newborn, *Transfusion Med Rev* 3(1):39-54, 1989.

Sell E, Gaines J, Gluckman C, et al: Early identification of learning problems in neonatal intensive care graduates, *Am J Dis Child* 139:460-463, 1985.

Sheftel D, Hustead V, and Friedman A: Hypertension screening in the follow-up of premature infants, *Pediatrics* 71:763-766, 1983.

Vohr BR and Coll CTG: Neurodevelopmental and school performance of very-low-birth-weight infants: A seven-year longitudinal study, *Pediatrics* 76:345-350, 1985.

Volpe JJ: *Neurology of the newborn,* ed 2, Philadelphia, 1987, WB Saunders.

26 *Prenatal Cocaine Exposure*

Elizabeth A. Kuehne and *Marianne Warguska*

ETIOLOGY

The problem of substance abuse during pregnancy is a long-standing one within our society (Chasnoff, 1989b). However, it was not until 1973, when the term fetal alcohol syndrome was first used to describe a distinctive pattern of malformations in infants born to alcoholic mothers (Jones et al., 1973), that these problems began to receive attention from health care professionals and the general public.

Since this time the effects of alcohol, opiates, marijuana, and other noncocaine substances on the developing fetus have been studied and described extensively. A summary of these effects is shown in the box on p. 466. Over the past 10 years the patterns of use of these drugs have changed very little (Chasnoff, 1988), while cocaine has emerged as society's present drug of choice.

An estimated 22 million Americans have tried cocaine once, and 6 million are believed to use it on a regular basis (National Institute on Drug Abuse, 1990). With cocaine's rise in popularity among the general public has come a rise in use by women of childbearing age (Chasnoff et al., 1985). In New York City cocaine is now the illicit substance most frequently used by pregnant women (Lowe, 1989).

Cocaine can be administered in a variety of ways: intranasal snorting, intravenous (IV) injection, and smoking (Hawks and Chiang, 1986). Currently the most popular form of cocaine is "crack." Crack consists of alkaloid crystals of cocaine that are smoked in a water pipe. Crack became available in the mid-1980s, and its popularity shows no signs of diminishing.

Crack differs from cocaine hydrochloride (the preparation used intranasally) in three ways. First, because it is smoked and not sniffed, the "high" is reached within 10 seconds and lasts approximately 5 to 15 minutes. Second, crack is absorbed more effectively from the highly vascular surface of the lung, creating a more intense and powerful high. Third, crack is relatively inexpensive, costing roughly $5 to $10 per "rock" (Gold, 1987; Howard, 1989a). These factors and elimination of the need for IV injection are believed to contribute to crack's popularity among both young people and women of childbearing age.

Because of crack's dramatic effects on users, a few patterns of use have emerged. Many women use crack to abort an unwanted pregnancy, or they use it in the belief that it will ease their deliveries. Some women use crack to induce labor thinking that early delivery will prevent further fetal exposure to cocaine. In addition, many women addicted to crack turn to prostitution for themselves or their children to support their habit (Lowe, 1989). This situation has many grave social and public health implications, which include sexually transmitted diseases (STDs), congenital infections, unwanted pregnancy, and the abandonment and physical and sexual abuse of children.

Crack has become popular very quickly and

EFFECTS OF DRUG USE ON FETAL DEVELOPMENT

Cocaine

Cocaine causes placental and uterine vasoconstriction, resulting in fetal hypoxia. Associated problems include prematurity, low birth weight, hypertonicity, irritability, tremors, central nervous system (CNS) abnormalities, neurodevelopmental problems, and congenital anomalies.

Heroin

Newborns undergo a true withdrawal syndrome that includes irritability, tremors, hypertonicity, and fever. Infants have an increased risk of sudden infant death syndrome (SIDS) and are vulnerable to many neonatal infections, including human immunodeficiency virus (HIV).

Alcohol

Infants undergoing withdrawal from alcohol may have tremors, irritability, hypertonicity, muscle twitching, and restlessness. The term fetal alcohol syndrome is used to describe a similar pattern of malformations noted in the offspring of alcohol-abusing women. Features of this syndrome include intrauterine growth retardation, slow postnatal growth, microcephaly, mental retardation, and craniofacial abnormalities.

Marijuana

Infants may have tremors, altered visual responses, low birth weight, growth retardation, and neurobehavioral abnormalities. Severity of symptoms is probably related to the quantity of drug used by the mother.

Barbiturates

Severe and prolonged withdrawal syndrome may occur. Symptoms include hyperactivity, restlessness, excessive crying, and hyperreflexia. Sudden withdrawal by the mother or infant can result in seizures.

Tobacco

Smoking in pregnancy is associated with spontaneous abortion, low birth weight, prematurity, and increased perinatal mortality.

---

additional types of illicit drugs can be anticipated in the future. New forms of amphetamines and heroin are two such possibilities. A smokable form of methamphetamine known as "ice" is becoming popular in Hawaii and on the West Coast. The effects of "ice" are reported to last 24 to 48 hours, and in certain areas the cost is cheaper than that of crack. The IV use of heroin has increased recently among crack users seeking to come down from the intense high of the crack. In addition, a smokable heroin-crack combination known as "crank" or "speedball" has become popular among women and teenagers who are often reluctant to use needles to inject heroin (Elvik, 1990; Falco, 1989). Little is known about the long-term effects of these drugs; however, the potential adverse health implications for women and infants are alarming.

INCIDENCE

According to a survey by the National Association for Perinatal Addiction Research and Education (NAPARE), an estimated 375,000 newborns are affected by drugs each year, with the rates varying from 0.4% to 27% (Chasnoff, 1989a). Similarly, the percentages of drug-exposed infants ranged from 2% to 18% in a recent U.S. House of Representatives subcommittee national survey of 18 hospitals (Miller, 1989). Variations in these studies were attributed primarily to the thoroughness of the substance abuse assessment at each hospital and secondarily to regional variations in drug use.

The NAPARE study revealed that 11% of the women delivering infants had used illegal drugs during their pregnancies. In other prevalence reports, evidence of cocaine use was found in 8% of women giving birth at a Chicago hospital (Neerhof et al., 1989) and 17% of women in a prenatal care program in Boston (Frank et al., 1988). A Rhode Island survey detected illicit drug use in 7.5% of women sampled, with cocaine found in 2.6% of that group (Hollinshead et al., 1990).

The study conducted in Rhode Island (Hollinshead et al., 1990) showed that cocaine was detected more often in women who were nonwhite, were classified as living in poverty, used public health insurance, and delivered in a regional perinatal center. In contrast, Chasnoff (1989c) reported the overall prevalence of illicit drug use by pregnant women in Pinellas County, Florida to be 14.8%, with a rate of 16.3% among women using public clinics and a rate of 13.1% for women in the private health care sector. Moreover, he found similar percentages of positive toxicologic results among black women and white women (14.1% versus 15.4%).

It is prudent to address illicit drug use with all pregnant women. Drug use is often denied by users. Accordingly, the clinician can expect an underestimation of drug use when relying entirely on maternal self-report (Frank et al., 1988). Other maternal factors that may assist the clinician in identifying children who have been exposed to cocaine in utero are history of drug use, previous birth of a drug-exposed infant, STD, signs of intoxication, lack of prenatal care, physical indications of drug use, and suspicious or erratic behavior.

Screening for cocaine and its metabolites can be performed using a variety of methods. Thin layer chromatography is the least sensitive method and has the possibility of producing false-negative results. Techniques such as the enzyme immunoassay (EIA) or the radioimmunoassay (RIA) are widely used and can detect benzoylecgonine (a cocaine metabolite) for 24 to 48 hours after use. Gas chromatography/mass spectroscopy provide the most specific and unchallengable information; they are also the most expensive (Hawks and Chiang, 1986; Udell, 1989).

Since urine toxicologic screening of newborns is feasible only during the immediate postpartum period, primary care practitioners will find its usefulness limited. For those clinicians working in the newborn nursery, toxicologic screening must be performed within institutional policy and protocol. Because of the rapid metabolism and excretion of cocaine, it is important to remember that a negative urine toxicologic result is in no way conclusive evidence of lack of prenatal exposure. Neonatal hair and nail sample tests for identification of long-term drug use by the mother are being tested.

CLINICAL MANIFESTATIONS AT TIME OF DIAGNOSIS
Pharmacology and physiologic effects of cocaine

Cocaine is benzoylmethylecgonine, a local anesthetic and CNS stimulant prepared from the extract of the leaves of the coca plant *(Erythroxylon coca)*

(Ritchie and Greene, 1980). It readily crosses from maternal to fetal circulation, and because of metabolic differences, it may remain in the fetal system long after it has been excreted by the mother. It is absorbed from all sites of application and is metabolized by liver and plasma cholinesterases into two major metabolites that are excreted in the urine: benzoylecgonine and ecgoine methyl ester (Hawks and Chiang, 1986; Kennedy and Haddox, 1986; Ritchie and Greene, 1980). Cocaine metabolites are detectable in the urine of adults for 48 to 72 hours and, because of liver immaturity and lower cholinesterase activity, may be detectable in newborns for up to 2 weeks (Hawks and Chiang, 1986; Jones, 1984; Udell, 1989).

Another metabolite, norcocaine, has been identified in humans and is believed to be biologically active (Jones, 1984). Norcocaine is water soluble with a high level of CNS penetration. Because of these characteristics, norcocaine does not easily reenter the maternal circulation, and theoretically the fetus may continue to be exposed to this metabolite by ingestion of the amniotic fluid (Chasnoff and Lewis, 1988).

Cocaine is a CNS stimulant that can cause feelings of well-being, euphoria, restlessness, and excitement. Overdosage can lead to convulsions, CNS depression, and respiratory failure (Kennedy and Haddox, 1986; Ritchie and Greene, 1980).

Cocaine inhibits the reuptake of neurotransmitters at the adrenergic nerve terminals, producing increased levels of norepinephrine and dopamine. These elevated levels of catecholamines result in increased blood pressure, tachycardia, and vasoconstriction. Cocaine also causes elevations in body temperature. Large doses are directly toxic to the myocardium and may result in cardiac failure (Kennedy and Haddox, 1986; Ritchie and Greene, 1980).

Prenatal effects of cocaine

Because cocaine readily crosses the placenta, its physiologic effects, such as CNS stimulation, vasoconstriction, tachycardia, and blood pressure elevations, are believed to occur in both the mother and the fetus. In animal studies the fetal complications of cocaine use have included cardiovascular changes and changes in fetal oxygenation resulting from reduced uterine blood flow and impaired oxygen transfer (Woods, Plessinger, and Clark, 1987).

Prenatal manifestations of maternal cocaine use are abruptio placenta, fetal death, spontaneous abortion, preterm labor, precipitous labor, fetal distress, meconium staining, and in utero cerebrovascular accidents (Bingol et al., 1987; Chasnoff, Burns, and Burns, 1987; Chasnoff et al., 1986; Chasnoff, MacGregor, and Chisum, 1988; Hadeed and Siegel, 1989; MacGregor et al., 1987; Ryan, Ehrlich, and Finnegan, 1987).

Manifestations at birth

Abundant literature describes the manifestations of intrauterine cocaine exposure exhibited at birth, including (1) prematurity, intrauterine growth retardation, microcephaly, and low birth weight*; (2) CNS abnormalities such as irritability, tremors, seizures, electroencephalogram (EEG) abnormalities, hypertonicity, and cerebral infarct (Chasnoff et al., 1986; Chasnoff, MacGregor, and Chisum, 1988; Doberczak et al., 1988); (3) irregular sleep patterns (Newald, 1986); (4) poor suck swallow response (Udell, 1989); (5) poor feeding (Newald, 1986); and (6) dilated iris vasculature (Isenberg, Spierer, and Inkelis, 1987).

Controversy exists over whether the adverse effects manifested in cocaine-exposed infants actually are indicative of a true withdrawal syndrome as seen with infants exposed to narcotics or are representative of another phenomenon. Some believe that these signs of cocaine exposure represent either CNS hyperexcitability due to the direct effects of cocaine or indications of permanent CNS damage. The answer to this question is unknown at this time.

TREATMENT

Infants who have been exposed to cocaine in utero can be identified based on maternal history, urine toxicologic screening, and clinical presentation.

Although pharmacologic therapy, including the use of phenobarbital, paragoric, and diazepam, has been advocated for narcotic withdrawal (Besunder

and Blumer, 1990), most infants who have been prenatally exposed to cocaine do not require such therapy. Pacification techniques such as swaddling and decreasing environmental stimuli are used in the nursery to treat the symptoms of irritability and tremors found with cocaine exposure.

Details of discharge planning for infants with prenatal exposure to cocaine will depend on who their caretakers will be after discharge. Planning for discharge is generally done in conjunction with hospital social service staff and in some cases child protective workers. Once the caretaker has been identified, he or she must be provided with routine discharge information, as well as information regarding behavioral patterns to expect and pacification techniques. A referral to or consultation with a primary care provider who is familiar with drug addiction and its associated problems is also important. These infants should be seen often, perhaps monthly, by the same provider.

PROGNOSIS

Conclusive information regarding the prognosis for children with prenatal exposure to cocaine is unavailable at this time. Birth certificate data collected between 1985 and 1987 in New York City show the mortality rate for infants exposed to cocaine in utero to be 35.4 per 1,000 compared with a citywide infant mortality rate of 13.1 per 1,000. Factors contributing to this increased rate were low birth weight, sudden infant death syndrome (SIDS), and acquired immune deficiency syndrome (AIDS) (Lowe, 1989). Currently no data are available to describe the long-term prognosis for children exposed to cocaine in utero. Further studies are needed to clarify issues surrounding the prognosis for these children.

ASSOCIATED PROBLEMS
Prematurity

Infants exposed to cocaine in utero are often born prematurely and consequently require appropriate neonatal intervention and long-term follow-up (see Chapter 25).

Congenital infections and infectious diseases

The general use of illicit drugs has become increasingly associated with infectious diseases, STDs (Centers for Disease Control, 1988;

---

*Bingol et al (1987), Cherukuri et al (1988), Chouteau, Namerow, and Leppert (1988), Fulroth, Phillips, and Durand (1989), Hadeed and Siegel (1989), Kaye et al (1989), and Zuckerman et al (1989).

Chasnoff, 1987; Lowe, 1989), and AIDS (Schoenbaum et al., 1989). Accordingly, the offspring of women using drugs can be expected to have increased rates of congenitally acquired infections.

In New York City the incidence of female primary and secondary syphilis rose 204% between 1986 and 1988 (Lowe, 1989). As would be expected, a concomitant rise in congenital syphilis has been reported. At the Children's Aid Society, among the cocaine-exposed infants entering foster care, 25% have congenital syphilis.

Many crack users will exchange sex for drugs; this frequent sexual activity with multiple partners is believed to be responsible for the recent explosion in the number of syphilis cases. This pattern of behavior also places the mother and the infant at increased risk for HIV infection. Many users of crack also inject cocaine or may use heroin to bring themselves down from periods of prolonged cocaine use, thus increasing their risk of HIV infection from contaminated needles.

In addition to syphilis and HIV infection, the practitioner must consider infectious diseases such as hepatitis B, tuberculosis, and TORCH (toxoplasmosis, rubella, cytomegalovirus, herpes) infections, as well as other STDs such as gonorrhea and chlamydia, when assessing the health status of an infant or child of a cocaine-abusing mother.

Growth patterns

Growth retardation in cocaine-exposed infants has been well documented and is believed to be related to chronic uterine and placental hypoxia secondary to cocaine-induced vasoconstriction. Poor maternal nutrition is probably also a factor, especially in light of the anorectic effects of cocaine.

Microcephaly

A particularly worrisome finding of prenatal cocaine exposure is that of microcephaly. Currently the causes for this manifestation remain speculative. The clinician must recognize that children with microcephaly may be at risk for serious long-term problems such as cerebral palsy, mental retardation, and learning deficits (Udell, 1989).

Congenital malformations

Cocaine may be a teratogen. Bingol and associates (1987) found the malformation rate among infants of cocaine users to be significantly higher than the rate among a control group not using drugs. Malformations included congenital heart disease and skull defects. An increased rate of genitourinary tract malformations among infants exposed to cocaine in utero has been reported (Chasnoff, Chisum, and Kaplan, 1988; Chavez, Mulinare, and Cordero, 1989). Malformations reported included prune belly syndrome, hypospadias, hydronephrosis, and female pseudohermaphrodism. Hoyme and co-workers (1990) described cocaine-exposed infants with limb reduction defects, cardiac anomalies, and intestinal atresia. It is thought that vascular compromise or fetal hypoxia resulting from cocaine-induced vasoconstriction may be responsible for the apparently increased rate of congenital malformations in these infants (Bingol et al., 1987; Hoyme et al., 1990).

Sudden infant death syndrome

At this juncture it is not clear whether infants exposed to cocaine prenatally are at an increased risk for SIDS. Chasnoff and colleagues (1989) described a retrospective review of 66 cocaine-exposed infants. They discovered 10 deaths which were attributed to SIDS, for an overall incidence of 15%. This incidence is significantly greater than that among the general population and greater than the risk previously described for narcotic-exposed infants. A subsequent prospective study by the same authors revealed no deaths from SIDS (Chasnoff, et al., 1989). Bauchner and associates (1988) studied 175 infants exposed to cocaine in utero and also found no deaths as a result of SIDS.

Neurologic and developmental effects

The effects of intrauterine cocaine exposure on the developing CNS that have been reported include seizures, perinatal cerebral infarction, and EEG abnormalities. Numerous neurodevelopmental abnormalities described include irritability, tremulousness, and hypertonicity. In addition, these infants demonstrate depressed interactive abilities and poor state control when compared with drug-free infants of the same ages (Chasnoff et al., 1985; Schneider, Griffith, and Chasnoff, 1989). Four common behavioral patterns have been described in cocaine-exposed infants: (1) a deep sleep state, (2) an agitated sleep state, (3) vacillating extremes of state during handling, and (4) a panicked awake state (Schneider, Griffith, and Chasnoff, 1989). These unusual patterns of behavior, combined with inconsolability and irritability, may interfere with appropriate care giver–infant interactions, potentially hindering the process of bonding and attachment.

Motor behavior in these infants is characterized by an increase in extensor tone, which interferes with children's ability to explore the environment and their own bodies. When supine, these children will often lie in an extended posture, and when held upright, they will stiffen and extend their ankles, knees, and hips, resulting in a weight-bearing position on their toes. These children have difficulty bringing their arms to midline and are poorly coordinated. Children with truncal hypertonicity often have difficulty with balance and may not be able to sit. These motor findings are mild or transient in some children and persistent in others, making general predictions of long-term outcome difficult.

In one study (Howard et al., 1989) the intellectual functioning, quality of play, and security of attachment to parent or parent figure of 18-month-old drug-exposed children were compared with those of a matched control group. The investigators found the drug-exposed toddlers to have significantly lower developmental scores, to engage in significantly less representational play, with play efforts being sparse and disorganized, and to be unable to show strong feelings of pleasure, anger, or distress. The authors express concern over the emotional, social, and cognitive toll that prenatal drug exposure may take on children in addition to the physical problems that have already been noted.

Van Baar, Fleury, and Ultee (1989) studied two groups of infants of drug-dependent mothers and a contrast group of 37 infants of drug-free mothers. They concluded that at 12 months of age there were no significant differences between groups on the Bayley Infant Scales of Development. Bauman and Dougherty (1983) studied preschoolers of mothers on methadone maintenance and mothers who were not drug addicted. They found that mothers on methadone maintenance were less adaptive on measures of parenting behavior and that their children performed poorly on measures of intelligence, development, and socially adaptive behavior. Similar

studies with cocaine-exposed infants are needed.

At this juncture, it can only be speculated as to what the long-term neurodevelopmental outcome of these children may be. More information will be needed to completely describe the cognitive, interactive, and motor abilities of children exposed to cocaine in utero.

Feeding difficulties

Feeding difficulties and gastrointestinal (GI) symptoms such as poor suck-swallow response, vomiting, diarrhea, and constipation have been reported among infants exposed to cocaine in utero (Newald, 1986; Udell, 1989). From our experience at the Children's Aid Society, we have noted another feeding characteristic of these children—a voracious appetite. Caretakers will report that an infant will take a full feeding every 2 hours around the clock. The infants are unable to be consoled by anything other than food; they seem genuinely hungry.

Postnatal exposure to cocaine

Children of cocaine-using parents can potentially be exposed to cocaine after birth as well as before. Cocaine and its metabolites are detectable in breast milk, and infants can be exposed to large doses of cocaine by breast-feeding. Irritability, tremulousness, and other signs of CNS stimulation are seen in infants who ingest cocaine via breast milk (Chasnoff, Douglas, and Squires, 1987).

In addition, children who have been passively exposed to the smoke of crack have manifested such neurologic symptoms as seizures, drowsiness, and unsteady gait (Bateman and Heagarty, 1989). The possibilities for later cocaine exposure via breast-feeding, passive inhalation, and accidental ingestion should be considered when one is caring for the children of drug-using parents.

Parenting issues

Parents dealing with their own addiction may have multiple medical and social problems that interfere with their ability to care for their children. They themselves may have been children of substance-abusing parents (Howard, 1989b). These parents, often single, may have had few positive parenting experiences in their own lives. If interventions such as preventive social service supports prove to be inadequate, the courts may move to terminate parental rights so that a permanency plan can be made for the young child. Many of these infants are at risk for double jeopardy—biologic vulnerability from intrauterine drug exposure exacerbated by inadequate parenting (Parker, Greer, and Zuckerman, 1988; Weston et al., 1989).

PRIMARY CARE MANAGEMENT
Growth and development

It is imperative that the primary care provider closely monitor the physical growth of these infants and young children. Monthly evaluations are prudent in the infancy period. Accurate measurements for weight, length, and head circumference require using the same scale and measuring tools at each visit. It is especially important that head size be measured accurately because of the high incidence of microcephaly. Data should be plotted on a standard National Center for Health Statistics growth chart. Data of infants with a history of prematurity should be plotted using the corrected age.

To date no long-term studies report on the growth of infants exposed prenatally to cocaine. It is known that in general infants who are small for gestational age (SGA) remain small. However, it has been reported that head size of preschoolers who have heroin-addicted, methadone-treated mothers did not differ significantly from that of children who have drug-free mothers. Head size at birth was related to maternal nutritional status and birth weight (Lifschitz et al., 1985).

Developmental assessment of an infant exposed to cocaine poses a challenge to the primary care provider. Routine office screening tools such as the Denver Developmental Screening Test may or may not be helpful. Their validity will depend on the stability of the infant's state control during testing. In addition, these infants may exhibit problems with motor development.

It is useful to assess the infant's development at monthly intervals during the first 6 months of life and every 2 months during the second 6 months of life. Frequent assessments by the same provider offer valuable information about the child's developmental progress. Early referrals for a more detailed assessment by a developmental psychologist may also prove useful.

For some infants simultaneous visual and voice stimuli may prove to be too stressful and may interfere with parent-infant interaction. Without appropriate guidance, bonding and attachment may be seriously jeopardized. Parents should be advised to make full use of the infant's quiet and alert states. They also need to know that the attainment of developmental milestones can be unpredictable and is generally slower in these fragile infants.

When the cocaine-exposed infant is evaluated, a complete physical assessment is essential. Abnormal neurologic findings are common in these young children. The examiner should observe for irritability, tremors, extended postures, limb stiffness, hyperreflexia, clonus, persistence of primitive reflexes, subtle signs of infantile spasms, jerky eye movements, the inability to track visually, and the inability to respond to sound.

A neurologic consultation is necessary if seizures or other withdrawal symptoms such as persistent hypertonicity, irritability, or disturbance in the sleep-wake state are noted in the newborn period. Moreover, early assessment and intervention by a neurodevelopmentally trained physical therapist can provide the parent with helpful advice about handling and positioning "stiff" infants.

Immunizations

No reports have yet been published with regard to immunizing children who have been exposed to cocaine prenatally. Until such recommendations are available, the practitioner must assess each child's health status, social situation, and immunization needs on an individual basis. In general the recommendations published by the American Academy of Pediatrics (AAP) should be followed.

Oral polio virus vaccine. Children born with prenatal drug exposure are at an increased risk for congenital HIV infection, and the AAP guidelines should be followed with regard to the administration of the live oral polio vaccine. In a child whose HIV status is seronegative or unknown but who is living with an immunocompromised caretaker, the inactivated polio virus (IPV) is recommended (Committee on Infectious Diseases, 1991). If there is any question as to the immune status of the parent, the IPV is the prudent choice.

Measles. For children living in areas where measles epidemics are likely to occur, such as large urban areas or areas with high concentrations of unimmunized children, it may be prudent to give the measles, mumps, and rubella vaccine at 12 months of age and again before entry to school. Immunogenicity among children immunized at the earlier age has been shown to be adequate (Committee on Infectious Diseases, 1991).

Pertussis. Children who have been exposed to cocaine in utero often show CNS manifestations of this exposure, and a small number of these children may have seizures. Infants and children with a history of seizures have an increased risk of seizures after receipt of pertussis-containing vaccines (Committee on Infectious Diseases, 1991). Because seizure activity in cocaine-exposed infants is limited generally to the early neonatal period, it is recommended that the pertussis component of the diphtheria, pertussis, tetanus vaccine be given to all of these infants except those who have persistent seizures. Consultation with the child's neurologist is recommended for those cocaine-exposed children whose neurologic status is not yet clearly understood.

Haemophilus influenzae type b conjugate vaccines. *Haemophilus influenzae* type b conjugate vaccine, 3 dose series, should be initiated at 2 months of age as recommended by the Immunization Practices Advisory Committee (1991).

Hepatitis. Hepatitis B infection is a problem common among cocaine-using parents (Chasnoff, 1988). Generally mothers are tested during the prenatal or immediate postpartum period, and in infants needing vaccination the series is started during the neonatal period. The primary care practitioner should be prepared to follow up with hepatitis vaccine according to the AAP guidelines.

Unfortunately a child's health care maintenance may not be a high priority for a drug-using parent. Every effort should be made to encourage the parent to keep the child's immunizations up to date and to keep the immunization record intact and in a safe place. The clinician may choose to administer several immunizations when the child is seen for health care because there may be no guarantee of compliance with follow-up visits. The AAP guidelines should be followed in doing this.

Screening

Vision. Routine screening is recommended.

Hearing. Routine screening is recommended unless there is a speech delay, in which case a complete audiologic evaluation is warranted.

Dental. Routine screening is recommended.

Blood pressure. Routine screening is recommended.

Hematocrit. Routine screening is recommended.

Urinalysis. Routine screening is recommended after it has been ascertained that no urinary tract abnormalities exist. An IV pyelogram, renal ultrasonogram, or a voiding cystourethrogram to evaluate the urologic system may initially be ordered by the consulting urologist.

Tuberculosis. There is a higher incidence of tuberculosis among the drug-using population, especially if the users are HIV infected. Yearly screening with purified protein derivative (PPD), 0.1 ml intradermally, is recommended beginning at age 12 months.

Condition-specific screening

TOXICOLOGY SCREENS. If a mother is a suspected substance abuser or has not received prenatal care, the newborn's urine is screened for drugs using one of the laboratory methods previously described.

INFECTIONS. Because substance abusers are also at high risk for contracting infectious diseases, obtaining TORCH titers to rule out congenital infections such as cytomegalovirus and a syphilis serologic test to rule out congenital syphilis may be prudent (Hurt, 1989).

CARDIAC ABNORMALITIES. The cardiologist may recommend an electrocardiogram (ECG) and echocardiogram (ECHO) to evaluate for heart disease.

NEUROLOGIC ABNORMALITIES. The neurologist may recommend any of the following studies: brainstem auditory evoked response (BAER), magnetic resonance imaging (MRI), EEG, and skull X-ray studies to evaluate the nervous system.

Drug interactions

If a child is taking anticonvulsants for seizure activity, the same precautions as outlined in Chapter 15 should be followed.

DIFFERENTIAL DIAGNOSIS AND MANAGEMENT OF COMMON PEDIATRIC CONDITIONS
Infections

During the first 3 months of life it is often difficult to diagnose illness because of the subtle signs and symptoms the newborn exhibits when ill. A change in behavior is often a key factor in the assessment of the child. This complicates diagnosing illness in infants exposed to cocaine in utero because of the great variability in their sleep-wake state control. The primary care provider should carefully assess the irritable or deeply sleeping infant for signs of concomitant illness.

Parents should be taught how to take temperatures. They should be encouraged to call the pediatric office or clinic with any concerns. Frequent telephone contact will help the parent manage the child at home. If the parent is a poor historian or seems overly concerned on the telephone, the child should be seen in the office or the clinic.

The practitioner needs to be aware of the increased risk of HIV infection in this population. Accordingly, frequent infections may warrant an immunologic consultation.

Gastrointestinal symptoms

Gastrointestinal symptoms such as poor feeding, vomiting, diarrhea, or constipation are common in the first 6 to 9 months of life (Lewis, Bennett, and Schmeder, 1989). Parents should be advised to report any GI symptoms to their primary care provider. Once serious illness is ruled out, routine advice for handling these problems is helpful. The diarrhea described by most parents consists of loose stools with a water ring; dietary changes usually help to control the consistency of the stool. Small frequent feedings are usually well tolerated. For relief of constipation, 1 tablespoon of white corn syrup (Karo Syrup) in 4 ounces of formula for the young infant and prune juice for the older infant may be recommended.

Neurologic symptoms

As mentioned earlier, seizures may occur in the neonatal period. Parents need to be advised about injury prevention when the child is having a seizure and the importance of having the child evaluated by the provider immediately (see Chapter 15).

Child abuse

These potentially difficult children are at increased risk for child abuse. The practitioner should be alert to this possibility and thoroughly examine the skin for marks or bruises. Parents who did not have appropriate parenting role models may have difficulty knowing how to care for themselves and may have no understanding of how to care for an irritable infant.

Parental drug use

The practitioner should also keep in mind that a parent who is high may not follow directions appropriately. Therefore, any potentially serious condition warrants an office visit, and children who are ill may need to be hospitalized or placed in temporary foster care to assure appropriate medical management.

DEVELOPMENTAL ISSUES
Safety

Because the chronic use of mind-altering drugs by the parent can interfere with memory, attention, and perception, safety of the child is a major concern for the provider (Howard et al., 1989). Home visits by health or social service professionals will help provide assessment of the home situation and limited parental supervision for these vulnerable children.

Often the primary interest of parents who are addicted, especially those using crack, is the drug, not their children. When they are high, they may be completely unaware of their child's presence. In addition, the children may be living in unstable, dangerous environments with parents who are unable to function as protectors. Because of this, it is important to keep the child visible in the community. Social service case workers can recommend infant stimulation programs, day-care programs, and after-school and weekend recreational programs that are appropriate for these children and that will allow community workers to assess the child's health and emotional status on a regular basis.

Substance-abusing parents should also be warned about the danger of passive inhalation or accidental ingestion of the drugs by their children.

Child care

Working parents often place children in day-care and preschool nursery programs; however, drug-exposed children may have trouble adjusting in these settings. Although conclusive studies are not available, reports in the literature suggest that behavior problems may persist into the preschool years. Kantrowitz and associates (1990) reported that these children have difficulty playing and even talking with their peers. In a comparison of two groups of toddlers who came from single-parent homes with similar ethnicity and socioeconomic status, Howard and colleagues (1989) found that drug-exposed children, whether securely attached or not, were more sparse and disorganized in their play.

These reports suggest that therapeutic settings would be more appropriate than preschool nurseries for many of these children. Unfortunately, few such programs are available, especially for the poor. It is important that the primary care provider assist the parent in identifying appropriate programs within the community. Public Law 99-457, which provides for early identification of developmental disabilities and comprehensive family-focused preventive intervention, may be useful in those states where it has been implemented.

Diet

As mentioned earlier, breast-feeding is not recommended for women using cocaine because the metabolites remain in the breast milk 12 to 60 hours after the last use (Hurt, 1989).

Because cocaine-exposed infants often have low birth weights, careful monitoring of caloric intake and feeding behavior is required. In addition, care takers may tend to overfeed the irritable infant. These infants tend to have poor coordination of sucking and swallowing reflexes, tongue thrusting, and tongue tremors, as well as general oral hypersensitivity (Lewis et al., 1989; Schneider et al., 1989).

Parents need continued support in introducing solid foods because the tongue thrust and oral hypersensitivity may persist beyond 6 months. Forced feeding is not appropriate and should be avoided. The practitioner should encourage the parent to give food and fluids that are tolerated well.

Proper positioning and handling are essential for satisfactory feeding. A gentle, calm approach with a soothing voice while maintaining the infant in a relaxed, flexed posture will assist with feeding. If vomiting or spitting up occurs after feeding, frequent feedings of small amounts may be better tolerated. A side-lying swaddled or prone position after feeding is recommended.

Discipline

Behavior in these infants and young children may be characterized by irritability, excessive crying, and hyperactivity. The practitioner can suggest techniques for pacifying these children such as swaddling, offering pacifiers, and decreasing environmental distractions. Older children, especially slow learners, require patient limit setting, and discipline must be developmentally appropriate. To date, few resources exist with expertise in managing these children's difficult behaviors. The primary care provider will need to assess mental health and developmental services in their home communities for appropriate referrals.

Toileting

Persistent motor delays, hyperactivity, and behavioral problems may cause difficulty with toilet training. Parents need a great deal of patience and support for their efforts with the child. Early counseling with the parents may help to avoid potential difficulties.

Children with persistent enuresis may require urologic evaluation because of the increased incidence of urinary tract anomalies found in cocaine-exposed children.

Sleep patterns

Because of these infants' variable sleep-wake control state patterns, establishing regular sleeping patterns is difficult. Techniques that assist parents with sleep problems include swaddling, slow rhythmic rocking, offering a pacifier, and holding the infant in a relaxed, flexed position. In addition, keeping the lights low and reducing noise in the environment are helpful. Fortunately, few sleep problems are reported after the first year.

School issues

Children who experience drug exposure during the neonatal period are at high risk for learning problems. It is prudent to make early referrals into a Head Start or preschool nursery program to give these children every opportunity to succeed.

If the child remains small on entering school, the child may feel unaccepted by peers, and this may contribute to poor self-esteem. Parents should be encouraged to assist the child in recognizing his or her strengths. In addition, these parents may benefit from programs that help them to increase their own self-esteem.

The long-term educational needs of these children have not been determined. Any child performing below grade level should be evaluated for learning disabilities, and a specialized educational program should be developed to meet their needs.

Sexuality

Besides giving routine advice to adolescents, the practitioner must be aware of the potential for desperate drug users to prostitute their children for drugs. In addition, there is the added risk of sexual abuse in these highly dysfunctional families. The practitioner should be alert to any physical or psychologic indications of sexual abuse and, if suspected, report the situation to the appropriate authorities.

SPECIAL FAMILY CONCERNS

The family court system may deem parents "unfit." In some areas, a neonatal drug screen test result that is positive for illicit drugs triggers a report to the Child Welfare Bureau as evidence of neglect. This situation forces relatives, often elderly grandparents, to assume full responsibility for these drug-addicted infants and their siblings while the parents seek treatment in the limited number of available programs that were surveyed. Few drug treatment programs will accept pregnant addicts. A recent survey of 78 programs in New York City showed that 87% had no services available for pregnant addicts using Medicaid; of the programs that were surveyed, only two had provisions for the care of children (Chavkin, 1989).

Before being placed in either a kinship or temporary foster home, these infants may stay in the hospital for 60 to 90 days as boarder infants or may be moved to a congregate care facility. In other cases children are moved quickly to preadoptive homes. There is now a growing movement among health and social service professionals to have family assessments made early to improve the potential for family recovery.

Foster and kinship foster parents need respite. The social service agency responsible for the child should be contacted. In addition, foster parents need ongoing positive reinforcement. As practitioners, we must empower them with the strength and resources to cope with these needy children. Professionals also need to examine their own feelings of attachment to the children of substance-abusing parents. It may be difficult to maintain empathy and concern for these parents without becoming judgmental. As Weston and associates (1989) have noted, "Stereotypes can blind us to the unique characteristics that both infants and mothers bring to their relationship, despite the impact of drugs."

Substance-abusing parents who continue to use illicit drugs must be warned about the possibility of losing custody of their children if they fail to adequately care for them or if they endanger them in any way.

Despite careful counseling by health care professionals, adoptive parents will often have expectations about the infant or child that they accept into their home. Since long-term outcomes are unknown in the cocaine-exposed population, adoptive parents must be advised accordingly. Many of these infants who have had a difficult first few months look "normal" to adoptive parents who so eagerly want a child. It is important to follow the child's progress with the adoptive parents while remaining objective and realistic about the outcome.

SUMMARY OF PRIMARY CARE NEEDS FOR THE CHILD WITH PRENATAL COCAINE EXPOSURE

Growth and development

Growth parameters, particularly weight and head circumference, should be monitored monthly for the first 6 months and every 2 months for the next 6 months.

Attainment of developmental milestones is unpredictable and generally slower than normal.

Motor problems are common.

Immunizations

Routine immunizations are recommended.

If the child tests HIV seropositive, the guidelines in Chapter 23 should be followed.

Infants with limited history of seizures in the neonatal period can receive the pertussis vaccine. Infants with persistent seizures require consultation with a pediatric neurologist.

Hepatitis B vaccine is given if the mother is infected.

Drug-using parents may not be compliant with well child care visits; the clinician may choose to give several immunizations at one visit.

Screening
Vision

Routine screening is recommended.

Hearing

Routine office screening is recommended unless there is a speech delay, in which case a complete audiologic evaluation is warranted.

Dental

Routine screening is recommended.

Blood pressure

Routine screening is recommended.

Hematocrit

Routine screening is recommended.

Urinalysis

Routine screening is recommended. The high incidence of urologic abnormalities in these children may require referral to a urologist for testing.

Tuberculosis

Yearly screening with PPD beginning at 12 months is recommended.

Condition-specific screening
   Toxicology

Urine toxicologic screening should be done if the mother is a suspected substance abuser or did not receive prenatal care.
   Infections

Syphilis serologic testing and TORCH titers should be considered.
   Cardiac screening

Both ECG and ECHO may be obtained if a heart murmur is detected.
   Neurologic screening

If neurologic problems are suspected, BAER, MRI, EEG and skull films may be obtained.

Drug interactions

No routine medications are prescribed. If the child is taking seizure medication, see Chapter 15.

Differential diagnosis
Infections

The irritable or deeply sleeping infant should be carefully assessed.

Parents should be taught to take temperatures.

An office visit should be scheduled if any questions exist about the child's condition.

These children are at high risk for contracting congenital infections, including HIV.

Gastrointestinal problems

Gastrointestinal symptoms such as vomiting, diarrhea, and constipation may persist for the first 6 to 9 months. Other illnesses need to be ruled out.

Neurologic problems

The child should be evaluated immediately if a seizure occurs.

Child abuse

Behavior should be observed and the skin checked closely for signs of abuse.

SUMMARY OF PRIMARY CARE NEEDS FOR THE CHILD WITH PRENATAL COCAINE EXPOSURE — cont'd

Parental drug use

If the parents are abusing drugs, the child may need to be hospitalized or placed in temporary foster care during periods of illness to assure medical management.

Developmental issues
Safety

Home visits are recommended if parents are suspected substance abusers.

Social service involvement and referrals to after school and recreational programs are recommended to keep the child visible in the community.

Parents should be warned about the dangers of passive inhalation of crack fumes and the potential for accidental ingestion of drugs by the children.

Child care

Drug-exposed children may have behavior problems that require a special therapeutic setting.

Diet

Breast-feeding is not recommended for cocaine-using women because cocaine metabolites are present in breast milk.

Caloric intake and feeding behavior should be monitored.

To enhance feeding, parents should be taught proper positioning and handling techniques.

Discipline

Behavior problems are common and begin in infancy with irritability and excessive crying.

Parents should be encouraged to be consistent, firm, and patient in their disciplinary efforts.

Sexuality

These children are at high risk for sexual abuse.

Special family concerns

Foster and kinship foster parents need respite.

Adoptive parents require cautious, ongoing counseling because long-term outcomes are generally unknown.

Health care providers must try to remain empathetic and nonjudgmental.

Toileting

Persistent motor delays, hyperactivity, and behavior problems may interfere with toilet training.

Children with persistent enuresis may need genitourinary work-up.

Sleep patterns

Trouble with regulation of the sleep-wake state is common in the first year of life.

Pacification techniques, low lighting, and a relatively quiet environment are helpful.

School issues

These children are at high risk for learning problems.

Early identification and referrals to programs such as Head Start are helpful.

Small-stature children require special attention to enhance self-esteem.

RESOURCES

Across the nation communities are responding to the devastating problems associated with drug addiction. NAPARE provides information on the dangers of substance abuse during pregnancy and on treatment options. In addition, many government and private agencies have substance abuse hotlines.

Organizations

National Association for Perinatal Addiction Research and Education (NAPARE)
11 E Hubbard St
Suite 200
Chicago, IL 60611
(312) 329-2512

> *This national organization is a resource center for individuals and groups concerned with perinatal addiction.*

The Family Center
Thomas Jefferson University Hospital
11th and Chestnut Sts
Suite 6105
Philadelphia, PA 19107
(215) 928-8850

> *This center provides pregnant addicts and their children with medical, psychiatric, and social services, as well as a variety of clinical assessments.*

National Institute on Drug Abuse (NIDA)
US Department of Health and Human Services
5600 Fishers Ln, Room 10-A-43
Rockville, MD 20852
(301) 443-6500 (NIDA hotline: 800-662-HELP)

American Council on Drug Education (ACDE)
5820 Hubbard Dr
Rockville, MD 20852
(301) 984-5700

Cocaine Helpline
(800) COCAINE

REFERENCES

American Academy of Pediatrics: *Report of the Committee on Infectious Diseases,* Evanston, Ill, 1988, The American Academy of Pediatrics.

American Academy of Pediatrics, Committee on Infectious Diseases 1990-1991: *Haemophilus influenzae* type b conjugate vaccine: Recommendations for immunizations of infants and children 2 months of age and older: Update issued January 1991.

Bateman DA and Heagarty MC: Passive freebase cocaine ('crack') inhalation by infants and toddlers, *Am J Dis Child* 143:25-27, 1989.

Bauchner H, Zuckerman B, McLain M, et al: Risk of sudden infant death syndrome among infants with in utero exposure to cocaine, *J Pediatr* 113:831-834, 1988.

Bauman P and Dougherty F: Drug addicted mother's parenting and their children's development, *Int J Addict* 18:291-302, 1983.

Besunder JB and Blumer JL: Neonatal drug withdrawal syndromes. In Koren G, ed: *Maternal-fetal toxicology: A clinician's guide,* New York, 1990, Marcel Dekker, pp 161-190.

Bingol N, Fuchs M, Diaz V, et al: Teratogenicity of cocaine in humans, *J Pediatr* 110:93-96, 1987.

Centers for Disease Control: Syphilis and congenital syphilis— United States, 1985-1988, *MMWR* 37:486-489, 1988.

Chasnoff IJ: Cocaine and methodone exposed infants: A comparison, *Nat Inst Drug Abuse Res Monogr Ser* 76:278, 1987.

Chasnoff IJ: Drug use in pregnancy: Parameters of risk, *Pediatr Clin North Am* 35:1403-1412, 1988.

Chasnoff IJ: Drug use and women: Establishing a standard of care, *Ann NY Acad Sci* 562:208-210, 1989a.

Chasnoff IJ: Drug use in pregnancy, NY State J Med 89:255, 1989b.

Chasnoff IJ: The incidence of cocaine use. In *Special currents: Cocaine babies,* Columbus, Ohio, 1989c, Ross Laboratories.

Chasnoff IJ, Burns KA and Burns WD: Cocaine use in pregnancy: Perinatal morbidity and mortality, *Neurotoxicol Teratol* 9:291-293, 1987.

Chasnoff IJ, Burns WJ, Schnoll SH, et al: Cocaine use in pregnancy, *N Engl J Med* 313:666-669, 1985.

Chasnoff IJ, Bussey ME, Savich R, et al: Perinatal cerebral infarction and maternal cocaine use, *J Pediatr* 108:456-459, 1986.

Chasnoff IJ, Chisum GM, and Kaplan WE: Maternal cocaine use and genitourinary tract malformations, *Teratology* 37:201-204, 1988.

Chasnoff IJ, Douglas EL, and Squires L: Cocaine intoxication in a breast-fed infant, *Pediatrics* 80:836-838, 1987.

Chasnoff IJ, Hunt CE, Kletter R, et al: Prenatal cocaine exposure is associated with respiratory pattern abnormalities, *Am J Dis Child* 143:583-587, 1989.

Chasnoff IJ and Lewis DE: Cocaine metabolism during pregnancy, *Pediatr Res* 23:257a, 1988 (abstract).

Chasnoff IJ, MacGregor S and Chisum G: Cocaine use during pregnancy: Adverse perinatal outcome. *Nat Inst Drug Abuse Res Monogr Ser* 81:265, 1988.

Chavez GF, Mulinare J, and Cordero JF: Maternal cocaine use during early pregnancy as a risk factor for congenital urogenital anomalies, *JAMA* 262:795-798, 1989.

Chavkin W: Testimony presented to the House Select Committee on Children, Youth and Families, Washington, DC, April 1989.

Cherukuri R, Minkoff H, Feldman J, et al: A cohort study of alkaloidal cocaine ("crack") in pregnancy, *Obstet Gynecol* 72:147-151, 1988.

Chouteau M, Namerow PB, and Leppert P: The effect of cocaine abuse on birthweight and gestational age, *Obstet Gynecol* 72:351-354, 1988.

Doberczak TM, Shanzer S, Senie RT, et al: Neonatal neurologic and electroencephalographic effects of intrauterine cocaine exposure, *J Pediatr* 113:354-358, 1988.

Elvik S: Effects of maternal substance abuse: Prenatal to preschool. Paper presented at the meeting of the National Association of Pediatric Nurse Associates and Practitioners, San Francisco, March 1990.

Falco M: *The substance abuse crisis in New York City: A call to action,* New York, 1989, New York Community Trust.

Frank DA, Zuckerman BS, Amaro H, et al: Cocaine use during pregnancy: Prevalence and correlates, *Pediatrics* 82:888-895, 1988.

Fulroth R, Phillips B, and Durand DJ: Perinatal outcome of infants exposed to cocaine and/or heroin in utero, *Am J Dis Child* 143:905-910, 1989.

Gold M: Crack abuse: Its implications and outcomes, *Resident and Staff Physician* 33:45-52, 1987.

Hadeed AJ and Siegel SR: Maternal cocaine use during pregnancy: Effect on the newborn infant, *Pediatrics* 84:205-210, 1989.

Hawks R and Chiang CN: Examples of specific drug assays, *Nat Inst Drug Abuse Res Monogr Ser* 73:84-114, 1986.

Hollinshead WH, Griffin JF, Scott HD, et al: Statewide prevalence of illicit drug use by pregnant women—Rhode Island. *MMWR* 39:225-227, 1990.

Howard J: Cocaine and its effects on the newborn. *Dev Med Child Neurol* 31:255-257, 1989a.

Howard J: Long term development of infants exposed prenatally to drugs, In *Special currents: Cocaine babies,* Columbus, Ohio, 1989b, Ross Laboratories pp 1-2.

Howard J, Beckwith L, Rodning C, et al: The development of young children of substance abusing parents: Insights from seven years of intervention and research, *Zero to Three: Bulletin of National Center for Clinical Infant Programs* 9:8-12, 1989.

Hoyme HE, Jones KL, Dixon SD, et al: Prenatal cocaine exposure and fetal vascular disruption, *Pediatrics* 85:743-747, 1990.

Hurt H: Medical controversies in evaluation and management of cocaine exposed infants, In *Special currents: Cocaine babies,* Columbus, Ohio, 1989, Ross Laboratories pp 3-4.

Isenberg SJ, Spierer A, and Inkelis SH: Ocular signs of cocaine intoxication in neonates, *Am J Ophthalmol* 103:211-214, 1987.

Jones KL, Smith DW, Ulleland CN, et al: Pattern of malformation in offspring of chronic alcoholic mothers, *Lancet* 1:1267-1271, 1973.

Jones RT: The pharmacology of cocaine, *Nat Inst Drug Abuse Res Monogr Ser* 50:34-53, 1984.

Kantrowitz B, Wingert P, De La Pena N, et al: The crack children, *Newsweek,* Feb 12, 1990, pp 62-63.

Kaye K, Elkind L, Goldberg D, et al: Birth outcomes for infants of drug abusing mothers, *NY State J Med* 89:256-261, 1989.

Kennedy RL and Haddox JD: Local anesthetics. In Craig CR and Stitzel RE, eds: *Modern pharmacology,* ed 2, Boston, 1986, Little, Brown, pp 480-490.

Lewis KD, Bennett B, and Schmeder NH: Care of infants menaced by cocaine use, *MCN* 14:324-329, 1989.

Lifschitz MH, Wilson GS, Smith OE, et al: Factors affecting head growth and intellectual functioning in children of drug addicts, *Pediatrics* 75:269-274, 1985.

Lowe C, ed: Maternal drug abuse—New York City, *City Health Information* 8:1-4, 1989.

MacGregor SN, Keith LG, Chasnoff IJ, et al: Cocaine use during pregnancy: Adverse perinatal outcome, *Am J Obstet Gynecol* 157:686-690, 1987.

Miller G: Addicted infants and their mothers, *Zero to Three: Bulletin of National Center for Clinical Infant Programs* 9:20-23, 1989.

National Institute on Drug Abuse: 1990 National Household Survey on Drug Abuse, U.S. Dept. of Health and Human Services (unpublished).

Neerhof MG, MacGregor SN, Retzky SS, et al: Cocaine abuse during pregnancy: Peripartum prevalence and perinatal outcome, *Am J Obstet Gynecol* 161:633-638, 1989.

Newald J: Cocaine infants: A new arrival at hospital's step? *Hospitals* 60:96, 1986.

Parker S, Greer S, Zuckerman B: Double jeopardy: The impact of poverty on early childhood development in children at risk. In Zuckerman B, Weitzman M, and Alpert J, eds: *Pediatric Clinics of North America,* WB Saunders, Vol 35, 1227-1240, 1988.

Ritchie JM and Greene NM: Local anesthetics. In Gilman AG, Goodman LS, and Gilman A, eds: *The pharmacological basis of therapeutics,* New York, 1980, MacMillan, pp 300-308.

Ryan L, Ehrlich S, and Finnegan LP: Cocaine abuse in pregnancy: Effects on the fetus and newborn, *Nat Inst Drug Abuse Res Monogr Ser* 76:280, 1987.

Schneider JW, Griffith DR, and Chasnoff IJ: Infants exposed to cocaine in utero: Implications for developmental assessment and intervention, *Infants Young Child* 2:25-36, 1989.

Schoenbaum EE, Hartel D, Selwyn PA, et al: Risk factors for human immunodeficiency virus infection in intravenous drug users, *N Engl J Med* 321:874-879, 1989.

Udell B: Crack cocaine. In *Special currents: Cocaine babies,* Columbus Ohio, 1989, Ross Laboratories, pp 5-8.

Van Baar AL, Fleury P, and Ultee CA: Behaviour in the first year after drug dependent pregnancy, *Arch Dis Child* 64:241-245, 1989.

Weston DR, Ivins B, Zuckerman B, et al: Drug exposed babies: Research and clinical issues, *Zero to Three: Bulletin of the National Center for Clinical Infant Programs* 9:1-7, 1989.

Woods JR, Plessinger MA, and Clark KE: Effect of cocaine on uterine blood flow and fetal oxygenation, *JAMA* 257:957-961, 1987.

Zuckerman B, Frank DA, Hingson R, et al: Effects of maternal marijuana and cocaine use on fetal growth, *N Engl J Med* 320:762-768, 1989.

27 *Chronic Renal Failure*

Elizabeth San Luis

ETIOLOGY

Although renal disease is uncommon in pediatrics, early recognition and management are essential to minimize the potentially devastating consequences of uremia. Chronic renal failure (CRF) is an irreversible reduction in glomerular filtration rate (GFR) to less than 25% of normal. The marked decline in renal function leads to metabolic abnormalities such as metabolic acidosis, renal osteodystrophy, anemia, and hypertension. The goal of therapy at this stage is prevention of metabolic complications.

End-stage renal disease (ESRD) is that degree of CRF requiring renal replacement therapy by either dialysis or transplantation. Residual renal function will be decreased to less than 12% of normal.

The etiologies of chronic renal disease are varied and can be broadly categorized as congenital, genetic, acquired, or metabolic diseases (see the box on p. 481).

It is important to establish the exact etiology of CRF in a child whenever possible, because (1) disorders may require different treatments and have varying prognoses; (2) genetic counseling and early diagnosis and treatment of similarly affected siblings should be initiated if a hereditary or metabolic disease is involved, and (3) the timing of renal transplantation may be altered in those diseases with a high incidence of recurrence in renal allografts.

INCIDENCE

The precise incidence and prevalance of CRF in children is unknown. Estimates are derived from the incidence of ESRD in children. Current available data from several surveys suggest an incidence of ESRD from 3 to 8 children per 1 million population and a prevalance of CRF from 18.5 to 32.4 per 1 million children (Foreman and Chan, 1988).

CLINICAL MANIFESTATIONS AT TIME OF DIAGNOSIS

Presenting symptoms at the time of diagnosis vary depending on the primary renal disease. Certain common clinical signs become overt, however, when renal function deteriorates to less than 30% of normal. The box on p. 481 presents a summary of the clinical manifestations of CRF in children.

Initially the child with CRF may have a loss of normal energy and increased fatigue on exertion. Such fatigue often develops gradually and goes unnoticed. The child may prefer sedentary activities rather than active play. Physical examination may reveal a slightly listless, pale child whose blood pressure is frequently elevated.

With further worsening of renal function, fatigue becomes more pronounced. The child will be disinterested in play, and schoolwork may deteriorate as attention span diminishes and memory becomes erratic. The child's appetite decreases. Polyuria and polydypsia, as well as secondary enuresis,

480

CAUSES OF RENAL FAILURE IN CHILDREN

Congenital disease: 11%-25%

Renal hypoplasia
Renal dysplasia
Reflux nephropathy
Obstructive uropathy
Congenital nephrosis

Acquired disease: 20%-43%

Glomerulonephropathies
Hemolytic uremic syndrome
Henoch-Schönlein purpura
Lupus nephritis
Minimal change nephrotic syndrome

Genetic disease: 16%-20%

Alport's syndrome
Polycystic disease
Juvenile nephrophthisis
Juene's syndrome

Metabolic disease: 5%-14%

Cytinosis
Oxalosis

COMMON CLINICAL MANIFESTATIONS OF CHRONIC RENAL FAILURE IN CHILDREN

Growth retardation
Electrolyte imbalance (sodium retention, hyperkalemia)
Metabolic acidosis
Anemia
Renal osteodystrophy

Anorexia
Hypertension
Congestive heart failure
Hyperlipidemia
Peripheral neuropathy
Delayed sexual development

---

may occur. The child develops a characteristic pallor because of anemia and urochrome pigment deposition. Secondary amenorrhea is common in adolescent girls.

Electrolyte abnormalities

Salt and water retention, edema, and hypertension can occur secondary to impaired sodium excretion. However, congenital renal abnormalities, such as hypoplasia and dysplasia, can produce a "salt-wasting" state requiring sodium chloride supplementation (Rodriguez-Soriano et al., 1986). Yet in children with salt-losing nephropathy, serum sodium levels may remain within normal limits because of volume contraction. Dietary sodium restrictions may lead to further deterioration in GFR as a result of decreased renal perfusion.

Hyperkalemia occurs as a result of catabolism, acidosis, and reduced renal excretion. Hypokalemia, although less common, can result from diuretic therapy (hydrochlorothiazide and furosemide [Lasix]) or dietary restriction in a child with polyuria (Fine, 1990). Metabolic acidosis caused by decreased ammonia production, decreased bicarbonate reabsorption, and secondary hyperparathyroidism is a feature of CRF when the GRF falls to less than 50% of normal (Rodriguez-Soriano et al., 1986). Acidosis manifests as tachycardia, hyperpnea, increased hyperkalemia, and possibly growth impairment.

Metabolic factors

Glucose intolerance is seen in CRF, as evidenced by abnormal glucose tolerance test results. Hypertriglyceridemia and hypercholesterolemia occur as CRF progresses. Anorexia can lead to signs of calorie malnutrition, such as reduced physical activity, reduced skinfold thickness, and overt wasting.

Uremia

Uremic toxicity is characterized by anorexia, nausea, somnolence, and malaise (Papadopoulou, 1990). If untreated, the child's symtoms can progress to vomiting, gastrointestinal (GI) bleeding, convulsions, and coma. Pericarditis, congestive heart failure, and arrhythmias are not uncommon.

TREATMENT
Electrolyte abnormalities

Therapy is directed at restoring and maintaining the child's health and preventing the metabolic consequences of CRF. Electrolyte disturbances are probably the most common abnormalities found in renal failure. Early recognition and prophylactic treatment with supplemental sodium chloride can prevent the hyponatremia and volume contraction associated with salt-wasting nephropathy (Fine, 1990). Hyperkalemia can be avoided through dietary counseling to limit foods high in potassium, as well as oral administration of sodium bicarbonate to prevent acidosis. Polystyrene sulfonate (Kayexalate), 1 g/kg once or twice daily, can also be given to maintain a serum potassium level of less than 6.0 mEq/L (Fine, 1990).

Diuretic-induced hypokalemia can be prevented with the concurrent use of potassium-sparing diuretics such as spironolactone (Aldactone) or triamterene (Dyrenium). Oral administration of potassium-containing medications such as potassium chloride and dietary counseling are also effective.

Anemia

Treatment options for anemia caused by CRF and ESRD include blood transfusions and oral iron supplementation if the serum ferritin or serum iron levels (or both) fall to less than 20 ng/L or 50 μg/dl, respectively. Washed leukocyte-poor red blood cell (RBC) mass instead of whole blood transfusion may be preferred, depending on local availability and transplant protocol. Children requiring frequent transfusion are at risk for iron overload, as defined by a serum ferritin level of more than 300 ng/ml

(Eschbach and Adamson, 1985). This can result in acquired hemochromatosis, which leads to tissue damage and dysfunction in the liver, pancreas, heart, and pituitary gland (Korbet, 1989).

The exciting discovery of epoetin alfa, a recombinant DNA form of erythropoietin, ends the transfusion dependency of children on hemodialysis (Cotton and Holochek, 1989; Sinai-Trieman, Salusky, and Fine, 1989). Epoetin alfa therapy corrects the anemia of CRF, improves ones' sense of well-being, and increases exercise tolerance. Hypertension caused by the increased hematocrit value has been a major side effect of this therapy (Casati et al., 1987). The dose must be carefully titrated to prevent a rapid rise in hematocrit value that could lead to a hypertensive crisis or thrombotic event.

Hypertension

The medical management of hypertension associated with CRF depends on the underlying etiology, the degree of renal impairment, the relative contributions of extracellular fluid (ECF) volume overload, and the renin-angiotensin system. Hypertensive control must be done in consultation with a nephrologist. Pre-ESRD treatment consists of dietary sodium restrictions, diuretics, antihypertensive agents, or a combination thereof (Dillon, 1987b). β-Adrenergic blockers, α-adrenergic agonists, peripheral vasodilators, calcium channel blockers, and angiotensin-converting enzyme inhibitors are the different groups of drugs available for the treatment of hypertension associated with CRF. Management of hypertension in children on dialysis includes salt and water restriction and removal of extra ECF by ultrafiltration on dialysis.

Calcium homeostasis

Control of calcium and phosphorus homeostasis is essential to prevent secondary hyperparathyroidism and renal osteodystrophy. Dietary phosphorus restriction and phosphate binders help to keep the serum phosphorus concentration within the normal range. Calcium carbonate is the phosphorus binder of choice rather than aluminum hydroxide because of aluminum-induced aplastic bone disease and possible deleterious effects of aluminum on brain development (McGraw and Haka-Ikse, 1985). Vitamin D replacement therapy with calcitriol (Ro-caltrol) or dihydrotachysterol (DHT) and calcium supplements (calcium carbonate) help to maintain serum calcium levels in the high-normal range, thereby preventing secondary hyperparathyroidism.

Dialysis

Indications for initiating dialysis vary and are dependent on the child's clinical state. Factors to be considered include the child's age, mental state, psychosocial state, and primary renal disease (Fine, Salusky, and Ettenger, 1987). Absolute indications include congestive heart failure, uncontrollable hypertension, pericarditis, uremic encephalopathy, and peripheral neuropathy (Fine, 1990). For the infant with CRF, additional important indications include growth failure, especially of the head, and failure to attain developmental milestones. Other relative indications for dialysis include failure to achieve optimal nutritional intake and impaired ability to conduct normal activities on conservative medical management.

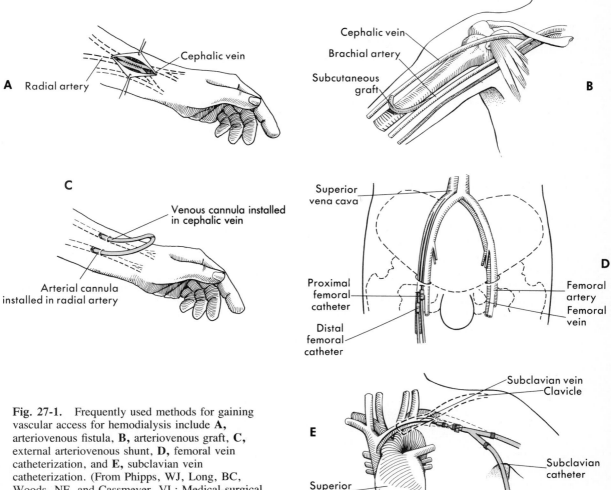

Fig. 27-1. Frequently used methods for gaining vascular access for hemodialysis include **A,** arteriovenous fistula, **B,** arteriovenous graft, **C,** external arteriovenous shunt, **D,** femoral vein catheterization, and **E,** subclavian vein catheterization. (From Phipps, WJ, Long, BC, Woods, NF, and Cassmeyer, VL: Medical-surgical nursing: concepts and clinical practice, ed. 4, St. Louis, 1991, Mosby–Year Book.

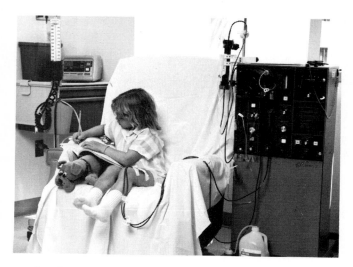

Fig. 27-2. Child undergoing hemodialysis. (From Whaley, LF and Wong, DL: Nursing care of infants and children, ed. 4, St. Louis, 1991, Mosby–Year Book.

Surgical insertion of a dialysis access, vascular or peritoneal, should be considered when the GFR (creatinine clearance) approaches 5 ml/min/1.73 m^2 (Fine, 1990).

Dialysis therapy involves the use of a semipermeable membrane to clear metabolic waste products. Hemodialysis uses an artificial membrane, whereas peritoneal dialysis uses the peritoneal membrane. Hemodialysis is performed 3 times per week for 3 to 4 hours in a dialysis center (Fig. 27-1). It requires a vascular access large enough to provide a blood flow rate of 150 to 300 ml/min. The first choice of vascular access in children is an internal arteriovenous fistula (Donckerwolcke and Chantler, 1987) (Fig. 27-2). Dialyzers or artificial kidneys are chosen with blood volume and clearance characteristics tailored to the specific child's needs. The total extracorporeal blood volume of the dialyzer and blood lines should not exceed 10% of the child's blood volume, calculated as 70 ml/kg (Donckerwolcke and Chantler, 1987).

Two types of peritoneal dialysis, continuous ambulatory peritoneal dialysis (CAPD) and continuous cyclic peritoneal dialysis (CCPD), are also used. Continuous ambulatory peritoneal dialysis is a less complex procedure and requires no elaborate machinery. In CAPD, four to six dialysate bag exchanges are performed each day, with a volume of 30 to 50 ml/kg of body weight per exchange.

The glucose concentration of the dialysate is adjusted according to the child's ultrafiltration needs. The child or parents perform daily CAPD exchanges at home or at school. The CCPD dialysis regimen involves five 2-hour cycles using an automated cycler, administered each night.

Several factors influence the type of dialytic therapy best suited for a child. These factors include the child's age, weight, anticipated length of time of dialysis, child's and parents' preference, and the ability to be trained for home dialysis. Although it is technically possible to use hemodialysis on infants less than 6 months of age, peritoneal dialysis remains the modality of choice for long-term dialysis of children weighing less than 20 kg (Fine et al., 1987). Peritoneal dialysis has several advantages over hemodialysis. It is a simple and safe procedure that can be carried out at home without the psychologic trauma associated with repeated fistula needle punctures. Near steady-state biochemical and fluid control is maintained, thereby avoiding the nausea, vomiting, and disequilibrium associated with hemodialysis. In addition, few restrictions, if any, are needed with regard to diet, fluid intake, or physical activity. Perhaps the most attractive feature of CAPD and CCPD is that they least interfere with normal daily activities. A child on peritoneal dialysis can attend school every day with little or no interruption. Family vacations are possible.

PROGNOSIS

Despite the encouraging outlook for children with ESRD as a result of improved dialysis techniques, growth retardation remains a problem. Early detection and treatment of CRF help to maximize growth and development and delay disease progression. Although CAPD and CCPD provide a more steady state of biochemical control and less restrictions for the child and family, they are not without problems. Children undergoing CAPD or CCPD tend to experience more complications than those on hemodialysis. Although most deaths are not a direct complication of dialysis treatment, peritoneal dialysis therapy is associated with a high mortality, morbidity, and failure rate. Fifty percent to 75% of children develop peritonitis after 3 to 12 months on peritoneal dialysis, with one episode of peritonitis occurring every 7.4 patient months. Potter (1987) reported a 54% 5-year survival rate for children on CAPD versus 95% for children on hemodialysis. The final outcome for these children is determined by the success of renal transplantation (see Chapter 22) (Gruskin et al., 1986).

ASSOCIATED PROBLEMS
Intercurrent illness

Children with ESRD develop frequent and various intercurrent illnesses. Infection is a frequent complication, especially infection of the vascular access and peritoneum (Lindholm and Bergstrom, 1989). Heart failure, pericarditis, pulmonary edema, and GI disease, such as peptic ulcer, are also frequent with uremia.

Growth failure

Growth failure usually occurs in children with kidney function less than 30% of normal (Broyer, 1982). More than half of the children with ESRD are greater than 2 SDs below mean height for age (Barratt et al., 1986). Age of onset of CRF appears to be an important variable affecting growth. The lowest growth rates and the greatest loss of growth potential occur in infants whose CRF occurred either at or shortly after birth (Rizzoni et al, 1986). Kleinknecht, Broyer, and Huot (1983) reported a fall in height with as low as 0.6 SD per month in infants with CRF in the first years of life.

Factors associated with poor growth in CRF are protein and calorie malnutrition, anorexia, electrolyte imbalance, uremic toxicity, and renal osteodystrophy (Rizzoni et al, 1986). Studies have shown that the combination of impaired renal function and calorie intake of less than the recommended daily allowance (RDA) have a profound effect on the infant's growth and development (Claris-Appiani et al., 1989; Rotundo, Nevins, and Lipton, 1982). Dietary manipulations to avoid exacerbation of uremic symptoms, such as protein restrictions, can further compromise growth. Using recombinant human growth hormone, Koch and associates (1989) demonstrated the potential for improving the stature of children with growth retardation caused by CRF.

Anemia

Anemia (hematocrit $< 30\%$) associated with CRF is normocytic, normochromic, and has a low reticulocyte index. Contributing factors of anemia in CRF include: (1) decreased RBC production caused by decreased production and release of erythropoietin (Adamson, Eschbach, and Finch, 1968), (2) shorter RBC life span because of hemodialysis (Lancaster, 1984), (3) retention of uremic toxins that inhibit erythropoiesis (Wallner and Vautrin, 1981), (4) blood loss as a result of platelet defects associated with uremia (Castaldi, Rozenberg, and Steward, 1966), (5) microcytic anemia caused by aluminum toxicity and folate deficiency (Korbet, 1989), and (6) blood loss associated with hemodialysis treatments (Paganini, 1989). Infection, malnutrition, and nephrectomy may further aggravate the decreased erythropoietin production (Papadopoulou, 1990). Of these factors, decreased erythropoietin, brought on by ESRD itself, is considered the primary mechanism leading to anemia (Paganini, 1989).

Bone disease

Renal osteodystrophy (ROD) is common, occurring in approximately 60% to 80% of children with uremia (Papadopoulou, 1990). This is a significant complication in growing children because of their open epiphyses and rapid bone mineralization and remodeling. The two most common types of bone disease are osteitis fibrosa and osteomalacia (Fine, 1990). Osteitis fibrosa is secondary to hyperparathyroidism, hyperphosphatemia, and high serum alkaline phosphatase activity. Osteomalacia is caused by vitamin D deficiency, resulting from the kidney's inability to convert 25-hydroxyvitamin A to 1α, 25-dihydroxyvitamin D_3. Renal bone disease can also manifest as myopathy, which can be mistakenly interpreted as malaise or generalized weakness (Papadopoulou, 1990). These children will usually not complain of bone pain but often restrict their physical activity to protect a painful extremity. They may develop subtle gait abnormalities. Clinical manifestations of ROD include valgus deformities, fractures, rickets, and, in severe bone disease, epiphyseal slipping of the femoral head and metaphyseal fractures (Mehls and Ritz, 1987).

Cardiovascular disorders

Abnormal cardiac function associated with CRF can be attributed to hypertension, anemia, and uremia. Congestive heart failure can occur as a result of fluid overload, severe hypertension, or uremic myocardiopathy (Fine, 1990). The presence of anemia and arteriovenous shunting (vascular access) can increase the cardiac workload and contribute to congestive heart failure (Papadopoulou, 1990). Heart murmurs are common in children with CRF as a result of anemia, hypertension, and volume overload. Electrocardiographic abnormalities include left ventricular hypertrophy, elevated T waves, and widened QRS complexes.

Hypertension is common in children with moderate to severe CRF because of increased peripheral vascular resistance secondary to renin overproduction and volume expansion secondary to salt and water retention. Children with glomerular disease or reflux nephropathy tend to have higher blood pressures than children with congenital renal disorders (Dillon, 1987a). Persistent hypertension can accelerate the decline in renal function.

Uremic pericarditis is a late manifestation of CRF, with such presenting signs and symptoms as fever, precordial pain, friction rub, sudden drop of hemoglobin level, cardiomegaly, cardiac arrhythmias, and cardiac failure (Papadopoulou, 1990).

Neurologic disorders

A syndrome of progressive neurologic deterioration in children with CRF caused by aluminum toxicity has been reported (Geary, Fennel, and Andriola, 1980; McGraw and Haka-Ikse, 1985; Rotundo, Nevins, and Lipton, 1982). It is indistinguishable from the dialysis dementia seen in adults and is characterized by speech disorders, seizures, and dementia. Aluminum toxicity can result in mental retardation or death. Using calcium-containing phosphate binders instead of aluminum-containing agents will hopefully reduce the incidence of mental retardation and other neurologic dysfunction in the future.

Moderate to severe delays for gross motor and language development were reported to be correlated with CRF present from infancy, although they are not correlated with age and severity of CRF at time of diagnosis (Polinsky et al., 1987). Aluminum toxicity, hyperparathyroidism, undernutrition, and psychosocial problems may be contributing factors in the developmental delays. Fennel and associates (1990) found a deterioration in the verbal performance of children 6 to 11 years related to the length of time in renal failure, but it was not found in an older age group. Renal insufficiency may have deleterious effects on verbal development during this time of language skill acquisition.

Uremic neuropathy often affects the lower extremities and involves both motor and sensory function (Papadopoulou, 1990). Signs of neuropathy caused by uremia include muscle weakness; postural hypertension; loss of deep tendon reflexes (especially patellar and Achilles); and "restless legs" syndrome, including peculiar creeping, crawling, prickly sensations, and pruritus, loss in the sensation of pain, light touch, vibration, and pressure.

Encephalopathy may be seen in advanced renal failure. Early symptoms include headache, fatigue, and listlessness. The child may have memory loss, decreased attention span, drowsiness, and impaired speech with further deterioration of renal function.

PRIMARY CARE MANAGEMENT
Growth and development

Attention to the child's growth is extremely important in the identification and management of children with CRF, especially those with congenital renal disease. Children with renal disease may not have any clinical signs other than retarded growth. Most children referred to pediatric nephrologists are already growth retarded at the time of the first visit (Gruskin et al., 1986). Despite advances in dialytic therapy for children with ESRD, inadequate growth is still a problem (Gruskin et al., 1986). Poor growth in children undergoing dialysis has been related to caloric intake that was less than 70% of the RDAs (Simmons et al., 1971). Improved growth rates and lean body mass in children on chronic peritoneal dialysis over those on chronic hemodialysis have been reported (Baum et al., 1982; Conley et al., 1982; Kohaut, 1982) as well as adequate growth in infants on CAPD treated with aggressive nutritional therapy (Conley et al., 1982).

Accurate growth measurements should be taken at each visit and at least every 6 months thereafter and plotted on National Center for Health Statistics growth charts. The weight/height index provides a measure of muscle and adipose tissue relative to height. A low weight/height index may be an indication of malnutrition. Caution should be paid to true values that may be obscured by an increase in ECF volume. Skinfold thickness at the biceps and subscapular sites should be obtained at least every 6 months and with any major change in the mode of treatment (Barratt and Chantler, 1987; Papadopoulou, 1989). It should also be noted that the child's height may be altered because of renal osteodystrophy and the development of rickets.

Neurologic status should be carefully ascertained. Head circumference should be obtained on all children less than 3 years of age and must be accurately recorded at 3- to 6-month intervals. The impact of the disease process on the child's psychologic status, school attendance, intellectual performance, and social development should be assessed every 6 to 9 months. Developmental assessments must be done with the onset of CRF and repeated at 2- to 9-month intervals, depending on the child's age and disease severity. The Denver Developmental Screening Test can be used as a screening tool, but the infant with CRF should be referred to a child psychologist for thorough evaluation. Pubertal staging using the Tanner scale should be determined yearly.

Immunizations

Routine immunizations should be given to children with CRF except for a few specific disease con-

ditions and therapies. Immunosuppressive therapy, used in treating responsive types of chronic glomerulonephritis, is an indication for withholding live virus immunizations (Weiss, 1988). Immunizations should be withheld until the child is in remission and off therapy for 6 months. Exceptions to this recommendation are those children who do not respond to therapy or who have frequent relapses. Then risks must be weighed against the benefits of immunizing the child. Diphtheria-pertussis-tetanus, measles-mumps-rubella, or oral polio vaccines may precipitate an exacerbation in a child with minimal change nephrotic syndrome (Travis, Brouhard, and Kalia, 1984) and therefore should not be given.

Pneumococcal and influenza vaccines are recommended for children with CRF and children with active nephrotic syndrome because of their increased susceptibility to infections (Committee on Infectious Disease, 1991; Travia, Brouhard, and Kalia, 1984). Given the high risk of hepatitis B exposure, hepatitis surface antigen and antibody status should be ascertained in children before starting hemodialysis (Shusterman and Singer, 1987). If a child is hepatitis B surface antigen negative, he or she should be immunized with the hepatitis vaccine as soon as possible. Because the antibody response to the hepatitis B vaccine may be diminished, these children may require repeated doses until seroconversion is achieved (Committee on Infectious Disease, 1991; Drachman et al., 1987). Serum antibody concentrations should be measured every 6 months because protection from the vaccine may be less complete.

Screening

Vision. In addition to routine vision screening, a yearly eye examination by pediatric ophthalmologist is recommended. The eyes should be examined for scleral calcification caused by hypercalcemia or uncontrolled hyperphosphatemia. The fundus should be examined for arterial narrowing, hemorrhages, exudates, and papilledema secondary to hypertension.

Hearing. Children with CRF should be referred to an audiologist for annual assessment. High-frequency sensorineural deafness is characteristic of Alport's syndrome (Barratt and Chantler, 1987).

Hearing loss can also result from the use of ototoxic drugs such as furosemide and gentamicin (Garamycin).

Dental. Routine dental care is recommended for children with CRF. Dental procedures can release microorganisms into the bloodstream and cause infective endocarditis or colonization of the vascular access. The pediatric nephrologist should be consulted regarding the use of prophylactic antibiotics before these procedures (Chow and Peterson, 1979) (see Chapter 11). Children with congenital renal disease will frequently have enamel defects. Poor nutritional intake may lead to poor mineralization of teeth.

Blood pressure. Blood pressure measurements should be taken at 1- to 3-month intervals, depending on the clinical condition. Most of the children with CRF develop some degree of hypertension during the course of their illness, with about 79% requiring antihypertensive therapy (Scharer and Ulmer, 1987). Initiation and follow-up of antihypertensive therapy should be done in consultation with the pediatric nephrologist.

Hematocrit. Routine screening may be deferred if a recent complete (CBC) blood count is included with the other renal function tests. Anemia is a chronic problem and is usually followed by the nephrology team.

Urinalysis. Routine screening is not necessary because of the frequent urine analysis done by the renal team.

Tuberculosis. Routine screening is recommended.

Condition-specific screening

BLOOD WORK. The nephrology team will regularly monitor the CBC, serum ferritin levels, RBC folate serum electrolytes levels, urea nitrogen values, creatinine clearance, and calcium, phosphorus, alkaline phosphatase, and serum protein (transferrin and albumin) levels. Metabolic acidosis needs to be identified and treated promptly to prevent bone demineralization. Parathyroid hormone levels should be monitored every 3 months with radiologic signs of bone disease and to assess the effectiveness of therapeutic interventions. These can be done in consultation with the nephrologist. Fasting triglyceride and cholesterol levels should be measured at 3- to 6-month intervals.

CARDIAC SCREENING. A chest radiograph and baseline electrocardiogram should be performed initially and at 6- to 12-month intervals to assess the cardiovascular status of children with CRF.

RADIOGRAPHIC BONE STUDIES. Radiographic studies of the hand and wrist or knee should be obtained at 3- to 6-month intervals for evaluation of renal osteodystrophy. Bone age should also be evaluated annually to assess growth.

Drug interactions

The most important factors to consider in pharmacokinetics is the extent to which the drug is excreted by the kidney and the degree of renal impairment. Drug dose regimens are altered with GFRs less than 30 to 40 ml/min (Trompeter, 1987). The initial loading dose of drugs excreted by the kidneys, however, is the same as it is for children without renal failure. Maintenance doses must be adjusted by either lengthening the interval between doses or by reducing individual doses. Cardiac glycosides or aminoglycoside antibiotics are examples of drugs that are almost entirely dependent on renal excretion for elimination, thus requiring dosage adjustment even in mild renal failure. Penicillin G with its wide therapeutic index and excretion by renal and hepatic metabolism requires no dose adjustments until renal function decreases to very low levels without dialysis therapy. Other penicillins such as carbenicillin (Geopen), ticarcillin (Ticar), and ampicillin, are cleared almost entirely by the kidney and thus require dosage adjustment (Adelman and Sinaiko, 1987). Cephalosporins are similar in many ways to penicillins and thus require dosage adjustments. Anticonvulsants, particularly phenobarbital, may also require dosage adjustments. The nephrologist should be consulted for appropriate dosage adjustments. If antacids are indicated, calcium-containing phosphate binders instead of aluminum-containing agents must be ordered to avoid aluminum toxicity with CRF.

DIFFERENTIAL DIAGNOSIS AND MANAGEMENT OF COMMON PEDIATRIC CONDITIONS
Fever

Peritonitis is the most frequent complication of CAPD. Symptoms include fever, abdominal pain, and cloudy dialysate. Early diagnosis and treatment are essential to avoid negative sequelae, such as the need to remove the peritoneal catheter because of intractable infection or catheter tunnel infection. The child should be immediately referred to the nephrologist for signs of peritonitis.

Vascular access of children on hemodialysis should be checked for signs of infection. The nephrologist should be consulted for the appropriate antibiotic therapy.

If infection of the dialysis access has been ruled out and the child has other symptoms compatible with a common pediatric childhood illness, the practitioner should consult with the nephrologist about existing protocols. Hydration for febrile illness will depend on the child's renal status. Selected antibiotics must be compatible with the child's renal function and diagnosed condition. The nephrologist may need to make temporary alterations in the child's dialysis program during periods of illness.

Gastrointestinal symptoms

Nausea and vomiting are common symptoms in childhood. Worsening renal function must be ruled out in children with mild renal failure, especially in the absence of associated fever.

Headaches and facial palsy

Uncontrolled hypertension should be ruled out in children with CRF complaining of frequent headaches or facial palsy.

DEVELOPMENTAL ISSUES
Safety

Physical activities should be limited only by the child's endurance. Children on CAPD are encouraged to become active in sports except for tackle football, wrestling, and gymnastics involving the uneven parallel bars, which have the potential for trauma to the abdomen and dislodgement of the peritoneal catheter. Swimming is encouraged as a safe form of exercise.

Children with hemodialysis arm vascular accesses must be cautioned against wearing restrictive clothing or accessories that can lead to venostasis and clotting. Children should be encouraged to wear a Medic-Alert bracelet or necklace to alert other health care providers of their CRF status, medication needs, and other possible complications.

Child care

Children with CRF are not restricted from day care. Those children with active nephrosis who are receiving corticosteroid therapy are much more susceptible to infections and would benefit from home care or small group child care. When child care is used, the care giver must be taught about the child's dietary restrictions and drug regimen. Specific instructions on proper administration of medications must be given (e.g., antacids used as phosphate binders must be given during meals to be effective). Children on CAPD and their parents are encouraged by the nephrology team to arrange the dialysis schedule around the child care hours whenever possible. If changes in dialysis schedules are necessary, the nephrology team should be consulted.

Diet

Dietary intake should be assessed for adequacy of calories, sodium, potassium, calcium, phosphorus, and protein intake at 1- to 3-month intervals. Normal growth velocity can be achieved by assuring the RDA of calories appropriate for age and size (Rizzoni, Basso, and Setari, 1984). Dietary restrictions will vary depending on the degree of renal function and the disease etiology. Water-soluble vitamins are frequently recommended to supplement dietary restrictions. The active form of vitamin D, 1α, 25-dihydroxcholecalciferol, is also given to prevent vitamin D deficiency related to renal failure.

The primary care provider should obtain the dietary management plan from the nephrology team to reinforce family education. Children who do not require dialysis should receive the RDA for energy and protein for a child the same height, but it may be necessary to limit the dietary intake of sodium, potassium, and phosphorus. Infants requiring special formulas are followed closely by the nephrology team, with changes made by them based on renal function, growth rates, fluid status, and ability to tolerate the formula. Children on dialysis are followed by the renal dietician monthly.

Discipline

Parental anxiety and despondency over their child's chronic condition may lead to ambivalent feelings toward child rearing or the treatment program, resulting in child behavior problems or nonadherence with the treatment regimen (Grupe et al., 1986). Parents should be encouraged to express their ambivalence and frustrations. They must be supported and encouraged to set appropriate limits and expectations for behavior. Parents must be counseled against being overprotective because of their own fears and concerns about their child's health.

Children on hemodialysis can have difficulty accepting the painful procedure of venipuncture required for each treatment. Management techniques for pain associated with procedures, such as guided imagery, hypnosis, and progressive muscle relaxation to help reduce anxiety, have been successfully taught to children and their parents.

Toileting

Toilet training for urinary continence may not be possible when the child is diagnosed with CRF, especially when the child is oliguric or anuric. Bowel training should be initiated when the toddler is developmentally ready. When urine production is reestablished after kidney transplantation, training for urine continence can be initiated (see Chapter 22).

Sleep patterns

Infants and young children, even those using CAPD or CCPD, should be encouraged to assume a normal sleeping pattern at night. Most children are able to sleep undisturbed using nocturnal CCPD treatment. An increased need for sleep and lethargy may be indications of worsening renal failure and should be reported to the nephrology team.

School issues

Every effort must be made to encourage the school-aged child to attend school full time. The CAPD exchanges should be scheduled around school activities whenever possible. The parents, child, and nephrology team should work together to identify a treatment plan and schedule that meets everyone's needs. Changes in schedules to accommodate after-school activities will need to be discussed with the nephrology team. Pediatric hemodialysis units should include a school teacher to assist children with missed schoolwork. Poor school performance must be evaluated for contributing factors, because several studies have demonstrated cognitive deficits with more advanced CRF and with congenital etiologies.

Sexuality

Delayed sexual development is common among children with CRF as a result of insufficient production of gonadal steroids and elevated gonadotropin levels (Fine, 1990). More than half of female adolescents with ESRD have delayed development of secondary sex characteristics and menarche. There are large individual variations in the time course of menstrual bleedings and the occurrence of amenorrhea and irregular bleeding among adolescent girls with CRF (Scharer et al., 1989). Although menstrual abnormalities (amenorrhea, oligomenorrhea, and menorrhagia) and infertility have been described, successful pregnancies in women who were on dialysis have been reported (Scharer et al., 1989). Adolescent males with ESRD may show delayed development of genitalia or pubic hair. Testicular size may also be reduced. These adolescents need to be counseled about birth control, sexually transmitted diseases, and acquired immune deficiency syndrome, as do their healthy counterparts.

The practitioner must explore with the adolescent issues related to delayed development, such as poor body image because of short stature, surgical scars from dialysis accesses, peritoneal catheters, malformed extremities caused by large vascular fistulas, and delayed pubertal development.

SPECIAL FAMILY CONCERNS

Chronic renal failure can lead to psychologic problems in some children. Conflicts can arise between the child and parents when the child has to adhere to a strict treatment regimen (e.g., diet restrictions, complex drug therapy, and dialysis). Families are also faced with the tremendous emotional and financial burden associated with renal failure. Therapy for ESRD is very costly. Parents continually worry about vascular access infections, peritonitis, and blood transfusions.

SUMMARY OF PRIMARY CARE NEEDS FOR THE CHILD WITH CHRONIC RENAL FAILURE

Growth and development

Growth retardation is a major problem in children with chronic renal failure.

Variations in the degree of retardation depends on several factors, (e.g., age at onset of illness and nutritional status). About one half of the children with CRF will be below the third percentile for height and weight.

Anthropometric measurements should be obtained at least every 6 months and with any major change in the mode of treatment.

Sexual maturation is often delayed.

Acquisition of developmental milestones is delayed in the infant and young child with uremia.

Immunizations

Routine immunizations are recommended unless the child is receiving immunosuppressive therapy for glomerulonephritis.

Routine immunizations are withheld from a child with minimal change nephrotic syndrome until the child has been in remission and off therapy for 6 months.

Influenza vaccine is recommended.

Pneumococcal vaccine is recommended for children with nephrotic syndrome who are nonresponsive to therapy or who have frequent relapses.

Hepatitis B vaccine is recommended for children on dialysis.

Screening
Vision

Fundoscopic examination should be done each visit.

Hearing

Routine screening and a yearly examination by an audiometrist are recommended.

Dental

Routine screening is recommended. Prophylactic antibiotics may be ordered by the nephrologist before dental work.

Enamel defects and poor mineralization of teeth are common problems.

Blood pressure

Measurements should be taken at 1- to 3-month intervals. Many children require antihypertensive therapy.

Hematocrit

Anemia is a chronic problem. Nephrology team should assess CBC counts on a regular basis.

Urinalysis

Routine screening is not necessary because of frequent urinalysis by renal team.

Tuberculosis

Routine screening is recommended.

Condition-specific screening
Blood work
CBC and levels of serum electrolytes, calcium, phosphorus, and alkaline phosphatase should be checked monthly. Serum ferritin and RBC folate levels should be assessed monthly to determine the adequacy of iron and folic acid intake.
Cardiac screening
Chest x-ray studies and electrocardiogram should be done every 6 to 12 months.
Bone studies
X-ray studies of the hand, wrist, and knee should be done at 3- to 6-month intervals for assessment of skeletal maturity and renal osteodystrophy.

Drug interactions

Aminoglycoside antibiotics require dosage adjustment even in mild renal failure.

Most penicillins and cephalosporins require dosage adjustment during renal failure.

Therapeutic levels of anticonvulsants should be monitored.

Aluminum antacids can lead to aluminum intoxication in children with impaired renal function.

Differential diagnosis
Fever

Rule out peritonitis in children who are using CAPD or who have infection of the dialysis access.

Continued.

Gastrointestinal symptoms

Rule out peritonitis in children using CAPD.

Headaches and facial palsy

Rule out severe hypertension.

Developmental issues
Child care

The child with nephrotic syndrome is more susceptible to infections and may require home care.

The child care provider must be informed of diet restrictions and medication requirements.

Dialysis schedules should be made around day care.

Diet

Inadequate caloric intake is a common problem in CRF. Sodium, potassium, phosphorus, and protein intake may need adjustments depending on the degree of renal function.

Water-soluble vitamins and vitamin D analogs may be required.

Discipline

Noncompliance with dietary restrictions and medications are often sources of conflict between

parents and child. Behavior problems associated with hemodialysis and pain may be helped by guided imagery, hypnosis, or muscle relaxation.

Toileting

Toilet training for urinary continency may not be possible due to oliguria or anuria.

Bowel training should be initiated when child is developmentally ready.

School issues

Decreased school attendance because of the time demands of the therapeutic regimen may affect performance. Regular school attendance should be encouraged. In the dialysis units or during hospitalizations, tutors should be utilized to help keep up with schoolwork.

Special family concerns

Special family concerns include the emotional and financial impact of chronic dialysis on the entire family, prevention of infection, and frequent blood transfusions needed for children on hemodialysis.

RESOURCES

The cost of ESRD treatment is very expensive, ranging from $20,000 to $35,000 per year. In July 1973, the Social Security Act was amended to provide Medicare benefits for persons less than 65 years of age who have chronic kidney disease and require dialysis or kidney transplantation (HR-1, Public Law 92-603, section 2991). The family should be referred to the social worker on the nephrology team for assistance in accessing available services.

Individual states may have a specialized medical care and rehabilitation program for children less than 21 years of age diagnosed as having a severe, chronic, or disabling disorder. Additional financial assistance is available through National Kidney Foundation affiliates and the American Kidney Fund.

Summer camp programs, such as the Moncrief Mountain Ranch Camp in Colorado, that provide respite for the families are available. Pediatric nephrology centers will also have information on local camps, other recreation programs, and family support groups.

Organizations

American Association of Kidney Patients
(813) 251-0725

American Kidney Fund
6110 Executive Blvd, No 1010
Rockville, MD 20852
(301) 881-3052 or (800) 638-8299

American Nephrology Nurses Association
North Woodbury Rd, Box 56
Pitman, NJ 08071
(609) 589-2187

End Stage Renal Disease Networks
They are divided into geographic regions. They are assigned to coordinate and review dialysis and transplant facilities to ensure the best possible care.

National Association of Patients on Hemodialysis and Transplantation (NAPHT)
211 E 43rd St, No 301
New York, NY 10017
(212) 867-6374

National Kidney Foundation
2 Park Ave
New York, NY 10016
(212) 889-2210
It has local chapters; contact them for summer camps.

Renal Physicians Association
1101 Vermont Ave, NW, No 500
Washington, DC 20005-3547
(202) 289-1700

REFERENCES

Adamson J, Eschbach J, and Finch C: The kidney and erythropoiesis, *Am J Med* 44:725-731, 1968.

Adelman RD and Sinaiko AR: Drugs and the kidney. In Holliday
MA, Barratt TM, and Vernier RL, eds: *Pediatric nephrology,*
ed 2, Baltimore, 1987, Williams & Wilkins, pp 252-271.

Barratt TM, Broyer M, Chantler C, et al: Assessment of growth,
Am J Kidney Dis 7:340-346, 1986.

Barratt TM and Chantler C: Clinical evaluation. In Holliday
MA, Barratt TM, and Vernier RL, eds: *Pediatric nephrology,*
ed 2, Baltimore, 1987, Williams & Wilkins, pp 275-281.

Baum M, Powell D, Calvin S, et al: Continuous ambulatory
peritoneal dialysis in children, *N Engl J Med* 307:1537-1542,
1982.

Broyer M: Growth in children with renal insufficiency, *Pediatr
Clin North Am* 29:991-1001, 1982.

Casati S, Passerini P, Campise M, et al: Benefits and risks of
protracted treatment with human recombinant erythropoietin
in patients having hemodialysis, *Br Med J* 295:1017-1020,
1987.

Castaldi P, Rozenberg M and Stewart J: The bleeding disorder
of uraemia, *Lancet* 2:66-69, 1966.

Chow MH and Peterson DS: Dental management for children
with chronic renal failure undergoing hemodialysis therapy,
Oral Surg 48:34-37, 1979.

Claris-Appiani A, Bianchi ML, Bini P, et al: Growth in young
children with chronic renal failure, *Pediatr Nephrol* 3:301-
304, 1989.

Committee on Infectious Diseases: *Report of the Committee on
Infectious Diseases,* ed 22, Elk Grove Village, Ill, 1991,
The American Academy of Pediatrics.

Conley SB, Brewer ED, Gandy S, et al: Normal growth in very
small children on peritoneal dialysis: 18 month experience,
Am J Kidney Dis, suppl 8, December 1982, p 8.

Cotton SL and Holechek MJ: Management of anemia using
recombinant human erythropoietin in patients on chronic

hemodialysis, *Am Assoc Nurse Anesth J* 16:463-468, 1989.

Dillon MJ: Clinical aspects of hypertension. In Holliday MA,
Barratt TM, and Vernier RL, eds: *Pediatric nephrology,* ed
2, Baltimore, 1987a, Williams & Wilkins, pp 743-757.

Dillon MJ: Drug treatment of hypertension. In Holliday MA,
Barratt TM, and Vernier RL, eds: *Pediatric nephrology,* ed
2, Baltimore, 1987b, Williams & Wilkins, pp 758-765.

Donckerwolcke RA and Chantler C: Dialysis therapy: Hemo-
dialysis. In Holliday MA, Barratt TM, and Vernier RL, eds:
Pediatric nephrology, ed 2, Baltimore, 1987, Williams &
Wilkins, pp 799-827.

Drachman R, Isachsohn M, Rudensky B, et al: Vaccination
against hepatitis B in children and adolescent patients on
dialysis, *Nephrol Dial Transplant* 4:372-374, 1987.

Eschbach JW and Adamson JW: Anemia of end-stage renal
disease, *Kidney Int* 28:1-5, 1985.

Fennel RS, Fennell EB, Carter RL, et al: Association between
renal function and cognition in childhood chronic renal failure, *Pediatr Nephrol* 4:16-20, 1990.

Fine RN: Recent advances in the management of the infant,
child, and adolescent with chronic renal failure, *Pediatr Rev*
11:277-283, 1990.

Fine RN, Salusky IB, and Ettenger RB: The therapeutic approach to the infant, child, and adolescent with end-stage
renal disease, *Pediatr Clin North Am* 34:789-801, 1987.

Foreman JW and Chan JCM: Chronic renal failure in infants
and children, *J Pediatr* 113:793-800, 1988.

Geary DF, Fennel RS, and Andriola M: Encephalopathy in
children with chronic renal failure, *J Pediatr* 96:41-45, 1980.

Grupe WE, Greifer I, Greenspan SI, et al: Psychosocial development in children with chronic renal insufficiency. *Am
J Kidney Dis* 7:324-328, 1986.

Gruskin AB, Alexander SR, Baluarte J, et al: Issues in pediatric
dialysis, *Am J Kidney Dis* 7:306-311, 1986.

Kleinknecht C, Broyer M, and Huot D: Growth and development
of non-dialysed children with chronic renal failure, *Kidney
Int* 24(suppl 15):40-47, 1983.

Koch VH, Lippem BM, Nelson PA, et al: Accelerated growth
after recombinant human growth hormone treatment of children with chronic renal failure, *J Pediatr* 115:365-371, 1989.

Kohaut EC: Growth in children with end-stage renal disease
with CAPD for at least one year, *Periton Dial Bull* 2:159-
160, 1982.

Korbet SM: Comparison of hemodialysis and peritoneal dialysis
in the management of anemia related to chronic renal disease,
Semin Nephrol 9(suppl 1):9-15, 1989.

Lancaster L: End stage renal disease: Pathophysiology, assessment and intervention. In Lancaster L, ed: *The patient with
end stage renal disease,* New York, 1984, John Wiley &
Sons, pp 1-28.

Lindholm B and Bergstrom J: Nutritional management of patients undergoing peritoneal dialysis. In Nolph KD, ed: *Peritoneal dialysis,* ed 3, Norwell, Mass, 1989, Kluwer Academic Publishers, pp 230-260.

McGraw ME and Haka-Ikse K: Neurologic-developmental sequelae of chronic renal failure in infancy, *J Pediatr* 106:579-583, 1985.

Mehls O and Ritz E: Renal osteodystrophy. In Holliday MA, Barratt TM, and Paganini EP, eds: Overview of anemia associated with chronic renal disease: Primary and secondary mechanisms, *Semin Nephrol* 9(suppl 1):3-8, 1989.

Paganini EP: Overview of anemia associated with chronic renal disease: primary and secondary mechanisms. *Semin Nephrol* 9(1 suppl 1): 1-3, 1989.

Papadopoulou ZL: Chronic renal failure. In Barakat AY, ed: *Renal disease in children,* New York, 1989, Springer-Verlag, New York.

Polinsky MS, Kaiser BA, Stover JB, et al: Neurologic development of children with severe chronic renal failure from infancy, *Pediatr Nephrol* 1:157-165, 1987.

Potter DE: Comparison of CAPD and hemodialysis in children. In Fine RN, ed: *Chronic ambulatory peritoneal dialysis and chronic cycling peritoneal dialysis in children,* Boston, 1987, Martinus Nijhoff Publishing, pp 297-306.

Rizzoni G, Basso T, and Setari M: Growth in children with chronic renal failuire on conservative treatment, *Kidney Int* 26:52-58, 1984.

Rizzoni G, Broyer M, Guest G, et al: Growth retardation in children with chronic renal disease: Scope of the problem, *Am J Kidney Dis* 7:256-261, 1986.

Rodriguez-Soriano J, Arant BS, Bordehl J, et al: Fluid and electrolyte imbalances in children with chronic renal failure, *Am J Kidney Dis* 7:268-274, 1986.

Rotundo A, Nevins TE, and Lipton M: Progressive encephalopathy in children with chronic renal insufficiency in infancy, *Kidney Int* 21:486-491, 1982.

Scharer K, Schaefer F, Trott M, et al: Pubertal development in children with chronic renal failure. In Scharer K, ed: *Growth and endocrine changes in children and adolescents with chronic renal failure,* New York, 1989, Karger, vol 20, pp 151-168.

Scharer K and Ulmer H: Cardiovascular complications. In Holliday MA, Barratt TM, and Vernier RL, eds: *Pediatric nephrology,* ed 2, Baltimore, 1987, Williams & Wilkins, pp 887-896.

Shusterman N and Singer I: Infectious hepatitis in dialysis patients, *Am J Kidney Dis* 6:447-455, 1987.

Simmons JM, Wilson CJ, Potter DE, et al: Relation of calorie deficiency to growth failure in children on hemodialysis and the growth response to calorie supplementation, *N Engl J Med* 285:635-656, 1971.

Sinai-Trieman L, Salusky IB, and Fine RN: Use of subcutaneous recombinant human erythropoietin in children undergoing continuous cycling peritoneal dialysis, *J Pediatr* 114:550-554, 1989.

Travis LB, Brouhard BH, and Kalia A: Overview with special emphasis on epidemiologic considerations. In Tune BM and Mendoze SA, eds: *Pediatric nephrology: Contemporary issues in nephrology,* New York, 1984, Churchill Livingstone, vol 12, pp 1-19.

Trompeter RS: A review of drug prescribing in children with end-stage renal failure, *Pediatr Nephrol* 1:183-194, 1987.

Wallner S and Vautrin R: Evidence that inhibition of erythropoiesis is important in the anemia of chronic renal failure, *J Lab Clin Med* 97:170-178, 1981.

Weiss R: Management of chronic renal failure, *Pediatr Ann* 17:584-589, 1988.

28 *Sickle Cell Disease*

Maryann E. Lisak

ETIOLOGY

Sickle cell disease is a term used to describe several inherited sickling hemoglobinopathy syndromes, including sickle-β-thalassemia (HgbS-B° thal or HbgS-B⁺ thal), sickle-C disease (Hgb SC), and most commonly sickle cell anemia (Hgb SS). Hemoglobin contains two pairs of polypeptide chains, α and β. Each of the hemoglobinopathy syndromes has sickle hemoglobin (Hgb S), which differs from normal hemoglobin (Hgb A) by the substitution of a single amino acid; in Hgb S, valine replaces glutamic acid at the sixth position of the β-chain.

A red blood cell (RBC) containing normal hemoglobin is a very pliable, biconcave disc and has a life span of approximately 120 days. Red blood cells containing predominantly Hgb S will, under certain conditions, develop a distorted sickle, or crescent, shape. In this form the cell is rigid and friable. Hypoxia and acidosis, which may be caused by fever, infection, dehydration, or other factors, are known to induce this change in shape (Fig. 28-1). Many times, however, the RBC changes shape without apparent provocation. To a limited degree this change in shape is reversible, though not indefinitely. Eventually the cells become irreversibly sickled cells (ISCs) with a life span of approximately 10 to 20 days. The fragility and shortened life span of these RBCs leads to chronic anemia. This serves as a stimulus to the bone marrow, resulting in an elevated reticulocyte count.

The sickle "prep" is a solubility test often used to screen infants and children for sickle cell disease.

It is inexpensive and rapidly performed but is not very specific. A sickle prep result will be positive for sickle cell trait, sickle cell anemia, and other sickle hemoglobinopathies but will not distinguish between them. The definitive diagnosis of sickle cell disease is made by performing a complete blood

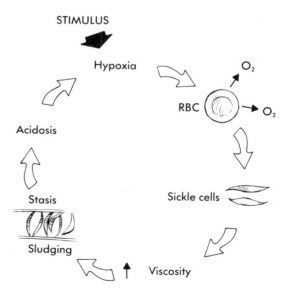

Fig. 28-1. Cycle causing vasoocclusive episodes in sickle cell anemia. (From Hockenberry, M and Coody, D (Eds.): Pediatric oncology and hematology: perspectives on care, St. Louis, 1986, CV Mosby.)

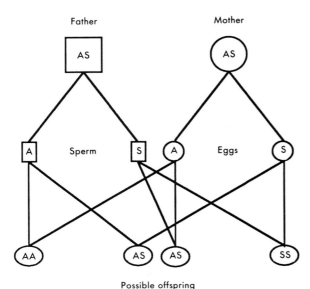

Fig. 28-2. Genetics of sickle cell anemia. Both parents possess one gene for normal hemoglobin *(A)* and one for sickle hemoglobin *(S)*. With each pregnancy, there is a 25% statistical chance that the child will have normal hemoglobin *(AA)* and a 25% chance of sickle cell anemia *(SS)*. 50% will have sickle cell trait. (From Miller, D and Baehner, R: Blood diseases of infancy and childhood: in the tradition of C.H. Smith, ed. 6, St. Louis, 1990, Mosby–Year Book.)

count (CBC), peripheral blood smear, and, most importantly, a quantitative hemoglobin electrophoresis. Occasionally it is helpful to perform hematologic studies on a child's parents to confirm the diagnosis.

Sickle cell disease has an autosomal recessive inheritance pattern. Both parents must carry some type of abnormal hemoglobin—one or both of them must carry sickle hemoglobin—for the disease to be manifested in their offspring. Carriers of sickle cell disease are described as having sickle cell trait (Hgb AS). When two individuals, each of whom has sickle cell trait, elect to have a child, there is a 25% chance of having a child with sickle cell anemia (Hgb SS), a 50% chance of having a child with sickle cell trait (Hgb AS), and a 25% chance of having a child with entirely normal hemoglobin (Hgb AA) with each pregnancy (Fig. 28-2).

In an effort to decrease morbidity and mortality through early identification and prophylactic treatment, many states are now performing routine newborn screening for hemoglobinopathies. Electrophoresis or high-performance liquid chromatography (HPLC) can be performed on cord blood or heel stick blood, usually at the same time that blood is obtained for other newborn screening tests (phenylketonuria, thyroid function, etc.). The hemoglobin electrophoresis of the newborn demonstrates 70% to 80% fetal hemoglobin, with the remaining 20% to 30% reflective of the infant's eventual adult hemoglobin pattern. The level of fetal hemoglobin usually falls gradually over the course of the first 6 months of life, with the infant's adult hemoglobin pattern becoming more apparent (Pearson, 1989). It is unusual to find clinical manifestations of the disease in the presence of significant amounts of fetal hemoglobin. Therefore, the disease may not be clinically apparent until 4 to 6 months of age or later.

INCIDENCE

Sickle cell disease is one of the most common genetic diseases. It is seen most often in individuals of African descent but is also found in other ethnic groups, including those from the Caribbean, Mediterranean, the Arabian Peninsula, and India (Pearson, 1987). In the United States, 1 in 12 black Americans is a carrier of sickle cell disease and 1 in 500 actually has the disease.

Prenatal diagnosis is available to those couples where each partner is known to be a carrier for a hemoglobinopathy. Diagnosis may be accomplished via chorionic villi sampling during the first trimester or amniocentesis during the second trimester. The choice of method is dependent on the risks and benefits of the techniques involved; both are adequate to determine the diagnosis.

CLINICAL MANIFESTATIONS

The majority of children with sickle cell anemia are symptomatic by the time they reach 1 year of age, with musculoskeletal pain as the most common symptom. Many children have dactylitis, a painful swelling of the hands and feet. It occurs as a manifestation of infarction in the metatarsals and the metacarpals; the infarction is a result of vasooc-

Table 28-1. Differential diagnosis of common hemoglobinopathies

Diagnosis	Clinical severity	Hemoglobin (g/dl)	Hematocrit (%)	Mean corpuscular volume (μ³)	% of reticulocytes	RBC morphology*	Solubility test	Electrophoresis (%)	Distribution of fetal hemoglobin
SS	Moderate-severe	7.5 (6-10)	22 (18-30)	93	11 (4-30)	Many ISCs, target cells, nucleated RBCs	Positive	80-90 S / 2-20 F / <3.6 A₂	Uneven
SC	Mild-moderate	10 (9-14)	30 (26-40)	80	3 (1.5-6)	Many target cells, rare ISCs	Positive	45-55 S / 45-55 C	Uneven
S/B° thal	Moderate-severe	8.1 (7-12)	25 (20-36)	69	8 (3-18)	Marked hypochromia, microcytosis and target cells, variable ISCs	Positive	0.2-8 F / 50-85 S / 2-30 F / >3.6 A₂	Uneven
S/B + thal	Mild-moderate	11 (8-13)	32 (25-40)	76	3 (1.5-6)	Mild microcytosis, hypochromia, rare ISCs	Positive	55-75 S / 15-30 A / 1-20 F / >3.6 A₂	Uneven
S/HPFH†	Asymptomatic	14 (11-15)	40 (32-48)	84	1.5 (.5-3)	No ISCs, occasional target cells, and mild hypochromia	Positive	60-80 S / 15-35 F / 1-3 A₂	Even
AS	Asymptomatic	Normal	Normal	Normal	Normal	Normal	Positive	38-45 S / 60-55 A / 1-3 A₂	Uneven

From Vichinsky EP and Lubin BH: *Pediatr Clin North Am 27:429-447, 1980.*
*ISCs, irreversibly sickled cells.
†S/HPFH, sickle hereditary persistence of fetal hemoglobin.

clusion caused by collections of sickled RBCs (Vichinsky and Lubin, 1980).

Other children have anemia, which is detected during routine screening or during evaluation of an acute illness (Table 28-1). This anemia may be the child's baseline state or may be a result of one of the associated problems of sickle cell disease, such as aplastic crisis, hyperhemolytic crisis, or splenic sequestration. Recurrent or unusually severe infection may be a manifestation of sickle cell disease and its concomitant functional asplenia.

TREATMENT

There is no cure for sickle cell disease. Despite the thorough understanding that exists regarding the inheritance, diagnosis, and pathophysiology of sickle cell disease, treatment is essentially supportive and symptomatic. The current focus of treatment is on prevention by providing genetic counseling to those individuals with sickle trait, prenatal diagnosis for pregnant women who are at risk for delivering a child with sickle cell disease, and education for parents of children newly diagnosed.

An important aspect of treatment is the prevention of the sickling process whenever possible by preventing hypoxia and acidosis. This includes the aggressive treatment of infection, maintenance of optimal hydration and body temperature, and, when necessary, transfusion.

Research is currently being done to develop treatments and cures for sickle cell disease. The limited use of vasodilators has been studied, with potential for expanding their use. A prospective study was done using hydroxyurea to improve the solubility of the hemoglobin of adults with sickle cell disease by increasing the concentration of fetal hemoglobin (Rodgers et al., 1990). There is also research being done to develop antisickling agents. Bone marrow transplantation has beeen accomplished with a small number of selected individuals, but as yet the benefits are largely outweighed by the risks associated with the procedure. Genetic engineering may hold the potential for ultimately curing this disease.

PROGNOSIS

In a classic study done nearly 20 years ago, a group of adults and children was followed longitudinally to determine the natural history of sickle cell disease. It was determined that the disease effects in the adult tended to be chronic and organ related and that the problems during childhood were acute and often infectious. Overall there was a 10% expected death rate during the first decade of life and 5% or less during any subsequent decade (Powars, 1975).

In a large prospective study that followed nearly 3,000 children and adolescents for varying periods of time, the following information was obtained:

1. For all hemoglobinopathies the proportion of individuals expected to survive to age 20 years was approximately 89%.
2. Most of the deaths were in children with Hgb SS.
3. Peak incidence of death was between 1 and 3 years of age.
4. The major cause of death in children aged 1 to 3 years was infection.
5. In children greater than 10 years of age, cerebrovascular accident (CVA) and traumatic events were the major causes of death.
6. The survival of children with sickle cell disease is improving (Leikin, et al., 1989).

This improved survival has been attributed to newborn screening coupled with extensive follow-up and parent education (Vichinsky et al., 1988), and the initiation of antibiotic prophylaxis in early infancy (Gaston et al., 1986).

ASSOCIATED PROBLEMS

Associated problems primarily result from (1) blockage of small blood vessels secondary to the clumping of sickled RBCs that cause tissue ischemia, and (2) hemolytic anemia and its sequelae (Fig. 28-3).

Functional asplenia

Splenic function is normal at birth, but by 6 months of age a state of splenic dysfunction develops, most likely as a result of massive infarction (Pearson, 1987). With the absence of adequate splenic function, children with sickle cell disease are at high risk for infection. Intervention should be threefold: (1) aggressive management of infectious episodes; (2) timely immunization including pneumococcal and *Haemophilus influenzae* type b (Hib) vaccines; and (3) antibiotic prophylaxis.

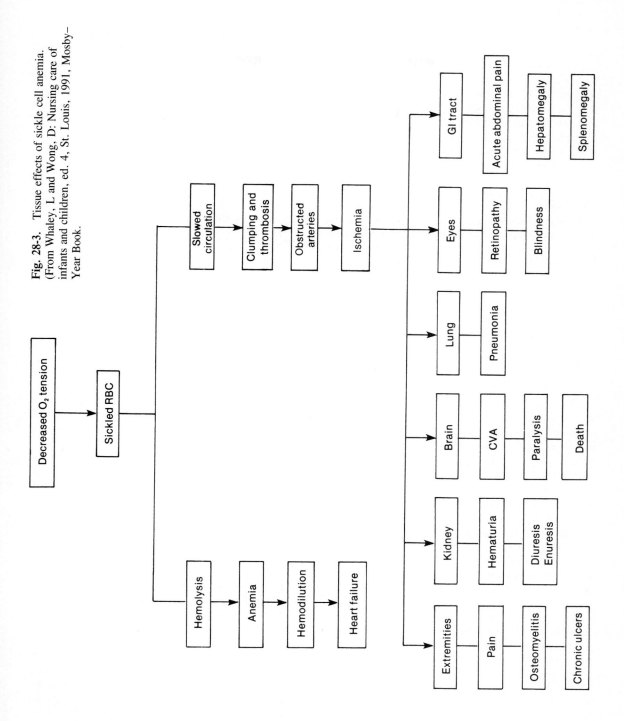

Fig. 28-3. Tissue effects of sickle cell anemia. (From Whaley, L and Wong, D: Nursing care of infants and children, ed. 4, St. Louis, 1991, Mosby–Year Book.

Because pneumococcal vaccines do not cover all pathogenic strains, antibiotic prophylaxis is the standard of care for all young children with sickle cell disease. It should be started at or before 2 months of age, and it is frequently easiest if started as soon as the diagnosis is made. The usual doses are as follows: penicillin, 125 mg twice daily for children less than age 3 years and 250 mg twice daily for those greater than 3 years of age. For children who are not compliant with oral antibiotic therapy at home, 500,000 to 1.2 million U of a long-acting penicillin may be given intramuscularly each month (Charache, Lubin, and Reid, 1989). For those children older than 5 years of age, the American Academy of Pediatrics Committee of Infectious Diseases suggests that strong consideration be given to continuing prophylaxis (Katz and Fernbach, 1988). The use of antibiotic prophylaxis in older children is currently being studied prospectively. As with other children taking antibiotics, the potential for monilial infections, gastrointestinal (GI) upset, and/or allergy exists. In the presence of penicillin allergy, other antibiotics may be used.

Splenic sequestration

In this condition blood flow into the spleen is adequate, but the vascular outflow system from the spleen to the systemic circulation is occluded. This results in a large collection of blood pooling in the spleen, causing significant enlargement. The systemic circulation may then be deprived of its needed blood volume, causing shock and cardiovascular collapse. The hemoglobin and hematocrit values fall, sometimes rapidly. Children with Hgb SS are susceptible to this at an early age (<5 years). Those with other variants of the disease may continue to be at risk for this until their teenage years because they maintain splenic circulation longer than children with Hgb SS.

Management requires hospitalization with immediate therapy, including transfusion. If shock is present, it will be necessary to support the systemic circulation with fluids. Once adequate circulation is reestablished, however, the volume of fluid previously sequestered in the spleen is returned to the circulation and circulatory overload must be avoided. For children who experience recurrent or severe episodes, splenectomy is indicated. Splenectomy, however, places the child at an increased risk of infection. It is optimal to splenectomize the child after the age of 2 years and after pneumococcal vaccine has been received. Children younger than 2 years of age who experience recurrent or severe episodes of splenic sequestration may be given regular transfusions in an effort to suppress the body's production of Hgb S and prevent further episodes of sequestration until splenectomy can safely be performed. A recent report suggests, however, that regular transfusions are of limited benefit to prevent recurrent episodes of sequestration (Kinney et al., 1990).

Neurologic problems

The vasculature of the brain is subject to vasoocclusive episodes in children with sickle cell disease; the frequency varies from 6% to 34% (Katz and Fernbach, 1988). When a blood vessel is partially occluded by a small embolus or vessel spasm, the manifestations may be focal and last less than 48 hours without residual deficit. This would be classified as a transient ischemic attack. When the affected vessel is completely occluded by thrombus or embolus with or without narrowing of the vessel lining, a CVA, or stroke, occurs. Intracranial hemorrhage is a rare but usually fatal complication that occurs when blood vessel walls are thinned by intravascular sickling then dilate and rupture (Charache, Lubin, and Reid, 1989). Acute treatment for CVA includes exchange transfusion, stabilization of cardiorespiratory function, and treatment of seizures, if present (see Chapter 15). After the acute phase a lengthy rehabilitation process may be needed. Some children have few or no deficits; others are neurologically devastated. As yet there are not adequate predictors of which children will develop strokes. Early identification of those children with a predisposition towards stroke may be facilitated by recent radiologic developments such as transcranial Doppler ultrasound (Rubin, 1991). It is known, however, that the recurrence rate is nearly 70% and that regular transfusions to maintain the circulating level of Hgb S at less than 30% greatly reduces this risk (Charache, Lubin, and Reid, 1989). Repeated RBC transfusions suppress bone marrow production of new RBCs that contain sickle hemoglobin. This is beneficial because it results in a minimal number of circulating RBCs that have the potential to become sickled and create further occlusion in the vascular bed. The necessary duration for transfusion on a regular basis is not known and probably is variable depending on the individual and the vasculature involved. Centers may give individuals transfusions for several years or may continue indefinitely (Wang et al., 1991; Wiznitzer et al., 1990).

Vasoocclusive crisis

Many sources cite painful, vasoocclusive episodes as the most common cause of emergency room visits and hospital admissions for individuals with sickle cell disease. The pattern of vasoocclusive episodes is quite variable among individuals with sickle cell disease. "Approximately one third of patients have one crisis every few years and another third have monthly to weekly crises. Interspersed between painful crises, the patient may be completely free of symptoms" (Vichinsky and Lubin, 1980, p. 433). The painful episode has been described as "the sudden onset of severe gnawing, throbbing pain that cannot be attributed to other causes" (Rozzell, Hijazi, and Pack, 1983, p. 185). The duration of episodes is also quite variable, from 1 day to 2 weeks.

Many health care providers attempt to discriminate between genuine vasoocclusive pain and "a child who is faking it." This is not necessary. A trusting relationship among the child, parent, and health care provider is essential for optimal care, and a suspicious attitude on the part of the health care provider can be much more harmful than the brief provision of fluids and analgesia. There are no hematologic parameters, including hemoglobin level, hematocrit value, or reticulocyte count, that prove or disprove the presence of pain; the child's self-report and the parents' and clinician's knowledge of the child's baseline behavior are the best indicators of the presence of pain. This is not to say that all complaints of pain are genuine; the possibility of secondary gain must be considered. However, given the inability to differentiate with certainty, a child who reports pain and is unable to perform the basic activities of living that the child enjoys must be believed.

The optimal treatment for vasoocclusive crises is multimodal and includes treating any antecedent causes, improving circulation, and providing analgesia. The treatment of antecedent causes includes correcting fever, hypoxia, and acidosis, treating infection, and rehydration.

Hydration is an important part of improving circulation to the affected area. The child may be hydrated orally or intravenously with an electrolyte solution. Options for oral hydration include juice, milk, Gatorade, Pedialyte, or Lytren. Fluids given intravenously may include a normal saline bolus, taking care not to tax the cardiovascular system with too large or rapid a bolus. Maintenance fluids of 5% dextrose with 0.45% normal saline are then given; this solution will replace excess sodium lost in the urine as a result of renal dysfunction in individuals with sickle cell disease. Potassium is added as needed after urinary output is established. The rate of fluids given should be approximately 1.5 times the maintenance dosage, or 2500 ml/m² daily. Circulation to infarcted areas may also be improved by the local application of heat (heating pad, warm bath, or whirlpool). Once comfort has been established, passive range of motion and massage may be initiated. The child should be encouraged to be as active as possible.

Analgesia may take several forms, including nonpharmacologic agents, nonnarcotic medicines, oral narcotics, or parenteral narcotics. Nonpharmacologic forms of pain relief include self-hypnosis, biofeedback, and distraction. They tend to be most useful in children who are willing and able to fantasize. Nonnarcotic medicines include acetaminophen, aspirin (provided there is no concurrent viral process or other contraindication), and ibuprofen. These may be given at the usual suggested dosages.

There are multiple narcotic agents from which to choose, and each child, health care provider, and institution are likely to have their preferences. At no time are placebos appropriate because they erode the trusting relationship between health care provider and child. The dose given should begin at a standard therapeutic dose or a dose known to be therapeutic for a given child and then adjusted as needed. It is inappropriate to administer intramuscular injections to children for pain relief because they themselves can be quite painful, unless it is for a single dose and a longer half-life is desired (e.g., for outpatient management) or unless IV access has not been obtained.

Many narcotics have very brief half-lives, and care must be taken to administer them frequently enough. For example, when a medication whose half-life is 1½ hours is used, dosing should be approximately every 2 hours to maintain consistent pain relief. Early in the course of a vasoocclusive episode, the vascular occlusion is constant, not intermittent. Later in the course, collateral circulation may develop or the occlusion may have decreased, improving circulation to the infarcted area. Thus, early in the course of a painful episode, pro re nata (prn) dosing is inappropriate. It is preferable to control the child's pain early in the course of the illness and maintain control. Children who become significantly uncomfortable experience anxiety and subsequently a heightened perception of pain.

It is important for the child, family, and health care providers to have goals related to pain control that are realistically attainable. The goal of pain management should not be the complete absence of pain but the reduction of pain to a manageable level. The alleviation of pain provided by narcotics needs to be balanced against their known side effects, such as pruritus, nausea, and constipation.

Shapiro (1989) cites several studies that document the low prevalence of drug addiction within this population. Despite these studies, health care providers continue to believe that drug addiction is a major problem among people with sickle cell disease. This is unfortunate because this misperception can interfere with the provision of adequate health care. The causes of this misperception are multiple; they include but are not limited to the rampant illicit drug problems in our society, cultural differences between the health care providers who are often white and clients who are often black, and the desire of most individuals who have chronic conditions to control some aspects of their treatment.

Pulmonary complications

Acute chest syndrome is a life-threatening complication that results from occlusions in the pulmonary vasculature, resulting in areas of infarcted lung tissue. The occlusion may be caused by localized sickling, thromboembolism, or embolism with collections of sickled cells, bone marrow, or marrow fat. It is characterized by acute chest pain, fever, and respiratory distress. It may be difficult to differentiate from, and in fact may be concurrent with, pneumonia. Physical examination usually reveals tachypnea; there may also be evidence of pulmonary consolidation, pleural effusion, or pleural friction rub. Chest x-ray studies may be normal for the first few days especially if the child is dehydrated. Lung scans may be useful but often are equivocal because a baseline study is rarely available for comparison.

Acute chest syndrome may be a fulminant process; admission to the intensive care unit may be necessary for close monitoring. Arterial blood gas levels should be followed closely; supplemental oxygen and further respiratory support should be provided as needed. Early transfusion may be necessary to prevent progressive problems because hypoxia will induce further sickling; partial or complete exchange transfusion may be needed (Charache, Lubin, and Reid, 1989).

Aplastic crisis

Periodically the bone marrow does not respond to a fall in hemoglobin and hematocrit values caused by the rapid turnover of RBCs. The hemoglobin and hematocrit values drop, and there is a lack of compensatory rise in the reticulocyte count. This usually happens during or following a viral infection. Thus, children being cared for during a viral illness should be observed for unusual pallor or prolonged lethargy in the face of improvement of other viral symptoms. Therapy includes slow transfusion to a hemoglobin level slightly above the baseline hemoglobin level. Recovery is indicated by a return of reticulocytosis.

Hyperhemolytic crisis

Occasionally there is increased hemolysis of the RBCs, further shortening their life span. This is indicated by a fall in the hemoglobin and hematocrit values and a profound rise in the reticulocyte count; there may be an elevation of the serum bilirubin level, and urobilinogen may be evident in the urine and stool. This process may be triggered by bacterial infection, poisons, or glucose-6-phosphate dehydrogenase deficiency. Treatment includes transfusion until the level of hemolysis returns to baseline levels and any antecedent causes are eliminated.

Renal problems

The environment within the renal medulla is characterized by low oxygen tension, acidosis, and hypertonicity. As such, intravascular sickling occurs more rapidly in the kidney than in any other organ. This leaves the kidney with a relative inability to concentrate urine (hyposthenuria) or adequately acidify the urine. The relative inability to concentrate urine often leads to enuresis or nocturia. It also results in a relative inability to excrete potassium and uric acid. Gross hematuria may occur in those with sickle cell disease or sickle trait. As with all individuals who have gross hematuria, glomerulonephritis, tumor, renal stones, urinary tract infection, and bleeding disorders need to be excluded. When other diagnoses have been eliminated, hematuria is often attributed to areas of ischemia or necrosis caused by sickled cells (Charache, Lubin, and Reid, 1989).

Priapism

Males with sickle cell anemia are subject to episodes of priapism. Priapism occurs when an accumulation of sickled cells obstructs the venous drainage of the corpora cavernosa of the penis, causing a prolonged and exquisitely painful erection of the penis. In one study there was a history of at least one episode of priapism in 42% of males with sickle cell anemia, with a median age of onset of 21 years. Two general patterns of priapism are described: (1) the "short, stuttering" attacks were brief (<3 hours) and recurrent, with a return to normal sexual functioning between episodes; and (2) the "major" episodes were lengthy (>24 hours) and were followed by partial or complete impotence (Emond et al., 1980).

Orthopedic skeletal changes

Skeletal changes as a result of expansion of the bone marrow and recurrent infarction are often seen in children with sickle cell disease. Repeated infarction may lead to avascular necrosis. This most commonly involves the femoral head but may also

occur in the head of the humerus or fibula. Treatment initially includes bed rest or bracing of the joint. Eventually if the child is unable to use the joint without pain, intervention in the form of prostheses or grafting may be necessary. Surgical treatment is not always successful, and the child may be left with some residual deficit and an increased risk for osteomyelitis (Charache, Lubin, and Reid, 1989).

Ophthalmologic changes

Ophthalmologic complications are a direct result of the vasoocclusive process within the eye. These complications include nonproliferative retinopathy, proliferative retinopathy, or elevated intraocular pressure in the presence of hyphema. Nonproliferative retinopathy may not affect visual acuity. Proliferative sickle retinopathy can cause vitreous hemorrhage and subsequent retinal detachment and blindness. The incidence of proliferative sickle retinopathy is dependent on the person's age and type of hemoglobinopathy. It generally begins in the late teens to midthirties, becoming more likely with increasing age. It is more common in people with Hgb SC but also occurs in other forms of sickle cell disease. Individuals with sickle hemoglobinopathies who sustain blunt trauma and subsequent hyphema to the eye may quickly develop increased intraocular pressure, which is an ophthalmologic emergency (Charache, Lubin, and Reid, 1989).

Audiologic problems

Vasoocclusive episodes within the circulation of the inner ear may cause sensorineural hearing loss. This loss may be unilateral or bilateral; it is generally manifested as a high-frequency deficit (Katz and Fernbach, 1988).

Leg ulcers

Leg ulcers are experienced by a significant number of older children and adults with sickle cell disease. The ulcers usually begin as a bite or scratch on the lower portion of the leg or the medial or lateral side of the ankle. Possibly a consequence of anemia (Pearson, 1987), leg ulcers are more likely caused by impaired circulation as a result of edema of the tissue surrounding the small initial injury (Noel, 1983). The ulcers may take 6 weeks to 6 months to heal. Treatment includes bed rest and wound care with antibiotics for cellulitic areas; skin grafting and transfusion therapy may be needed. The specific type of wound care is controversial and should be directed by a consultant plastic surgeon. Recurrence is very common (Katz and Fernbach, 1988).

Preparation for anesthesia or contrast medium

General anesthesia and hyperosmolar contrast medium are both known to induce sickling. If an operative or diagnostic procedure using these agents is anticipated, many health care providers suggest that the child with sickle cell disease receive repeated transfusions until the percentage of circulating Hb S is less than 30%.

Cardiac problems

Over time the cardiovascular system accommodates chronic anemia. Cardiac enlargement is often apparent on chest radiograph and a low-grade systolic ejection murmur is often found. Exercise-related cardiac dysfunction has been documented in children with sickle cell disease. This dysfunction was demonstrated to be nonprogressive, and exercise tolerance was directly related to hemoglobin and hematocrit levels (Alpert et al., 1984).

Hepatobiliary problems

The ongoing elevated rate of RBC hemolysis generates an increase in bilirubin load for metabolism. An elevation of the serum alkaline phosphatase and lactic dehydrogenase levels as a result of bone metabolism and hemolysis is frequently seen. Gallstones made of bile or calcium bilirubinate are a common finding and are easily visualized by ultrasound. They are found in 23% to 30% of children with sickle cell disease and are most common in individuals with Hgb SS (Charache, Lubin, and Reid, 1989; Rennels et al., 1984).

Transfusion complications

Individuals with sickle cell disease may need transfusions emergently, episodically, or chronically. The complications of transfusion include possible exposure to bloodborne infectious agents, formation of alloantibodies, and, with chronic or multiple transfusion, iron overload. Individuals with iron overload experience progressive organ dysfunction. Iron chelation is a difficult process, and an efficient, easily administered chelating agent does not currently exist.

Psychosocial problems

Children with sickle cell disease must learn to accommodate chronic recurrent pain and the potential for sudden or premature death. In a study that examined anxiety, self-concept, and personal and social adjustment in children with sickle cell anemia, it was demonstrated that these children did not differ from their healthy peers in personal, social, and total adjustments. They did, however, demonstrate a lower self-concept. Interestingly, they were also found to be less acutely anxious than their healthy peers (Kumar et al., 1976).

PRIMARY CARE MANAGEMENT
Growth and development

Children with sickle cell disease, when matched with controls of similar socioeconomic status, have comparable physical parameters at birth, including weight, length, and head circumference, as well as similar 1- and 5-minute Apgar scores. Beginning at approximately 6 months of age, and clearly defined by the preschool years, these children demonstrate a pattern of physical growth that is divergent from that of their nonaffected peers. They are shorter, weigh less (Fig. 28-4), have a smaller percentage of body fat, and have delayed bone age. Muscle mass and head circumference, however, remain comparable with that of their nonaffected peers (Kramer et al., 1980). Weight is affected more than height (Platt, Rosenstock, and Espeland, 1984), and males are affected more than females (Phebus, Gloninger and Maciak, 1984).

These changes are coincident with the usual physiologic waning of fetal hemoglobin levels. It has also been noted that children who, for unknown reasons, persist in producing fetal hemoglobin are usually not as growth retarded as other children with sickle cell disease (Kramer et al., 1980). Nutritional factors alone do not explain growth delays in children with sickle cell disease (Finan et al., 1988).

As with standard well child care, physical growth parameters should be measured and plotted

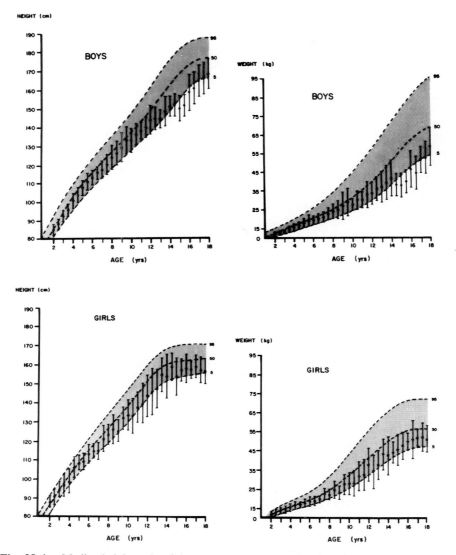

Fig. 28-4. Median height and weight measurements ($\pm$ 1 SD) in male and female patients with SCD at ages 2 to 18 years compared with National Center for Health Statistics growth percentiles. (From Phebus, CK, Gloninger, MF and Maciak, BJ: Growth patterns by age and sex in children with sickle cell disease, J Pediatr, 105:28-33, 1984.)

on standardized growth charts at regular intervals. If the pattern of growth begins to plateau or become otherwise abnormal, serial measurements should be obtained more frequently.

Longitudinal studies of the neuropsychologic development of children with sickle cell disease are needed. Chadorkoff and Whitten's study (cited in Swift et al., 1989), they concluded that sickle cell anemia did not affect intellectual or psychologic functioning. Another recent study suggested that children with sickle cell anemia have some degree of cognitive impairment but that academic achievement was comparable with intellectual ability. This study examined children aged 7 through 16 years without history of strokes. The data suggest that the onset of impairment occurred before 7 years of age (Swift et al., 1989).

Standardized tools such as the Denver Developmental Screening Test are helpful when one is screening for developmental delay. Children found to be at developmental risk should be referred for a more thorough developmental assessment. The involvement of a consistent care giver and the care giver's rapport with a consistent health care provider are invaluable tools for monitoring developmental progress in the child with sickle cell disease.

Immunizations

The conventional schedule may be used for diphtheria-pertussis-tetanus (DPT) vaccine, oral poliomyelitis vaccine (OPV), measles-mumps-rubella vaccine, and Hib vaccine. The risk of *H. influenzae* septicemia or meningitis is 4 times greater in this population (Committee on Infectious Disease, 1991; Katz and Fernbach, 1988). It is important to note that children younger than 6 years of age with sickle cell disease may not develop a reliably immunogenic response to the Hib vaccine (Rubin, Voulalas, and Carmody, 1989); therefore, even an immunized child may be vulnerable to infection by this organism.

Pneumococcal vaccine (Pneumovax) should be given at age 2 years to all children with sickle cell disease; booster immunization should be given every 3 to 5 years (Weintrub, et al., 1984). It is important to emphasize that even with vigilant immunization and antibiotic prophylaxis, episodes of pneumococcal septicemia have occurred (Buchanan and Smith, 1986).

Because the risk of contracting hepatitis B from blood transfusion is approximately 0.4% per unit (Sarnaik, Merline, and Bond, 1988), protection against hepatitis B is very important. Children with sickle cell disease respond normally to the vaccine (Sarnaik, Merline, and Bond, 1988). The usual schedule of immunization is an initial dose, a second dose 1 month later, and a final dose 6 months after the initial one. Serum conversion should be documented 1 month or more after the final dose. Because of the rather lengthy course of immunization and the relative lack of deleterious effects experienced with this vaccine, many centers empirically immunize their children against hepatitis B in infancy. It is expedient to begin the immunization series at the first clinic visit so that the series is likely to be completed before the infant is symptomatic from the disease. It may be given concurrently with the DPT, OPV, and Hib vaccine.

Children with hemoglobinopathies are identified as being at risk for influenza-related complications. Also, children with sickle cell disease are known to be at high risk for bacterial infection, and this risk could be further raised by concurrent viral infection (Glezen, Glezen, and Alcorn, 1983). Therefore it is recommended that all children with sickle cell disease receive influenza vaccine on an annual basis.

Opinions regarding the use of meningococcal vaccine are divergent. Some centers suggest administering the vaccine to children more than 2 years of age (Katz and Fernbach, 1988), but this is not uniform among all comprehensive care centers.

Screening

Vision. During the first decade of life, the child with sickle cell disease requires routine screening. Thereafter the child needs an annual retinal examination by an ophthalmologist to screen for sickle retinopathy.

Hearing. Yearly audiologic evaluations are optimal to screen for hearing loss related to vasoocclusion in the inner ear.

Dental. Routine screening is recommended.

Blood pressure. Blood pressure should be measured every 6 months after 2 years of age. This is especially important because of the occurrence of occult hypertension among black Americans.

Hematocrit. Hematocrit testing is deferred because a CBC is required every 6 months.

Urinalysis. Urinalysis is deferred because of annual renal function testing.

Tuberculin. Routine screening is recommended.

Condition-specific screening

HEMATOLOGIC SCREENING. A CBC with differential, RBC smear, and reticulocyte count is useful in establishing baseline data and ascertaining bone marrow function. It is very useful to determine the RBC phenotype and alloantibodies of a well child who has not had a transfusion to possibly expedite any future transfusions.

RENAL FUNCTION TESTING. A urinalysis should be done and the blood urea nitrogen (BUN) and creatinine levels checked annually to monitor renal function. An inability to concentrate or to acidify urine may be demonstrated in the urinalysis and would be commonly seen in children with sickle cell disease. Urobilinogen, as a by-product of bilirubin metabolism, would also be a frequent finding. Hematuria may be a manifestation of renal dysfunction secondary to sickle cell disease or other, unrelated, pathologic condition. The child should be referred to a nephrologist for further evaluation and treatment if the hematuria is severe or if casts are present in the urine.

LEAD POISONING. Determining erythrocyte protoporphyrin (EP) levels to screen children who may be at high risk for lead intoxication is not valid for children with sickle cell disease. Total EP levels may be elevated with iron deficiency, lead intoxication, or reticulocytosis. In a child with sickle cell disease, an elevated EP level may reflect the process of accelerated reticulocytosis rather than lead intoxication (Tigner-Weekes et al., 1979).

SCOLIOSIS. Scoliosis screening should be done through late adolescence because of the delayed growth spurt of the child with sickle cell disease.

CARDIAC FUNCTION. Electrocardiography (ECG) and echocardiography (ECHO) should be performed every 1 to 2 years to evaluate the impact of chronic anemia on ventricular function.

LIVER FUNCTION. Yearly liver function studies are helpful to evaluate RBC metabolism and liver function.

Drug interactions

Antihistamines and barbiturates given concurrently with narcotics may cause respiratory depression, hypoxia, and further sickling. Diuretics and some bronchodilators, which have a diuretic effect, may cause dehydration and sickling. They should be used with caution in children with sickle cell disease.

DIFFERENTIAL DIAGNOSIS AND MANAGEMENT OF COMMON PEDIATRIC CONDITIONS
Infections

As a result of functional asplenia, bacterial infection is a significant cause of morbidity and mortality in children with sickle cell disease. The incidence of bacteremia in children with sickle cell disease is highest among those less than 2 years of age, and it declines from age 2 to 6 years. The most common pathogen in children younger than 6 years is *Streptococcus pneumoniae.* The course of *S. pneumoniae* sepsis is often fulminant, with mortality reaching 24% to 50%. *Escherichia coli* bacteremia is often associated with urinary tract infection and *Salmonella* bacteremia with osteomyelitis (Pearson, 1987; Zarkowsky et al., 1986).

Fever is a common finding during vasoocclusive episodes, as well as during infectious episodes. There is no test or diagnostic tool to differentiate fever of an infectious origin from fever that results from inflammation secondary to infarction.

A child less than 5 years of age who has a low-grade temperature elevation (<38.5° C) may be given appropriate antibiotic coverage and treated as an outpatient, provided a probable cause of temperature elevation can be identified and the child is stable and looks well clinically. There should be careful follow-up by telephone or clinic visit in 24 to 48 hours. Research is being done to determine the feasibility of outpatient management of fever in the young child with sickle cell anemia, but currently a child less than 5 years of age with a temperature of more than 38.5° C must be admitted to the hospital (Rogers et al., 1990). An aggressive search for the cause should include a CBC count, blood culture, urinalysis, urine culture, chest radiograph, and possibly sinus radiographs. Lumbar puncture should be performed if there is any suspicion of meningitis. Intravenous antibiotic therapy with broad-spectrum antibiotics should be instituted. The course of treatment should be based on the child's clinical course and culture results; the child should be hospitalized for a minimum of 48 to 72 hours.

In children older than 5 years of age with temperatures more than 38.5° C, an aggressive search for the likely cause should be undertaken and antibiotics administered. The location of treatment, inpatient or outpatient, should depend on the following: the child's clinical condition, anticipated compliance with therapy, and ability to obtain follow-up over the upcoming 24 to 72 hours (Charache, Lubin, and Reid, 1989; Katz and Fernbach, 1988).

Even common infections such as otitis media or sinusitis may precipitate a vasoocclusive crisis if fluid intake is reduced and dehydration and acidosis result. During periods of illness, the child must be assessed frequently for early signs of crisis. Maintaining fluid intake and controlling fever are critical.

Urinary tract infections

Asymptomatic bacteriuria, symptomatic urinary tract infection, and pyelonephritis occur much more commonly in individuals with sickle cell disease than in the general population. In the presence of urinary tract infection or pyelonephritis, the child should have a blood culture obtained because bacteremia is present in at least 50% of those with urinary tract infection (Katz and Fernbach, 1988). Appropriate antibiotic therapy should be instituted and adequate follow-up arranged. Follow-up should include a repeat culture. Further diagnostic studies such as renal ultrasound or voiding cystourethrogram should be done to exclude treatable conditions in children with pyelonephritis or recurrent urinary tract infection.

Orthopedic symptoms

Areas of bone infarction may be easily confused with osteomyelitis or rheumatologic disorders. Even after the diagnosis of sickle cell disease is

made, it is important to differentiate areas of infarction from areas of infection because children with sickle cell disease have an increased incidence of osteomyelitis. In both pathologic processes the child may have an elevated white blood cell count, fever, and equivocal x-ray findings. Osteomyelitis, however, is more often associated with an increased number of immature granulocytes, bacteremia, and a purulent joint aspirate. Bone scans may be useful in differentiating osteomyelitis from areas of bone infarction. Bone marrow scans have also been used to further discriminate between areas of infection and infarction, especially when the bone scan is equivocal. Opinions regarding the use of the bone marrow scan are somewhat divergent, however, and are largely dependent on the level of expertise available at a given facility.

Acute gastroenteritis

Vomiting and diarrhea must be carefully evaluated and managed in children with sickle cell disease because these children lack the ability to concentrate urine to compensate for decreased fluid intake or excess losses. Significant dehydration may occur quickly and lead to metabolic acidosis and sickling. If the child's oral fluid intake is less than that needed to maintain hydration, the child must receive IV hydration, often as an inpatient.

Abdominal pain

Episodes of infarction of the abdominal organs such as the liver, spleen, and abdominal lymph nodes occur and may be quite painful. It is important to differentiate these abdominal crises from those problems that would require surgical intervention, such as appendicitis. Abdominal crises are associated with (1) little or no fever; (2) no significant hematologic changes; (3) persistence of peristaltic activity; and (4) response to symptomatic, supportive therapy (Miller and Baehner, 1989). If the abdominal pain is localized to the right upper quadrant and occurs with fever, jaundice, and an elevation of the conjugated bilirubin level, the possibility of cholecystitis must be considered and an abdominal ultrasound obtained. Most children find that their sickle cell pain has a unique quality or character and are often able to report whether or not the pain they are having is typical of their vasoocclusive pain.

Anemia

Virtually all children with sickle cell disease are anemic at baseline. Periodically a child with sickle cell disease may have acute lethargy and pallor. A CBC and reticulocyte count should be obtained. If these reveal a significant drop in the hemoglobin and hematocrit levels, it is likely that the child is experiencing an aplastic crisis, hyperhemolytic crisis, or splenic sequestration. Usually a fall in the hemoglobin and hematocrit values serves as a stimulus to the bone marrow, which then produces new RBCs in the form of reticulocytes. If the reticulocyte count is low in the presence of low hemoglobin and hematocrit levels, the child is experiencing an aplastic crisis. If the reticulocyte count is very high and there is evidence of an elevated bilirubin level, it is likely to be a hyperhemolytic episode. If the child's spleen is enlarged, he or she is likely to be experiencing splenic sequestration. Regardless of exact diagnosis, the child will require immediate hospitalization, with close observation and transfusion.

Respiratory distress

Increased respiratory rate and effort, chest pain, fever, rales, and dullness to percussion may indicate pneumonia or acute chest syndrome. Infiltrates on chest radiograph may reflect either process. With acute chest syndrome the chest radiograph may be clear in the first few days; a pleural effusion is frequently seen. The child should receive antibiotics, hydration, analgesics, and oxygen as needed. Transfusion or partial exchange transfusion may be indicated, depending on the degree of respiratory distress.

Neurologic changes

The child who has a seizure, hemiparesis, or changes in speech, gait, level of consciousness, or blurry or double vision should have expedient neurologic and radiologic evaluation for the presence of stroke. This is a medical emergency and requires exchange transfusion as soon as possible.

DEVELOPMENTAL ISSUES
Safety

Most children with sickle cell anemia regularly take medicines orally at home, such as folic acid, antibiotics, and narcotics. It is unlikely that the accidental ingestion of the folate or antibiotics would be dangerous, but ingestion of narcotics could lead to lethargy and respiratory depression or death. All medicines should be safely stored. Adolescents should be cautioned about driving a car or using machinery while taking narcotics and that substances such as alcohol may potentiate the depressant effects of narcotics. Alcohol should also be avoided because it can cause dehydration and subsequent sickling.

Recreational activities that involve prolonged exposure to cold, prolonged exertion, or exposure to high altitudes ($>$10,000 feet) in an unpressurized aircraft should be avoided. Sports injuries should not be treated with ice, because this can cause localized sickling. Adolescents with sickle cell disease often demonstrate the same limit-testing and risk-taking behaviors as other adolescents. Parents must balance their child's need for safety with the child's need to become self-sufficient. An information card or medical alert bracelet is often helpful in emergency situations.

Child care

Children with sickle cell disease can participate in normal day-care centers, although small group or home-centered day care may be preferable because it provides less exposure to infections. The care giver will need to be informed of the child's need for extra fluids and need to void frequently. They may also need to administer medications during day-care hours and must be instructed in this regard. The care giver needs to be able to contact the parent or seek medical care for the child quickly in the event of fever, severely painful vasoocclusive crisis, respiratory distress, or stroke, because these events may be life threatening.

Diet

The child's diet should be well balanced with a generous amount of fluid. Diet during illness or disease exacerbation may include whatever healthy solid foods the child desires with oral fluids at 1½ times his or her usual fluid intake. Supplemental folate requirements may be met by the administration of folate tablets, 1 mg daily. Children who are receiving chronic transfusions should limit their oral intake of vitamin C–rich foods, because the presence of vitamin C will enhance the GI absorption of iron and may worsen the iron overload inherent in the chronic transfusion process.

Discipline

The expectations regarding the behavior of children with sickle cell disease should vary little from the expectations held for their siblings or peers. These expectations should be clear and as consistent as possible. Likewise, the parent should strive to make discipline fair and consistent. Many parents are fearful of disciplining or setting limits for their children with sickle cell disease, especially because emotional stress is thought to possibly precipitate vasoocclusive crisis. The health care provider can point out to the parent that a lack of or inconsistently set limits may, in fact, be more stressful to the child than consistently set limits. It is also important to encourage the parent to learn which behaviors the child demonstrates consistently when in pain, such as a certain pitch to his or her cry, a change in activity level, or changes in appetite. This will help the parent discriminate episodes of pain from episodes when the parent is being manipulated.

Toileting

Toilet training should be initiated using the conventional guidelines to assess readiness for training. Bowel training usually progresses without difficulty. Bladder training, however, must take into account the fact that many children with sickle cell disease have difficulty concentrating urine and thus produce a large volume of dilute urine. They may need to be given the opportunity to use the bathroom every 2 to 3 hours during the day. At night the parent may initially choose to continue using diapers. By the time the child reaches preschool or school age, however, the use of diapers will often adversely affect the child's self-esteem and sense of mastery. Many families choose to wake the child once or twice during the night to urinate. It is not uncommon for enuresis to continue into the teenage years and is especially troublesome when the child requires extra fluids during a vasoocclusive episode.

Sleep patterns

Because of chronic anemia, some children with sickle cell disease may fatigue more easily than their nonaffected peers and desire extra sleep.

School issues

Some children with sickle cell disease have frequent school absences because of illness and may be reluctant to return to school for fear of having fallen behind during their absence. The absences are often not predictable. Tutoring, offered in the hospital, school, or home, is often quite helpful in maintaining performance and self-esteem.

While at school children with sickle cell disease need to have more access to fluids than their peers. They may carry a thermos with them or be excused to go to the water fountain. They also need to be given the opportunity to go to the restroom at least every 2 to 3 hours. Children with sickle cell disease should be encouraged to participate in mainstream physical education as much as possible. They may tire quickly but should be able to rejoin the activity after resting until they have returned to their baseline energy level. Those children who have sustained strokes, severe leg ulcers, avascular necrosis of bones with recurrent infarcts, or other debilitating consequences of their disease may need to have a physical education program modified to meet their special needs.

Sexuality

Children with sickle cell disease progress through the Tanner stages in an orderly and consistent manner but usually experience puberty several years later than their peers. This can have significant adverse effects on the adolescent's self-concept. Once sexual maturation has occurred, fertility and contraception become important issues that must be addressed by the health care provider.

For men, impotence is often a problem following a major episode of priapism. Even if sexual function is normal, infertility or subfertility as a result of alterations in the concentration, morphology, and motility of their sperm is common (Osegbe, Amaku, and Akinyanju, 1981). For female adolescents, menarche is often delayed by 2 to 2½ years, but fertility is normal. Decisions regarding contraception must take into account the attitudes, life-style, and maturity of the adolescent, as well as the hematologic ramifications of the method chosen. Sickle cell disease is not a contraindication for the use of oral contraceptives, but many health care providers encourage the use of low-dose estrogen or progesterone-only pills because estrogen is believed to induce sickling. Also, oral contraceptives are known to elevate plasma levels of triglycerides and phospholipids, which may increase the already elevated risk of stroke in individuals with sickle cell disease (Walters et al., 1983). Adolescents with sickle cell disease should receive careful, repeated genetic counseling before puberty and during adolescence. They need to understand the pattern of transmission of sickle cell disease and the availability of testing for partners before conceiving a child.

FAMILY CONCERNS

The families of children with sickle cell disease experience the same psychologic ramifications as do other families of children with chronic conditions. They bear the additional burden of knowing that this disease is genetically transmitted; this knowledge can prompt feelings of overwhelming guilt and responsibility. Exacerbations of the condition often occur without provocation, prompting feelings of helplessness. Many manifestations of the condition are not objectively visible or measurable; therefore, children with sickle cell disease can appear to be well when they are potentially extremely ill. Many parents are fearful that the therapeutic effects of narcotics and blood transfusions will be outweighed by their deleterious effects.

Genetic counseling should be offered to the parents of a child with sickle cell disease at the time of the child's diagnosis and when subsequent pregnancies are contemplated. It is also recommended that the child's siblings be screened to determine their carrier status.

SUMMARY OF PRIMARY CARE NEEDS FOR THE CHILD WITH SICKLE CELL DISEASE

Growth and development

These children tend to weigh less and be shorter than their peers; weight is affected more than height, and males are affected more than females.

Puberty is delayed for both sexes.

Developmental impairment varies.

Immunizations

Routine standard immunizations are recommended.

Haemophilus influenzae type b vaccine is given at 2, 4, and 6 months; immunogenic response is not reliable.

Pneumococcal vaccine is given at 24 months, with boosters given every 3 to 5 years thereafter.

Hepatitis vaccine is strongly recommended.

Influenza vaccine given annually is strongly recommended.

Screening
Vision

Routine screening is recommended until 10 years of age, then an annual retinal examination is recommended to rule out sickle retinopathy.

Hearing

Yearly audiologic examination is recommended.

Dental

Routine screening is recommended.

Blood pressure

Blood pressure should be measured every 6 months after 2 years of age.

Hematocrit

Hematocrit is deferred because of condition-specific screening.

Urinalysis

Urinalysis is deferred because of condition-specific screening.

Tuberculosis

Routine screening is recommended.

Condition-specific screening

Hematologic screening

A CBC with differential, reticulocyte count, and RBC smear should be checked every 6 months.

Renal function screening

The BUN and creatinine levels should be checked and a urinalysis done on a yearly basis.

Lead poisoning

Lead screening using the EP level is unreliable; the serum lead level must be determined.

Scoliosis

Screening should be extended to the late teens because of delayed puberty.

Cardiac function

Both ECG and ECHO should be used every 1 to 2 years after age 5.

Liver function

Serum liver function tests should be done yearly. The gallbladder should be assessed using ultrasound every 2 years after age 10.

Drug interactions

Antihistamines and barbiturates may potentiate narcotics.

Diuretics and bronchodilators, which may have diuretic effects, may cause dehydration and sickling.

Differential diagnosis
Fever

Age 5 years or less

TEMPERATURE LESS THAN 38.5°C

Outpatient management may be considered if the source of the fever can be identified, appropriate antibiotics are given, and follow-up is ensured.

TEMPERATURE MORE THAN 38.5°C

The child should be admitted to the hospital for fever work-up, parenteral antibiotics, and observation.

Age 5 years or more

The child's condition, compliance with therapy, and ability to obtain follow-up determine whether or not he or she should receive inpatient or outpatient care.

SUMMARY OF PRIMARY CARE NEEDS FOR THE CHILD
WITH SICKLE CELL DISEASE — cont'd

Acute gastroenteritis

Significant dehydration may occur quickly and lead to acidosis and sickling. If oral intake is inadequate, IV hydration is needed.

Abdominal pain

Abdominal pain crisis may be differentiated from surgical problems by evaluating fever, hematologic changes, peristalsis, and response to symptomatic, supportive therapy.

Anemia

Hemoglobin and hematocrit levels significantly lower than baseline levels may reflect aplastic crisis, hyperhemolytic crisis, or splenic sequestration. Splenic sequestration may be life threatening.

Respiratory distress

It is important to evaluate the patient for acute chest syndrome, which may be fulminant and require exchange transfusion.

Neurologic changes

Neurologic changes may indicate stroke. Rapid, thorough evaluation is critical. Exchange transfusion should be performed as quickly as possible if stroke occurs.

Developmental issues
Safety

Ingestion of narcotics could lead to respiratory depression.
Alcohol may dehydrate and potentiate narcotics.
Narcotics may impair driving or safe use of machinery.
Recreational activities that involve prolonged exposure to cold, prolonged exertion, or exposure to high altitudes should be avoided. Ice should not be used to treat injuries.
A medical alert bracelet may be helpful.

Diet

Diet should be well balanced with a generous amount of fluid; fluid intake should be in-creased during illness. Supplemental folate requirements may be met with folate tablets, 1 mg daily. Children who are receiving chronic transfusions should limit their oral intake of vitamin C-rich foods to limit iron overload.

Child care

The care giver needs to be mindful of fluid requirements and the importance of maintaining normal body temperature and must be able to administer medicines.

Discipline

Expectations should be consistent, fair, and similar to those of peers and siblings.

Toileting

Enuresis is frequently a long-term issue because of a large volume of dilute urine.
Nocturia may persist.

Sleep patterns

Routine care is recommended.

School issues

The child may have frequent, unpredictable absences. While at school, the child needs access to fluids and liberal bathroom privileges. He or she may participate in mainstream physical education.

Sexuality

Puberty may be delayed. Men may have fertility problems. Women usually have normal fertility but have some special contraceptive concerns.

Special family concerns

Because sickle cell disease is genetically transmitted, there is a need for genetic counseling, as well as support for feelings of guilt and responsibility.

RESOURCES
Organizations

National Association for Sickle Cell Disease, Inc
4221 Wilshire Blvd, Suite 360
Los Angeles, CA 90010-3506
(800) 421-8453 (outside California)
   This is a national organization with local community-based chapters. It offers education, counseling, and support services to families of children with sickle cell disease. Many local branches of this organization also coordinate a summer camp for children with sickle cell disease.

REFERENCES

Alpert BS, Dover EV, Strong WB, et al: Longitudinal exercise hemodynamics in children with sickle cell anemia, *Am J Dis Child* 138:1021-1024, 1984.

American Academy of Pediatrics: Policy statement: *Haemophilus influenzae* type b conjugated vaccines: Immunization of children at 15 months of age, *AAP News,* July 1990, p 10.

Buchanan GR and Smith SJ: Pneumococcal septicemia despite pneumococcal vaccine and prescription of penicillin prophylaxis in children with sickle cell anemia, *Am J Dis Child* 140:428-431, 1986.

Charache S, Lubin B, and Reid CD: *Management and therapy of sickle cell disease,* NIH publication No 89-2117, Washington, DC, 1989, US Government Printing Office.

Emond AM, Holman R, Hayes RJ, et al: Priapism and impotence in homozygous sickle cell disease, *Arch Internal Med* 140:1434-1437, 1980.

Finan AC, Elmer MA, Sasanow SR, et al: Nutritional factors and growth in children with sickle cell disease, *Am J Dis Child* 142:237-240, 1988.

Gaston MH, Verter JI, Woods G, et al: Prophylaxis with oral penicillin in children with sickle cell anemia: A randomized trial *N Engl J Med* 314:1593-1599, 1986.

Glezen WP, Glezen LS, and Alcorn R: Trivalent, inactivated influenza virus vaccine in children with sickle cell disease, *Am J Dis Child* 137:1095-1097, 1983.

Hockenberry M and Coody D, eds: *Pediatric oncology and hematology: Perspectives on care,* St Louis, 1986, CV Mosby.

Katz JA and Fernbach DJ: *Guidelines for management of pediatric patients with sickle cell anemia,* Houston, 1988, Texas Children's Hospital.

Kinney TR, Ware RE, Schultz WH, et al: Long-term management of splenic sequestration in children with sickle cell disease, *J Pediatr* 117:194-199, 1990.

Kramer MS, Rooks Y, Washington LA, et al: Pre- and postnatal growth and development in sickle cell anemia, *J Pediatr* 96:857-860, 1980.

Kumar S, Powars D, Allen J, et al: Anxiety, self-concept and personal and social adjustments in children with sickle cell anemia, *J Pediatr* 88:859-863, 1976.

Leikin SL, Gallagher D, Kinney TR, et al: Mortality in children and adolescents with sickle cell disease, *Pediatrics* 84:500-508, 1989.

Miller DR and Baehner RL, eds: *Blood diseases of infancy and childhood,* St Louis, 1989, CV Mosby.

Noel C: Leg ulcers, *Nurs Clin North Am* 18:155-159, 1983.

Osegbe DN, Amaku EO, and Akinyanju O: Fertility in males with sickle cell disease, *Lancet* 2:275-276, 1981.

Pearson HA: Sickle cell diseases: Diagnosis and management in infancy and childhood, *Pediatr Rev* 9:121-130, 1987.

Pearson HA: Neonatal testing for sickle cell diseases—a historical and personal review, *Pediatrics* 83:815-818, 1989.

Phebus CK, Gloninger MF, and Maciak BJ: Growth patterns by age and sex in children with sickle cell disease, *J Pediatr* 105:28-33, 1984.

Platt OS, Rosenstock W, and Espeland MA: Influence of sickle hemoglobinopathies on growth and development, *New Engl J Med* 311:7-12, 1984.

Powars DR: Natural history of sickle cell disease—the first ten years, *Semin Hematol* 12:267-281, 1975.

Rennels MB, Dunne MG, Grossman NJ, et al: Cholelithiasis in patients with major sickle hemoglobinopathies, *Am J Dis Child* 138:66-67, 1984.

Rodgers GP, Dover GJ, Noguchi CT, et al: Hematologic responses of patients with sickle cell disease to treatment with hydroxyurea, *N Engl J Med* 322:1037-1045, 1990.

Rogers ZR, Morrison RA, Vedro DA, et al: Outpatient management of febrile illness in infants and young children with sickle cell anemia, *J Pediatr* 117:736-739, 1990.

Rozzell MS, Hijazi M and Pack B: The painful episode, *Nurs Clin North Am* 18:185-199, 1983.

Rubin LG, Voulalas D, and Carmody L: Immunization of children with sickle cell disease with *Haemophilus influenzae* type b polysaccharide vaccine, *Pediatrics* 84:509-513, 1989.

Rubin W: Doppler may help assess stroke risk in sickle cell, *Pediatric News,* March 1991, p. 2.

Sarnaik SA, Merline JR, and Bond S: Immunogenicity of hepatitis b vaccine in children with sickle cell anemia, *J Pediatr* 112:429-430, 1988.

Shapiro B: The management of pain in sickle cell disease, *Pediatr Clin North Am* 36:1029-1044, 1989.

Swift AV, Cohen MJ, Hynd GW, et al: Neuropsychologic impairment in children with sickle cell anemia, *Pediatrics* 84:1077-1085, 1989.

Tigner-Weekes L, Pegelow C, Lee S, et al: Lead screening in sickle cell disease, *J Pediatr* 95:738-740, 1979.

Vichinsky E, Hurst D, Earles A, et al: Newborn screening for sickle cell disease: Effect on mortality, *Pediatrics* 81:749-755, 1988.

Vichinsky EP and Lubin BH: Sickle cell anemia and related hemoglobinopathies, *Pediatr Clin North Am* 27:429-447, 1980.

Walters I, Baysinger M, Buchanan I, et al: Complication of sickle cell disease, *Nurs Clin North Am* 18:139-184, 1983.

Wang WC, Kovnar EH, Tonkin IL, et al: High risk of recurrent stroke after discontinuance of 5 to 12 years of transfusion therapy in patients with sickle cell disease, *J Pediatr,* 118:377-382.

Weintrub PS, Schiffman G, Addiego JE, et al: Long-term follow-up and booster immunization with polyvalent pneumococcal polysaccharide in patients with sickle cell anemia, *J Pediatr* 105:261-263, 1984.

Whaley LF and Wong DL: *Nursing care of infants and children,* ed 3, St Louis, 1988, CV Mosby.

Wiznitzer M, Ruggieri PM, Masaryk TJ, et al: Diagnosis of cerebrovascular disease in sickle cell anemia by magnetic resonance angiography, *J Pediatr* 117:551-555, 1990.

Zarkowsky HS, Gallagher D, Gill FM, et al: Bacteremia in sickle hemoglobinopathies, *J Pediatr* 109:579-585, 1986.

Appendix — Additional Resources

··

AboutFace
99 Crowns Lane, 3rd Floor
Toronto, Ontario
Canada M5R 3P4
(416) 944-3223

The goals of the organization are to link and educate affected individuals, their families, and professionals; educate professionals and the public; and assist in providing advocacy services for those with facial disfigurement.

Allergy Information Center
54 Tromley Drive, Suite 10
Etobicoke, Ontario
Canada M9B 5Y7

This organization is designed to help individuals gain control over their allergy symptoms, thus improving their overall health. A variety of services including periodic reports, a quarterly magazine, and allergy cookbooks (designed for individuals with food allergies) are all published by this organization.

The Alliance of Genetic Support Groups
38th and R Streets, NW
Washington, DC 20057
(202) 331-0942

This alliance is a resource for consumers seeking genetic support groups as well as for genetic counselors and other professionals. Instruction on initiating support groups and advocacy services and a variety of published literature are available.

American Juvenile Arthritis Organization
  (AJAO)
Arthritis Foundation
1314 Spring Street, NW
Atlanta, GA 30309
(404) 872-7100

AJAO is a national membership association of the Arthritis Foundation that serves the special needs of young people with arthritis or rheumatic diseases and their families. Videotapes, quarterly newsletters, educational materials for children, parents, and health professionals, as well as information about summer camps, pen pal clubs, and family support groups are available through the national office.

American Society for Deaf Children
814 Thayer Avenue
Silver Spring, MD 20910
(301) 585-5400

This society provides support to families through referrals, networking deaf individuals with each other, publishing informational materials, and representing the needs of the deaf to legislative bodies. Sign language is supported.

American Trauma Society
1400 Mercantile Lane
Suite 188
Landover, MD 20785
(301) 925-8811
(800) 556-7890

This association focuses its activities on public awareness and education. It conducts a yearly symposium and disseminates printed educational materials.

Association for Brain Tumor Research
3725 North Talman Avenue
Chicago, IL 60618
(312) 286-5571

This organization compiles and distributes relevant information to medical specialists, treatment facilities, and brain tumor support groups. Printed materials including information about diagnosis and treatment options and a triannual newsletter are available. Research support is also provided.

Association for Retarded Citizens
2501 Avenue J
Arlington, TX 76006
(817) 640-0204

This organization is dedicated to improving the welfare of mentally retarded children and adults. Services regarding employment, training, education, and independent living to individuals with mental retardation and their families are provided. Extensive public education (print and nonprint media), research support, and advocacy efforts are also provided.

Autism Society of America
8601 Georgia Avenue, Suite 503
Silver Spring, MD 20910
(301) 565-0433

This society has approximately 160 chapters nationwide. Activities include providing information about referral services, publishing of selected materials, and lobbying for reform at the local, state, and federal levels.

Beach Center on Families and Disability
University of Kansas
Bureau of Child Research
3111 Haworth Hall
Lawrence, KA 66045
(913) 864-7600

This is the only federally funded national research and training center with an exclusive focus on families with members with disabilities. Research findings are disseminated to families and the professionals that serve them through teleworkshops, a newsletter, conferences, training workshops, and publications.

Boy Scouts of America
Scouting for the Handicapped
1325 Walnut Hill Lane
Irving, TX 75062-1296
(214) 659-2127

A program of Boy Scouts of America, it operates in cooperation with numerous national agencies that provide services to youth with chronic conditions. Various services and materials are available to assist in mainstreaming boys into regular scouting events or establishing units for boys who share similar disabilities.

Cancer Information Service
Office of Cancer Communications
National Cancer Institute
Bethesda, MD 20892
(800) 4-CANCER

This service, supported by the National Cancer Institute, provides support and information on cancer prevention, early detection, treatment, and continuing care. Much of this information is available through the cancer hot line, (800) 4-CANCER. Database searches are also available using the PDQ (Physician Data Query). Publications for children and family members may also be obtained.

Candlelighter's Childhood Cancer Foundation
1312 18th Street, NW
Suite 200
Washington, DC 20036
(202) 659-5136
(800) 366-2223

Candlelighters is a worldwide network of over 400 peer-support groups for parents of children with cancer. Other relatives and professionals working in the field of cancer also belong. Support, information, and socialization opportunities are provided. A newsletter, bibliography, and other print materials are published.

Children in Hospitals, Inc.
31 Wilshire Park
Needham, MA 02192
(617) 482-2915

This organization for parents and professionals seeks to educate concerned individuals about the needs of children and parents when either is hospitalized. It encourages hospitals to adopt family-centered policies whenever possible. Some literature is available.

Children's Defense Fund
122 C Street, NW
Washington, DC 20015
(202) 628-8787

This organization serves as a strong voice for children who cannot effectively lobby or speak for themselves. Efforts are made to educate the public about preventive investment in children. Specific attention is paid to poor, minority, and disabled children. Technical assistance is provided to other organizations.

Clearinghouse on Disability Information
Office of Special Education and Rehabilitative
  Services
U.S. Department of Education
Room 3132 Switzer Building
Washington, DC 20202-2524
(202) 732-1241

Created by the Rehabilitation Act of 1973, the Clearinghouse responds to inquiries, researches, and documents information in areas of federal program funding, legislation, and programs serving disabled people. Knowledgeable about a variety of information sources, the Clearinghouse refers inquiries as appropriate. A wide variety of publications is also available.

Cleft Palate Foundation
1218 Grandview Avenue
Pittsburgh, PA 15211
(412) 481-1376
(800) 24-CLEFT

The foundation's primary purpose is to educate and assist the public about cleft lip and palate and other craniofacial anomalies and to encourage research in the field. CLEFTLINE, a toll-free service, provides information and referral to parents of newborns born with these problems. Parent support groups, patient and public educational activities, and research grants are also sponsored.

The Council for Exceptional Children
1920 Association Drive
Reston, VA 22091-1589
(703) 620-3660

This organization's primary goal is to advance the education of handicapped and gifted youth. CEC Information Services is an information broker for educators, students, and parents. In part, this is done through sponsoring the ERIC Clearinghouse on Handicapped and Gifted Children (see ERIC) and the Exceptional Child Education Resources (ECER) data base. Other activities include monitoring and analyzing governmental policies concerning exceptional children, conducting policy research, and disseminating information through conferences, academies, symposia, and other training activities.

Dystonia Medical Research Foundation
8383 Wilshire Boulevard
Suite 800
Beverly Hills, CA 90211
(213) 852-1630

This organization supports research directed toward finding the causes of generalized dystonia, spasmodic torticollis, writer's cramp, blepharospasm and other focal dystonias. Support for this endeavor is provided through research grants, specialty workshops, and physician-patient education.

Easter Seal Society
70 East Lake Street
Chicago, IL 60601
(312) 726-6200

Dedicated to increasing the independence of people with disabilities, Easter Seal Society offers a wide range of services, research initiatives, educational programs, and advocacy assistance through a national network of 170 affiliates. Specific services include occupational, physical, and speech therapies; vocational evaluation, training, and placement; camping and recreation; and psychological counseling. Prevention and screening programs are also sponsored.

Epilepsy Foundation of America
4351 Graden City Drive
Landover, MD 20785
(301) 459-3700
(800) EFA-1000

This foundation works toward curing epilepsy through a broad range of programs including education, advocacy, research support, and service delivery. An extensive library and resource center with an in-house data base is maintained to answer individualized requests. In addition, the foundation is affiliated with approximately 100 local organizations nationwide.

ERIC Clearinghouse on Handicapped and Gifted Children
1920 Association Drive
Reston, VA 22091-1589

Information from special education documents is collected and abstracted. To date, the data base contains over 700,000 items. The Clearinghouse provides database searches, printed materials, and referral assistance to agencies and individuals (see Council for Exceptional Children).

FACE
The Friends for Aid, Correction, Education of Craniofacial Disorders
PO Box 1424
Sarasota, FL 34230
(813) 955-9250

The purpose of FACE is to provide emotional support and referrals for corrective treatment to individuals with craniofacial disorders. Print and audiovisual materials are also available for educational purposes to help dispel prejudice.

FACES
The National Association for the Craniofacially Handicapped
Box 11082
Chattanooga, TN 37401
(615) 266-1632

The three purposes are this organization are to (1) provide families with travel money when seeking treatment at comprehensive medical centers, (2) provide information and support to families who have a member with a craniofacial abnormality, and (3) increase public awareness and understanding about facial disfigurement.

Federation for Children with Special Needs
95 Berkeley Street
Suite 104
Boston, MA 02116
(617) 482-2915

A coalition of parent groups, this organization represents children with a variety of disabilities by providing advocacy and information services. Various special projects are sponsored and a wide array of literature is published.

Forward Face
Institute of Reconstructive Surgery, H-148
New York University Medical Center
560 1st Avenue
New York, NY 10016
(212) 263-5205
(800) 422-FACE

This organization provides a comprehensive support system for families through referral to self-help groups, networking services, newsletter subscriptions, and other print and audiovisual materials.

Foundation for the Faces of Children
PO Box 505
Weston, MA 02193-0505
(617) 891-0325

This foundation supports families of children with craniofacial deformities. Support for educational information, clinical work at Boston Children's Hospital, and some financial assistance for families are provided.

Girl Scouts of America
830 Third Avenue
New York, NY 10022

The national organization offers an informal educational program designed to help girls with disabilities develop their own values and sense of individual self-worth. Girls with disabilities participate in the same program as others; mainstreaming is encouraged whenever possible.

Handicapped Adventure Playground Association
Central Office, Fulham Palace
Bishops Avenue
London, England SW6 6EA

This organization offers advice and information to individuals and organizations interested in designing playgrounds for children with disabilities.

The Heartline Group, Inc.
10500 Noland Road
Overland Park, KS 66215
(913) 492-6317

A national newsletter is published for parents of children with complex congenital heart disease.

Hemifacial Microsomia Family Support Network
6 Country Way
Philadelphia, PA 19115
(215) 677-4787

This organization supports the families of children with hemifacial microsomia/Goldenhar syndrome by providing information, presenting treatment options, and advocating for involved children. A newsletter, family directory, resource directory, information library, and newborn outreach program are services provided.

Joseph P. Kennedy, Jr. Foundation
1350 New York Avenue, NW
Suite 500
Washington, DC 20005-4709
(202) 393-1250

This foundation funds research, diagnosis, treatment, and education of children and adults with mental retardation. It also meets the physical education and recreational needs of persons with mental retardation through the Special Olympics program.

Juvenile Diabetes Foundation, International
432 Park Avenue South
New York, NY 10016-8013
(212) 889-7575

The purpose of this organization is to support research into the causes, treatment, prevention, and cure of diabetes and its complications. Support for this mission is provided through research grants, career development awards, fellowships, and new training for established scientists.

Learning Disabilities Association of America
4156 Library Road
Pittsburgh, PA 15234

Dedicated to defining and finding solutions for the broad spectrum of learning problems, this association has more than 775 local chapters throughout the United States. Activities of this association include providing a wide range of materials, serving as a referral center, working with school systems to improve assessment and implementation programs, lobbying for children's rights, and conducting international and state conferences.

The Library of Congress
Division for the Blind and Physically
  Handicapped
Washington, DC 20542
(202) 707-5100

An extensive program of braille and recorded materials for blind and physically disabled individuals is provided. Books, periodicals, children's publications, music services, and supportive equipment are provided.

Mainstream, Inc.
1030 15th Street, NW
Suite 1010
Washington, DC 20005
(202) 833-1162

This organization works with employers and service providers to increase employment opportunities for persons with disabilities. Services include print materials, an annual conference, and job placement programs for selected cities.

March of Dimes Birth Defects Foundation
National Headquarters
1275 Mamaroneck Avenue
White Plains, NY 10605
(914) 428-7100

The mission of this organization is to prevent birth defects and related problems of low birth weight and infant death through ongoing programs of research (basic, applied, and clinical), health services, professional and public education, and public affairs.

Muscular Dystrophy Association
810 Seventh Avenue
New York, NY 10019
(212) 586-0808

This organization provides comprehensive medical services for individuals with a wide range of neuromuscular diseases through a network of nationwide clinics. In addition, research activities, public and professional education, a wide variety of print and audiovisual materials are supported.

National Addison's Disease Foundation
505 Northern Boulevard
Suite 200
Great Neck, NY 11021
(516) 487-4992

This foundation is dedicated to serving the needs of those with Addison's disease through education, a newsletter, support groups, and, where possible, arranging contact with others with the disease.

National Alopecia Areata Foundation
714 C Street
San Rafael, CA 94901
(415) 456-4644

This foundation acts as the international center for alopecia areata information. Funding of research, service to individuals with the disease, and ongoing public awareness programs are sponsored. Specific activities include a newsletter, yearly conference, support groups, and print and audiovisual materials.

National Association for Sickle Cell Disease
3345 Wilshire Boulevard
Suite 1106
Los Angeles, CA 90010-1880
(213) 736-5455
(800) 431-8453

The NASCD prepares and distributes educational materials; trains sickle cell trait counselors; conducts patient, professional, and public education programs; and provides technical assistance for national, state, and local programs. In addition, support is provided for research and screening activities.

National Association for the Visually
  Handicapped
22 West 21st Street
6th Floor
New York, NY 10010
(212) 889-3141

This organization provides public and professional education, client counseling, and a wide array of large print books and visual aids to the partially seeing. It serves as a clearinghouse for related services from public and private sources. Some materials are available in languages other than English.

National Brain Tumor Foundation
323 Geary Street
Suite 510
San Francisco, CA 94102
(415) 296-0404

This foundation raises funds for research and provides information and support services to brain tumor survivors and their families. A resource guide, newsletter, and biannual conference are all sponsored.

National Center for Education in Maternal and
    Child Health (NCEMCH)
38th and R Streets, NW
Washington, DC 20057
(202) 625-8400

This organization serves as a national resource for information, educational services, and technical assistance to organizations, agencies, and individuals with maternal and child health interests.

National Center for Learning Disabilities
99 Park Avenue
New York, NY 10016
(212) 687-7211

This organization provides legislative advocacy, publications, and training seminars to assist parents, educators, social workers, psychologists, and health care providers in the United States and abroad. Publications and referrals are provided for American families overseas through the Family Liaison Office, US Department of State.

National Coalition for Cancer Survivorship
323 Eighth Street SW
Albuquerque, NM 87102
(505) 764-9956

This organization identifies and addresses issues that affect the quality of living for survivors. Activities include publications, national assemblies and conferences, a speakers' bureau, and advocacy

efforts on such issues as insurance coverage and employment rights.

National Committee for Citizens in Education
10840 Little Patuxent Parkway
Suite 301
Columbia, MD 21044-3199
(301) 997-9300

The mission of this organization is to improve the quality of public schools through parent involvement. Services provided include a toll-free help line, printed resource materials, and technical assistance for school-based improvement and parent involvement.

National Down Syndrome Congress
1800 Dempster Street
Park Ridge, IL 60068-1146
(312) 823-7550
(800) 232-6372

This organization for parents and professionals is dedicated to improving education, fostering research, and improving the quality of life for individuals with Down syndrome. It also serves as a clearinghouse for information about Down syndrome.

National Down Syndrome Society
666 Broadway
New York, NY 10012
(212) 460-9330
(800) 221-4602

The major goals of this society are to promote a better understanding of Down syndrome, to support research about this genetic disorder, and to provide services for families and individuals. A variety of print and audiovisual materials is available.

The National Easter Seal Society for Crippled
    Children & Adults
70 East Lake Street
Chicago, IL 60601
(312) 726-6200

A wide variety of services is provided, including physical, occupational, and speech therapies; vocational evaluation, training, and placement; camping and recreation; and psychological counseling. Prevention and screening programs are also sponsored. Services are delivered through a network of 170 nationwide affiliates.

National Foundation for Facial Reconstruction
317 East 34th Street
New York, NY 10016
(212) 340-6656
(800) 422-FACE

The major purposes of this organization are to (1) provide facilities for the treatment and nonsurgical assistance of individuals unable to afford private reconstructive surgical care, (2) assist in training and education of health care personnel involved in reconstructive plastic surgery, and (3) conduct a public education program.

The National Fragile X Foundation
1441 York Street
Suite 215
Denver, CO 80206
(303) 333-6155
(800) 688-8765

The National Fragile X Foundation was established to educate parents, professionals, and the lay public regarding the diagnosis and treatment of fragile X syndrome and other forms of X-linked mental retardation. In addition, the foundation promotes research pertaining to fragile X syndrome in the areas of biochemistry, genetics, and clinical applications.

National Gaucher Foundation
1424 K Street, NW
Washington, DC 20005
(202) 393-2777

This foundation is primarily devoted to funding research for Gaucher disease. A bimonthly newsletter is published and a yearly conference is held for affected individuals and their families.

National Hemophilia Foundation
Soho Building
110 Green Street, Room 406
New York, NY 10012
(212) 219-8180

This foundation is dedicated to the treatment and cure of hemophilia, related bleeding disorders, and complications (including HIV infection) and to improving the quality of life for those affected. Services provided include research support, educational programs for professionals and the public, and promotion of beneficial public policies, including the establishment of the comprehensive hemophilia diagnostic and treatment centers. HANDI, the Hemophilia and AIDS/HIV Network for the Dissemination of Information, makes referrals and disseminates resources and materials to those requesting information.

National Hydrocephalus Foundation
22427 South River Road
Joliet, IL 60436
(815) 467-6548

This organization seeks to educate the lay public and affected individuals about hydrocephalus, lobbies for effective legislation, and has support groups throughout the United States. A wide array of services are provided to its members including numerous publications, videos, and a referral network.

National Information Center for Children and
    Youth with Handicaps
PO Box 1492
Washington, DC 20013
(703) 893-6061

NICHCY provides free information to assist parents, educators, caregivers, advocates, and others to help children and youth with disabilities become participating members of the community. NICHCY provides personal responses to specific questions, prepared information packets, publications on current issues, technical assistance to parents and professional groups, and referrals to other organizations/sources of help.

National Neurofibromatosis Foundation, Inc.
141 Fifth Avenue
Suite 7-S
New York, NY 10010
(212) 460-8980
(800) 323-7938

The four purposes of this organization include (1) sponsoring research aimed at finding the cause of and cure for neurofibromatosis, (2) promoting the development of diagnostic protocols, (3) increasing public awareness of the disease through education, and (4) assisting patients and their families by providing information, support, and referrals to specialists.

National Organization for Rare Disorders
PO Box 8923
New Fairfield, CT 06812-1783
(203) 746-6518

This agency is composed of national health organizations, researchers, health care personnel, and interested others dedicated to the identification, control, and cure of rare debilitating disorders. It serves as a clearinghouse for information, encourages research, and accumulates and disseminates information about orphan drugs and devices.

National Rehabilitation Information Center
  (NARIC)
8455 Colesville Road
Suite 935
Silver Spring, MD 20910-3319
(301) 588-9284
(800) 346-2742

NARIC is a library and information center on disability and rehabilitation. Funded by the National Institute on Disability and Rehabilitation Research (NIDRR), NARIC collects and disseminates the results of federally funded research projects. The collection also includes commercially available materials.

National Tay-Sachs & Allied Diseases
  Association, Inc.
2001 Beacon Street, Room 304
Brookline, MA 02146
(617) 277-4463

This association is committed to the elimination of Tay-Sachs and allied diseases, to be accomplished through several avenues: (1) public and professional education, (2) carrier testing, (3) family services, and (4) research support.

ODPHP National Health Information Center
PO Box 1133
Washington, DC 20013-1133
(800) 336-4797

This center serves as a clearinghouse for specialty organizations. It maintains an on-line directory of over 1000 health-related organizations that provide health information. Federal and state agencies, private associations, professional societies, and self-help and support groups are all indexed. A special component, the National Information Center for Orphan Drugs and Rare Diseases (NICODARD), responds to inquiries on rare diseases (under 200,000 cases) and little-known drugs.

Osteogenesis Imperfecta Foundation
PO Box 14087
Clearwater, FL 34629-4807
(813) 855-7077

This organization is dedicated to helping people cope with osteogenesis imperfecta. Services offered include literature for lay and professional individuals, a quarterly newsletter, a parent contact network, and a biennial national conference. Some research is also funded.

Phoenix Society for Burn Survivors
11 Rust Hill Road
Levittown, PA 19056
(215) 946-BURN
(800) 888-BURN

Services provided by this society are peer counseling, reentry programs to school, information services, and legislative monitoring. Public education programs, seminars, and conferences for survivors, their families, and professionals are offered. A limited number of scholarships is available to send children who have been burned to specialty camps.

Pike Institute for the Handicapped
Boston University School of Law
765 Commonwealth Avenue
Boston, MA 02215
(617) 353-2904

This institute provides services in the areas of individualized and systems advocacy, public policy and legal research, educational seminars about the rights of the disabled, and a variety of publications on these issues.

Prader-Willi Syndrome Association
6490 Excelsior Boulevard, E-102
St. Louis Park, MN 55426
(612) 926-1947

This organization promotes communication among parents, professionals, and other interested people through a bimonthly newsletter and a wide variety of publications. Research and selected family services are also supported.

RP Foundation Fighting Blindness
1401 Mt. Royal Avenue
Baltimore, MD 21217-4245
(301) 255-9409
(800) 638-2300

The RP Foundation supports research into the cause, prevention, and treatment of retinitis pigmentosa and allied inherited retinal degenerative diseases. In addition, related literature is made available to professionals and the public. Services are also provided to affected individuals and their families. A postmortem retina donor program for research is sponsored.

Scleroderma Association
PO Box 910
Lynnfield, MA 01940
(508) 535-6600

The major thrust of this organization is to provide education and support for persons with scleroderma and their families. Activities include providing print information, physician referral, peer counseling and increasing the public's awareness. In addition, medical information, meetings and patient education seminars are presented annually. Research into the cause of, and cure for, scleroderma is also supported.

SEFAM Family Support Program
Merry Wood School
16120 NE Eighth Street
Bellevue, WA 98008
(206) 747-4004

SEFAM (Supporting Extended Family Members) provides services for fathers of children with developmental disabilities. Activities include outreach training, technical assistance on how to integrate fathers into patterns of service delivery, curriculum development, and a newsletter.

Sibling Information Network
Connecticut's University Affiliated Program
991 Main Street
Suite 3A
East Hartford, CT 06108
(203) 282-7050

This network assists families and professionals, with an emphasis on siblings, interested in the welfare of individuals with disabilities. It serves as a clearinghouse of information, ideas, projects, literature, support groups, and research regarding siblings and other related issues. The network also publishes a quarterly newsletter.

Siblings for Significant Change
United Charities Building
105 East 22nd Street
New York, NY 10010
(212) 420-0776

This organization eases the strain of helping individuals with disabilities by providing support and information to their siblings and other caregivers. Conferences, workshops, advocacy training, and counseling services are provided.

SKIP (Sick Kids Need Involved People)
216 Newport Drive
Severna Park, MD 21146

This organization is dedicate to assisting families raising children with special needs by helping them identify and connect with available resources.

Spina Bifida Association of America
1700 Rockville Pike
Suite 540
Rockville, MD 20852-1654
(800) 621-3141

This association provides information and referral, adult services, advocacy, and public awareness; supports research into the cause of spina bifida; and publishes a quarterly newsletter.

Sturge-Weber Foundation
PO Box 460931
Aurora, CO 80015
(303) 693-2986
(800) 627-5482

This foundation serves as a clearinghouse for information regarding Sturge-Weber syndrome, acts as support group for interested parties, disseminates materials to professionals and the lay public, and facilitates related research.

TASH: The Association for Persons with Severe
   Handicaps
7010 Roosevelt Way, NE
Seattle WA 98115
(206) 523-8446

TASH is concerned with the human dignity, education, and independence for individuals traditionally classified as severely cognitively impaired. Ongoing activities include advocacy services, dissemination of research findings specific to education and rehabilitation, and other educational initiatives.

Tourette Syndrome Association, Inc.
Dennis Hirshfelder, Executive Director
42-40 Bell Boulevard
Bayside, NY 11361-2861
(718) 224-2999

This association develops and disseminates a wide range of print and nonprint educational material to individuals, professionals, and agencies in the fields of health care, education, and the government; operates support groups and other services; and stimulates and funds research toward finding a cure and seeking to improve treatment for Tourette syndrome.

Treacher Collins Foundation
PO Box 5
Concord, NH 03302-0005
(802) 649-3020

The mission of this foundation is to serve affected individuals and their families through providing support, referrals, resources, and networking opportunities.

United Cerebral Palsy Associations, Inc.
1522 K Street
Suite 1112
Washington, DC 20005
(202) 842-1266
(800) USA-5UCP

This organization is a national network of over 170 local affiliates in 45 states. The mission—to improve the quality of life for individuals with cerebral palsy—is operationalized in several ways. A variety of information services about laws and regulations as well as appropriate programs and services are provided. Other services are also offered but may vary among local affiliates.

United Scleroderma Foundation
Robert Harrison, Executive Director
PO Box 350
Watsonville, CA 95077
(408) 728-2202

This foundation publishes numerous handbooks, brochures, and newsletters for individuals with scleroderma. A network of local chapters provide workshops and personal contact. Physician referrals are also made from the national office.

Index

A

Abdomen
  Down syndrome and, 248
  hydrocephalus and, 311-312
Abdominal pain
  arthritis and, 346
  hemophilia and, 94
  inflammatory bowel disease and, 329
  sickle cell disease and, 508
  transplant and, 401
ABO blood type, transplant and, 394
Abscess, gastrointestinal, 326
Absolute neutrophil count, 138
  fever and, 140
Abuse
  child, 473
  cocaine, 465-479; *see also* Cocaine exposure, prenatal
  sexual, 409
Acetaminophen
  cancer and, 139
  DTP vaccination in epilepsy and, 277
Acetylsalicylic acid, 340; *see also* Aspirin
Acid
  folic
    cancer chemotherapy and, 139
    myelodysplasia and, 373
  valproic
    as antiepileptic agent, 274
    aspirin and, 278
    toxicity of, 277
Acidifier, urinary, 365-366
Acidosis, renal failure and, 481
Acquired immunodeficiency syndrome; *see also* Human immunodeficiency virus infection

Acquired immunodeficiency syndrome—cont'd
  associated problems with, 413-415
  clinical manifestations of, 410-412
  developmental issues in, 419-421
  differential diagnosis of, 418-419
  etiology of, 408
  family and, 421
  incidence of, 409-410
  management of, 415-418
  prognosis for, 413
  treatment of, 412-413
ACTH
  as antiepileptic agent, 274
  hypothalamus and, 169
Actinomycin-D, 125
Acuity, visual; *see* Vision
Acute chest syndrome in sickle cell disease, 502
Acute lymphoblastic leukemia, 118
  bone marrow transplantation for, 129
  central nervous system prophylaxis and, 132
  Down syndrome and, 252
Acute nonlymphoblastic leukemia, 118
  Down syndrome and, 252
Acyanotic heart defects, 191
Acyclovir
  herpes infection and, 140
  human immunodeficiency virus infection and, 419
Adaptive Behavior School, 34
Adaptive equipment
  arthritis and, 346-347
  myelodysplasia and, 381, 383
Adjuvant radiation therapy, 128

Adolescent
  adrenal hyperplasia and, 181, 182
  bleeding disorder and, 95-96
  cerebral palsy and, 164
  cystic fibrosis and, 216, 218-219, 223
  developmental tasks of, 28-29
  diabetes mellitus and, 233, 234
    eating disorders and, 238
    sexuality and, 240
  Down syndrome and, 262
  drug abuse and, 474-475
  epilepsy and, 280, 282
  heart disease and, 204
  human immunodeficiency virus infection and, 409-410, 421
  hydrocephalus and, 314
  inflammatory bowel disease and, 331
  learning disabilities and, 366
  myelodysplasia and, 384
  perception of medical procedures and, 31
  phenylketonuria and, 437-439
  renal failure and, 490
  safety and
    electrical equipment and, 72
    medications and, 73
  sickle cell disease and, 509, 510
  transplant and, 403
  understanding of death by, 31-32
Adrenal hyperplasia
  associated problems with, 175-176
  clinical manifestations of, 172-173
  developmental issues in, 180-182
  differential diagnosis of, 178-180
  etiology of, 169-171
  family and, 182-183
  gender of infant and, 173
  incidence of, 171-172
  management of, 176-178, 184
  prognosis of, 175
  treatment of, 173-175
Adrenal insufficiency, 175, 179-180
Adrenocorticotropic hormone
  as antiepileptic agent, 274
  hypothalamus and, 169
Advocacy, 41-42
Aerosolized antibiotics, 216
Age
  bone, 175
  developmental tasks and, 27-29

Air travel for child with heart disease, 202
Airway
  bronchopulmonary dysplasia and, 105
  cystic fibrosis and, 211
Alcohol
  cystic fibrosis and, 219
  diabetes mellitus and, 233
  epilepsy and, 280
  fetus and, 466
Aldosterone regulation, 169, 171
Alkalinizer, urinary, 365-366
Alkaloid, plant, 124-125
Alkylating agents for cancer, 123
Allen Picture Card Test of Visual Acuity, 37
Allergic reaction
  adrenal hyperplasia and, 178-179
  asthma and, 67, 71
  myelodysplasia and, 377
Altitude, heart disease and, 202
Aluminum toxicity, renal failure and, 486
Alveolus, Down syndrome and, 251
Ambiguous genitalia, 173, 175-176
Ambulatory dialysis, 484
Amiloride, 216
Aminoglycoside, 488
5-Aminosalicylic acid, 321
Amoxicillin, 195
Analgesia
  for dying child, 22
  sickle cell disease and, 501-502
Anastomosis, ileal pouch–anal, 324
Anemia
  arthritis and, 342
  heart disease and, 195
  hemophilia and, 90
  human immunodeficiency virus infection and, 414, 417
  inflammatory bowel disease and, 327
  premature infant and, 450
  renal failure and, 482, 485
  sickle cell disease and, 498, 509
Anesthesia, sickle cell disease and, 504
Ankylosing spondylitis, 325
Anomalous venous return, 190
Anomaly, congenital; *see* Congenital *entries*
Anorexia
  cancer and, 131
  diabetes mellitus and, 238
  heart disease and, 201

Antacid
  bronchopulmonary dysplasia and, 107
  renal failure and, 488
Antenatal diagnosis; *see* Prenatal diagnosis
Anti-inflammatory drug
  asthma and, 66-67
  nonsteroidal
    arthritis and, 340
    respiratory symptoms and, 346
    Reye's syndrome and, 344
Antibiotic
  arthritis and, 344
  as cancer chemotherapy, 125-126
  cystic fibrosis and, 216
    respiratory infection and, 215
  diabetes mellitus and, 235
  heart disease and, 195
  hydrocephalus and, 305
  myelodysplasia and, 378
  renal failure and, 488
  sickle cell disease and, 500
Antibody
  to clotting factor concentrate, 86
  hepatitis B, 93
Anticholinergic agent
  asthma and, 67
  myelodysplasia and, 378
Anticonvulsant drugs, 274, 275
  drug interactions with, 277-278
  myelodysplasia and, 378
  renal failure and, 488
Antidepressant
  antiepileptic drugs and, 278
  learning disabilities and, 361
Antiemetic, cancer and, 131
Antiepileptic drugs; *see* Anticonvulsant drugs
Antifibrinolytic agent
  drug interactions and, 93
  hemophilia and, 89
Antigen
  histocompatibility leukocyte, 229
  P24, 410
Antihistamine
  asthma and, 71
  bronchopulmonary dysplasia and, 109
Antimetabolite, 123-124
Antineoplastic therapy; *see* Chemotherapy
Antinuclear antibodies, arthritis and, 344
Antispasmodic agent, 323

Anxiety, heart disease and, 197
Aorta
  coarctation of, 189
  fragile X syndrome and, 293
Apgar score, cerebral palsy and, 149
Aplastic crisis, 502
Apnea
  breath-holding spells and, 278
  premature infant and, 451-452
Appetite, cocaine exposure and, 470
Aqueductal stenosis, 303
Arnold-Chiari II malformation, 375, 379
Arrhythmia, 278-279
Arthritis
  inflammatory bowel disease and, 325
  juvenile rheumatoid, 336-354
    associated problems with, 342-343
    clinical manifestations of, 337-339
    developmental issues in, 346-349
    differential diagnosis of, 345-346
    etiology of, 336-337
    family and, 349
    management of, 343-345
    prognosis of, 339, 342
    treatment of, 339
Artificial airway, 105
Artificial sweetener
  diabetes mellitus and, 238
  phenylketonuria and, 435
L-Asparaginase, 126
Aspartame, 435
Asphyxia, cerebral palsy and, 149
Aspiration pneumonia, 159
Aspirin
  antiepileptic drugs and, 278
  bleeding disorders and, 93
  heart disease and, 200
  intolerance to, 346
Asplenia
  heart disease and, 195, 200
  sickle cell disease and, 498, 500
Asthma, 63-80
  associated problems with, 67-68
  clinical manifestations of, 64
  developmental issues of, 72-76
  differential diagnosis of, 72
  etiology of, 63
  family and, 76
  incidence of, 63-64

Asthma—cont'd
  management of, 68-71, 77-78
  prognosis of, 67
  treatment of, 64-67
Astrocytoma, supratentorial, 118-119
Ataxic cerebral palsy, 148
Atlantoaxial instability, 250, 259
Atresia
  biliary, 393
  tricuspid, 190
Atrial catheter, 130
Atrial septal defect, 189
Atropine for asthma, 67
Attention deficit disorder, 355-372; see also Learning
    disabilities
Auditory perceptual deficit, 358, 359
Auranofin, 340
Aurothioglucose, 340
Austitic-like tendencies in fragile X syndrome, 294
Autoimmune disease, 336
5-Azacytidine, 123
AZT, 412
  anemia and, 417
Azulfidine, inflammatory bowel disease and, 321, 322

B

Bacterial infection
  adrenal hyperplasia and, 179
  bronchopulmonary dysplasia and, 105
  endocarditis and, 305
  human immunodeficiency virus infection and, 412-
      413
  transplant and, 401
Bacteruria in sickle cell disease, 508
Balloon, gastrostomy tube and, 107
Bankson Language Screening Test, 38
Barbiturate
  adrenal hyperplasia and, 178
  fetus and, 466
Bayley Infant Scales, 34
Behavior
  cocaine exposure and, 470
  Down syndrome and, 260
  fragile X syndrome and, 294
  inflammatory bowel disease and, 330
Behavior Style Questionnaire, 35
Benzolmethylecgonine; see Cocaine exposure, prenatal
Bereavement, 22-23
Beta-adrenergic agent for asthma, 65

Biliary tract, cystic fibrosis and, 212
Bineland Adaptive Behavior Scales, 37
Bineland Social Maturity Scale, 37
Birth defect; see Congenital entries
Birth order, 17
Birth weight
  bronchopulmonary dysplasia and, 103
  cerebral palsy and, 149
  growth and development and, 452
  prematurity and, 446
Bladder, myelodysplasia and, 377
Bladder training; see Toileting
Bleeding, gastrointestinal, 346
Bleeding disorder, 81-100
  associated problems with, 90-92
  clinical manifestations of, 82-83
  developmental issues with, 94-96
  differential diagnosis of, 93-94
  etiology of, 81-82
  family and, 96
  heart disease and, 195
  human immunodeficiency virus infection and, 414
  management of, 92-93, 97-98
  prognosis of, 90
  treatment of, 84-90
Bleomycin, 125-126
Blindness
  bronchopulmonary dysplasia and, 106
  diabetes mellitus and, 234
Block grants for child health, 50-54
Blood
  antineoplastic therapy and, 134
  human immunodeficiency virus infection and, 410
  inflammatory bowel disease and, 319
  universal precautions for, 419
Blood cell count
  antiepileptic drugs and, 277
  human immunodeficiency virus infection and, 417
Blood cells
  human immunodeficiency virus infection and, 414
  sickle cell disease and, 495
Blood disorder
  bleeding, 81-100; see also Bleeding disorder
  leukemia as, 118
    bone marrow transplantation for, 129
    central nervous system prophylaxis and, 132
    Down syndrome and, 251-252, 260
  sickle cell disease as, 495-515; see also Sickle cell
      disease

Blood glucose
    diabetes mellitus and, 232, 233
    ketoacidosis and, 236
Blood pressure
    adrenal hyperplasia and, 177
    arthritis and, 344
    asthma and, 70
    bronchopulmonary dysplasia and, 109
    cancer patient and, 139
    diabetes mellitus and, 235
    Down syndrome and, 259
    epilepsy and, 277
    heart disease and, 199
    human immunodeficiency virus infection and, 416-
        417
    hydrocephalus and, 310
    inflammatory bowel disease and, 327
    learning disabilities and, 365
    myelodysplasia and, 378
    portal hypertension and, 393
    premature infant and, 455
    pulmonary hypertension and, 251
    renal failure and, 488
    sickle cell disease and, 507
    transplant and, 400
Blood test
    myelodysplasia and, 378
    phenylketonuria and, 434
    renal failure and, 488
Blood transfusion
    human immunodeficiency virus infection and, 409
    platelets and, 131-132
    sickle cell disease and, 504
Blood vessels in sickle cell disease, 500
Blue Cross–Blue Shield, 45-46
Body, perception of, 30
Body fluid, universal precautions for, 419
Bone
    antineoplastic therapy and, 135
    bronchopulmonary dysplasia and, 106
    cancer of, prognosis of, 129-130
    phenylketonuria and, 429
    renal failure and, 485-486, 488
    tumors of, 121
Bone age, adrenal hyperplasia and, 175, 178
Bone marrow
    antineoplastic therapy and, 131-132, 134
    transplantation of, 129
Bordetella pertussis, 309

Bottle-feeding; *see also* Feeding of infant
    cystic fibrosis and, 221
    heart disease and, 202
    premature infant and, 457-458
        formula for, 451, 458
Bowel management; *see* Toileting
Brain
    cerebral palsy and, 148
    epilepsy and, 275
    hemophilia and, 90
    human immunodeficiency virus infection and,
        413
    hydrocephalus and, 303-317; *see also* Hydro-
        cephalus
Brain tumor
    headache and, 141
    ventriculoperitoneal shunt and, 312
Breast-feeding
    cystic fibrosis and, 221
    Down syndrome and, 261
    heart disease and, 202
Breast milk
    bronchopulmonary dysplasia and, 104
    cocaine and, 470
    premature infant and, 451, 457
Breath-holding spells, 278
Bronchiolitis, 63
Bronchodilator
    bronchopulmonary dysplasia and, 105, 109
    cystic fibrosis and, 216
Bronchopulmonary dysplasia, 101-117
    associated problems with, 105-108
    clinical manifestations of, 103
    developmental issues in, 110-113
    differential diagnosis of, 109-110
    etiology of, 101-103
    family concerns in, 113
    incidence of, 103
    premature infant and, 451
    primary care management and, 108-109
    prognosis for, 104-105
    treatment of, 103-104
Bronchospasm, bronchopulmonary dysplasia and,
    105
Bulimia, diabetes mellitus and, 238
Bulk-forming agent, myelodysplasia and, 378
Burn from humidifier, 72
Bzoch-League Receptive Expressive Emergent Lan-
    guage Scale, 38

C

Calcium
   arthritis and, 347
   bronchopulmonary dysplasia and, 106
   renal failure and, 482-483
Calcium channel blocker, 397
Calculus
   cholelithiasis and, 106
   renal
      bronchopulmonary dysplasia and, 106
      inflammatory bowel disease and, 326
Caloric requirements
   bronchopulmonary dysplasia and, 104
   cystic fibrosis and, 215
   diabetes mellitus and, 232
   heart disease and, 202
Cancer, 117-147
   associated problems with, 130-132
   clinical manifestations of, 117, 122
   developmental issues in, 141-143
   differential diagnosis of, 139-141
   etiology of, 117
   family and, 143
   incidence of, 117
   leukemia and, 118
      bone marrow transplantation for, 129
      central nervous system prophylaxis and, 132
      Down syndrome and, 251-252, 260
   management of, 137-139, 144-145
   prognosis for, 129-130
   treatment of, 122-129
   ventriculoperitoneal shunt and, 312
Candidal infection
   bronchopulmonary dysplasia and, 110
   cancer and, 140
   diabetes mellitus and, 233
   human immunodeficiency virus infection and, 414
Captopril, 397
Car seat
   cerebral palsy and, 160
   hydrocephalus and, 312
Carbamazepine
   as antiepileptic agent, 274
   erythromycin and, 278
   fragile X syndrome and, 296
   toxicity of, 277
Carbohydrate in phenylketonuria, 433
Carbohydrate meal plan, 238
Cardiac disorder; see Heart entries

Cardiac glycoside, 488
Cardiomyopathy
   antineoplastic therapy and, 133
   heart transplant and, 390-391
   medical treatment of, 393-394
   prognosis of, 395
   transplant and, 392
Cardiovascular system; see also Heart entries
   antineoplastic therapy and, 133
   renal failure and, 486, 488
Carey Infant Temperament Questionnaire, 34
Caries, cerebral palsy and, 153
Carmustine, 127
Carrier of hemophilia, 81
Case management, 9
Cataract, arthritis and, 344
Catheterization
   atrial, 130
   cardiac, 194-195
   urinary, 382
Cell-cycle phase chemotherapy agents, 128
Centers for Disease Control, HIV infection and,
         409
   classification of, 411
Central nervous system
   antineoplastic therapy and, 136-137
   cancer and, treatment effects and, 132
   cancer of, 118-119
   cocaine and, 467
   epilepsy and, 268; see also Epilepsy
   heart disease and, 196
   hemophilia and, 88
   myelodysplasia and, 373-388; see also Myelodys-
         plasia
Cerebral hemisphere, epilepsy and, 275
Cerebral palsy, 148-168
   associated problems with, 153-155
   clinical manifestations of, 150-152
   developmental issues in, 159-164
   differential diagnosis of, 158-159
   etiology of, 148-149
   family and, 164
   incidence of, 149-150
   management of, 155-158, 165
   treatment of, 152-153
Cerebrospinal fluid, hydrocephalus and, 303; see also
         Hydrocephalus
Cerumen, 259
Cervical spine, arthritis and, 342

CHAMPUS; *see* Civilian Health and Medical Program
    of the Uniformed Services
Chart, growth, Down syndrome and, 252-256
Chemotherapy
    adverse effects of, 133-137
    bone marrow suppression and, 131-132
    for cancer, 122-128
    human immunodeficiency virus infection and,
        412
    sexuality and, 143
Chest
    asthma and, 68
    bronchopulmonary dysplasia and, 101, 103, 109
    Down syndrome and, 248
Chest pain in cystic fibrosis, 220
Chest physiotherapy
    bronchopulmonary dysplasia and, 105
    cystic fibrosis and, 215-216
Chest syndrome in sickle cell disease, 502
Chickenpox
    cancer and, 138
    cystic fibrosis and, 220
    human immunodeficiency virus infection and, 418-
        419
    transplant and, 399
Child Behavior Checklist, 35, 40-41
Child care
    adrenal hyperplasia and, 180
    arthritis and, 347
    asthma and, 73-74
    bleeding disorder and, 95
    bronchopulmonary dysplasia and, 111-112
    cancer patient and, 142
    cerebral palsy and, 160
    cocaine exposure and, 474
    cystic fibrosis and, 221
    diabetes mellitus and, 236-237
    Down syndrome and, 260-261
    epilepsy and, 280
    fragile X syndrome and, 296
    heart disease and, 202
    human immunodeficiency virus infection and, 419-
        420
    hydrocephalus and, 312-313
    inflammatory bowel disease and, 329-330
    learning disabilities and, 366-367
    myelodysplasia and, 381
    phenylketonuria and, 436
    premature infant and, 457

Child care—cont'd
    renal failure and, 489
    sickle cell disease and, 509
    transplant and, 401-402
Child development; *see* Development
Children's Depression Inventory, 35
Chlamydia, premature infant and, 456
Chlorambucil chemotherapy, 123
Cholangitis, 393
Cholelithiasis, 106
Choline magnesium trisalicylate, 340
Choline salicylate, 340
Cholinergic agent in Down syndrome, 260
Chromosome 12, 426-428
Chromosome 21, 245; *see also* Down syndrome
Chronic illness, definition of, 3, 13
Chronic renal failure, 480-494; *see also*
        Renal failure
Cigarette smoking, fetus and, 466
Ciprofloxacin, 220
Circumcision, bleeding disorder and, 95
Circumference of head; *see* Head circumference
Cirrhosis, 134
Cisplatin, 127-128
Civilian Health and Medical Program of the Uni-
    formed Services, 48
Classical 21-hydroxylase deficiency, 171
Clean intermittent catheterization, 382-383
Clinical Linguistic and Auditory Scale, 156
Clitoris, adrenal hyperplasia and, 172
Clonazapam, 274
Clonidine, 291
Clonopin, 274
Clotrimazole, 414
Clotting factors in bleeding disease, 81-82
    hemophilia and, 84, 86, 88-89
Coarctation of aorta, 189
Cocaine exposure, prenatal, 465-479
    associated problems with, 468-471
    clinical manifestations of, 467-468
    developmental issues and, 473-475
    differential diagnosis of, 473
    etiology of, 465-466
    family and, 475
    incidence of, 466-467
    management of, 471-472
    prognosis for, 468
    treatment of, 468
Cognitive development, 69

Cognitive function; *see also* Intelligence
    epilepsy and, 276
    myelodysplasia and, 377, 383
    phenylketonuria and, 430
    transplant and, 399
Colitis, ulcerative; *see* Ulcerative colitis
Collagen hemostatic fibers, 89
Communicating hydrocephalus, 303-304
Communication disorder in cerebral palsy, 154
Compensating hydrocephalus, 305
Complex partial seizure, 270, 271
Compression of nerve, 94
Confirming Second Surgical Opinion, 46
Congenital adrenal hyperplasia, 169-186; *see also* Adrenal hyperplasia
Congenital anomaly
    cocaine exposure and, 469
    phenylketonuria and, 438
Congenital heart disease, 187-209
    bronchopulmonary dysplasia and, 106
    clinical manifestations of, 190-192
    developmental issues in, 201-204
    differential diagnosis of, 200-201
    etiology of, 187
    family and, 204
    heart transplant and, 391
    incidence of, 187, 190
    management of, 198-200, 205-206
    problems associated with, 195-197
    prognosis for, 195
    treatment of, 192-195
Congenital obstructive hydrocephalus, 303
Congestive heart failure, 190-191
    clinical manifestations of, 392-393
Connective tissue disorder, fragile X syndrome and, 293, 295
Conners Teacher Rating Scale, 368
Constant carbohydrate meal plan, 238
Constipation
    cerebral palsy and, 154
    cystic fibrosis and, 217-218
Continence
    inflammatory bowel disease and, 330-331
    myelodysplasia and, 382
Continuous dialysis, renal failure and, 484
Contraception
    arthritis and, 349
    cystic fibrosis and, 224
    diabetes mellitus and, 240

Contraception—cont'd
    heart disease and, 204
    sickle cell disease and, 510-511
    transplant patient and, 403
Contracture in cerebral palsy, 154-155, 158
Contrast medium, sickling and, 504
Convulsive seizure, 270-271; *see also* Seizure
Cord, spinal
    cancer and, 141
    tethering of, 379
Corpus callostomy, epilepsy and, 275
Cortef, 178
Cortex, adrenal, 169
Corticosteroid
    arthritis and
        glaucoma and, 344
        growth and, 343
        nutrition and, 347
    asthma and, 66-67
    cancer and, 126
        nutrition and, 142
    cystic fibrosis and, 216
    inflammatory bowel disease and, 321, 322, 323
        drug interactions and, 328
        sleep disturbance and, 331
    prematurity and, 447
    sexual development and, 76
    transplant and
        growth and, 398
        school and, 403
Corticotropin-releasing factor, 169
Cortisol, 169
Cost of health care; *see* Financial concerns
Cough
    asthma and, 64
    bronchopulmonary dysplasia and, 105-106
    cystic fibrosis and, 220-221
Cough suppressant
    asthma and, 71
    bronchopulmonary dysplasia and, 109
Counseling
    genetic
        Down syndrome and, 249, 262
        Maternal and Child Health Block Grant for, 54
        sickle cell disease and, 511
    primary care provider's role in, 42
Crack baby, 465-479; *see also* Cocaine exposure, prenatal
Cranial nerve, myelodysplasia and, 379

Cranium, hemophilia and, 90-91
Crawling, cerebral palsy and, 152
CRF; *see* Corticotropin-releasing factor
Crisis
    family, 13-14
    sickle cell disease and, 502, 502-503
Crohn's disease, 318-335
    associated problems with, 324-327
    clinical manifestations of, 319-321
    developmental issues in, 329-332
    differential diagnosis of, 328-329
    etiology of, 318
    family and, 332
    incidence of, 318-319
    management of, 327-328
    treatment of, 321-324
Cromolyn sodium for asthma, 66
Crying
    breath-holding spells and, 278
    heart disease and, 198
Cryoprecipitate, 89
Cryotherapy for retinopathy of prematurity, 450
Cryptic 21-hydroxylase deficiency, 171
Culture
    human immunodeficiency virus infection and, 410
        fever and, 418
    vascular access device and, 139
Cyanosis
    breath-holding spells and, 278
    heart disease and, 191-192
Cyclic peritoneal dialysis, 484
Cyclophosphamide, hemorrhagic cystitis and, 139
Cyclophosphamide chemotherapy, 123
Cyclosporine
    drug interactions and, 400
    inflammatory bowel disease and, 323-324
    transplant and, 396
        blood levels of, 400
        growth and, 398
Cylert, 360
Cystic fibrosis, 210-228
    clinical manifestations of, 212-215
    developmental issues in, 221-224
    differential diagnosis of, 220-221
    etiology of, 210-212
    family and, 224
    incidence of, 212
    management of, 218-220, 225-226
    problems associated with, 217-218

Cystic fibrosis—cont'd
    treatment of, 215-217
Cystitis, hemorrhagic
    antineoplastic therapy and, 135
    cyclophosphamide and, 139
Cytomegalovirus
    cancer and, 132, 140
    transplant and, 394
Cytosine arabinoside, 123

D

D-Penicillamine, arthritis and, 341
Dacarbazine, 127
Dactylitis, 496, 498
Daunorubicin, 125
Day care; *see* Child care
Death; *see also* Mortality
    child's understanding of, 31-32
    primary care provider's role and, 448, 452
Decannulation, 110
Decongestant, 200
Deductible, insurance, 46
Dehydration, 217
Dementia, dialysis, 486
Dental care
    arthritis and, 344
    bleeding disorders and, 93
    bronchopulmonary dysplasia and, 109
    cancer patient and, 138-139
    cerebral palsy and, 153, 157-158
    cystic fibrosis and, 219
    Down syndrome and, 251, 259
    epilepsy and, 277
    fragile X syndrome and, 295
    heart disease and, 198-199
    human immunodeficiency virus infection and, 416
    hydrocephalus and, 310
    inflammatory bowel disease and, 327
    phenylketonuria and, 433
    premature infant and, 455
    renal failure and, 488
    transplant and, 400
Denver Articulation Screening Exam, 38
Denver Developmental Screening Test, 33, 35
    cerebral palsy and, 155-156
    hydrocephalus and, 309
    premature infant and, 453-454
    renal failure and, 487
    sickle cell disease and, 506

Denver Eye Screening Test, 37
Depakene, 277
Depokote, 274
Dermatitis, diaper, HIV infection and, 420
Dermatologic disorder; *see* Skin
Desmopressin, 89
Development, 26-44
  adrenal hyperplasia and, 177
  arthritis and, 343-345
  asthma and, 68-69, 72-76
  bleeding disorders and, 92
  bronchopulmonary dysplasia and, 107-108
  cancer and, 137
  cerebral palsy and, 155-156
  characteristics of child and, 27-29
  cocaine and, 469-472
  cystic fibrosis and, 218-219
  diabetes mellitus and, 234
  Down syndrome and, 248, 252, 257, 258
  epilepsy and, 276-278
  family and social networks and, 29-30
  fragile X syndrome and, 294
  heart disease and, 197, 198
  human immunodeficiency virus infection and, 413, 415
  hydrocephalus and, 307-308
  inflammatory bowel disease and, 327
  learning disabilities and, 365
  myelodysplasia and, 377
  natural history of condition and, 26-27
  perspectives of body, illness, and death, 30-32
  phenylketonuria and, 432-433
  premature infant and, 452-454
  primary care provider's role in, 32-33, 41-43
  renal failure and, 486-487
  of sibling of chronically ill child, 16-17
  sickle cell disease and, 504-506
  transplant and, 398-399
Developmental Disabilities Services and Facilities Construction Act, 55
Developmental disability, federal programs for, 54-56
Developmental Profile II, 35
Dexamethasone, 341
Dextroamphetamine
  drug interactions and, 365-366
  learning disabilities and, 360, 361, 364, 365-366
Di-Atro, inflammatory bowel disease and, 323
Diabetes mellitus, 229-244
  clinical manifestations of, 229-231

Diabetes mellitus—cont'd
  developmental issues in, 236-240
  etiology of, 229
  family and, 240-241
  management of, 235-236
  problems associated with, 233
  prognosis of, 232-233
  treatment of, 231-232
Diagnosis-related groups, Medicaid and, 49
Dialysis dementia, 486
Dialysis for renal failure, 393, 483-484
Diaper dermatitis with HIV infection, 420
Diarrhea
  asthma and, 72
  cancer and, 140-141
  cerebral palsy and, 159
  heart disease and, 201
  inflammatory bowel disease and, 319, 329
  myelodysplasia and, 380
  sickle cell disease and, 508
  transplant and, 401
Diet
  adrenal hyperplasia and, 180-181
  arthritis and, 347
  asthma and, 74
  bleeding disorder and, 95
  bronchopulmonary dysplasia and, 102-103, 104, 112
  cancer patient and, 142
  cerebral palsy and, 153-154, 160-161
  cocaine exposure and, 474
  cystic fibrosis and, 215, 218, 221-223
  diabetes mellitus and, 232, 237-238
  Down syndrome and, 261
  elemental, inflammatory bowel disease and, 324
  epilepsy and, 280
  fragile X syndrome and, 296-297
  heart disease and, 202-203
  human immunodeficiency virus infection and, 420
  hydrocephalus and, 313
  inflammatory bowel disease and, 330
  ketogenic, epilepsy and, 275
  learning disabilities and, 362-363, 367
  myelodysplasia and, 381
  phenylketonuria and, 430-431, 435, 436-437
  premature infant and, 450-451, 457-458
  renal failure and, 489
  sickle cell disease and, 509-510
  transplant and, 402

Diffuse alterations, 358-359
Diflunisal, 340
Digoxin
   cardiomyopathy and, 393-394
   drug interactions and, 200
   safe use of, 201
   sulfasalazine and, 328
   toxicity of, 197
Dilantin
   aspirin and, 278
   dental care and, 277
     gingival hyperplasia and, 157-158
   dosage and side effects of, 274
   sulfasalazine and, 328
   toxicity of, 277
Diphenoxylate, 323
Diphtheria, tetanus, and pertussis vaccine
   cancer and, 138
   cerebral palsy and, 156-157
   epilepsy and, 277
   hydrocephalus and, 309
   transplant and, 399
Diphtheria vaccine in HIV infection, 415
Diplegia in cerebral palsy, 148
Discipline
   adrenal hyperplasia and, 181
   arthritis and, 347
   asthma and, 74
   bleeding disorder and, 95
   bronchopulmonary dysplasia and, 112
   cancer patient and, 142
   cerebral palsy and, 161
   cocaine exposure and, 474
   cystic fibrosis and, 223
   diabetes mellitus and, 238
   Down syndrome and, 261
   epilepsy and, 281
   fragile X syndrome and, 297
   heart disease and, 203
   human immunodeficiency virus infection and, 420
   hydrocephalus and, 313
   inflammatory bowel disease and, 330
   learning disabilities and, 367
   myelodysplasia and, 381-382
   phenylketonuria and, 437
   premature infant and, 459
   renal failure and, 489-490
   sickle cell disease and, 510
   transplant and, 402

Dislocation, hip
   cerebral palsy and, 154-155, 158
   Down syndrome and, 250, 259
Distance Visual Acuity Screening Test for Young
     Children, 37
Diuretic
   bronchopulmonary dysplasia and, 104
   cardiomyopathy and, 393-394
   digoxin and, 197
Divorce, 20
Down syndrome, 245-267
   clinical manifestations of, 246, 248-249
   developmental issues in, 260-262
   differential diagnosis of, 260
   etiology of, 245
   family and, 262-263
   incidence of, 245-246
   management of, 252-260, 264-265
   problems associated with, 250-252
   treatment of, 249-250
Doxorubicin, 125
Driving, learning disabilities and, 366
Drooling, cerebral palsy and, 152, 154
Drug abuse
   child abuse, 473
   cocaine, 465-479; *see also* Cocaine exposure, pre-
     natal
   human immunodeficiency virus infection and, 415
Drug interactions
   adrenal hyperplasia and, 178
   arthritis and, 345
   asthma and, 71
   bleeding disorders and, 93
   bronchopulmonary dysplasia and, 109
   cancer and, 139
   cerebral palsy and, 158
   cystic fibrosis and, 219-220
   diabetes mellitus and, 235
   Down syndrome and, 259-260
   epilepsy and, 277-278
   fragile X syndrome and, 296
   heart disease and, 200
   human immunodeficiency virus infection and, 417-
     418
   inflammatory bowel disease and, 328
   learning disabilities and, 365-366
   myelodysplasia and, 378
   phenylketonuria and, 434-436
   renal failure and, 488

Drug interactions—cont'd
  sickle cell disease and, 507
  transplant and, 400-401
Drug toxicity screening, epilepsy and, 277
Dual organ transplant, 390
Dying child; *see also* Mortality
  child's understanding of death and, 31-32
  family of, 21-23
  primary care provider's role with, 42-43
Dyskinetic cerebral palsy, 148
Dysmorphology in phenylketonuria, 438
Dysplasia, bronchopulmonary, 101-117, 451; *see also*
    Bronchopulmonary dysplasia
Dysrhythmia, 196-197
Dysuria, 94

E

Ear; *see also* Hearing
  bronchopulmonary dysplasia and, 105
  cerebral palsy and, 158
  fragile X syndrome and, 287, 295, 296
  human immunodeficiency virus infection and, 416,
    418
Early Intervention Program for Infants and Toddlers
    with Handicaps, 9
Eating problems; *see also* Diet; Feeding of infant
  cerebral palsy and, 153-154
  diabetes mellitus and, 238
Education; *see* School
Education of All Handicapped Children Act, 56-57
Electrical safety
  arthritis and, 347
  heart disease and, 201
  oxygen therapy and, 111
  prevention of burns and, 72
Electroencephalography, 432
Electrolytes in renal failure, 481, 482
Elemental diet
  inflammatory bowel disease and, 324
  phenylketonuria and, 430-431, 435-437
Embryoma, renal, 121
Emergent Language Milestone Scale, 38
Encephalopathy
  human immunodeficiency virus infection and, 413
  renal failure and, 486
End-stage disease
  liver, 391-392
  renal
    Medicare's program for, 50

End-stage disease—cont'd
  renal—cont'd
    renal failure and, 480
    transplant and, 390
Endocarditis, 195-196
  dental care and, 199
  fever and, 200-201
  hydrocephalus and, 305
Endocrine system, antineoplastic therapy and, 135-
    136
Endosclerosis, esophageal, 393
Enema, retention, 321
Enteral feeding, 324
Enteritis, 134
Enterocolitis, necrotizing, 451
Enzyme
  adrenal hyperplasia and, 169
  cancer therapy and, 126
  cystic fibrosis and, 221-223
  phenylketonuria and, 431
Ependymoma, 118
Epilepsy, 268-285
  associated problems with, 276
  classification of seizures and, 269, 271, 273
  clinical management of, 276-278
  developmental issues in, 279-282
  differential diagnosis of, 278-279
  etiology of, 268
  family and, 282
  incidence of, 268
  manifestations of, 268, 271, 273
  prognosis for, 275-276
  treatment of, 273-275
Epistaxis, 86, 87
Epoetin alfa for renal failure, 482
Epstein-Barr virus
  immunosuppressive therapy and, 397
  transplant and, 394
Equipment
  adaptive
    arthritis and, 346-347
    myelodysplasia and, 381, 383
  monitoring
    bronchopulmonary dysplasia and, 112
    for premature infant, 457
Erythema nodosum, inflammatory bowel disease and,
    326
Erythrocyte protoporphyrin, sickle cell disease and,
    507

Erythrocyte sedimentation rate, inflammatory bowel disease and, 328

Erythromycin
  antiepileptic drugs and, 278
  cystic fibrosis and, 220

Erythropoietin, premature infant and, 450

Escherichia coli
  premature infant and, 456
  sickle cell disease and, 507

Esophageal endosclerosis, 393

Estrogen, von Willebrand's disease and, 89

Ewing's sarcoma, 121

Exchange system, dietary, diabetes mellitus and, 237-238

Exercise
  cystic fibrosis and, 216
  diabetes mellitus and, 239
  epilepsy and, 280
  transplant and, 401

Extremity
  arthritis and, toileting and, 348
  cerebral palsy and, 148
  Down syndrome and, 248
  sickle cell disease and, 503-504

Eye; *see* Vision

Eyeglasses
  cerebral palsy and, 157
  Down syndrome and, 258

F

Facial dysmorphology in phenylketonuria, 438

Facial palsy, renal failure and, 489

Factor VIII, 86, 88-89

Failure to thrive
  cystic fibrosis and, 213
  heart disease and, 197
  human immunodeficiency virus infection and, 413

Fallot's tetralogy, 189

Family, 12-25
  adrenal hyperplasia and, 182-183
  arthritis and, 349
  asthma and, 76
    self-management and, 64-65
  bleeding disorders and, 96
  bronchopulmonary dysplasia and, 113
  cancer patient and, 143
  cerebral palsy and, 164
  child development and, 29-30
  cocaine exposure and, 475

Family—cont'd
  crisis in, 13-14
  cystic fibrosis and, 224
  diabetes mellitus and, 240-241
  Down syndrome and, 262-263
  dying child and, 21-23
  epilepsy and, 282
  fragile X syndrome and, 297-298
  heart disease and, 204
    anxiety and, 197
  human immunodeficiency virus infection and, 421
  hydrocephalus and, 314
  inflammatory bowel disease and, 332
  learning disabilities and, 369
  long-term adaptation by, 19-21
  myelodysplasia and, 384
  phenylketonuria and, 439-440
  premature infant and, 460
  reaction to diagnosis and, 14
  renal failure and, 490
  responses to treatment and, 14-19
  sickle cell disease and, 511
  transplant and, 403

Fecal occult blood test, 328

Fee-for-service plans, 45-46

Feeding of infant
  cerebral palsy and, 161
  cocaine exposure and, 470
  cystic fibrosis and, 221
  Down syndrome and, 261
  heart disease and, 202-203
  myelodysplasia and, 381
  premature, 450-451, 457-458

Feingold diet, 362-363

Female patient; *see also* Menstruation; Pregnancy
  adrenal hyperplasia and, 172-173
    genital surgery and, 182
  cystic fibrosis and, 224
  epilepsy and, 282
  fragile X syndrome and, 289-290
  phenylketonuria and, 438-439
  sexuality and
    fragile X syndrome and, 297
    myelodysplasia and, 384

Fenamates, 340

Fenoprofen, 340

Ferric chloride reaction, 434

Fertility
  adrenal hyperplasia and, 176, 182

Fertility—cont'd
   fragile X syndrome and, 297
   inflammatory bowel disease and, 331-332
   phenylketonuria and, 439
Fetal alcohol syndrome, 465
Fetus
   adrenal hyperplasia and, 175-176
   cocaine exposure of, 465-479; see also Cocaine
      exposure, prenatal
Fever
   adrenal hyperplasia and, 179
   arthritis and, 345
   asthma and, 72
   bronchopulmonary dysplasia and, 110
   cancer and, 139-140
   cerebral palsy and, 158
   cystic fibrosis and, 220
   DTP vaccine and, epilepsy and, 277
   epilepsy and, 279
   heart disease and, 200
   human immunodeficiency virus infection and,
      418
   hydrocephalus and, 310-311
   myelodysplasia and, 380
   renal failure and, 488-489
   sickle cell disease and, 507-508
   transplant and, 401
Fibroplasia, retrolental, 449-450
Fibrosis
   cystic, 210-228; see also Cystic fibrosis
   hepatic, chemotherapy and, 134
   pulmonary, antineoplastic therapy and, 133
Financial concerns, 45-59
   as barrier to health care, 4-5
   bronchopulmonary dysplasia and, 112
   cancer and, 143
   effect on family of, 18
   future needs for, 57-58
   government programs and, 47-57
   private health insurance and, 45-47
Fire, oxygen and, 110-111
Fistula, inflammatory bowel disease and, 326
FK 506 for transplant patient, 395-396, 400
Flagyl, 322
Flammability of oxygen, 110-111
Florinef, 178
Fluid
   bronchopulmonary dysplasia and, 104
   cancer and, 140-141

Fluid—cont'd
   cerebrospinal, hydrocephalus and, 303; see also Hy-
      drocephalus
   heart disease and, 201
   ketoacidosis and, 236
   renal failure and, 481
   synovial, 91
   transplant and, 401
   universal precautions for, 419
Focal seizure, 269-270
Folic acid
   cancer chemotherapy and, 139
   fragile X syndrome and, 291
   myelodysplasia and, 373
Formula, infant
   cystic fibrosis and, 221
   heart disease and, 202
   premature infant and, 451, 458
Foster care, 18
Fragile X syndrome, 286-302
   associated problems with, 293-294
   clinical manifestations of, 287-290
   development issues in, 296-297
   etiology of, 286
   family and, 297-298
   incidence of, 286-287
   management of, 294-296
   otitis media and, 296
   treatment of, 290-293
Functional status evaluation, 32-33
Functional Status Index, 40
Funeral, planning of, 22
Fungal infection, 414
Furazolidone, 365
Furosemide, 106

G
Gait, 94
Gallstone
   bronchopulmonary dysplasia and, 106
   inflammatory bowel disease and, 326
Gamma globulin, 412
Gastroesophageal reflux
   asthma and, 67-68
   bronchopulmonary dysplasia and, 107
   premature infant and, 458
   seizure versus, 278
Gastrointestinal system
   antineoplastic therapy and, 134

Gastrointestinal system—cont'd
  arthritis and, 346
  asthma and, 72
  bronchopulmonary dysplasia and, 110
  cancer and, 140-141
  cerebral palsy and, 159
  cocaine exposure and, 470, 473
  cystic fibrosis and, 211, 220
    obstruction and, 217-218
  Down syndrome and, 249, 260
  heart disease and, 201
  hemophilia and, 88, 91
  hydrocephalus and, 311-312
  myelodysplasia and, 380
  premature infant and, 452
  renal failure and, 489
  sickle cell disease and, 508
Gastrostomy stoma, 107
Gender of sibling, 17
Gene therapy for phenylketonuria, 430
Generalized seizure, 270-271, 273
Genetic counseling
  bleeding disorders and, 96
  block grant for testing and, 54
  Down syndrome and, 262
  fragile X syndrome and, 292
  sickle cell disease and, 511
Genetic disease
  bleeding disorder as, 81-100; *see also* Bleeding disorder
  cystic fibrosis and, 210, 212
  Down syndrome and, 249
  fragile X syndrome as, 286-302; *see also* Fragile X syndrome
  phenylketonuria as, 426; *see also* Phenylketonuria
  sickle cell disease as, 495-515; *see also* Sickle cell disease
Genitalia
  adrenal hyperplasia and, 172-173, 175, 175-176, 182
  fragile X syndrome and, 287
Genitourinary system
  hemophilia and, 88, 91-92
  premature infant and, 452
Germinal matrix, 448
Gestational age, 446, 447; *see also* Prematurity
Gilles de la Tourette's syndrome, 364
Gingival hyperplasia, 157-158

Gland
  adrenal, 169-186; *see also* Adrenal hyperplasia
  salivary, 212
  sweat, 211
  thyroid
    antineoplastic therapy and, 135
    diabetes mellitus and, 235
    Down syndrome and, 251, 259
Glasses
  cerebral palsy and, 157
  Down syndrome and, 258
Glaucoma, corticosteroid-induced, 344
Globulin
  gamma, 412
  immune, varicella zoster
    cancer and, 138
    premature infant and, 454
    transplant and, 399
Glucocorticoid
  adrenal hyperplasia and, 169
  arthritis and, 341
Glucose
  energy and, 230
  ketoacidosis and, 236
Glycosylated hemoglobin, 235
Gold sodium thiomalate, 340
Gonad, antineoplastic therapy and, 136
Government health care programs, 47-57
  Civilian Health and Medical Program of the Uniformed Services as, 48
  Education of All Handicapped Children Act and, 56-57; *see also* Public Law *entries*
  future needs in, 57-58
  Indian Health Service and, 48
  Maternal and Child Health Blood Grant as, 50-54
  Medicaid as, 48-50
  Medicare as, 50
  mental retardation and, 54-56
Granulation, tracheostomy stoma and, 107
Great vessels, transposition of, 189
Grief
  of parents, 22-23
  of siblings, 23
Group B streptococcal infection, 456
Growth
  adrenal hyperplasia and, 175, 176-177
    bone age and, 178
  arthritis and, 343-345
  asthma and, 68

Growth—cont'd
  bleeding disorders and, 92
  bronchopulmonary dysplasia and, 107-109
  cancer and, 137
  cerebral palsy and, 155-156
  chemotherapy and, 132
  cocaine exposure and, 469, 471-472
  cystic fibrosis and, 218-219
  diabetes mellitus and, 234
  Down syndrome and, 248, 252-256
  epilepsy and, 276-278
  fragile X syndrome and, 294
  heart disease and, 197, 198
  human immunodeficiency virus infection and, 415
  hydrocephalus and, 307-308
  inflammatory bowel disease and, 325, 327, 330
  learning disabilities and, 365
  myelodysplasia and, 377
  phenylketonuria and, 432-433
  premature infant and, 452-454
  renal failure and, 485, 486-487
  sickle cell disease and, 504-506
  transplant and, 398-399

H

Haemophilus influenzae, premature infant and, 456
Haemophilus influenzae type b vaccine
  cancer and, 138
  cerebral palsy and, 157
  cocaine exposure and, 472
  human immunodeficiency virus infection and, 416
  hydrocephalus and, 309
  sickle cell disease and, 506
  transplant and, 399
Hair loss, chemotherapy and, 132
Handedness, cerebral palsy and, 152
Haplotypes, phenylketonuria, 427
Head circumference
  bronchopulmonary dysplasia and, 108
  cocaine exposure and, 472
  human immunodeficiency virus infection and, 415
  hydrocephalus and, 307, 310
  premature infant and, 452-453
  renal failure and, 487
Head injury
  bleeding disorder and, 93-94
  epilepsy and, 279
Headache
  asthma and, 72

Headache—cont'd
  bleeding disorder and, 93-94
  cancer and, 141
  hydrocephalus and, 312
  renal failure and, 489
  seizure versus, 278
Health insurance, private, 45-47
Health maintenance organization, 47
Hearing
  arthritis and, 344, 346
  bronchopulmonary dysplasia and, 109
  cancer patient and, 138
  cerebral palsy and, 153, 157
  cystic fibrosis and, 219
  Down syndrome and, 251, 258-259
  fragile X syndrome and, 295
  human immunodeficiency virus infection and, 416
  hydrocephalus and, 310
  learning disabilities and, 365
  myelodysplasia and, 378
  premature infant and, 455
  renal failure and, 487-488
  sickle cell disease and, 503, 506-507
  transplant and, 399-400
Hearing aid, Down syndrome and, 259
Heart
  bronchopulmonary dysplasia and, 106
  catheterization of, 194-195
  cocaine exposure and, 472
  fragile X syndrome and, 293
  renal failure and, 486, 488
  sickle cell disease and, 504, 507
Heart block, postoperative, 197
Heart disease, 187-209
  clinical manifestations of, 190-192, 392-393
  developmental issues in, 201-204
  differential diagnosis of, 200-201
  etiology of, 187
  family and, 204
  incidence of, 187, 190
  management of, 198-200, 205-206
  problems associated with, 195-197
  prognosis for, 195
  treatment of, 192-195
Heart failure, congestive, 190-191
Heart transplant
  etiology of, 389-390
  growth and, 399
  incidence of, 391-392

Heart transplant — cont'd
  prognosis of, 395
  rejection of, 398
Height
  adrenal hyperplasia and, 177
  arthritis and, 343
  cerebral palsy and, 155
  hydrocephalus and, 307
  phenylketonuria and, 429
  renal failure and, 487
  sickle cell disease and, 505
Helmet, epilepsy and, 279
Hemarthrosis, 91
Hematocrit
  antiepileptic drugs and, 277
  arthritis and, 344
  bleeding disorders and, 93
  bronchopulmonary dysplasia and, 109
  cancer patient and, 139
  cystic fibrosis and, 219
  heart disease and, 195, 199-200
  inflammatory bowel disease and, 327-328
  phenylketonuria and, 434
  premature infant and, 450, 455
  renal failure and, 488
Hematologic disorder
  heart disease and, 195
  hemophilia and von Willebrand's disease as, 81-
      100; *see also* Bleeding disorder
  human immunodeficiency virus infection and, 414
  sickle cell disease as, 495-515; *see also* Sickle cell
      disease
Hematologic screening for sickle cell disease,
    507
Hematopoietic system, 134
Hematuria
  bleeding disorder and, 94
  hemophilia and, 92
Hemiparesis, 152
Hemispherectomy, 275
Hemodialysis, 484
Hemoglobin
  cancer and, 132
  glycosylated, 235
  heart disease and, 199-200
  premature infant and, 450
Hemophilia
  clinical manifestations of, 82-83
  etiology of, 81

Hemophilia — cont'd
  treatment of, 84-89, 97-98
Hemoptysis, 218
Hemorrhage; *see also* Bleeding disorder
  gastrointestinal, 346
  periventricular-intraventricular, 448-449
Hemorrhagic cystitis
  antineoplastic therapy and, 135
  cyclophosphamide and, 139
Hemostatic agent, 89
Hepatic fibrosis, 134
Hepatitis B vaccine
  bleeding disorders and, 93
  cocaine exposure and, 472
  Down syndrome and, 258
  premature infant and, 454
  renal failure and, 487
  sickle cell disease and, 506
  transplant and, 399
Hepatobiliary disorder
  inflammatory bowel disease and, 326
  sickle cell disease and, 504
Hernia
  fragile X syndrome and, 293
  inguinal, premature infant and, 452
  premature infant and, 455-456
Heroin, 466
Herpes simplex virus
  cancer and, 140
  premature infant and, 456
Herpes zoster virus, 416
Hib vaccine; *see Haemophilus influenzae* type b
    vaccine
Hip dislocation
  cerebral palsy and, 154-155, 158
  Down syndrome and, 250, 259
Hirschsprung's disease, Down syndrome and,
    260
Histocompatibility leukocyte antigen, 229
HLA system
  arthritis and, 337
  diabetes mellitus and, 229
  transplant and, 394
HMO; *see* Health maintenance organization
Hodgkin's disease, 120
  Haemophilus influenzae and, 138
Home care, 18
  bleeding disorder and, 95
  for dying child, 43

Hormone
    adrenal, 169
    adrenocorticotropic, 169
    as cancer therapy, 126
Human immunodeficiency viral infection
    hemophilia and, 85
Human immunodeficiency virus infection, 408-425
    associated problems with, 413-415
    bleeding disorder and
        hemophilia treatment center and, 85
        polio immunization and, 92-93
        prognosis of, 90
        sexuality and, 96
    clinical manifestations of, 410-412
    cocaine exposure and, 469
    developmental issues in, 419-421
    differential diagnosis of, 418-419
    etiology of, 408-409
    family and, 421
    incidence of, 409-410
    management of, 415-418
    prognosis for, 413
    treatment of, 412-413
Human leukocyte antigen
    arthritis and, 337
    diabetes mellitus and, 229
    transplant and, 394
Humidifier, safety of, 72
Humulin, 231
Hyaline membrane disease, 101
Hydration
    sickle cell disease and, 501
    transplant and, 401
Hydrocephalus, 303-317
    associated problems with, 306-307
    clinical manifestations of, 304
    developmental issues in, 312-314
    differential diagnosis of, 310-312
    etiology of, 303-304
    family and, 314
    incidence of, 304
    management of, 307-310
    myelodysplasia and, 375-376, 379-380
    prognosis of, 306
    treatment of, 304-306
Hydrocortisone
    adrenal hyperplasia and, 173-174
        child care and, 180
        growth and, 176

Hydrocortisone—cont'd
    adrenal hyperplasia—cont'd
        immunizations and, 177
        vomiting and, 179
    adrenal insufficiency and, 179-180
Hydronephrosis, 326
21-Hydroxylase deficiency, 171; see also Adrenal hyperplasia
Hydroxyurea, 127
Hygiene, oral; see also Dental care
    cancer patient and, 138-139
    cerebral palsy and, 158
    Down syndrome and, 259
Hyperactivity, 355-372; see also Learning disabilities
    fragile X syndrome and, 288-289
Hyperalimentation, parenteral, 324
Hyperglycemia, 232-233
Hyperhemolytic crisis, 502-503
Hyperkalemia, 481, 482
Hyperphenylalaninemia, 426; see also Phenylketonuria
Hyperplasia
    adrenal, 169-186; see also Adrenal hyperplasia
    gingival, phenytoin and, 157-158
Hypersensitivity, oral, in premature infant, 458
Hypertension
    portal, liver disease and, 393
    premature infant and, 455
    pulmonary, Down syndrome and, 251
    renal failure and, 482, 486
    transplant and, 397
Hypertonic cerebral palsy, 150
Hypertrophic cardiomyopathy, 393
    treatment of, 394
Hypoglycemia, 233
    sleep and, 239
Hypokalemia, 481, 482
Hyponatremia, 217
Hypothalamus, 169
Hypothermia for retinopathy of prematurity, 450
Hypotonia
    cerebral palsy and, 150
        sleeping position and, 163
    fragile X syndrome and, 293
Hypoxemia, 191-192
Hypoxia, 106

I

Iatrogeny, developmental, 27
Ibuprofen, arthritis and, 340

"Ice," 466
IEP; *see* Individualized educational plan
Ileal pouch–anal anastomosis, 324
Ileus, meconium, 213, 217-218
Illiterate E test, 157
Immune complex, arthritis and, 336
Immune globulin, varicella zoster
  cancer and, 138
  premature infant and, 454
  transplant and, 399
Immune system
  antineoplastic therapy and, 134
  Down syndrome and, 251, 260
  hemophilia and, 91
  human immunodeficiency virus infection and,
    412
Immunization
  adrenal hyperplasia and, 177
  arthritis and, 343-344
  asthma and, 69-70
  bleeding disorders and, 92-93
  bronchopulmonary dysplasia and, 108
  cancer and, 137-138
  cerebral palsy and, 156-157
  cocaine exposure and, 471-472
  cystic fibrosis and, 219
  diabetes mellitus and, 234
  Down syndrome and, 258, 261
  epilepsy and, 276-277
  fragile X syndrome and, 295
  heart disease and, 198
  human immunodeficiency virus infection and, 415-
    416
  hydrocephalus and, 309
  inflammatory bowel disease and, 327
  myelodysplasia and, 377-378
  phenylketonuria and, 433
  premature infant and, 454
  renal failure and, 487
  sickle cell disease and, 506
  transplant and, 399
Immunologic markers in human immunodeficiency
    virus infection, 417
Immunosuppressant
  arthritis and, 341
  drug interactions and, 400-401
  pregnancy and, 403
  renal failure and, 487
Immunosuppressant—cont'd

  transplant and, 395-397
    child care and, 401-402
  tuberculosis and, 139
Immunotherapy for cancer, 128-129
Imodium, 323
Impotence with diabetes, 240
Inactivated poliomyelitis vaccine, 415-416
Incontinence; *see also* Toileting
  inflammatory bowel disease and, 330-331
  myelodysplasia and, 382
Indian Health Service, 48
Individualism, 29
Individualized educational plan
  learning disabilities and, 367-368
  myelodysplasia and, 383
Indoleacetic acids, 340
Infant
  adrenal hyperplasia and
    genitalia of, 172-173
    screening for, 171-172
  bronchopulmonary dysplasia and, 101; *see also*
    Bronchopulmonary dysplasia
  cerebral palsy and, 149-152
    Denver Developmental Screening Test and, 156
    feeding of, 161
    sleep and, 163
  cystic fibrosis and
    respiratory infection and, 213
    salt depletion and, 216
  developmental tasks of, 28
  diabetes mellitus and, 239
  diagnosis of chronic condition in, 14
  Down syndrome and, 248, 249-250
    feeding and, 261
    hearing and, 259
  Education of All Handicapped Children Act and, 56
  epilepsy and, 268
  feeding of; *see* Feeding of infant
  heart disease and
    congestive heart failure and, 190-191
    feeding and, 202-203
    infection and, 200
    surgery for, 192-194
  hemophilia and, 83
  human immunodeficiency virus infection and,
    408
    neurologic disorder and, 413
  hydrocephalus and, 304, 307, 309; *see also* Hydro-
    cephalus shunt for, 306, 311

hypoglycemia and, 233
infantile spasms and, 273
weight gain and, 280
myelodysplasia in, 373-388; *see also* Myelodysplasia
perspectives on body and illness of, 30-31
phenylketonuria and; *see* Phenylketonuria
premature, 446-464; *see also* Prematurity
prenatal cocaine exposure and, 465-479; *see also* Cocaine exposure, prenatal
safety with medications for, 73
seizure and, 278-279
Infantile spasms, 273
Infection
adrenal hyperplasia and, 178-179
cancer and, 131, 139
candidal
bronchopulmonary dysplasia and, 110
cancer and, 140
diabetes mellitus and, 233
human immunodeficiency virus infection and, 414
cocaine exposure and, 468-469, 472, 473
Down syndrome and, 261
heart disease and, 195, 200
day care and, 202
human immunodeficiency virus, 408-425; *see also* Human immunodeficiency virus infection
hydrocephalus and, 312-313
premature infant and, 456
respiratory tract; *see* Respiratory tract infection
shunt for hydrocephalus and, 305-306
sickle cell disease and, 498, 500, 507-508
transplant and, 398, 401
urinary tract
arthritis and, 346
cerebral palsy and, 154, 159
myelodysplasia and, 378, 380
sickle cell disease and, 508
vascular access site and
cancer and, 130-131
dialysis and, 489
viral; *see* Viral infection
Inflammatory bowel disease, 318-335
associated problems with, 324-327
clinical manifestations of, 319-321

Inflammatory bowel disease—cont'd
developmental issues and, 329-332
differential diagnosis of, 328-329
etiology of, 318
family and, 332
incidence of, 318-319
management of, 327-328
treatment of, 321-324
Influenza vaccine
arthritis and, 344
asthma and, 69
bronchopulmonary dysplasia and, 108
cerebral palsy and, 157
cystic fibrosis and, 219
diabetes mellitus and, 234
Down syndrome and, 258
human immunodeficiency virus infection and, 416
renal failure and, 487
sickle cell disease and, 506
Infusion, at home, 95
Inguinal hernia, 452
Inhaler
for asthma, 65-67
safety of, 73
Injectable hydrocortisone
adrenal hyperplasia and, 174
adrenal insufficiency and, 179-180
child care and, 180
Injury
adrenal hyperplasia and, 179
bleeding disorder and, 93-94
epilepsy and, 276
helmet for prevention of, 279
learning disabilities and, 366
Insulin-dependent diabetes mellitus, 229-244; *see also* Diabetes mellitus
Insurance, 4-5
private, 45-47
Integrative processing, 358, 359
Integument; *see* Skin
Intelligence
cerebral palsy and, 153
cocaine and, 470
Down syndrome and, 250
fragile X syndrome and, 291
hydrocephalus and, 305
learning disabilities and, 355-372; *see also* Learning disabilities
myelodysplasia and, 376, 377

Intelligence—cont'd
  phenylketonuria and, 429, 430, 432
  transplant and, 399
Intestinal disorder; *see* Gastrointestinal system
Intracranial pressure, seizure and, 307
Intrauterine exposure to cocaine, 468; *see also* Cocaine exposure, prenatal
Intubation of premature infant, 455
Ipratropium, 67
Iridocyclitis, 342
Iron for premature infant, 458-459

J

Joint
  arthritis and, 337, 339; *see also* Arthritis
  hemophilia and, 86, 87, 88, 91
  inflammatory bowel disease and, 325
Joint laxity, fragile X syndrome and, 293
Juvenile myoclonic epilepsy, 273
Juvenile periodontitis, 251
Juvenile rheumatoid arthritis, 336-354
  associated problems with, 342-343
  clinical manifestations of, 337-339
  developmental issues in, 346-349
  differential diagnosis of, 345-346
  etiology of, 336-337
  family and, 349
  management of, 343-345
  prognosis of, 339, 342
  treatment of, 339

K

Ketoacidosis, diabetic, 233
  prevention of, 235-236
Ketogenic diet, 275, 280-281
Kidney; *see* Renal *entries*
Kinesthetic-proprioceptive ability, 307
Kock pouch, 324

L

L-asparaginase, 126
Labeling
  child development and, 33, 41
  of learning disabled child, 363-364
Lactose intolerance, 327, 330
Language
  fragile X syndrome and, 291-292, 295
  renal failure and, 486
  testing of, 38-39

Lannox-Gastaut syndrome, 273
Lead poisoning, 507
Leakage of gastrostomy stoma, 107
Learning disabilities, 355-372
  associated problems with, 363-364
  asthma and, 75
  clinical manifestations of, 357-359
  developmental issues in, 366-369
  differential diagnosis of, 366
  etiology of, 355-357
  family and, 369
  incidence of, 357
  management of, 364-366
  premature infant and, 459-460
  treatment of, 359-363
Leg ulcer, 503-504
Leukemia, 118
  bone marrow transplantation for, 129
  central nervous system prophylaxis and, 132
  Down syndrome and, 251-252, 260
Leukopenia, 131
Liver
  antineoplastic therapy and, 134
  sickle cell disease and, 504, 507
Liver disease
  clinical manifestations of, 391-392
  transplant and, 393
Liver function test
  inflammatory bowel disease and, 328
  pemoline and, 364
Liver transplant
  etiology of, 389
  growth and, 399
  incidence of, 390
  prognosis of, 395
  rejection of, 398
Local seizure, 269-270
Lomustine, 127
Loperamide, inflammatory bowel disease and, 323
Low birth weight
  bronchopulmonary dysplasia and, 103
  cerebral palsy and, 149
  growth and development and, 452
  prematurity and, 446
Lower extremity
  cerebral palsy and, 152
  Down syndrome and, 248
  sickle cell disease and, 503-504

Lumbar puncture, headache and, 141

Lung
  cystic fibrosis and, 211, 215-216
  premature infant and, 451

Lymphoblastic leukemia, 118
  bone marrow transplantation for, 129

Lymphoid interstitial pneumonitis, human immunodeficiency virus and, 414

Lymphoma
  Hodgkin's, 120; *see also* Hodgkin's disease
  non-Hodgkin's, 119-120

Lymphoproliferative disease, immunosuppressive
    therapy and, 397

M

McCarthy Scales of Children's Abilities, 35

Magnet, pacemaker and, 201

Magnetic resonance imaging, phenylketonuria and,
    432

Mainstreaming; *see* Public Law *entries*

Major histocompatibility complex, 337

Major medical expense insurance, 46

Malabsorption, 213, 215

Male patient
  adrenal hyperplasia and, 173
  cystic fibrosis and, 224
  Down syndrome and, 249
  fragile X syndrome and, 287-289
  hemophilia and, 83
  myelodysplasia and, 384
  priapism and, 503
  sickle cell disease and, 503

Malignant disease, 117-147; *see also* Cancer

Malnutrition, arthritis and, 347

Marijuana, fetus and, 466

Marital relations, 20

Mass, cancer and, 117

Masturbation, fragile X syndrome and, 297

Maternal and Child Health block grants, 50-54, 57

Maternal phenylketonuria syndrome, 428, 438

Maternity and Infant Act, 51

Matrix, germinal, 448

Maturational alterations, 26-27

Meal plans for diabetes mellitus, 237-238

Measles, mumps, and rubella vaccine
  cancer and, 138
  cocaine exposure and, 472
  human immunodeficiency virus infection and,
    416

Measles vaccine
  cerebral palsy and, 157
  epilepsy and, 277
  hydrocephalus and, 309

Mechanical ventilation
  bronchopulmonary dysplasia and,
    101, 102, 104
  premature infant and, 451

Mechlorethanine chemotherapy, 123

Meclofenamate sodium, 340

Meconium ileus, 213

Meconium ileus equivalent, 217-218

Medicaid, 4-5
  eligibility and services for, 48-50

Medical identification emblem, 95

Medicare, 50

Medulloblastoma, 118

Megacolon, toxic, 326-327

Megavitamins, 362

Melanin spots, 435

Membrane, hyaline, 101

Meningocele, 374; *see also* Myelodysplasia

Meningococcal vaccine, 506

Menstruation
  adrenal hyperplasia and, 182
  cystic fibrosis and, 218-219
  Down syndrome and, 262
  epilepsy and, 282
  renal failure and, 490

Mental Health Centers Construction Act, 55

Mental retardation
  Down syndrome and, 345-367; *see also* Down syn-
    drome
  federal programs for, 54-56
  fragile X syndrome and, 286-287; *see also* Frag-
    ile X syndrome

Mental status with ketoacidosis, 236

Mercaptopurine, 123, 322, 323

Metabolic disorder
  renal failure and, 481
  transplant and, 401

Metabolic pathway for phenylalanine, 426

Metaclopramide, 107

Metal detector, pacemaker and, 201

Metastasis via ventriculoperitoneal shunt, 312

Metered dose inhaler, 65-67
  safety of, 73

Methadone maintenance, 470

Methamphetamine, 466

Methotrexate
  arthritis and, 341
  for cancer, 124
Methylphenidate, 360, 364, 365
Methylprednisone, 105
Metronidazole
  drug interactions with, 328
  inflammatory bowel disease and, 322
Microcephaly
  cocaine exposure and, 469
  human immunodeficiency virus infection and, 413, 415
Microcytosis, 342
Micrognathia, 342
Microotoscopy, 259
Microwave oven, pacemaker and, 201
Migraine headache, 278
Milk; *see also* Feeding of infant
  breast, cocaine and, 470
  premature infant and, 451
Mineralocorticoid, 175
Minerals, bronchopulmonary dysplasia and, 103
Minnesota Child Development Inventory, 36
Minnesota Infant Development Inventory, 36
Mitral valve prolapse, 293, 295
MMR vaccine; *see* Measles, mumps, and rubella vaccine
Mobility in cerebral palsy, 153
Monilial infection; *see* Candidal infection
Monitoring equipment
  bronchopulmonary dysplasia and, 112
  for premature infant, 457
Monoamine oxidase inhibitor
  dextroamphetamine and, 366
  phenylketonuria and, 435
Morning headache, 141
Mortality
  adrenal hyperplasia and, 175
  asthma and, 67
  bronchopulmonary dysplasia and, 104
  cancer and, 132
  diabetes mellitus and, 232
  hypertrophic cardiomyopathy and, 393
  Periventricular-intraventricular hemorrhage and, 449
  premature infant and, 448, 452
  prenatal cocaine exposure and, 469
Motor-expressive performance alterations, 358, 359
Motor function
  arthritis and, 343

Motor function—cont'd
  cerebral palsy and, 148
  cocaine and, 470
  Down syndrome and, 250
  hydrocephalus and, 307, 309
  myelodysplasia and, 376
  renal failure and, 486
Motor neuron, cerebral palsy and, 148
Mouth; *see* Dental care; Oral cavity
Mouth bleeding in hemophilia, 94
Mucolytic agent, 216
Mumps vaccine
  cancer and, 138
  cocaine exposure and, 472
Muscle, hemophilia and, 86, 87
Muscle tone
  cerebral palsy and, 150
  Down syndrome and, 248
  epilepsy and, 279
  premature infant and, 453
Musculoskeletal system
  arthritis and, 342
  cystic fibrosis and, 220
  Down syndrome and, 248, 250, 260
  hemophilia and, 91
  inflammatory bowel disease and, 325, 329
  myelodysplasia and, 376
  sickle cell disease and, 496, 498
Mycelex, 414
Mycobacterium avium intracellulare, 417
Myelodysplasia, 373-388
  associated problems with, 375-377
  clinical manifestations of, 374-375
  developmental issues in, 380-384
  differential diagnosis of, 378-380
  etiology of, 373
  family and, 384
  incidence of, 374
  management of, 377-378
  prognosis of, 375
  treatment of, 375
Myelomeningocele, 374; *see also* Myelodysplasia
  hydrocephalus and, 304
Myopathy, renal failure and, 486
Myosline, as antiepileptic agent, 274

N

Naproxen, 340
Narcotic agent, sickle cell disease and, 501-502

Nasal polyps, 217

Nasogastric tube, 161

National Center for Health Statistics growth charts, 252-256

National Clearinghouse for Human Genetic Diseases, 54

Nausea
  cancer and, 131, 140-141
  hydrocephalus and, 311
  myelodysplasia and, 380

Nebulized treatment for asthma, 65-67

Neck, Down syndrome and, 248

Necrotizing enterocolitis, premature infant and, 451

Neonate
  adrenal hyperplasia and, 171-172, 175-176
  bronchopulmonary dysplasia and, 101; see also
Bronchopulmonary dysplasia
  diagnosis of chronic condition in, 14
  Down syndrome and, 248
  hemophilia and, 83
  phenylketonuria screening of, 428, 440

Nephritis, radiation, 134-135

Nephroblastoma, 121

Nerve, cranial, myelodysplasia and, 379

Nerve compression, bleeding disorder and, 94

Nervous system; see Central nervous system

Network, social, 29-30

Neural tube defect, 373-388; see also Myelodysplasia

Neuroblastoma, 120-121
  prognosis of, 129

Neurogenic bladder, 377

Neurologic disorder
  cerebral palsy and, 150-152
  cocaine exposure and, 469-470, 472, 473, 4712
  heart disease and, 201
  hemophilia and, 90-91
  human immunodeficiency virus infection and, 413
  myelodysplasia and, 379
  phenylketonuria and, 432
  renal failure and, 486
  sickle cell disease and, 500-501, 509

Neuromotor therapy in cerebral palsy, 153

Neuromuscular disorder in premature infant, 453-454

Neuron, cerebral palsy and, 148

Neuropathy, 486

Neurophysiologic retraining, 362

Neuropsychologic development in sickle cell disease, 506

Neurotoxicity of cancer treatment, 132

Neurotransmitter enzymes, 259-260

Neutrophil count, 131

Newborn; see Infant; Neonate

Nightmares, hypoglycemia and, 239

Nitrogen balance, 435

Nitrosurea, 127

Nonclassic 21-hydroxylase deficiency, 171

Nonconvulsive seizure, 270-271

Nondisfunction of chromosome 21, 245, 247

Non-Hodgkin's lymphoma, 119-120
  prognosis of, 129

Non-insulin-dependent diabetes mellitus, 229; see also
    Diabetes mellitus

Nonlymphoblastic leukemia, 118
  Down syndrome and, 252

Nonsteroidal anti-inflammatory drug
  arthritis and, 340
  respiratory symptoms and, 346
  Reye's syndrome and, 344

Norcocaine, 467

Normalization of family life, 16

Nose
  Down syndrome and, 248
  hemophilia and, 86, 87

Numbness, bleeding disorder and, 94

Nutrasweet, phenylketonuria and, 435

Nutrition; see Diet

Nystatin, 414

O

Obesity
  diabetes mellitus and, 234
  fragile X syndrome and, 296-297

OBRA; see Omnibus Budget Reconciliation Act

Obstruction
  hydrocephalus and, 303
  intestinal, cystic fibrosis and, 217-218

Occult blood, 328

Occupational therapy, 292

Ocular disorder; see Vision

Odor in phenylketonuria, 429

Omnibus Budget Reconciliation Act, 49, 50, 51
  mental retardation and, 55

Ophthalmic corticosteroid, 341

Ophthalmologic disorder; see Vision

Opistonic posturing, 152

Opportunistic infection, 414

Optometric visual training, 362

Oral antifibrinolytic agent, 89
  drug interactions and, 93

Oral cavity
    bleeding disorder and, 94
    Down syndrome and, 248, 251
    fragile X syndrome and, 294
    hemophilia and, 88
Oral contraceptive
    antiepileptic drugs and, 278
    arthritis and, 349
    cystic fibrosis and, 224
    diabetes mellitus and, 240
    heart disease and, 204
    sickle cell disease and, 510-511
Oral hygiene; *see also* Dental care
    cancer patient and, 138-139
    cerebral palsy and, 158
    Down syndrome and, 259
Oral hypersensitivity in premature infant, 458
Oral polio vaccine; *see* Poliomyelitis vaccine
Oral thrush, 414
Organ transplant, 389-407; *see also* Transplant
Orotracheal intubation, 455
Orthomolecular therapy, 362
Orthopedic disorder
    arthritis as, 336-354; *see also* Arthritis
    bronchopulmonary dysplasia and, 106
    cerebral palsy and, 153
    Down syndrome and, 250
    sickle cell disease and, 503, 508
Orthotic appliance, 346-347
Osteitis fibrosa, 485-486
Osteodystrophy, renal, 485
Osteomalacia, 486
Osteomyelitis, 508
Osteosarcoma, 121
Otitis media
    bronchopulmonary dysplasia and, 105, 109
    cerebral palsy and, 158
    fragile X syndrome and, 293, 296
    human immunodeficiency virus infection and, 418
Otorhinolaryngologic disorder, 105-106
Over-the-counter medication
    bleeding disorders and, 93
    diabetes mellitus and, 235
Oxicams, 340
Oxygen therapy, 101, 102, 103
    safety of, 110-111

P

P24 antigen, 410

Pacemaker, 201
Pain
    abdominal
        arthritis and, 346
        bleeding disorder and, 94
        sickle cell disease and, 508
        transplant and, 401
    cancer and, 141
    cystic fibrosis and, 220
    inflammatory bowel disease and, 329
    respiratory infection and, cerebral palsy and, 158-159
    sickle cell disease and, 496, 498, 501-502
Pain control
    bleeding disorder and, 89
    for dying child, 22
Palate, fragile X syndrome and, 294
Palliative heart surgery, 193
Palsy
    cerebral, 148-168; *see also* Cerebral palsy
    facial, 489
Pancreas in cystic fibrosis, 211
Pancreatic enzyme deficiency, 215
Pancytopenia, 414
Pansinusitis, 217
Parenteral nutrition
    bronchopulmonary dysplasia and, 104
    inflammatory bowel disease and, 324
    premature infant and, 451
Parenting, cocaine abuse and, 470-471
Parents; *see* Family
Partial seizure, 269-270, 271, 273
Patent ductus arteriosus, 188
Patterning, 362
Pauciarticular arthritis, 339
Peabody Picture Vocabulary Test, Revised, 39, 40
Peak expiratory flow rate, 70-71
Pedigree in fragile X syndrome, 292
Pemoline, 360, 361
    side effects of, 364
Penicillin
    renal failure and, 488
    sickle cell disease and, 500
Penis
    adrenal hyperplasia and, 176
    sickle cell disease and, 503
Peptic ulcer
    arthritis and, 346
    phenylketonuria and, 432

Perceptual deficit, 358, 359
   myelodysplasia and, 376
Pericardiotomy, 200
Pericarditis
   antineoplastic therapy and, 133
   renal failure and, 486
Perinatal transmission of human immunodeficiency
      virus, 408-409, 410
Periodontitis, 251
Peripheral arthritis, 325
Peritoneal cavity, shunt and, 304-305
Peritoneal dialysis, 393, 484
   peritonitis and, 485
Periventricular-intraventricular hemorrhage, 448-449
Pertussis vaccine
   bronchopulmonary dysplasia and, 108
   cocaine exposure and, 472
   epilepsy and, 277
   hydrocephalus and, 309
Pharyngitis, 94
Phenistix test, 434
Phenobarbital
   as antiepileptic agent, 274
   heart disease and, 200
Phenomenism, 31
Phenylalanine, 426; *see also* Phenylketonuria
Phenylalanine ammonia lyase, 431
Phenylalanine tolerance testing, 434
Phenylketonuria, 426-445
   associated problems with, 432-433
   clinical manifestations of, 429
   developmental issues in, 436-439
   differential diagnosis of, 435-436
   etiology of, 426-427
   family and, 439-440
   incidence of, 427-428
   management of, 432-435
   prognosis of, 432
   treatment of, 429-431
Phenytoin
   aspirin and, 278
   dental care and, 277
     gingival hyperplasia and, 157-158
   dosage and side effects of, 274
   sulfasalazine and, 328
   toxicity of, 277
Phosphorus, renal failure and, 482
Photosensitive skin reaction, arthritis and, 346
Physical education for cerebral palsy, 163
Physical therapy for bleeding disorder, 90

Physician's Developmental Quick Screen for Speech
    Disorders, 39
Physiotherapy, chest
   bronchopulmonary dysplasia and, 105
   cystic fibrosis and, 215-216
Picture Care Test, 38
Pigmentation, phenylketonuria and, 435
Pilocarpine iontophoresis, 214
Pirocicam, 340
PKU; *see* Phenylketonuria
Placenta, cocaine and, 467-468
Plant alkaloid, 124-125
Plastic surgery for Down syndrome, 249
Platelets
   cancer and, 131-132, 141
   human immunodeficiency virus and, 414
Pneumococcal vaccine
   asthma and, 69-70
   cystic fibrosis and, 219
   diabetes mellitus and, 234
   Down syndrome and, 258
   Hodgkin's disease and, 138
   human immunodeficiency virus infection and,
     416
   renal failure and, 487
   sickle cell disease and, 506
Pneumocystis carinii
   AIDS and, 414
   cancer and, 140
Pneumonia
   asthma and, 64
   cerebral palsy and, 159
   Pneumocystis carinii, 414
Pneumonitis
   antineoplastic therapy and, 133
   Pneumocystis carinii, 140
Poisoning, lead, 507
Poliomyelitis vaccine
   bleeding disorders and, 92-93
   cancer and, 138
   cocaine exposure and, 471
   human immunodeficiency virus infection and, 415-
     416
   premature infant and, 454
   transplant and, 399
Polyarticular arthritis, 339
Polycose, 202
Polymerase chain reaction, 410
Polyps, nasal, 217

Polyvalent pneumococcal vaccine; *see* Pneumococcal vaccine
Portal hypertension, 393
Positioning in cerebral palsy, 152
    for sleep, 163
Positive airway pressure, 451
Positive pressure ventilation, 101
Postpericardiotomy syndrome, 200
Posturing in cerebral palsy, 152
Potassium
    digoxin and, 197
    renal failure and, 481, 482
Pouch, Kock, 324
Pre-Hospital Admission Review, 46-47
Precautions, universal, HIV infection and, 419
Precocious puberty
    hydrocephalus and, 307
    myelodysplasia and, 377
Prednisolone, 341
Prednisone
    arthritis and, 341
    bronchopulmonary dysplasia and, 105
    cancer and, 126
    cystic fibrosis and, 216
    inflammatory bowel disease and, 321, 322, 323
Preferred Provider Option, 46
Pregnancy
    adrenal hyperplasia and, 182
    cocaine and, 465-479; *see also* Cocaine exposure, prenatal
    cystic fibrosis and, 224
    diabetes mellitus and, 240
    epilepsy and, 282
    heart disease and, 204
    inflammatory bowel disease and, 331-332
    myelodysplasia and, 384
    phenylketonuria and, 438-440
    prematurity and, 446-464; *see also* Prematurity
    transplant and, 403
Prematurity, 446-464
    associated problems with, 448-452
    bronchopulmonary dysplasia and, developmental problems and, 108
    clinical manifestations of, 446-447
    cocaine and, 468
    developmental issues and, 456-460
    enteral feeding and, 451
    etiology of, 446
    family and, 460

Prematurity—cont'd
    incidence of, 446
    infection and, 456
    management of, 452-456
    prognosis for, 447-448
    treatment of, 447
Prenatal diagnosis
    cystic fibrosis and, 212
    fragile X syndrome and, 292-293
    myelodysplasia and, 375
    phenylketonuria and, 427-428
Prenatal drug exposure
    to cocaine, 465-479; *see also* Cocaine exposure, prenatal
    human immunodeficiency virus infection and, 415
Prepaid health plan, 47
Preschool-aged child
    developmental tasks of, 28
    perspectives on body and illness of, 30, 31
Pressure
    intracranial, 307
    positive airway, 451
Priapism, 503
Primary care for chronically ill child, 3-11
    barriers to optimal care and, 4-6
    case management and, 9
    child development and, 32-33, 41-43
    family and, 14-15
    role of, 6-9
Primidone, 274
Private health insurance, 45-47
Procarbazine, 127
Proctocolectomy, 324
Prolapse
    mitral valve, 293, 295
    rectal, 217, 223
Proliferative sickle retinopathy, 503
Prophylaxis
    arthritis and, 344
    endocarditis and, 196
    heart disease and, 195
    hydrocephalus and, 305
    myelodysplasia and, 378
    sickle cell disease and, 500
    varicella, cancer and, 138
Proprionic acid derivatives, 340
Protein
    clotting factor concentrates and, 86
    transmembrane regulator, 210

Proteinuria, 235
Pseudoseizure, 279
Psychologic disorder
    Down syndrome and, 260
    epilepsy and, 276, 281
    fragile X syndrome and, 294
    learning disabilities and, 363-364
    sickle cell disease and, 504, 505
Pterin excretion test, 433
Puberty
    arthritis and, 348-349
    cystic fibrosis and, 218-219
    Down syndrome and, 262
    precocious
        hydrocephalus and, 307
        myelodysplasia and, 377
    sickle cell disease and, 510
Public Law 94-142
    human immunodeficiency virus infection and, 420
    learning disabilities and, 367-368
    myelodysplasia and, 381
    provisions of, 56-57
Public Law 99-457
    myelodysplasia and, 381
    provisions of, 56-57
Pulmonary disease; see Respiratory system
Pulmonary fibrosis, 133
Pulmonary function test
    asthma and, 70-71
    bronchopulmonary dysplasia and, 109
    cystic fibrosis and, 219
    human immunodeficiency virus infection and, 417
Pulmonary hypertension, 251
Puncture, lumbar, 141
Pyelonephritis, 508
Pyloric stenosis
    Down syndrome and, 260
    phenylketonuria and, 433
Pyoderma gangrenosum, 326

Q

Quadriplegia, 148

R

Radiation therapy, 128
    adverse effects of, 134-137
Radiologic evaluation
    bone age in adrenal hyperplasia and, 178
    bronchopulmonary dysplasia and, 101, 103, 109

Rales, 103
Ranitidine, 107
Rapid Developmental Screening Checklist, 36
Rash, arthritis and, 345-346
Rectal prolapse, 217, 223
Red blood cells
    cancer and, 132
    human immunodeficiency virus infection and, 414
    sickle cell disease and, 495, 500-501
Reflex, cerebral palsy and, 151
Reflux
    gastroesophageal
        asthma and, 67-68
        bronchopulmonary dysplasia and, 107
        premature infant and, 458
    urinary, 380
Rejection of transplanted organ, 397-398
Renal disease
    bleeding disorder and, 94
    bronchopulmonary dysplasia and, 106
    cancer as, 121
    clinical manifestations of, 391
    cyclosporine and, 397
    end-stage
        Medicare's program for, 50
        transplant and, 390
    inflammatory bowel disease and, 326
    medical management of, 393
    sickle cell disease and, 503, 507
Renal embryoma, 121
Renal failure
    associated problems with, 485-486
    clinical manifestations of, 480-482
    developmental issues and, 489-490
    differential diagnosis of, 488-489
    etiology of, 480
    family and, 490
    incidence of, 480
    management of, 486-488
    prognosis of, 485
    treatment of, 482-484
Renal system
    antineoplastic therapy and, 134
    bronchopulmonary dysplasia and, 106
Renal transplant
    etiology of, 389
    prognosis of, 395
    rejection of, 397-398, 398
Reproductive system; see Sexuality

Reservoir, shunt, 305
Respiratory distress
 bronchopulmonary dysplasia and, 101
 human immunodeficiency virus infection and, 418
 sickle cell disease and, 509
Respiratory system
 antineoplastic therapy and, 133
 arthritis and, 346
 asthma and, 63-79; *see also* Asthma
 bronchopulmonary dysplasia and, 101-117; *see also*
  Bronchopulmonary dysplasia
 cerebral palsy and, 154
 cystic fibrosis and, 211, 215-216
 Down syndrome and, 251
 hemophilia and, 91
 human immunodeficiency virus infection and,
  417
 premature infant and, 451-452
 sickle cell disease and, 502
Respiratory tract infection
 adrenal hyperplasia and, 178-179
 asthma and, 63, 72
 bronchopulmonary dysplasia and, 109-110
 cerebral palsy and, 158-159
 cystic fibrosis and, 213, 215
 Down syndrome and, 251, 260
 heart disease and, 201
 premature infant and, 456
Restriction fragment length polymorphism,
  phenylketonuria and, 426-427
Retardation
 growth; *see also* Growth
  cerebral palsy and, 155
  cystic fibrosis and, 218
  heart disease and, 197
  inflammatory bowel disease and, 330
  renal failure and, 485
 mental
  Down syndrome and, 245-267; *see also* Down
   syndrome
  fragile X syndrome and, 286-287; *see also* Fragile X syndrome
Retention enema, 321
Reticulocyte count, 509
Retinoblastoma, 122
Retinopathy
 diabetic, 234
 of prematurity, 449-450
  bronchopulmonary dysplasia and, 106

Retinopathy—cont'd
 proliferative sickle, 503
Retrolental fibroplasia, 449-450
Retrovir, 412
Reye's syndrome
 aspirin and, 346
 nonsteroidal anti-inflammatory drugs and, 344
Rhabdomyosarcoma, 121
 prognosis of, 129
Rheumatoid arthritis, 336-354; *see also* Juvenile rheumatoid arthritis
Rheumatoid rash, 345-346
Rickets, 106
Rifampin, 178
Right atrial catheter, 130
Riley Motor Problems Inventory, 39
Riley Preschool Developmental Inventory, 40
Rubber allergy in myelodysplasia, 377
Rubella vaccine
 cancer and, 138
 cocaine exposure and, 472

S

Sacroileitis, 325
Safety
 adrenal hyperplasia and, 180
 arthritis and, 346
 asthma and, 72-73
 bleeding disorder and, 94-95
 bronchopulmonary dysplasia and, 110-111
 cancer and, 141
 cerebral palsy and, 159-160
 cocaine exposure and, 473
 cystic fibrosis and, 221
 diabetes mellitus and, 236
 Down syndrome and, 260
 epilepsy and, 279-280
 fragile X syndrome and, 296
 heart disease and, 201-202
 human immunodeficiency virus infection and, 419
 hydrocephalus and, 312
 inflammatory bowel disease and, 329-330
 learning disabilities and, 366
 myelodysplasia and, 380-381
 phenylketonuria and, 436
 premature infant and, 456-457
 renal failure and, 489
 sickle cell disease and, 509
 transplant and, 401

Salicylates, arthritis and, 340
    dental care and, 344
Salicylsalicylic acid, 340
Salivary gland, cystic fibrosis and, 212
Salk polio vaccine, cancer and, 138
Salmonella, sickle cell disease and, 507
Salt
    cystic fibrosis and, 217
    renal failure and, 481
Salt-losing adrenal hyperplasia, 170, 171; *see also*
        Adrenal hyperplasia
    gender of infant, 173
Sandimmune; *see* Cyclosporine
Sarcoma, 121
School
    adrenal hyperplasia and, 181
    arthritis and, 348
    asthmatic child and, 75
    bleeding disorder and, 95
    bronchopulmonary dysplasia and, 113
    cancer patient and, 142-143
    cerebral palsy and, 163-164
    cocaine exposure and, 474-475
    cystic fibrosis and, 223-224
    diabetes mellitus and, 239
    Down syndrome and, 262
    epilepsy and, 281-282
    family and, 19-20
    fragile X syndrome and, 297
    heart disease and, 203
    human immunodeficiency virus infection and, 420-
        421
    hydrocephalus and, 313-314
    inflammatory bowel disease and, 331
    learning disabilities and, 367-368
    myelodysplasia and, 383
    phenylketonuria and, 437
    premature infant and, 459-460
    readiness tests for, 39-40
    renal failure and, 490
    sickle cell disease and, 510
    transition to, 42
    transplant and, 402-403
School-age child
    developmental tasks of, 28
    safety with electrical equipment and, 72
    safety with medications for, 73
Scleroderma, 436
Sclerotherapy, 393

Scoliosis
    arthritis and, 342
    cerebral palsy and, 154-155, 158
    fragile X syndrome and, 293
    myelodysplasia and, 378
    sickle cell disease and, 507
Screening
    adrenal hyperplasia and, 171-172, 177-178
    arthritis and, 344-345
    bronchopulmonary dysplasia and, 109
    cancer and, 138-139
    cerebral palsy and, 156-158
    cocaine exposure and, 472
    cystic fibrosis and, 219
    diabetes mellitus and, 234-235
    Down syndrome and, 258-259
    epilepsy and, 277
    fragile X syndrome and, 295-296
    heart disease and, 198-200
    human immunodeficiency virus infection and, 416-
        417
    hydrocephalus and, 310
    inflammatory bowel disease and, 327-328
    language development, cerebral palsy and, 156
    learning disabilities and, 365
    myelodysplasia and, 378
    phenylketonuria, 428, 440
    phenylketonuria and, 433-434
    premature infant and, 454-456
    renal failure and, 487-488
    sickle cell disease and, 506-507
    transplant and, 399-401
Screening tests
    asthma and, 70-71
    bleeding disorders and, 93
Seizure
    bronchopulmonary dysplasia and, 106
    cerebral palsy and, 154
        safety concerns and, 160
    cyclosporine and, 397
    epilepsy and
        associated problems with, 276
        classification of seizures and, 269, 271, 273
        clinical manifestations of, 268, 271, 273
        developmental issues in, 279-282
        differential diagnosis of, 278-279
        family and, 282
        management of, 276-278
        prognosis for, 275-276

Seizure—cont'd
  epilepsy and—cont'd
    treatment of, 273-275
  etiology of, 268
  fragile X syndrome and, 293-294, 295-296
  hydrocephalus and, 307
    pertussis vaccine and, 309
  incidence of, 268
  myelodysplasia and, 375-376, 381
Self-care
  asthma and, 64-65
  catheterization and, 382
  diabetes mellitus and, 240
Self-monitored blood glucose, 232, 233
Sensory function in myelodysplasia, 376
Sensory integration, 362
  fragile X syndrome and, 294
Sensory-receptive intake, 358
Septal defect
  atrial, 189
  ventricular, 188
Sequestration, splenic, 500
Serum 17-OHP, 177-178
Sexual abuse, 409
Sexuality
  adrenal hyperplasia and, 181-182
  arthritis and, 348-349
  asthma and, 75-76
  bleeding disorder and, 95-96
  bronchopulmonary dysplasia and, 112
  cancer patient and, 143
  cerebral palsy and, 164
  cystic fibrosis and, 224
  diabetes mellitus and, 240
  Down syndrome and, 262
  drug abuse and, 474-475
  epilepsy and, 282
  fragile X syndrome and, 297
  heart disease and, 204
  human immunodeficiency virus infection and, 421
  hydrocephalus and, 314
  inflammatory bowel disease and, 331-332
  learning disabilities and, 369
  myelodysplasia and, 384
  phenylketonuria and, 438-439
  prematurity and, 460
  renal failure and, 490
  sickle cell disease and, 510
  transplant and, 403

Sheppard-Towner Act, 51
Short stature, 177
Shunt
  hydrocephalus and, 304-305
    infection and, 311
  myelodysplasia and, 381
Sibling
  of chronically ill child, 16-18
  of dying child, 23
  learning disabilities and, 369
Sickle cell disease, 495-515
  associated problems with, 498, 500-504
  clinical manifestations of, 496, 498
  developmental issues and, 509-511
  differential diagnosis of, 509-509
  etiology of, 495-496
  family and, 511
  genetic testing and counseling for, 54
  incidence of, 496
  management of, 504-507
  treatment of, 498
Sickle prep test, 495-496
Simple partial seizure, 269, 271, 273
Sinusitis
  asthma versus, 72
  bronchopulmonary dysplasia and, 105-106
  cystic fibrosis and, 217
  human immunodeficiency virus infection and, 418
Skeletal system
  antineoplastic therapy and, 135
  arthritis and, 342
  inflammatory bowel disease and, 329
  sickle cell disease and, 503
Skin
  arthritis and, 345-346
  Down syndrome and, 248
  inflammatory bowel disease and, 326
  myelodysplasia and, 375
  phenylketonuria and, 435
  tracheostomy stoma and, 106-107
Skinfold measurements
  cerebral palsy and, 155
  renal failure and, 487
Skull, Down syndrome and, 248
Sleep
  adrenal hyperplasia and, 181
  arthritis and, 348
  asthma and, 74-75
  bronchopulmonary dysplasia and, 112

Sleep—cont'd
  cerebral palsy and, 162-163
  cocaine exposure and, 474
  cystic fibrosis and, 223
  diabetes mellitus and, 239
  Down syndrome and, 262
  epilepsy and, 281
  fragile X syndrome and, 297
  heart disease and, 203
  human immunodeficiency virus infection and, 420
  hydrocephalus and, 313
  inflammatory bowel disease and, 331
  learning disabilities and, 367
  myelodysplasia and, 383
  phenylketonuria and, 437-438
  premature infant and, 459
  renal failure and, 490
  sickle cell disease and, 510
  transplant and, 402
Slow-acting antirheumatic drug, 340-341
Small-for-gestational-age infant; *see also* Prematurity
  bronchopulmonary dysplasia and, 108
Smoking
  asthma and, 76
  of crack, 470
  fetus and, 466
Snellen Illiterate E Test, 38
Social Security Act, 55
Social Security supplemental income program, 53-54
Sodium
  adrenal hyperplasia and, 180-181
    salt-losing, 170, 171, 173
  cystic fibrosis and, 217
  renal failure and, 481
Somatic gene therapy, 431
Somogyi phenomenon, 234
Sore throat, 94
Spastic cerebral palsy, 148
  sleep position and, 163
Speech and language
  fragile X syndrome and, 287, 291-292, 295
  renal failure and, 486
  testing of, 38-39
Sperm banking, 143
Spina bifida occulta, 374
Spine
  arthritis and, 342
  cancer and, 141
  cerebral palsy and, 154-155, 158

Spine—cont'd
  hemophilia and, 91
  myelodysplasia and, 373; *see also* Myelodysplasia
  tethering of cord and, 379
Splenic sequestration, 500
Splint, arthritis and, 346-347
Spondylitis, ankylosing, 325
Sports
  adrenal hyperplasia and, 180
  bleeding disorder and, 94-95
  for child with asthma, 69
  diabetes mellitus and, 239
  Down syndrome and, 260
  hydrocephalus and, 313-314
  transplant and, 401
Spots, melanin, 436
Staining of teeth, 109
Staphylococcal infection
  premature infant and, 456
  shunt for hydrocephalus and, 306
Status epilepticus, 273
Stenosis
  aqueductal, 303
  pyloric
    Down syndrome and, 260
    phenylketonuria and, 433
  subaortic, 188
Sterility, 224; *see also* Fertility
Sterilization, Down syndrome and, 262
Steroid, adrenal, 169, 171; *see also* Corticosteroid
    hyperplasia and, 175, 178
Stiffness in cerebral palsy, 148
Stimulant drugs for learning disabilities, 361-362, 364, 365-366, 366
Stimulation program
  fragile X syndrome and, 291
  human immunodeficiency virus infection and, 415
Stoma, 106-107
Stone
  cholelithiasis and, 106
  renal
    bronchopulmonary dysplasia and, 106
    inflammatory bowel disease and, 326
Stool softener, 378
Strabismus
  bronchopulmonary dysplasia and, 106
  fragile X syndrome and, 293
Streptococcal infection
  premature infant and, 456

Streptococcal infection—cont'd
  sickle cell disease and, 507
Subaortic stenosis, 188
Subluxation, Down syndrome and, 250
Substance abuse
  cocaine, 465-479; *see also* Cocaine exposure, prenatal
  fetal alcohol syndrome and, 465
  human immunodeficiency virus and, 415
Subviron influenza vaccine, 108; *see also* Influenza vaccine
Suctioning, bronchopulmonary dysplasia and, 105
Sudden death
  cocaine exposure and, 469
  hypertrophic cardiomyopathy and, 393
  premature infant and, 452
Sulfasalazine
  arthritis and, 341
  drug interactions with, 328
  inflammatory bowel disease and, 321, 322, 331
Sulindac, 340
Sun exposure, chemotherapy and, 141
Supplemental Security Income, 53-54
Suppository for fungal infection, 414
Supratentorial astrocytoma, 118-119
Supraventricular tachycardia, 197
Surgery
  adrenal hyperplasia and, 175
  bleeding disorder and, 90
  congenital heart disease and, 193-194
  Down syndrome and, 249
  epilepsy and, 275
  inflammatory bowel disease and, 324
Sweat gland, cystic fibrosis and, 211
Sweat test for cystic fibrosis, 214-215
Sweetener, artificial
  diabetes mellitus and, 238
  phenylketonuria and, 434-435
Sympathomimetic agent, 378
Synovitis
  arthritis and, 337
  hemophilia and, 91
Syphilis, 469
Syringe, disposal of, 236

T

Tachycardia, supraventricular, 197
Tachypneic heart disease, 203
Tactile perception, 358

Tanner stages of development, 234
Task, developmental, 28-29
Teeth
  bronchopulmonary dysplasia and, 109
  Down syndrome and, 251
  premature infant and, 455
Tegretol
  aspirin and, 277
  dosage and side effects of, 274
  erythromycin and, 278
  toxicity of, 277
Temporomandibular joint, 342, 346
Testicle
  bleeding disorder and, 94
  fragile X syndrome and, 287
  hemophilia and, 91-92
  premature infant and, 455-456
  undescended, 452
Tetanus vaccine, 415; *see also* Diphtheria, tetanus, and pertussis vaccine
Tethering of spinal cord, 379
Tetralogy of Fallot, 189
Texas Pre-school Screening Inventory, 40
Theophylline
  asthma and, 66
    blood levels of, 71
  bronchopulmonary dysplasia and, 109
  cystic fibrosis and, 220
6-Thioguanine, 124
Thrombocytopenia
  cancer and, 131-132
  human immunodeficiency virus infection and, 414
Thrush, 414
Thyroid gland
  antineoplastic therapy and, 135
  diabetes mellitus and, 235
  Down syndrome and, 251, 259
Tingling, bleeding disorder and, 94
Tobacco, fetus and, 466
Toddler
  developmental tasks of, 28
  Education of All Handicapped Children Act and, 56
  safety with medications for, 73
Toileting
  adrenal hyperplasia and, 181
  arthritis and, 348
  asthma and, 74
  bronchopulmonary dysplasia and, 112
  cancer patient and, 142

Toileting—cont'd
  cerebral palsy and, 161-162
  cocaine exposure and, 474
  cystic fibrosis and, 223
  diabetes mellitus and, 238-239
  Down syndrome and, 261-262
  epilepsy and, 281
  fragile X syndrome and, 297
  heart disease and, 203
  human immunodeficiency virus infection and, 420
  hydrocephalus and, 313
  inflammatory bowel disease and, 330-331
  learning disabilities and, 367
  myelodysplasia and, 382
  phenylketonuria and, 437
  premature infant and, 459
  renal failure and, 490
  sickle cell disease and, 510
  transplant and, 402
Tolmetin sodium, 340
Tone, muscle
  cerebral palsy and, 150
  Down syndrome and, 248
  epilepsy and, 279
  premature infant and, 453
Topical hemostatic agent, 89
Total parenteral nutrition, 104
Tourette's syndrome, 364
Toxic megacolon, 326-327
Toxicity
  aluminum, 486
  aspirin, 346
  digoxin, 197
  drug, epilepsy and, 277
Toxicology screen, cocaine exposure and, 472
Toxoplasma, transplant and, 394
Trace elements, 434
Tracheostomy tube
  bronchopulmonary dysplasia and, 106-107
  safety concerns and, 110
Transfusion
  human immunodeficiency virus and, 414
  platelet, cancer and, 131-132
  sickle cell disease and, 500-501, 504
Translocation of chromosome 21, 245
Transmembrane regulator protein, 210
Transplant, 389-407
  associated problems with, 395-398
  biliary atresia, 393

Transplant—cont'd
  clinical manifestations of, 391-393
  developmental issues in, 401-403
  etiology of, 389-390
  family and, 403
  incidence of, 390-391
  management of, 398-401
  prognosis of, 394-395
  treatment of, 393-394
Transposition of great vessels, 189
Trauma
  adrenal hyperplasia and, 179
  epilepsy and, 276
    helmet for prevention of, 279
  head, bleeding disorder and, 93-94
  learning disabilities and, 366
Tricuspid atresia, 190
Tricyclic antidepressant, 361
Trimethoprim-sulfamethoxazole
  heart disease and, 195
  toxicity of, 417-418
Truncus arteriosus, 188
Tryptophan, 435
Tube
  gastrostomy, 107
  nasogastric, 161
  tracheostomy
    bronchopulmonary dysplasia and, 106-107
    safety concerns and, 110
Tuberculosis
  arthritis and, 344
  cancer patient and, 139
  cocaine exposure and, 472
  human immunodeficiency virus infection and, 417
  inflammatory bowel disease and, 328
  transplant and, 400
Tumor; *see* Cancer
Tyrosine, 434

U

Ulcer
  arthritis and, 346
  peptic, phenylketonuria and, 432
  sickle cell disease and, 503-504
Ulcerative colitis, 318-335
  associated problems with, 324-327
  clinical manifestations of, 319-321
  developmental issues in, 329-332
  differential diagnosis of, 328-329

Ulcerative colitis — cont'd
  etiology of, 318
  family and, 332
  incidence of, 318-319
  management of, 327-328
  treatment of, 321-324
Undescended testis, 452
Undifferentiated attention-deficit disorder, 355; *see also* Learning disabilities
Universal precautions, 419
Upper extremity, Down syndrome and, 248
Upper respiratory infection
  adrenal hyperplasia and, 178-179
  asthma and, 63, 64
  bronchopulmonary dysplasia and, 105
  heart disease and, 201
Uremia, 482
Uremic pericarditis, 486
Urinalysis
  arthritis and, 344
  asthma and, 70
  bleeding disorders and, 93
  cancer patient and, 139
  cocaine exposure and, 472
  cystic fibrosis and, 219
  diabetes mellitus and, 235
  human immunodeficiency virus infection and, 417
  inflammatory bowel disease and, 328
  myelodysplasia and, 378
  renal failure and, 488
  transplant and, 400
Urinary acidifier, 365-366
Urinary tract
  antineoplastic therapy and, 134-135
  Down syndrome and, 249
  hemophilia and, 88
  myelodysplasia and, 377
Urinary tract infection
  arthritis and, 346
  cerebral palsy and, 154, 159
  myelodysplasia and, 378, 380
  sickle cell disease and, 508
Urine
  bleeding disorder and, 94
  diabetes mellitus and, 239
  phenylketonuria and, 434
Uveitis, arthritis and, 342

V
Vaccination; *see* Immunization
Vaginal infection, diabetes mellitus and, 233
Valproic acid
  as antiepileptic agent, 274
  aspirin and, 278
  toxicity of, 277
Valve, mitral, 293, 295
Varicella
  cancer and, 138
  cystic fibrosis and, 220
  human immunodeficiency virus infection and, 416, 418-419
Varicella-zoster immune globulin
  premature infant and, 454
  transplant and, 399
Vascular access
  cancer and, 130-131
  for dialysis, 489
  fever and, 139
Vasoocclusion in sickle cell disease, 495, 500, 501-502
Venous access
  cancer and, 130
  fever and, 139
Venous return, anomalous, 190
Ventilation
  bronchopulmonary dysplasia and, 101, 102, 104
  premature infant and, 451
Ventricular septal defect, 188
Ventriculoperitoneal shunt, 304-305
  myelodysplasia and, 381
Very-low-birth-weight infant, 452
Vinblastine, 124
Vincristine, 124
Viral infection
  asthma and, 63
  bronchopulmonary dysplasia and, 105
  cancer and, 140
  cystic fibrosis and, 220
  Epstein-Barr
    immunosuppressive therapy and, 397
    transplant and, 394
  human immunodeficiency, 408-425; *see also* Human immunodeficiency virus infection
  premature infant and, 456
  respiratory syncytial, 110
  transplant and, 401
  varicella; *see* Varicella

Virilization, 172-173, 175-176, 181-182
Vision
　arthritis and, 342
　asthma and, 70
　bleeding disorder and, 93, 94
　bronchopulmonary dysplasia and, 106, 109
　cancer patient and, 138
　cerebral palsy and, 153, 157
　cystic fibrosis and, 219
　diabetes mellitus and, 234
　Down syndrome and, 248, 250-251, 258
　fragile X syndrome and, 293, 295
　human immunodeficiency virus infection and, 416
　hydrocephalus and, 305-306, 310
　inflammatory bowel disease and, 326, 327
　learning disabilities and, 365
　myelodysplasia and, 376, 378
　premature infant and, 454-455
　renal failure and, 487
　retinoblastoma of, 122
　retinopathy of prematurity and, 449-450
　sickle cell disease and, 503, 506
　tests for, 37-38
　transplant and, 399
Visual perceptual deficit, 358, 359
Vital signs, HIV infection and, 417
Vitamins
　cancer patient and, 142
　cystic fibrosis and, 215
Vomiting
　adrenal hyperplasia and, 179
　asthma and, 72
　cancer and, 131, 140-141
　cerebral palsy and, 159
　heart disease and, 201
　hydrocephalus and, 311
　inflammatory bowel disease and, 329
　myelodysplasia and, 380
　sickle cell disease and, 508
　transplant and, 401
von Willebrand's disease
　clinical manifestations of, 83, 85
　etiology of, 81-82
　treatment of, 89-90, 97-98
VP-16-213, 125

Vulnerable child syndrome
　heart disease and, 197
　premature infant and, 459

W
Weight
　arthritis and, 343
　birth, prematurity and, 446
　cancer and, 131
　cerebral palsy and, 155
　cystic fibrosis and, 218
　diabetes mellitus and, 234
　Down syndrome and, 252
　epilepsy and, 280
　hydrocephalus and, 307
　phenylketonuria and, 429-430
　renal failure and, 487
　sickle cell disease and, 504, 505
Wheel Guide to Normal Milestones of Development, 37
Wheelchair use, 160
　school and, 163-164
Wheezing
　asthma and, 64
　bronchopulmonary dysplasia as, 103
　cystic fibrosis and, 221
　differential diagnosis of, 72
White blood cells, cancer and, 131
Wide Range Achievement Test, 40
Wilms' tumor, 121
　prognosis of, 129

X
X chromosome, fragile X syndrome and, 286
X-linked disorder
　fragile X syndrome and, 292
　hemophilia as, 81

Z
Zantac, 107
Zidovudine
　human immunodeficiency virus infection and, 412
　　anemia and, 417
　toxicity of, 417-418

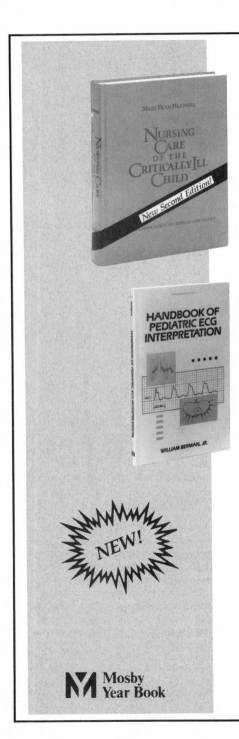